Rapid On-site Evaluation (ROSE)

Guoping Cai • Adebowale J. Adeniran
Editors

Rapid On-site Evaluation (ROSE)

A Practical Guide

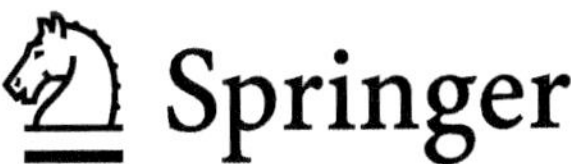

Editors
Guoping Cai
Department of Pathology
Yale University School of Medicine
New Haven, CT
USA

Adebowale J. Adeniran
Department of Pathology
Yale University School of Medicine
New Haven, CT
USA

ISBN 978-3-030-21801-0 ISBN 978-3-030-21799-0 (eBook)
https://doi.org/10.1007/978-3-030-21799-0

This Springer imprint is published by the registered company Springer Nature Switzerland AG
The registered company address is: Gewerbestrasse 11, 6330 Cham, Switzerland

Contents

Contributors

Rita Abi-Raad, MD Department of Pathology, Yale University School of Medicine, New Haven, CT, USA

Adebowale J. Adeniran, MD Department of Pathology, Yale University School of Medicine, New Haven, CT, USA

Tamar C. Brandler, MD, MS Department of Pathology, New York University Langone Health, New York, NY, USA

Marilyn M. Bui, MD, PhD Department of Anatomic Pathology, H. Lee Moffitt Cancer Center & Research Institute, Tampa, FL, USA

Guoping Cai, M.D. Department of Pathology, Yale University School of Medicine, New Haven, CT, USA

Joan F. Cangiarella, MD Department of Pathology, New York University Langone Health, New York, NY, USA

Evita B. Henderson-Jackson, MD Department of Anatomic Pathology, H. Lee Moffitt Cancer Center & Research Institute, Tampa, FL, USA

Andrea Hernandez, DO Department of Pathology, New York University Langone Health, New York, NY, USA

Angelique W. Levi, M.D. Department of Pathology, Yale University School of Medicine, New Haven, CT, USA

Part I
Introduction to Rapid On-Site Evaluation

Chapter 1
Overview

Guoping Cai and Adebowale J. Adeniran

The increasing use of minimally invasive procedures such as fine needle aspiration (FNA) and thin core needle biopsy has significantly improved patient's experience of medical care by providing the choice of more tolerable but informative procedures [1–3]. The material obtained from biopsies are not only for diagnostic purpose but can also provide information for treatment decisions in the era of personalized medicine [4–7]. Historically, cytopathology practice has focused on diagnosis which is based on morphology with or without the addition of routine immunocytochemistry. With more recent advances in molecular pathology and the detection of molecular targets for therapeutic management, cytological samples have been put in the spotlight as they are suitable and sometimes the preferred material for molecular testing [6, 8].

The expanded utilization of biopsied material in tailoring personalized therapy has heightened the importance of specimen acquisition and increased the need for obtaining adequate specimens. Rapid on-site evaluation (ROSE) is a laboratory service to assess the cytomorphologic features of FNA smears or biopsy touch imprints, which is often performed by cytopathologists or experienced general pathologists in the biopsy suite and can provide real-time feedback and guidance to the biopsy operator through rapid cytological evaluation of biopsy material. ROSE has been repeatedly shown to improve diagnostic yield of biopsy procedure and help secure sufficient material for ancillary testing [5, 9–12].

G. Cai (✉) · A. J. Adeniran
Department of Pathology, Yale University School of Medicine, New Haven, CT, USA
e-mail: guoping.cai@yale.edu; adebowale.adeniran@yale.edu

G. Cai, A. J. Adeniran (eds.), *Rapid On-site Evaluation (ROSE)*,
https://doi.org/10.1007/978-3-030-21799-0_1

Purposes of On-Site Evaluation

Rapid on-site evaluation (ROSE) is a central component of FNA biopsy procedure performed by pathologists and can also be carried out to assist imaging-guided FNA biopsy or small tissue biopsy. The true benefits of ROSE may vary in cases with or without imaging guidance, or with different imaging techniques, and may differ in different organ systems and different entities encountered [10, 13–15]. The scope of ROSE includes sampling adequacy assessment and proper specimen triage. ROSE also allows for a preliminary diagnosis so that additional material can be requested for ancillary studies such as flow cytometry, microbiology culture, and molecular tests.

Sampling Adequacy Assessment

Assessment of specimen adequacy is a major task that is performed during ROSE. There are however no well-established numeric criteria to define an adequate specimen in most organs and systems with thyroid being the only exception in which the adequacy is specifically defined [16]. In general, an adequate specimen is deemed sufficient to explain the underlying cause for the sampled lesion, the most common example being the presence of tumor cells in the FNA of a mass lesion. Identification of infectious microorganisms or granulomatous inflammation is more likely considered as adequate for nonneoplastic lesions although a tumor can coexist with an inflammatory or infectious process.

Surely, it is more difficult to define adequacy for the cases with uncertain clinical impression. For example, mediastinal or hilar lymph node sampling is frequently performed to stage lung cancers, which may or may not be involved by metastatic tumor. There are a few reports suggesting minimal numbers of lymphocytes required for a negative diagnosis; however, there are no consensus opinions about the exact numbers needed [17–20]. To avoid a false-negative biopsy, multiple passes should always be attempted. Ultimately, clinical correlation is recommended to address the issue of possible false-negative diagnosis. In cases with clinical suspicion of malignancy but negative cytology results, additional sampling including follow-up excisional biopsy may be indicated.

In cases with malignant diagnoses, additional samples are often needed for ancillary studies to support the diagnosis and further classification of tumors. In the era of precision and personalized medicine, molecular or biomarker testing has increasingly been requested to be performed on biopsy material in order to customize therapy for the individual patient [6–8]. Thus, the efforts should be focused on obtaining sufficient biopsy material. It should also be emphasized that as much material as possible should be preserved during ROSE, hence there is the need to balance the use of material for immediate diagnostic assessment with saving specimen for additional ancillary studies.

Besides cytopathologists or general pathologists, on-site adequacy assessment can be performed by certified cytotechnologists or trained physicians and similar efficacy can be achieved [10, 11, 21, 22].

Specimen Triage

The lesions subjected to biopsy may comprise of a variety of entities, ranging from inflammation, infections, and benign tumors to malignant neoplasms. The malignant neoplasms can be derived from diverse lineages of cells, including epithelial, hematopoietic, and mesenchymal tumors. To achieve a higher diagnostic yield, appropriate ancillary studies are crucial. During on-site evaluation, it is pivotal to recognize and classify the lesions into inflammation/infection, hematopoietic lesion and other tumors, and triage specimens accordingly (Fig. 1.1).

For a well-defined focal lesion by imaging studies, the possibility of an infectious etiology should be raised if the specimen shows (1) significant amount of inflammatory cells, (2) presence of necrosis, and (3) absence of overt malignant cells. For such cases, part of the specimen should be saved in a sterile container and sent for microbiology culture studies. Since inflammation with or without necrosis can accompany malignant tumors, additional sampling with at least three passes is generally recommended to rule out the possibility of a coexisting malignancy.

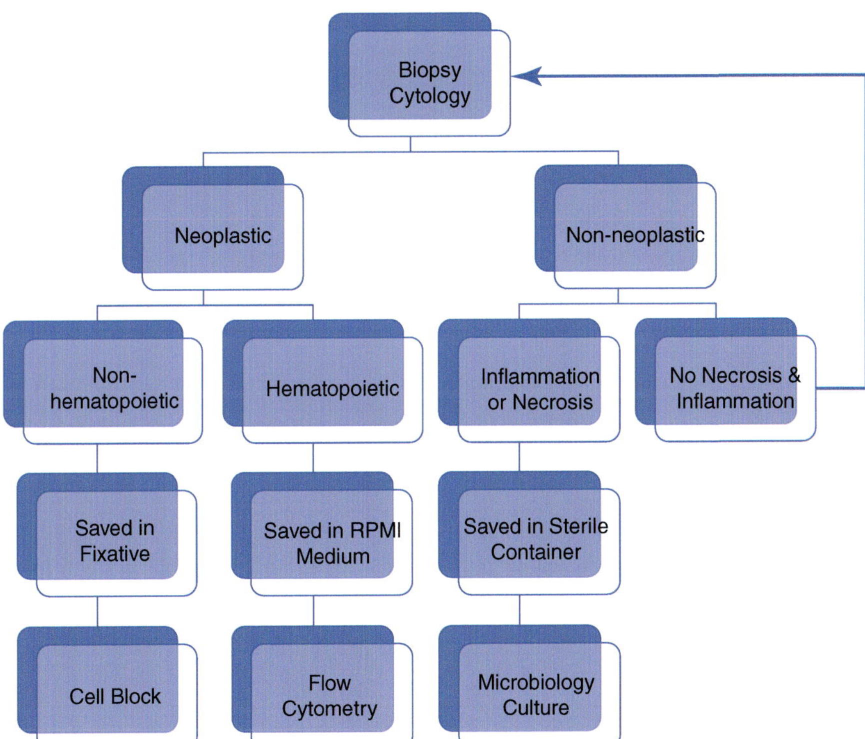

Fig. 1.1 Flowchart of specimen triage based on on-site cytological evaluation of biopsy specimens

Lymphoproliferative disorders can present as focal lesions in patients with or without prior history of hematopoietic malignancy. The following cytomorphologic features are helpful for recognizing lymphoid lesions during on-site evaluation: (1) single-cell distribution, (2) nuclear streaming artifact, and (3) lymphoglandular bodies. If a lymphoid lesion is suspected, part of specimen should be saved in RPMI preservative and sent for flow cytometry analysis.

In addition to direct smears used for on-site evaluation, the specimen should be saved as much as possible, including the cases suspected for infections and lymphoproliferation disorders. It is advised that only a portion of aspirates should be used for direct smears. If the aspirates are all expelled onto the glass slide, using another slide to pick up part of specimens for smearing is recommended and the remainder should be saved. The tissue fragments or blood clots found on the glass slide can also be saved by picking them up with a needle or a toothpick. The remainder of the specimens are saved in fixatives and processed for a cell block. The cell block material can be used for additional studies such as special stain, immunocytochemistry, and molecular testing. The results of these ancillary studies are crucial for substantiating diagnosis and/or providing prognostic and therapeutic information for better management of patients.

Decision to appropriately triage specimens requires expertise and extensive experiences, which might be best carried out by a cytopathologist or an experienced general pathologist or cytotechnologist. For indeterminate cases, part of the specimens should be sent for ancillary studies such as microbiology culture and flow cytometry analysis, even if those tests are eventually found to be unnecessary or noncontributory, as long as initial differential diagnosis includes the possibility of infections or lymphoproliferative disorders.

Preliminary Diagnosis

Based on the cytomorphologic analysis, a preliminary diagnosis can be rendered in most cases during on-site evaluation. Interpretation of cytomorphologic findings is critical in the process of specimen adequacy assessment and specimen triage determination.

Rendering a preliminary diagnosis can also help clinicians to manage patients in a timely manner. If a diagnosis of malignancy is provisionally rendered, additional biopsy procedures may be performed as such to determine nodal stage of the tumor or rule out a metastasis in a suspicious lesion in a nearby organ. In addition, imaging study-based metastasis work-up and oncologist counseling can also be initiated as early as possible. These measures may help ease the anxiety of patients when they are waiting for biopsy results and being offerred treatment options.

In rare cases in which urgent care or treatment is needed, preliminary diagnosis can serve as a guide for empirical or more specific treatment regimens. Clinical scenarios such as opportunistic infections in an immunocompromised patient, symptomatic brain metastasis in patients with small cell carcinoma of the lung, and mediastinal high-grade lymphoma with respiratory distress may warrant intiating treatment as early as possible.

In general, ROSE has a good correlation with final diagnosis [23–25]. Due to the potential impact on biopsy procedure and patient management, a preliminary diagnosis should be rendered with caution and with a more conservative approach [26]. Overinterpretation of the findings may lead to premature termination of the biopsy procedure, which often results in a repeat biopsy. An incorrect preliminary diagnosis may also cause unnecessary further work-up, inappropriate treatment, and patient's stress. Because of the diagnostic challenges and ramifications as well as associated legal and/or regulatory issues, preliminary diagnosis should only be rendered by experienced cytopathologists or general pathologists.

Applications of Rapid On-Site Evaluation

Rapid on-site evaluation (ROSE) can help improve diagnostic yield of FNA or biopsy procedures. ROSE is time-consuming and requires expertise and resources. Each institution may have to set its own policy to implement ROSE service through which the benefits of ROSE can be maximized, but the practice of ROSE is economically sounded.

Superficial Versus Deep-Seated Lesions

ROSE is very important in modern patient care because immediate feedback is often required for oncologic specimens in order to aid biopsy procedure and clinical management. ROSE is needed for FNAs performed on superficial lesions as well as deep-seated lesions. FNAs for superficial lesions are typically performed by radiologists and clinicians, under ultrasound guidance, while FNAs for deep-seated lesions are usually performed by interventional radiologists under CT scan or MRI guidance. Some of the superficial lesions may be palpable and as such do not require imaging guidance. Superficial organs whose aspiration may require ROSE include but not limited to the thyroid, parathyroid, lymph nodes, salivary gland, and breast, while deep-seated lesions that often require ROSE are commonly found in the lung, mediastinum, liver, kidney, adrenal gland, pancreas, bone, and soft tissue.

Endoscopic ultrasound-guided FNA (EUS-FNA) is now a well-established diagnostic technique in the assessment of lesions in the gastrointestinal tract and adjacent organs [27, 28]. The majority of the procedures are aimed at the pancreas and intra-abdominal lymph nodes. Likewise, endobronchial ultrasound-guided FNA (EBUS-FNA) is a highly effective procedure used in the sampling of lung and mediastinal lesions [29]. This provides real-time images, which allows easy view and access when compared with conventional mediastinoscopy. This technique was first used in the diagnosis and staging of lung cancer but is now being used for the diagnosis of lymphoma and other malignant conditions as well as benign conditions such as sarcoidosis and infectious conditions. Whether or not EBUS is employed for sampling a lesion depends on the size and location of the lesion. The accuracy and speed of EUS and EBUS is a direct reflection of ROSE, as pathologists are able to process and evaluate FNA samples and can request additional passes immediately if needed.

In case there are limited resources and also taking consideration of economic aspects, it is reasonable to take precedence of the deep-seated lesions over the superficial ones when providing ROSE service. The biopsies of deep-seated lesions often require more sophisticated imaging techniques such as CT and endoscopy, and longer procedure time, and are more costly. Also, the biopsies of deep-seated lesions may be associated with slightly higher risks of complications.

Sensitivity and Specificity

When FNAs are performed without ROSE, the average nondiagnostic rate is reported to be 20%, whereas it is 2–10% when ROSE is available [30–34]. There have been reported high sensitivity, specificity, and positive/negative predictive values in different organ sites when FNA findings have been correlated with histopathologic material and clinical follow-up [30, 31, 33, 35–40]. There are a number of issues that affect both sensitivity and specificity. One very important factor is the size of the lesion. Generally speaking, the smaller the size of the nodule, the higher the nondiagnostic rate and the lower the sensitivity of FNA [31]. ROSE tends to decrease the nondiagnostic rate by improving adequacy of the specimen, and in general, ROSE correlates well with final diagnosis [3, 5, 23, 40, 41]. However, there are other factors that are unrelated to the size of the lesion, which may affect sensitivity and specificity. A very classic example is the difficulty in differentiating well-differentiated hepatocellular carcinoma from benign reactive hepatocytes [38]. The very fact that the biopsy needle in most abdominal FNAs traverses the gut is a challenge as reactive cells in the gut can be misdiagnosed as well-differentiated adenocarcinoma. One other pitfall that may contribute to false-positive rates is the misdiagnosis of benign hepatocytes as oncocytic neoplasm in the biopsy of the right kidney [42]. Diagnosis of unusual neoplasms may also be challenging and can affect the sensitivity and specificity of FNA and ROSE. Another factor that may affect sensitivity and specificity is the fact that only air-dried smears stained with Diff-Quik stain are available at the time of ROSE.

Most simple cysts can be reliably diagnosed by imaging studies, in which ROSE has a very limited role in assisting the biopsy because the biopsy often yields very low cellularity. However, for cysts that display atypical radiologic features such as multilocularity, mural nodules, and irregularly thickened or calcified walls, the diagnosis is often much difficult and dependent on the areas of the cyst sampled. ROSE may offer some help in this setting. Overall, cystic lesions would still have relatively low sensitivity and specificity [43, 44].

The most common cause of false-negative interpretation in lymph node sampling is the presence of tingible-body macrophages [29]. Although a hallmark feature of reactive lymph node, this feature has also been seen to varying extent in mantle cell lymphoma, marginal zone lymphoma, and Burkitt's lymphoma. Many of these issues can be resolved when additional passes are obtained for ancillary studies such as immunocytochemical staining, flow cytometry, and molecular studies, ensuring that the final diagnosis is accurate and all-inclusive.

Advent of Telecytopathology

ROSE has not been uniformly implemented among institutions across the country and around the world due to variations in resources as well as reimbursement of associated costs. Technological advances in imaging transmission platforms have made it feasible to remotely assess cytological specimens. The advent of telecytopathology has added a new dimension to ROSE. Pathologists don't have to be physically present at the biopsy site or travel to different locations for the procedures; hence the wait time at the site of evaluation and traveling time to various locations to perform ROSE are eliminated [45].

References

1. Sharma A, Shepard JO. Lung cancer biopsies. Radiol Clin N Am. 2018;56(3):377–90.
2. Gonzalez MF, Akhtar I, Manucha V. Changing trends and practices in cytopathology. Acta Cytol. 2017;61(2):91–5.
3. da Cunha Santos G. ROSEs (rapid on-site evaluations) to our patients: the impact on laboratory resources and patient care. Cancer Cytopathol. 2013;121(10):537–9.
4. Eszlinger M, Lau L, Ghaznavi S, Symonds C, Chandarana SP, Khalil M, Paschke R. Molecular profiling of thyroid nodule fine-needle aspiration cytology. Nat Rev Endocrinol. 2017;13(7):415–24.
5. Jain D, Allen TC, Aisner DL, Beasley MB, Cagle PT, Capelozzi VL, Hariri LP, Lantuejoul S, Miller R, Mino-Kenudson M, Monaco SE, Moreira A, Raparia K, Rekhtman N, Roden AC, Roy-Chowdhuri S, da Cunha Santos G, Thunnissen E, Troncone G, Vivero M. Rapid on-site evaluation of endobronchial ultrasound-guided transbronchial needle aspirations for the diagnosis of lung cancer: a perspective from members of the Pulmonary Pathology Society. Arch Pathol Lab Med. 2018;142(2):253–62.
6. da Cunha Santos G, Saieg MA, Troncone G, Zeppa P. Cytological preparations for molecular analysis: a review of technical procedures, advantages and limitations for referring samples for testing. Cytopathology. 2018;29(2):125–32.
7. Brainard J, Farver C. The diagnosis of non-small cell lung cancer in the molecular era. Mod Pathol. 2019; https://doi.org/10.1038/s41379-018-0156-x. [Epub ahead of print].
8. Coley SM, Crapanzano JP, Saqi A. FNA, core biopsy, or both for the diagnosis of lung carcinoma: obtaining sufficient tissue for a specific diagnosis and molecular testing. Cancer Cytopathol. 2015;123(5):318–26.
9. Mehmood S, Jahan A, Loya A, Yusuf MA. Onsite cytopathology evaluation and ancillary studies beneficial in EUS-FNA of pancreatic, mediastinal, intra-abdominal, and submucosal lesions. Diagn Cytopathol. 2015;43(4):278–86.
10. Mohanty SK, Pradhan D, Sharma S, Sharma A, Patnaik N, Feuerman M, Bonasara R, Boyd A, Friedel D, Stavropoulos S, Gupta M. Endoscopic ultrasound guided fine-needle aspiration: what variables influence diagnostic yield? Diagn Cytopathol. 2018;46(4):293–8.

11. Pearson LN, Layfield LJ, Schmidt RL. Cost-effectiveness of rapid on-site evaluation of the adequacy of FNA cytology samples performed by nonpathologists. Cancer Cytopathol. 2018;126(10):839–45.
12. Stevenson T, Powari M, Bowles C. Evolution of a rapid onsite evaluation (ROSE) service for endobronchial ultrasound guided (EBUS) fine needle aspiration (FNA) cytology in a UK Hospital: a 7 year audit. Diagn Cytopathol. 2018; https://doi.org/10.1002/dc.23967. [Epub ahead of print].
13. Schmidt RL, Witt BL, Lopez-Calderon LE, Layfield LJ. The influence of rapid onsite evaluation on the adequacy rate of fine-needle aspiration cytology: a systematic review and meta-analysis. Am J Clin Pathol. 2013;139(3):300–8.
14. Kappelle WFW, Van Leerdam ME, Schwartz MP, Bülbül M, Buikhuisen WA, Brink MA, Sie-Go DMDS, Pullens HJM, Nikolakopoulos S, Van Diest PJ, Leenders M, Moons LMG, Bogte A, Siersema PD, Vleggaar FP. Rapid on-site evaluation during endoscopic ultrasound-guided fine-needle aspiration of lymph nodes does not increase diagnostic yield: a randomized, multicenter trial. Am J Gastroenterol. 2018;113(5):677–85.
15. Sehgal IS, Dhooria S, Aggarwal AN, Agarwal R. Impact of rapid on-site cytological evaluation (ROSE) on the diagnostic yield of transbronchial needle aspiration during mediastinal lymph node sampling: systematic review and meta-analysis. Chest. 2018;153(4):929–38.
16. Cibas ES, Ali SZ. The 2017 Bethesda system for reporting thyroid cytopathology. Thyroid. 2017;27(11):1341–6.
17. Alsharif M, Andrade RS, Groth SS, Stelow EB, Pambuccian SE. Endobronchial ultrasound-guided transbronchial fine-needle aspiration: the University of Minnesota experience, with emphasis on usefulness, adequacy assessment, and diagnostic difficulties. Am J Clin Pathol. 2008;130(3):434–43.
18. Nayak A, Sugrue C, Koenig S, Wasserman PG, Hoda S, Morgenstern NJ. Endobronchial ultrasound-guided transbronchial needle aspirate (EBUS-TBNA): a proposal for on-site adequacy criteria. Diagn Cytopathol. 2012;40(2):128–37.
19. Karunamurthy A, Cai G, Dacic S, Khalbuss WE, Pantanowitz L, Monaco SE. Evaluation of endobronchial ultrasound-guided fine-needle aspirations (EBUS-FNA): correlation with adequacy and histologic follow-up. Cancer Cytopathol. 2014;122(1):23–32.
20. Choi SM, Lee AR, Choe JY, Nam SJ, Chung DH, Lee J, Lee CH, Lee SM, Yim JJ, Yoo CG, Kim YW, Han SK, Park YS. Adequacy criteria of rapid on-site evaluation for endobronchial ultrasound-guided transbronchial needle aspiration: a simple algorithm to assess the adequacy of ROSE. Ann Thorac Surg. 2016;101(2):444–50.
21. Olson MT, Ali SZ. Cytotechnologist on-site evaluation of pancreas fine needle aspiration adequacy: comparison with cytopathologists and correlation with the final interpretation. Acta Cytol. 2012;56(4):340–6.
22. Bonifazi M, Sediari M, Ferretti M, Poidomani G, Tramacere I, Mei F, Zuccatosta L, Gasparini S. The role of the pulmonologist in rapid on-site cytologic evaluation of transbronchial needle aspiration: a prospective study. Chest. 2014;145(1):60–5.
23. Eloubeidi MA, Tamhane A, Jhala N, Chhieng D, Jhala D, Crowe DR, Eltoum IA. Agreement between rapid onsite and final cytologic interpretations of EUS-guided FNA specimens: implications for the endosonographer and patient management. Am J Gastroenterol. 2006;101(12):2841–7.
24. Fassina A, Corradin M, Zardo D, Cappellesso R, Corbetti F, Fassan M. Role and accuracy of rapid on-site evaluation of CT-guided fine needle aspiration cytology of lung nodules. Cytopathology. 2011;22(5):306–12.
25. Wangsiricharoen S, Lekawanvijit S, Rangdaeng S. Agreement between rapid on-site evaluation and the final cytological diagnosis of salivary gland specimens. Cytopathology. 2017;28(4):321–8.
26. Gupta N, Klein M, Chau K, Vadalia B, Khutti S, Gimenez C, Das K. Adequate at rapid on-site evaluation (ROSE), but inadequate on final cytologic diagnosis: analysis of 606 cases of endobronchial ultrasound-guided trans bronchial needle aspirations (EBUS-TBNA). Diagn Cytopathol. 2018; https://doi.org/10.1002/dc.24121. [Epub ahead of print].

27. Jhala NC, Jhala DN, Chhieng DC, Eloubeidi MA, Eltoum IA. Endoscopic ultrasound-guided fine-needle aspiration. A cytopathologist's perspective. Am J Clin Pathol. 2003;120(3):351–67.
28. Chang KJ, Albers CG, Erickson RA, Butler JA, Wuerker RB, Lin F. Endoscopic ultrasound-guided fine needle aspiration of pancreatic carcinoma. Am J Gastroenterol. 1994;89(2):263–6.
29. Jeffus SK, Joiner AK, Siegel ER, Massoll NA, Meena N, Chen C, Post SR, Bartter T. Rapid on-site evaluation of EBUS-TBNA specimens of lymph nodes: comparative analysis and recommendations for standardization. Cancer Cytopathol. 2015;123(6):362–72.
30. Williams DB, Sahai AV, Aabakken L, Penman ID, van Velse A, Webb J, Wilson M, Hoffman BJ, Hawes RH. Endoscopic ultrasound guided fine needle aspiration biopsy: a large single centre experience. Gut. 1999;44(5):720–6.
31. Jhala NC, Jhala D, Eltoum I, Vickers SM, Wilcox CM, Chhieng DC, Eloubeidi MA. Endoscopic ultrasound-guided fine-needle aspiration biopsy: a powerful tool to obtain samples from small lesions. Cancer. 2004;102(4):239–46.
32. Gress FG, Hawes RH, Savides TJ, Ikenberry SO, Lehman GA. Endoscopic ultrasound-guided fine-needle aspiration biopsy using linear array and radial scanning endosonography. Gastrointest Endosc. 1997;45(3):243–50.
33. Shin HJ, Lahoti S, Sneige N. Endoscopic ultrasound-guided fine-needle aspiration in 179 cases: the M. D. Anderson Cancer Center experience. Cancer. 2002;296(3):174–80.
34. Klapman JB, Logrono R, Dye CE, Waxman I. Clinical impact of on-site cytopathology interpretation on endoscopic ultrasound-guided fine needle aspiration. Am J Gastroenterol. 2003;98(6):1289–94.
35. Wiersema MJ, Vilmann P, Giovannini M, Chang KJ, Wiersema LM. Endosonography-guided fine-needle aspiration biopsy: diagnostic accuracy and complication assessment. Gastroenterology. 1997;112(4):1087–95.
36. Bentz JS, Kochman ML, Faigel DO, Ginsberg GG, Smith DB, Gupta PK. Endoscopic ultrasound-guided real-time fine-needle aspiration: clinicopathologic features of 60 patients. Diagn Cytopathol. 1998;18(2):98–109.
37. Chang KJ, Nguyen P, Erickson RA, Durbin TE, Katz KD. The clinical utility of endoscopic ultrasound-guided fine-needle aspiration in the diagnosis and staging of pancreatic carcinoma. Gastrointest Endosc. 1997;45(5):387–93.
38. Crowe DR, Eloubeidi MA, Chhieng DC, Jhala NC, Jhala D, Eltoum IA. Fine-needle aspiration biopsy of hepatic lesions: computerized tomographic-guided versus endoscopic ultrasound-guided FNA. Cancer. 2006;108(3):180–5.
39. Jiang D, Zang Y, Jiang D, Zhang X, Zhao C. Value of rapid on-site evaluation for ultrasound-guided thyroid fine needle aspiration. J Int Med Res. 2019;47(2):626–34.
40. Anila KR, Nayak N, Venugopal M, Jayasree K. Role of rapid on-site evaluation in CT-guided fine needle aspiration cytology of lung nodules. J Cytol. 2018;35(4):229–32.
41. Ali S, Hawes RH, Kadkhodayan K, Rafiq E, Navaneethan U, Bang JY, Varadarajulu S, Hasan MK. Utility of rapid onsite evaluation of touch imprint cytology from endoscopic and cholangioscopic forceps biopsy sampling (with video). Gastrointest Endosc. 2019;89(2):340–4. https://doi.org/10.1016/j.gie.2018.08.050. Epub 2018 Sep 5.
42. Adeniran AJ, Al-Ahmadie H, Iyengar P, Reuter VE, Lin O. Fine needle aspiration of renal cortical lesions in adults. Diagn Cytopathol. 2010;38(10):710–5.
43. Singhi AD, Zeh HJ, Brand RE, Nikiforova MN, Chennat JS, Fasanella KE, Khalid A, Papachristou GI, Slivka A, Hogg M, Lee KK, Tsung A, Zureikat AH, McGrath K. American Gastroenterological Association guidelines are inaccurate in detecting pancreatic cysts with advanced neoplasia: a clinicopathologic study of 225 patients with supporting molecular data. Gastrointest Endosc. 2016;83(6):1107–17.
44. Okasha HH, Ashry M, Imam HM, Ezzat R, Naguib M, Farag AH, Gemeie EH, Khattab HM. Role of endoscopic ultrasound-guided fine needle aspiration and ultrasound-guided fine-needle aspiration in diagnosis of cystic pancreatic lesions. Endosc Ultrasound. 2015;4(2):132–6.
45. Lin O, Rudomina D, Feratovic R, Sirintrapun SJ. Rapid on-site evaluation using telecytology: a major cancer center experience. Diagn Cytopathol. 2019;47(1):15–9.

Chapter 2
Facility, Equipment, Specimen Preparation, and Stains

Guoping Cai

Facility, Equipment, and Supplies

Facility

Fine needle aspiration (FNA) can be performed by palpation or under imaging guidance. Common locations for performing rapid on-site evaluation (ROSE) include FNA clinic, physician's office, ultrasound suite, computed tomography room, and bronchoscopy or endoscopy suite. ROSE may sometimes be performed in operating room. Depending on the frequency of service needs, there are several options for setting ROSE service. If there is a frequent need for ROSE service, a separate room adjacent to the biopsy suite or a designated area within the biopsy suite is preferred. A mobile station can be used as an alternative when the service is less frequently requested or requested only for rare occasions. Regardless which setting is chosen, the ultimate goal is to ensure the delivery of ROSE service in a timely manner.

Microscope and Accessories

Microscope is essential for on-site cytological evaluation. Due to time constraint of the service, a fully functional, high-quality microscope is required to relay reliable results to the biopsy physician, which may have significant impact on the biopsy procedure. A two-headed microscope is preferred which allows, if needed, pathologist to discuss the findings with the biopsy physician when reviewing the morphology together. Alternatively, a camera or video camera can be attached to the

G. Cai (✉)
Department of Pathology, Yale University School of Medicine, New Haven, CT, USA
e-mail: guoping.cai@yale.edu

G. Cai, A. J. Adeniran (eds.), *Rapid On-site Evaluation (ROSE)*,
https://doi.org/10.1007/978-3-030-21799-0_2

microscope, allowing the transfer of live images to the monitors. This setting also allows the biopsy physician to view live images without leaving the biopsy suite and/or allows pathologists to remotely evaluate the biopsy primarily or as a second opinion consultation [1–3]. Based on the need, image transfer can be accomplished via local cable connection or an internet-based approach.

Supplies

The supplies needed for on-site evaluation include needles, syringes, grass slides, staining reagents, and the containers with fixatives. Sterile containers may also need to be stocked for potential microbiology culture study. A temperature-adjustable electric heat plate should be equipped, which can help dry the slide quickly if the smears are thick and bloody.

Fixatives

Specimen fixatives may include 95% ethanol, other ethanol-/methanol-based fixatives, and 10% neutral buffered formalin solution. Some freshly prepared smear slides should be immediately fixated in 95% ethanol fixative for Papanicolaou staining later on. To achieve an optimal diagnostic yield, part of the aspirates should be saved for preparation of a cell block. The aspirates can be saved in formalin or ethanol-/methanol-based fixatives. The tissue or cellular material using ethanol-/methanol-based fixatives may or may not be ideal for immunohistochemical analysis since in most pathology labs, the test is optimized for formalin-fixed tissue including negative and positive controls [4–8]. However, ethanol-/methanol-fixated material is equivalent or superior to formalin-fixed tissue for molecular testing [9–14]. In addition, some ethanol/methanol fixatives such as CytoRich fixative have the capability to lyse red blood cells, which will be ideal for bloody specimens.

Cell preservatives such as Roswell Park Memorial Institute (RPMI) medium should also be stocked in case there is a need to send fresh specimen for flow cytometry analysis. RPMI solution should be kept in refrigerator until its use.

Specimen Preparation

On-site cytological evaluation can be applied to a variety of specimens including fine needle aspirates, core needle biopsy tissue fragments, forceps biopsy tissue fragments, and less frequently surgical excision/biopsy specimens. Among them, fine needle aspirates are the most common type of specimens submitted for on-site evaluation, from which direct smears are often made. Other forms of preparations for on-site evaluation include touch preparation and scrapping smear. During on-site evaluation, it is important to save adequate specimen for additional ancillary studies.

Smear Preparation

Direct smears are the primary preparations of fine needle aspiration biopsy. The aspirates obtained are expelled onto the glass slides usually by a syringe. In case the aspirates get clotted within the biopsy needle (often occurs when using longer biopsy needles during endoscopy- or bronchoscopy-guided biopsy), a stellate can be used to remove the aspirates. Smears are the preferred preparations for on-site evaluation because smearing process can make the cellular aspirates to be optimally distributed on slide. The organizational characteristics of cellular material on slide may offer cytomorphologic clues to determine the important issue with cell type. For example, the tumor cells of epithelial origin tend to cluster together, and different epithelial tumors may display specific arrangements such as sheets, papillary architecture, and acinar formation. Hematopoietic tumors and melanomas, on the other hand, have a dispersed single-cell distribution. The presence of smearing artifacts such as nuclear streaming and lymphoglandular bodies may also aid in the diagnosis of lymphoproliferative disorders [15, 16].

One-Slide Smearing Technique

This smearing technique can be used for slide preparation when the aspirates are scant. As illustrated in Fig. 2.1, the slide preparation consists of three steps: (1) expel the aspirates onto the slide at the spot above the middle portion; (2) place a second slide, the spreader slide, crosswise over the specimen slide; and (3) keep the specimen slide steady and pull gently the spreader slide back toward the end of the specimen slide. This smearing technique produces one single slide. The spreader slide often contains little or no cellular material and is discarded.

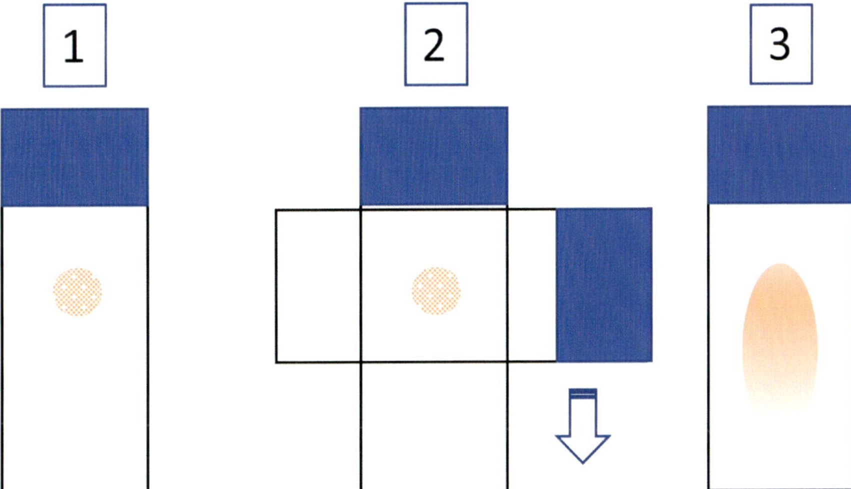

Fig. 2.1 On-slide smearing technique

Two-Slide Smearing Technique

This smearing technique can be used for slide preparation when there is a large amount of specimen. As illustrated in Fig. 2.2, the preparation consists of three steps: (1) expel the aspirates onto the slide at the spot slightly below the middle portion, (2) place a second slide inline over the specimen slide, and (3) pull gently the specimen slide and the second slide toward the opposite directions. This smearing technique produces two slides with similar amount of material. One slide can be air-dried, stained with Diff-Quik stain, and used for on-site evaluation. The second slide should be immediately fixed in 95% of alcohol and saved for Papanicolaou or hematoxylin-eosin stain later on.

Tips for Smearing Techniques

Timing is an important factor for the production of high-quality direct smears. How quickly should you start the smearing process after placing the second slide over the specimen slide depends upon the texture of aspirates. If the aspirates are thick, you should wait for a while before starting the smearing step so that the aspirates can spread out slightly by capillary action. By this way, the prepared smears are not too thick to be used for cytological evaluation. If the aspirates are watery, you have to act quickly and start the smearing step right after placing two slides over together. Otherwise, you will not be able to move the slides because too much tension force is formed between the slides.

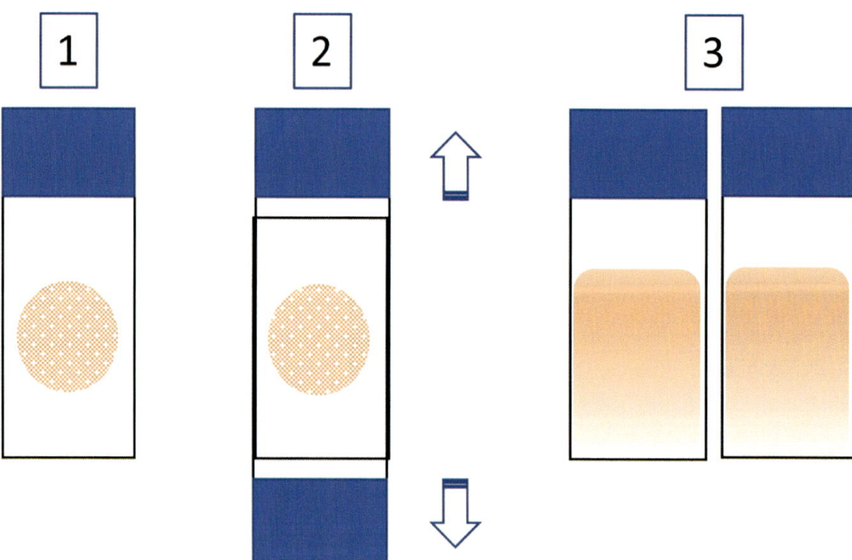

Fig. 2.2 Two-slide smearing technique

During the preparation of smearing slides, it is important to keep the smearing slide and the specimen slide parallel, which helps minimize the damage to the cells. Also, no additional force should be applied to the slides except for the force to gently pull the slides. The tension forces the aspirate creates in between two slides should be sufficient to spread out the aspirates.

Touch Preparation or Imprint

Touch preparation is primarily used for on-site evaluation of tissue obtained by core needle biopsy or forceps biopsy [17]. To prepare a touch preparation, the obtained tissue fragments are placed on the glass slide (Fig. 2.3). Then, a needle or toothpick is used to gently roll or flip the tissue over repeatedly toward close to the end of the slide. After preparation of the slide, the tissue fragments should be saved in formalin fixative and submitted for histopathological evaluation. Forceps should not be used to handle tissue becuase it may cause damage to the tissue. The rolling or flapping

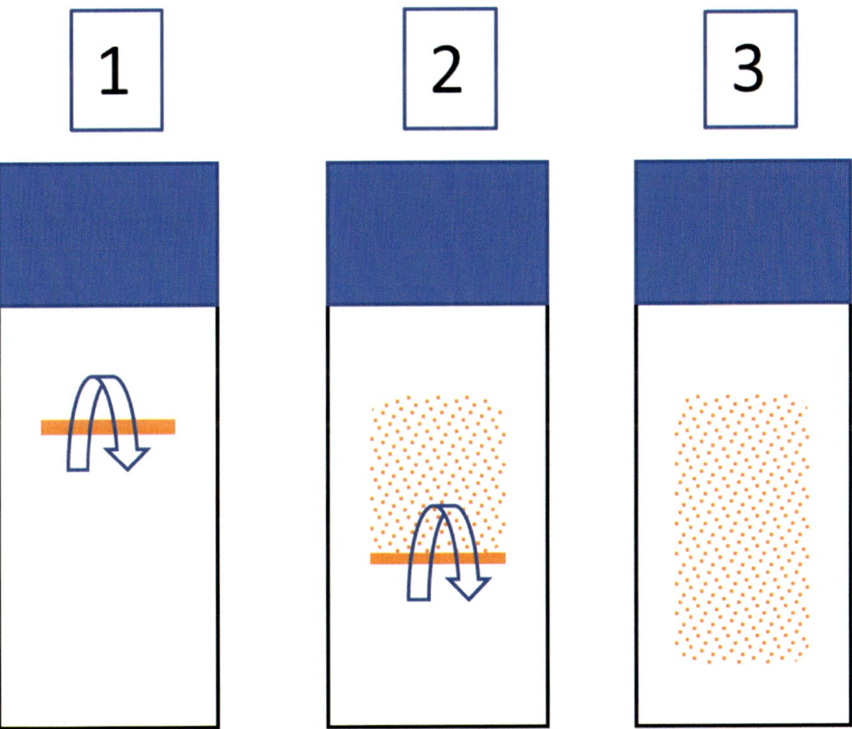

Fig. 2.3 Touch preparation of core biopsy tissue

process should be carried out with extreme caution. A recent study has shown that vigorous touch preparation might cause significant damage to tissue or loss of diagnostic material, which could lead to failure to render diagnosis and perform molecular testing [18].

During intraoperative consultation, touch imprint can be made from surgically removed tissue such as sentinel lymph node. Cytopathological evaluation of touch imprint can be used as a solely diagnostic evaluation or as an adjunction to frozen section [19–21].

It should be kept in mind that touch imprints are different from smears because no tension force is applied to cellular material when preparing touch preparations. Thus, touch imprints are not optimal to assess the cohesiveness of cells of interest and less reliable to classify cell types based on the organizational architectures seen on touch imprints.

Scrapping Smear

During intraoperative consultation, surgically removed specimens, if sizable, can also be used to prepare a scrapping smear for cytological evaluation [22, 23]. To make a scrapping smear, the specimens are sliced to reveal the lesion of interest. A scalpel blade is then used to collect superficial tissue fragments of the lesion by gently moving the blade back and forth along the cut surface of the lesion. The tissue fragments collected are transferred onto a glass slide. The one-slide smearing technique is often used to make a smear.

Similar to direct smears made from fine needle aspirates, scrapping smears provide, in addition to cell morphology, the information about cohesiveness of the cells. The organizational architectures of cell arrangement and smearing artifacts seen on scrapping smears may also provide diagnostic clues. Thus, scrapping smears are particularly useful and may be superior to touch imprints in cases such as tumors of an unknown cell lineage.

Stains Suitable for On-Site Evaluation

On-site cytological evaluation is time-sensitive and the staining process should be completed with a short period of time. Therefore, time is the most important issue for choosing appropriate staining reagents. Other factors to be considered include the preservation of cytomorphology and complexity of staining process. Whether staining reagents contain hazardous material should also be taken into consideration unless the staining process is performed in an environmentally safe setting such as in frozen section room. Selection of a specific staining protocol for laboratory use ultimately depends on the resources, experiences, and personal preferences.

Diff-Quik Stain

Diff-Quik stain is a commercially branded Romanowsky stain and is modified from the Wright Giemsa stain. With the modification, the staining time is reduced to less than 1 min. The staining reagents include: (1) fixative reagents containing methanol and triarylmethane dye, (2) eosinophilic solution (solution I) containing xanthene dye and sodium azide, and (3) basophilic solution (solution II) containing thiazine dye.

The details of Diff-Quik staining procedure:

(a) Slide preparation: completely air-dried
(b) Fixative solution: 10 dips
(c) Solution I: 10 dips
(d) Solution II: 10 dips
(e) Water: 10 dips

Due to its rapid staining process, Diff-Quik stain has become the stain of choice for on-site evaluation [24–27]. Cytoplasmic details such as intracytoplasmic mucin, fat droplets, and cytoplasmic granules can readily be visible on Diff-Quik stain. Extracellular substances such as mucin, colloid, and matrix can easily be stained and appear metachromatic (Figs. 2.4, 2.5, and 2.6). Diff-Quik can also stain some microorganisms such as bacteria and some fungal organisms [28].

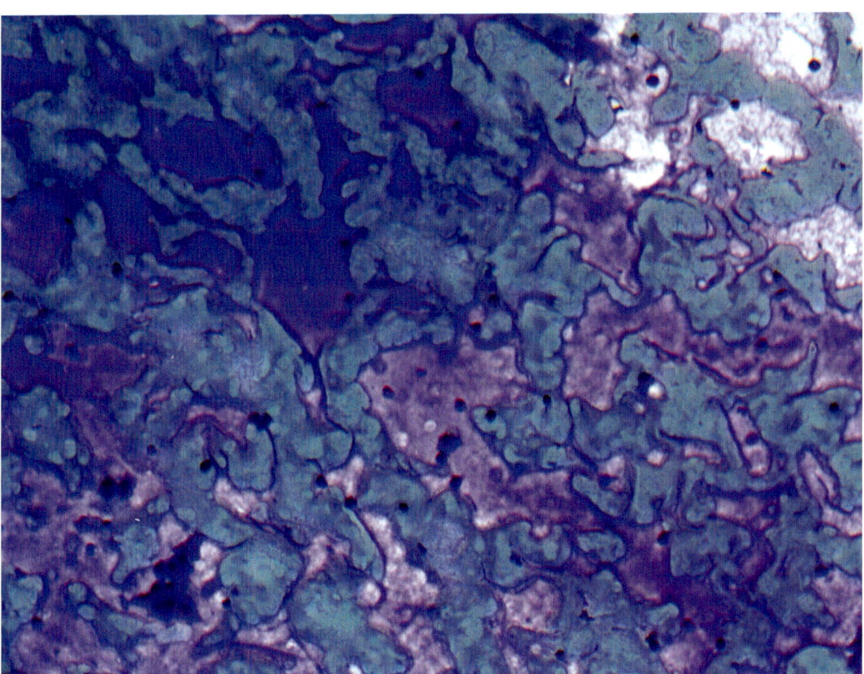

Fig. 2.4 Benign thyroid nodule showing abundant colloid as thick metachromatic material on Diff-Quik stain (original magnification, ×200)

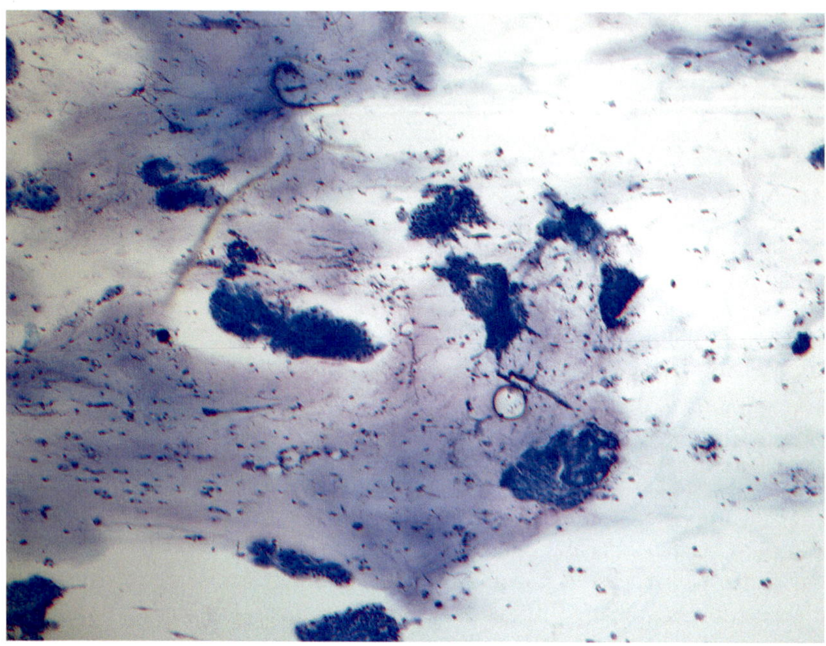

Fig. 2.5 Mucinous cyst of the pancreas showing clusters of epithelial cells in a background of mucinous material on Diff-Quik stain (original magnification, ×40)

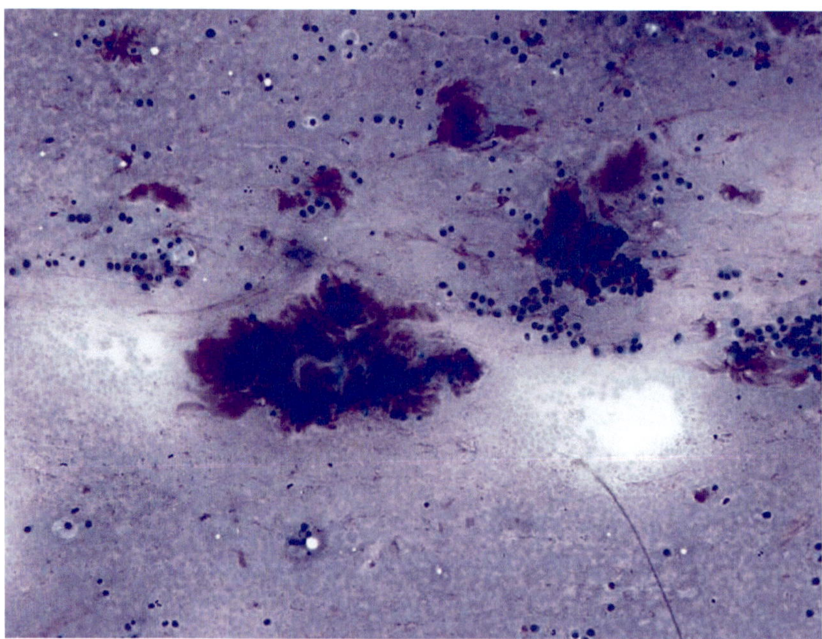

Fig. 2.6 Pleomorphic adenoma of the parotid gland showing dyscohesive epithelioid cells intermixed with metachromatic fibrillary matrix on Diff-Quik stain (original magnification, ×100)

Because air-dried slides are used for the staining, the cells on Diff-Quik-stained slides appear larger than those seen on other stains. It should be cautious to interpret cytological atypia, particularly related to cell size. Nuclear details such as nuclear membrane irregularity, chromatin pattern, and nucleoli are not well appreciated on Diff-Quik stain [29, 30].

Rapid Papanicolaou Stain

Papanicolaou (Pap) stain is the most commonly used staining technique in cytopathology practice. The stain is very reliable and can be applied to a variety of cytological preparations including smears and touch preparation. Cytological details, especially nuclear and chromatin features as well as cytoplasmic keratinization, are well illustrated on Pap-stained slides (Figs. 2.7 and 2.8). However, Pap staining process is lengthy and requires at least a half hour to complete. This has encouraged modifications to the standard protocol with lesser staining time but maintaining cell morphology, known as rapid Pap stain [29–34].

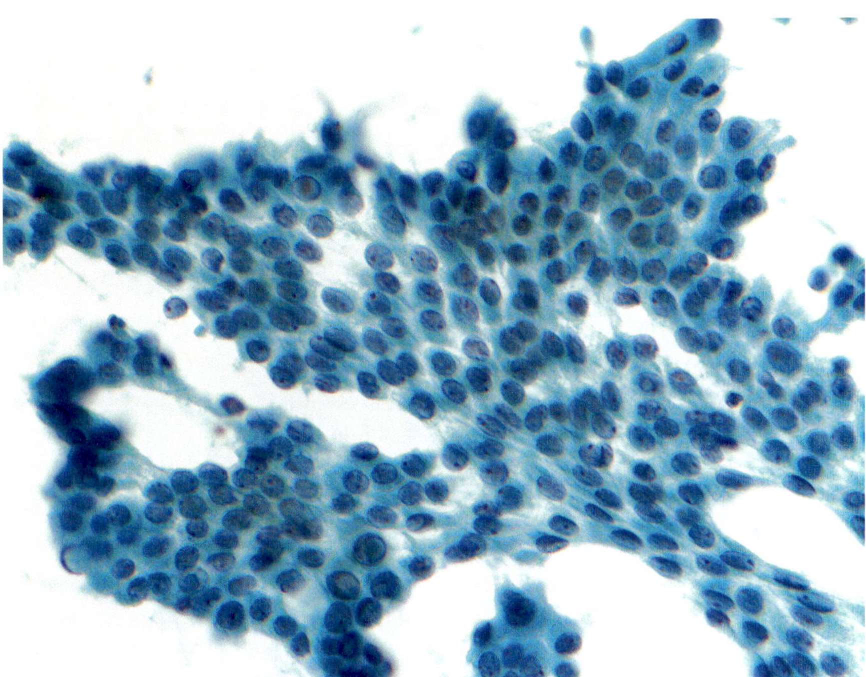

Fig. 2.7 Papillary thyroid carcinoma showing sheets of follicular cells with enlarged oval nuclei, washout chromatin, nuclear grooves, and intranuclear pseudoinclusions on Papanicolaou stain (original magnification, ×400)

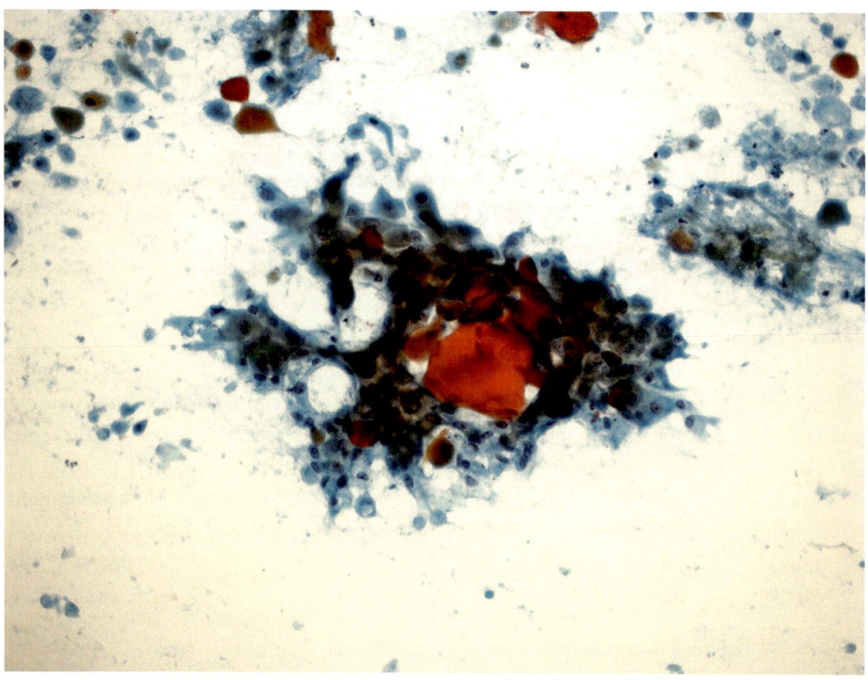

Fig. 2.8 Metastatic keratinizing squamous cell carcinoma of the neck showing clusters of epithelial cells with dense orangeophilic cytoplasm on Papanicolaou stain (original magnification, ×200)

The details of rapid Pap staining procedure:

(a) Fixed in 95% ethanol.
(b) Wash smear in water: 20 s.
(c) Stain in hematoxylin solution: 1–3 min.
(d) Wash in water.
(e) Bluing solution: 20 s.
(f) Wash in water.
(g) 95% ethanol: 20 s.
(h) Stain in Papanicolaou stain OG 6-EA: 1–3 min.
(i) 100% ethanol.
(j) 100% ethanol.
(k) Xylene.
(l) Xylene.
(m) Coverslip.

Further modification of the dehydration steps before and after Pap OG-6 with acetic acid instead of ethanol can further shorten the staining time [32, 34]. Rapid Pap stain can also be applied to air-dried smears with addition of a rehydration step at the beginning of staining process and minor revisions of staining reagents, known as Ultrafast Pap stain [29, 30, 35–38]. Ultrafast Pap stain may be superior to the standard rapid Pap stain in part due to short staining time [36, 38]. Some cytomorphologic features such as washout or clear chromatin pattern of papillary thyroid carcinoma and large nucleoli of Hodgkin lymphoma are better appreciated on Ultrafast Pap stain [36, 37].

Hematoxylin-Eosin Stain

Hematoxylin-eosin (H&E) stain is the standard staining for histopathological evaluation. Rapid protocols for H&E staining can be performed in about 3 min and are widely used for intraoperative frozen service, yielding excellent results. Rapid H&E stain has also been applied to evaluation of cytological specimens [29, 39–43]. Excellent nuclear details can be revealed on rapid H&E stain (Fig. 2.9).

The details of rapid H&E staining procedure:

(a) Wash in water: 20 dips
(b) Hematoxylin: 1 min
(c) Wash in water: 10 dips
(d) Bluing solution: 10 dips

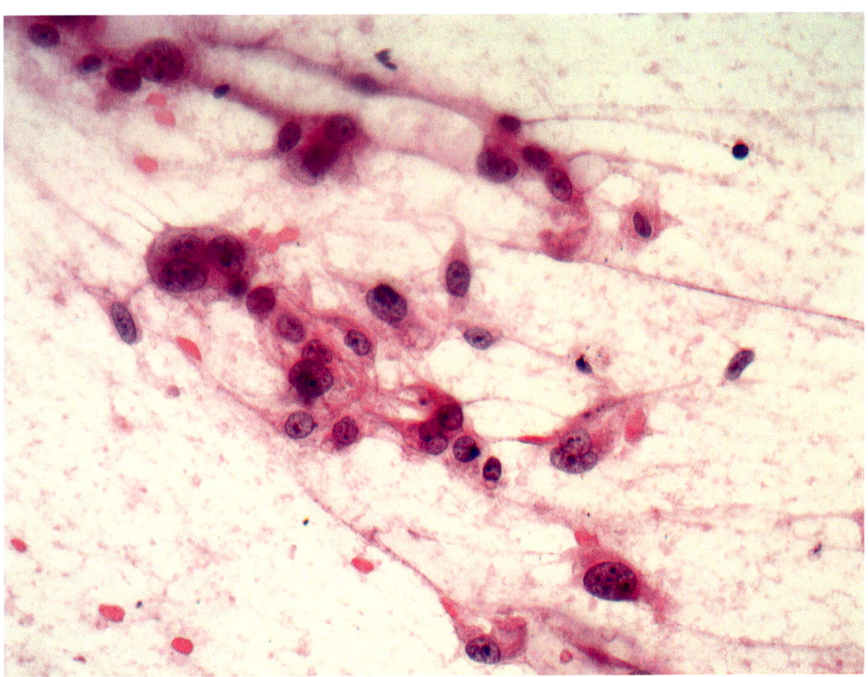

Fig. 2.9 Sarcomatoid carcinoma of the nasal cavity showing loosely cohesive groups of tumor cells with pleomorphic nuclei, irregular nuclear contours, and conspicuous nucleoli on hematoxylin-eosin stain (original magnification, ×400)

(e) Wash in water: 10 dips
(f) 95% ethanol: 10 dips
(g) Eosin: 3 s
(h) 95% ethanol: 10 dips
(i) 100% ethanol: 10 dips
(j) 100% ethanol: 10 dips
(k) Xylene: 10 dips
(l) Xylene: 10 dips

Toluidine Blue Stain

Toluidine blue is a basic thiazine metachromatic dye with high affinity for acidic tissue components. It stains nucleic acids blue and polysaccharides purple. In addition to its utility in forensic examination, renal pathology, and neuropathology, toluidine blue can also be used for on-site evaluation. The stain is prepared by dissolving 0.5 g of crystalline toluidine blue in 20 ml of 95% ethanol and then adding distilled water up to 100 ml. The prepared stain is filtered and saved in refrigerator till use.

Toluidine blue reagent can be directly applied to specimen-containing slide or to 95% ethanol fixed smear slide [44–46]. The specimen on the slide is mixed with a few drops of the stain reagent. The slide is then coverslipped and the wet film will be ready for microscopic evaluation in a few seconds. After the evaluation, the slide with its coverslip is saved in Coplin jar with 95% ethanol and can be used for routine Papanicolaou stain later on. Toluidine stain is a quick, economic staining but may probably not be the best stain for revelation of cytomorphologic details.

References

1. Buxbaum JL, Eloubeidi MA, Lane CJ, Varadarajulu S, Linder A, Crowe AE, Jhala D, Jhala NC, Crowe DR, Eltoum IA. Dynamic telecytology compares favorably to rapid onsite evaluation of endoscopic ultrasound fine needle aspirates. Dig Dis Sci. 2012;57(12):3092–7.
2. Kern I, Gabric S, Triller N, Pozek I. Telecytology for rapid assessment of cytological specimens. J Telemed Telecare. 2012;18(2):86–9.
3. Sirintrapun SJ, Rudomina D, Mazzella A, Feratovic R, Lin O. Successful secure high-definition streaming telecytology for remote cytologic evaluation. J Pathol Inform. 2017;8:33.
4. Sauter G, Lee J, Bartlett JM, Slamon DJ, Press MF. Guidelines for human epidermal growth factor receptor 2 testing: biologic and methodologic considerations. J Clin Oncol. 2009;27(8):1323–33.
5. Nietner T, Jarutat T, Mertens A. Systematic comparison of tissue fixation with alternative fixatives to conventional tissue fixation with buffered formalin in a xenograft-based model. Virchows Arch. 2012;461(3):259–69.
6. Maleki S, Dorokhova O, Sunkara J, Schlesinger K, Suhrland M, Oktay MH. Estrogen, progesterone, and HER-2 receptor immunostaining in cytology: the effect of varied fixation on human breast cancer cells. Diagn Cytopathol. 2013;41(10):864–70.

7. Pereira MA, Dias AR, Faraj SF, Cirqueira Cdos S, Tomitao MT, Nahas SC, Ribeiro U Jr, de Mello ES. Carnoy's solution is an adequate tissue fixative for routine surgical pathology, preserving cell morphology and molecular integrity. Histopathology. 2015;66(3):388–97.
8. Vohra P, Buelow B, Chen YY, Serrano M, Vohra MS, Berry A, Ljung BM. Estrogen receptor, progesterone receptor, and human epidermal growth factor receptor 2 expression in breast cancer FNA cell blocks and paired histologic specimens: a large retrospective study. Cancer Cytopathol. 2016;124(11):828–35.
9. van Hemel BM, Suurmeijer AJ. Effective application of the methanol-based PreservCyt(TM) fixative and the Cellient(TM) automated cell block processor to diagnostic cytopathology, immunocytochemistry, and molecular biology. Diagn Cytopathol. 2013;41(8):734–41.
10. Rosenblum F, Hutchinson LM, Garver J, Woda B, Cosar E, Kurian EM. Cytology specimens offer an effective alternative to formalin-fixed tissue as demonstrated by novel automated detection for ALK break-apart FISH testing and immunohistochemistry in lung adenocarcinoma. Cancer Cytopathol. 2014;122(11):810–21.
11. Gailey MP, Stence AA, Jensen CS, Ma D. Multiplatform comparison of molecular oncology tests performed on cytology specimens and formalin-fixed, paraffin-embedded tissue. Cancer Cytopathol. 2015;123(1):30–9.
12. Roy-Chowdhuri S, Goswami RS, Chen H, Patel KP, Routbort MJ, Singh RR, Broaddus RR, Barkoh BA, Manekia J, Yao H, Medeiros LJ, Staerkel G, Luthra R, Stewart J. Factors affecting the success of next-generation sequencing in cytology specimens. Cancer Cytopathol. 2015;123(11):659–68.
13. Hopkins E, Moffat D, Parkinson I, Robinson P, Jersmann H, Dougherty B, Birader MI, Francis K, Nguyen P. Cell block samples from endobronchial ultrasound transbronchial needle aspiration provide sufficient material for ancillary testing in lung cancer-a quaternary referral centre experience. J Thorac Dis. 2016;8(9):2544–50.
14. Hwang DH, Garcia EP, Ducar MD, Cibas ES, Sholl LM. Next-generation sequencing of cytologic preparations: an analysis of quality metrics. Cancer Cytopathol. 2017;125(10):786–94.
15. Stastny JF, Almeida MM, Wakely PE Jr, Kornstein MJ, Frable WJ. Fine-needle aspiration biopsy and imprint cytology of small non-cleaved cell (Burkitt's) lymphoma. Diagn Cytopathol. 1995;12(3):201–7.
16. Rodriguez EF, Sepah YJ, Jang HS, Ibrahim M, Nguyen QD, Rodriguez FJ. Cytologic features in vitreous preparations of patients with suspicion of intraocular lymphoma. Diagn Cytopathol. 2014;42(1):37–44.
17. Chandan VS, Zimmerman K, Baker P, Scalzetti E, Khurana KK. Usefulness of core roll preparations in immediate assessment of neoplastic lung lesions: comparison to conventional CT scan-guided lung fine-needle aspiration cytology. Chest. 2004;126(3):739–43.
18. Rekhtman N, Kazi S, Yao J, Dogan S, Yannes A, Lin O, Silk M, Silk T, Durack JC. Depletion of core needle biopsy cellularity and DNA content as a result of vigorous touch preparations. Arch Pathol Lab Med. 2015;139(7):907–12.
19. Sun L, Chen G, Zhou Y, Zhang L, Jin Z, Liu W, Wu G, Jin F, Li K, Chen B. Clinical significance of MSKCC nomogram on guiding the application of touch imprint cytology and frozen section in intraoperative assessment of breast sentinel lymph nodes. Oncotarget. 2017;8(44):78105–12.
20. Komenaka IK, Torabi R, Nair G, Jayaram L, Hsu CH, Bouton ME, Dave H, Hobohm D. Intraoperative touch imprint and frozen section analysis of sentinel lymph nodes after neoadjuvant chemotherapy for breast cancer. Ann Surg. 2010;251(2):319–22.
21. Krishnamurthy S, Meric-Bernstam F, Lucci A, Hwang RF, Kuerer HM, Babiera G, Ames FC, Feig BW, Ross MI, Singletary E, Hunt KK, Bedrosian I. A prospective study comparing touch imprint cytology, frozen section analysis, and rapid cytokeratin immunostain for intraoperative evaluation of axillary sentinel lymph nodes in breast cancer. Cancer. 2009;115(7):1555–62.
22. Kolte SS, Satarkar RN. Role of scrape cytology in the intraoperative diagnosis of tumor. J Cytol. 2010;27(3):86–90.
23. Alvarez-Rodríguez F, Jiménez-Heffernan J, Salas C, Pastrana M, Sanz E. Cytological features of ossifying fibromyxoid tumor of soft parts. J Cytol. 2012;29(3):205–7.

24. Baloch ZW, Tam D, Langer J, Mandel S, LiVolsi VA, Gupta PK. Ultrasound-guided fine-needle aspiration biopsy of the thyroid: role of on-site assessment and multiple cytologic preparations. Diagn Cytopathol. 2000;23(6):425–9.
25. Recine M, Kaw M, Evans DB, Krishnamurthy S. Fine-needle aspiration cytology of mucinous tumors of the pancreas. Cancer. 2004;102(2):92–9.
26. Hikichi T, Irisawa A, Bhutani MS, Takagi T, Shibukawa G, Yamamoto G, Wakatsuki T, Imamura H, Takahashi Y, Sato A, Sato M, Ikeda T, Hashimoto Y, Tasaki K, Watanabe K, Ohira H, Obara K. Endoscopic ultrasound-guided fine-needle aspiration of solid pancreatic masses with rapid on-site cytological evaluation by endosonographers without attendance of cytopathologists. J Gastroenterol. 2009;44(4):322–8.
27. Wu M, Idrees M, Zhang Z, Genden E, Burstein DE. Papanicolaou stain may not be necessary in majority of head and neck fine-needle aspirations: evidence from a correlation study between Diff-Quik-based onsite diagnosis and final diagnosis in 287 head and neck fine-needle aspirations. Diagn Cytopathol. 2010;38(11):846–53.
28. Allison DB, Simner PJ, Ali SZ. Identification of infectious organisms in cytopathology: a review of ancillary diagnostic techniques. Cancer Cytopathol. 2018;126(Suppl 8):643–53.
29. Jörundsson E, Lumsden JH, Jacobs RM. Rapid staining techniques in cytopathology: a review and comparison of modified protocols for hematoxylin and eosin, Papanicolaou and Romanowsky stains. Vet Clin Pathol. 1999;28(3):100–8.
30. Louw M, Brundyn K, Schubert PT, Wright CA, Bolliger CT, Diacon AH. Comparison of the quality of smears in transbronchial fine-needle aspirates using two staining methods for rapid on-site evaluation. Diagn Cytopathol. 2012;40(9):777–81.
31. Sato M, Taniguchi E, Kagiya T, Nunobiki O, Yang Q, Nakamura M, Nakamura Y, Mori I, Kakudo K. A modified rapid Papanicolaou stain for imprint smears. Acta Cytol. 2004;48(3):461–2.
32. Dighe SB, Ajit D, Pathuthara S, Chinoy R. Papanicolaou stain: is it economical to switch to rapid, economical, acetic acid, Papanicolaou stain? Acta Cytol. 2006;50(6):643–6.
33. Diacon AH, Koegelenberg CF, Schubert P, Brundyn K, Louw M, Wright CA, Bolliger CT. Rapid on-site evaluation of transbronchial aspirates: randomised comparison of two methods. Eur Respir J. 2010;35(6):1216–20.
34. Bhagat P, Susheilia S, Singh K, Sadhukhan S, Rajwanshi A, Dey P. Efficacy of modified rapid economic acetic acid-based Papanicolaou stain. Cytopathology. 2016;27(6):452–5.
35. Yang GC, Alvarez II. Ultrafast Papanicolaou stain. An alternative preparation for fine needle aspiration cytology. Acta Cytol. 1995;39(1):55–60.
36. Yang GC, Liebeskind D, Messina AV. Ultrasound-guided fine-needle aspiration of the thyroid assessed by Ultrafast Papanicolaou stain: data from 1135 biopsies with a two- to six-year follow-up. Thyroid. 2001;11(6):581–9.
37. Zu Y, Gangi MD, Yang GC. Ultrafast Papanicolaou stain and cell-transfer technique enhance cytologic diagnosis of Hodgkin lymphoma. Diagn Cytopathol. 2002;27(5):308–11.
38. Choudhary P, Sudhamani S, Pandit A, Kiri V. Comparison of modified ultrafast Papanicolaou stain with the standard rapid Papanicolaou stain in cytology of various organs. J Cytol. 2012;29(4):241–5.
39. Daskalakis A, Kostopoulos S, Spyridonos P, Glotsos D, Ravazoula P, Kardari M, Kalatzis I, Cavouras D, Nikiforidis G. Design of a multi-classifier system for discriminating benign from malignant thyroid nodules using routinely H&E-stained cytological images. Comput Biol Med. 2008;38(2):196–203.
40. Mueller JS, Schultenover S, Simpson J, Ely K, Netterville J. Value of rapid assessment cytology in the surgical management of head and neck tumors in a Nigerian mission hospital. Head Neck. 2008;30(8):1083–5.
41. Asioli S, Maletta F, Pacchioni D, Lupo R, Bussolati G. Cytological detection of papillary thyroid carcinomas by nuclear membrane decoration with emerin staining. Virchows Arch. 2010;457(1):43–51.
42. Pak HY, Yokota SB, Teplitz RL. Rapid staining techniques employed in fine needle aspirations. Acta Cytol. 1983;27(1):81–3.

43. Dekker A, Reyna EL, Fuhrman C. Usefulness of a near-total fine-needle aspiration biopsy retrieval method: a study of its use in 85 consecutive patients. Diagn Cytopathol. 1991;7(3):308–16.
44. Davenport RD. Rapid on-site evaluation of transbronchial aspirates. Chest. 1990;98(1):59–61.
45. Ammanagi AS, Dombale VD, Patil SS. On-site toluidine blue staining and screening improves efficiency of fine-needle aspiration cytology reporting. Acta Cytol. 2012;56(4):347–51.
46. Chandra S, Chandra H, Sindhwani G. Role of rapid on-site evaluation with cyto-histopathological correlation in diagnosis of lung lesion. J Cytol. 2014;31(4):189–93.

Part II
Biopsies of Superficially Located Organs With or Without Imaging Guidance

Chapter 3
Thyroid

Adebowale J. Adeniran

Introduction

Fine needle aspiration (FNA) is the procedure of choice for the evaluation of thyroid nodules. More recently, the implementation of ultrasonographic-guided FNAs of the thyroid has increased the overall diagnostic yield and accuracy of the procedure [1–4]. However, despite the improvement in diagnostic yield, a significant subset of thyroid FNAs continues to be inadequate for interpretation, and this leads to some uncertainty in the follow-up management for such patients.

The diagnostic yield for thyroid FNA may be affected by several factors such as the nature of the lesion (e.g., size, cystic vs. solid), needle size, skill and level of experience of the operator, as well as the level of experience of the cytopathologist [1]. Many of these factors fluctuate between different institutions; hence one would expect significant variation in FNA adequacy rates. The presence or absence of rapid on-site evaluation (ROSE) by a cytopathologist or a cytotechnologist to assess for specimen adequacy during the FNA procedure is a potential factor, which can greatly affect the yield and can be standardized between institutions. Numerous studies have been published regarding the influence of ROSE on thyroid FNA specimen adequacy, with most of the studies acknowledging that FNA is more likely to be adequate for interpretation with ROSE [2, 5, 6]. More so, ROSE has been shown to decrease the number of needle passes, increase diagnostic accuracy, and reduce the risk for a repeat procedure [7, 8]. Immediate evaluation of the material also allows the opportunity to obtain additional material for cell blocks and/or ancillary

A. J. Adeniran (✉)
Department of Pathology, Yale University School of Medicine, New Haven, CT, USA
e-mail: adebowale.adeniran@yale.edu

G. Cai, A. J. Adeniran (eds.), *Rapid On-site Evaluation (ROSE)*,
https://doi.org/10.1007/978-3-030-21799-0_3

studies [9]. This is especially important in suspected cases of medullary thyroid carcinoma, which require immunostaining for calcitonin, and in suspected cases of lymphoma, which require additional material for flow cytometry.

Specimen Adequacy Assessment

Recommendations for optimal specimen preparation include the use of air-dried and alcohol-fixed slides, prepared for Romanowsky and Papanicolaou staining, respectively, with supplemental combinations of liquid-based or cytospin preparations, cell blocks, and RPMI for flow cytometric evaluation where appropriate and possibly sterile material for microbiology. For cyst-fluid-only specimens, only one or two smears are recommended with the remainder being processed as either cytospin or liquid-based preparations.

Examination usually starts with the review of the slides under scanning magnification. This quickly gives significant information as most benign follicular nodules are sparsely cellular, consisting predominantly of colloid. Colloid can be thin and watery, thick and opaque with sharp outlines, or extremely thick and sticky. Smears that have a high ratio of colloid to follicular cells generally indicate a benign thyroid nodule [10]. Some features are generally nonspecific. For instance, macrophages can be seen in cyst contents, benign hyperplastic nodule with cystic degeneration, as well as cystic papillary thyroid carcinoma. In a similar fashion, multinucleated giant cells can be seen in granulomatous diseases, benign hyperplastic nodule with cystic degeneration, papillary carcinoma, and anaplastic carcinoma.

A thyroid FNA specimen is deemed to be satisfactory for evaluation if it has at least six groups of benign, well-visualized follicular cells, with each group consisting at least 10 follicular cells [11, 12]. Tissue fragments with multiple follicles can be split up and counted as separate and distinct groups [13]. Exceptions to this adequacy requirement include: abundance of colloid even in the absence of six follicular groups, abundance of lymphocytes necessitating the diagnosis of lymphocytic thyroiditis, and presence of atypia [14].

Cystic Lesions of the Thyroid

Diagnostic Consideration

Thyroid FNA specimens with abundant histiocytes having few to no follicular cells are interpreted as "fluid cyst only," under the category of "nondiagnostic" [15, 16] (Fig. 3.1). Numerous macrophages can be seen in a variety of hyperplastic and neoplastic benign and malignant thyroid nodules undergoing cystic degeneration.

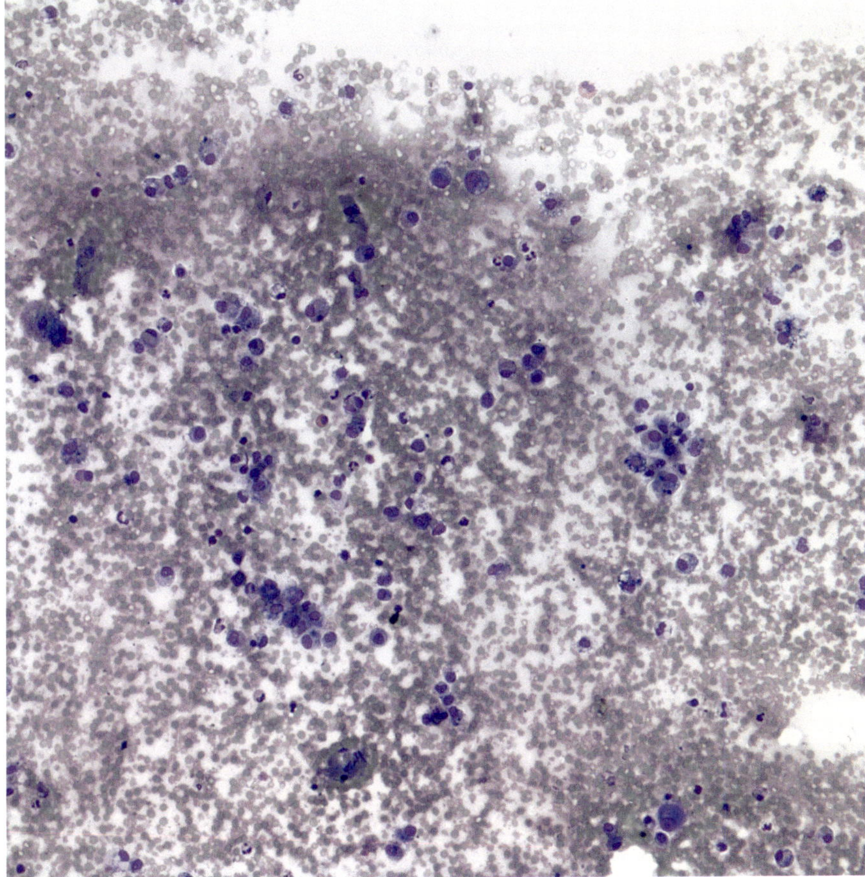

Fig. 3.1 Fluid cyst only. Abundant macrophages and no follicular cells (Diff-Quik stain, ×200)

Benign cysts arising from nodular goiters collapse after drainage. A small number may reaccumulate or bleed immediately following an FNA, necessitating reaspiration. Recurrence with hemorrhagic or chocolate-colored contents is a warning for the possibility of malignancy [17].

Cystic Degeneration in a Hyperplastic Nodule

Cytomorphologic Features

- Low cellularity.
- Abundant macrophages.
- Reactive follicular cell changes.

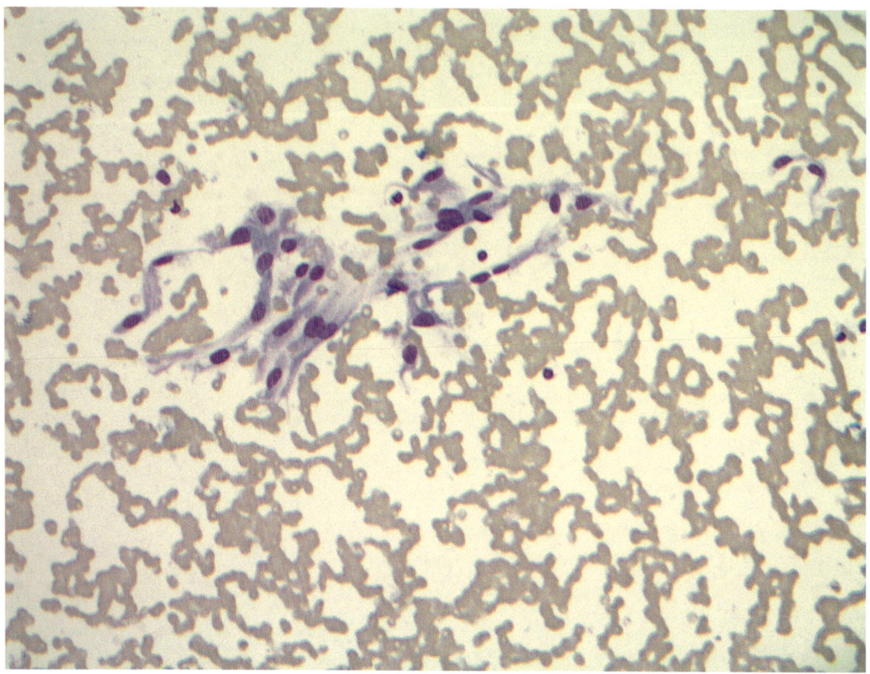

Fig. 3.2 Cystic degeneration in a hyperplastic nodule. Cyst lining cells with pulled-out appearance that mimics reparative epithelium (Diff-Quik stain, ×200)

Tips and Pitfalls

- Cyst lining cells typically show reactive changes. They have a pulled-out appearance that mimics reparative epithelium (Fig. 3.2).
- Cases may be diagnosed as FLUS/AUS because of the reparative changes.
- Dystrophic calcifications can mimic psammoma bodies.

Cystic Papillary Carcinoma

Cytomorphologic Features

- Tumor can be partially or totally cystic, unilocular or multilocular, or thin or thick walled and may contain residual tumor in the wall [18].
- Tissue fragments exhibit scalloped borders, and they are arranged in a cartwheel pattern with nuclei at the outside perimeter [17] (Fig. 3.3).

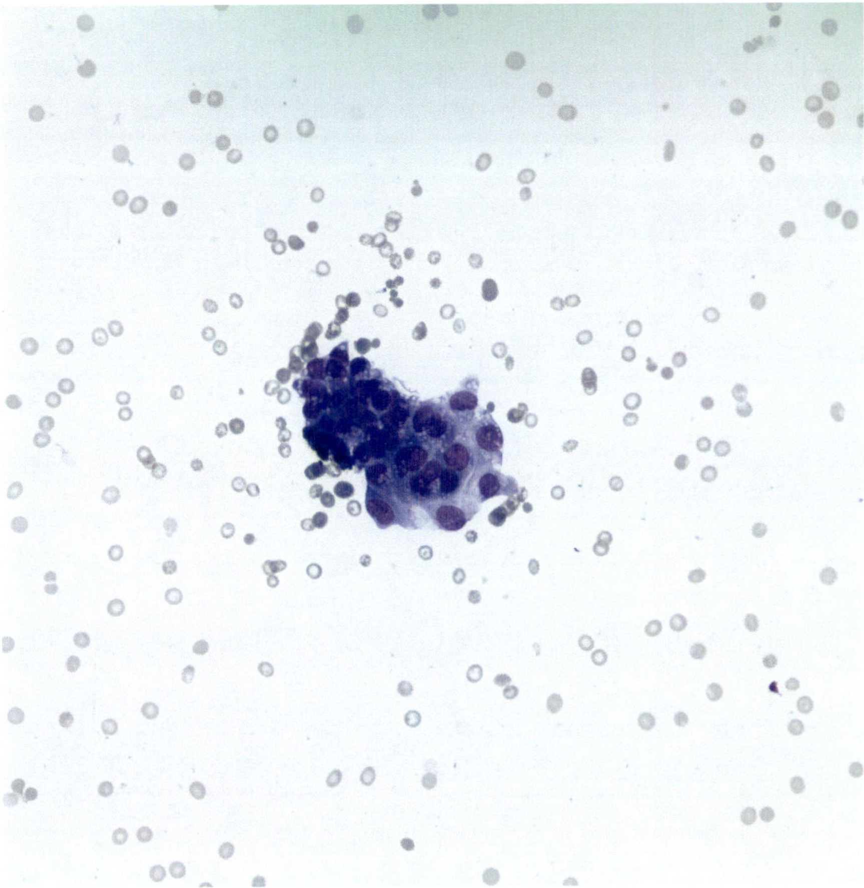

Fig. 3.3 Cystic papillary carcinoma. Tissue fragment showing scalloped borders with nuclei at the outside perimeter. Cytoplasm is vacuolated (Diff-Quik stain, ×400)

- Cytologic features commonly seen include three-dimensional fragments, anisonucleosis, nuclear crowding, nuclear enlargement, intranuclear inclusions, and cytoplasmic vacuoles [19, 20] (Fig. 3.4).

Tips and Pitfalls

- Fine, powdery chromatin of PTC may not be present because the chromatin tends to stain intensely due to degeneration.
- The combination of macrophages, hemosiderin, and cellular debris in the background may obscure distinction from cystic goiter.

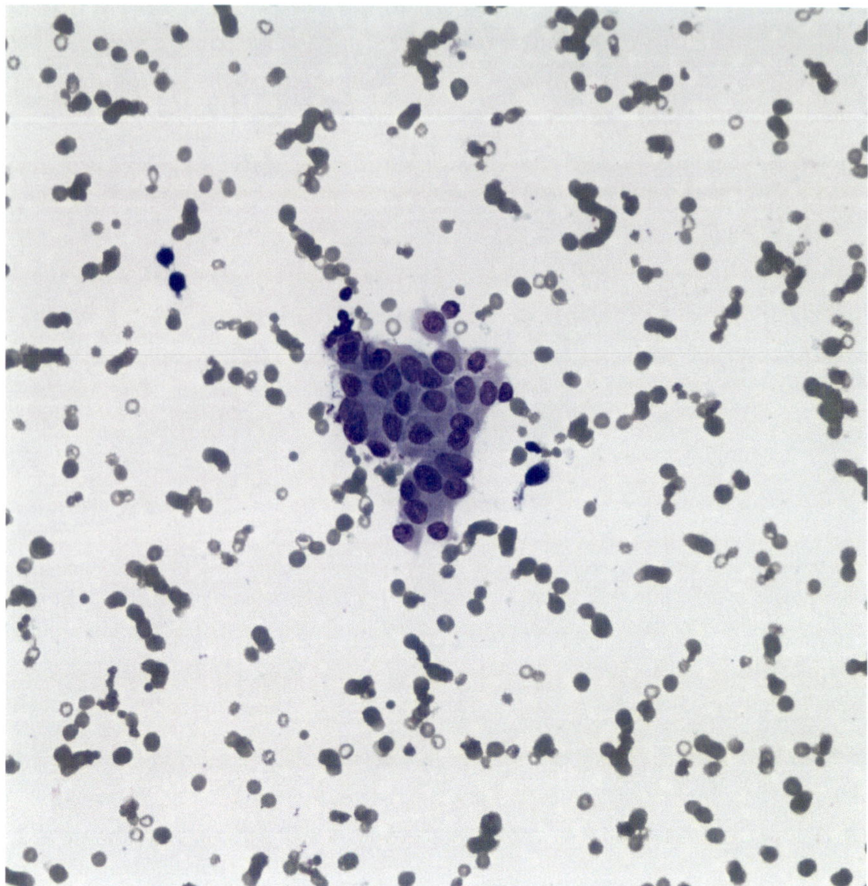

Fig. 3.4 Cystic papillary carcinoma. Cells show some of the nuclear features of papillary thyroid carcinoma, such as nuclear enlargement, nuclear elongation, and nuclear grooves (Diff-Quik stain, ×400)

- Atypical histiocytoid cells of cystic PTC may be difficult to distinguish from clusters of histiocytes with foamy cytoplasm and enlarged nuclei that are seen in cystic degeneration in goiters [21].

Lymphoepithelial Cysts

- Lymphoepithelial cysts in the thyroid bear close resemblance to their counterparts in the salivary gland.
- The cysts are lined predominantly by squamous epithelium and focally by columnar epithelium.
- The epithelium is bordered by a fibrous capsule and surrounded by lymphoid tissue, often with follicles and germinal centers [22].

Lymphocytes-Rich Lesions of the Thyroid

Diagnostic Consideration

Thyroid glands with Hashimoto thyroiditis usually show diffuse enlargement and the gland feels firm and rubbery. FNA is performed only if there is a suspicious nodule that raises the possibility of a coexisting malignancy.

Primary lymphoid neoplasms of the thyroid are uncommon. They are basically of two types: diffuse large B-cell lymphoma (DLBCL) and extranodal marginal zone B-cell lymphoma (ENMZBL) also referred to as MALT lymphomas. MALT lymphomas are low grade and often arise in a background of Hashimoto's thyroiditis.

Hashimoto Thyroiditis

Cytomorphologic Features

- Very cellular, with numerous lymphoid cells.
- The most characteristic feature is the presence of intense infiltration of the gland by polymorphous population of lymphocytes and plasma cells (Figs. 3.5 and 3.6).
- There may be occasional clusters of Hürthle cells.
- Normal follicular cells are infrequent or absent altogether.

Tips and Pitfalls

- The proportion of Hürthle cells varies widely from case to case. When it is present in abundance, the cells may proliferate to form nonneoplastic Hürthle cell nodules, with little to no lymphoid infiltrate, thereby making it difficult to distinguish from Hürthle cell neoplasm on cytologic preparations. The cells of Hürthle cell neoplasm, however, usually have more prominent nucleoli and they usually do not have a prominent lymphoid infiltrate [10].
- In florid Hashimoto thyroiditis with atrophy of the follicular cells, lymphocytes predominate, often forming follicles and germinal centers and may be difficult to distinguish from intrathyroidal lymph node sampling. Often this can also lead to a misdiagnosis of malignant lymphoma [23]. When in doubt, additional material should be collected at the time of ROSE for ancillary studies like flow cytometry.
- Occasionally, multinucleated giant cells are seen and this may lead to confusion with subacute thyroiditis.
- Syncytial tissue fragments of follicular epithelium with papillary-like architecture can often be seen in Hashimoto thyroiditis and can lead to a misdiagnosis of papillary carcinoma especially when the Hürthle cells display reactive nuclear changes like chromatin clearing, nuclear enlargement, and occasional grooves [18].

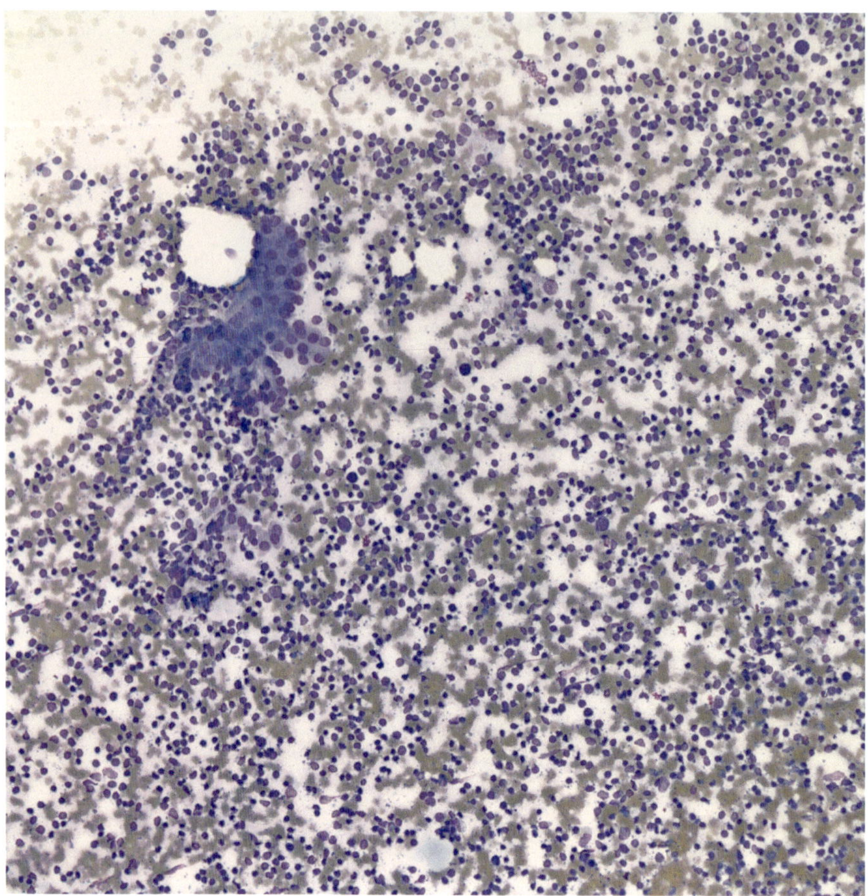

Fig. 3.5 Hashimoto thyroiditis. Polymorphous population of lymphocytes and cluster of Hurthle cells (Diff-Quik stain, ×200)

Lymphoid Neoplasms of the Thyroid

Cytomorphologic Features

Diffuse Large B-Cell Lymphoma

- Variable cellularity, usually very cellular.
- Dense and monomorphous population of poorly differentiated lymphoid cells, which are usually larger than the normal lymphocytes (Fig. 3.7).
- Cells are large, with high nuclear/cytoplasmic (N:C) ratio and finely granular chromatin.
- Nucleoli may be small or large.
- Mitotic activity is frequent and Karyorrhexis is a common feature.
- Cytomorphologic features of Hashimoto thyroiditis may be present on the smear.

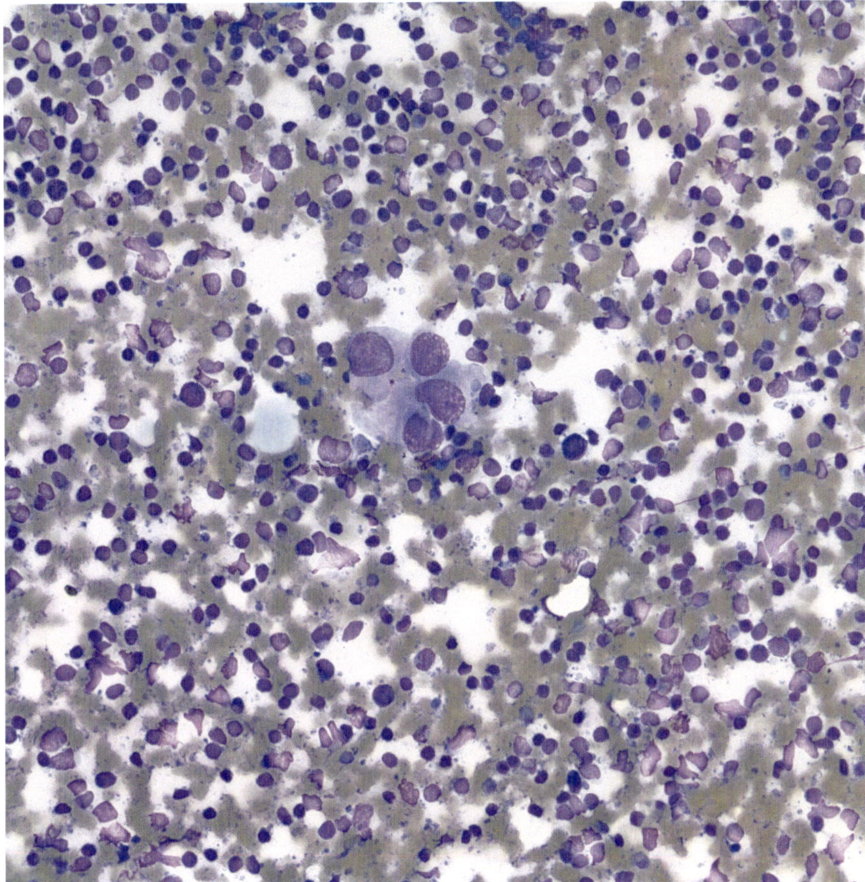

Fig. 3.6 Hashimoto thyroiditis. Polymorphous population of lymphocytes and rare Hurthle cells (Diff-Quik stain, ×400)

MALT Lymphoma

- Polymorphous population of lymphocytes and plasma cells (Fig. 3.8).

Tips and Pitfalls

- DLBCL cells are often seen in large aggregates and this may lead to misdiagnosis as an epithelial neoplasm, most notably anaplastic carcinoma and metastatic carcinoma.
- MALT lymphoma can be very difficult to differentiate from the florid lymphoid phase of Hashimoto thyroiditis because of the heterogeneous population of lymphocytes and both entities may coexist [23].
- Additional material should be obtained at the time of ROSE for immunohistochemical stains.
- Flow cytometry is an important ancillary study and additional material should be obtained at the time of ROSE in RPMI solution for flow cytometry.

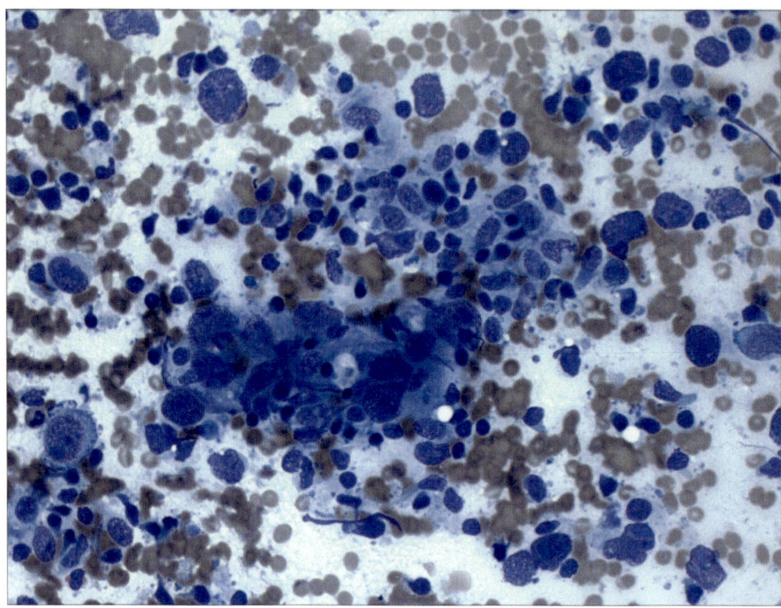

Fig. 3.7 Diffuse large B-cell lymphoma. Poorly differentiated, large lymphoid cells with high N:C ratio (Diff-Quik stain, ×400)

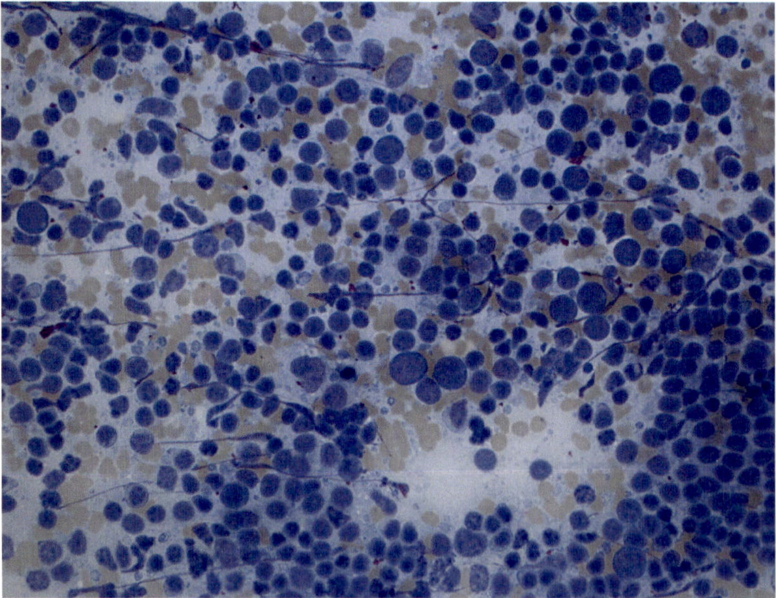

Fig. 3.8 MALT lymphoma. Polymorphous population of lymphocytes and plasma cells (Diff-Quik stain, ×400)

Papillary Thyroid Carcinoma

Diagnostic Consideration

Papillary thyroid carcinoma (PTC) is defined based on nuclear features. The classic PTC has true papillary architecture, but there are a large number of PTC variants with some having virtually no papillary architecture. It is important to be aware of these variants so that they are not confused with other neoplasms. Some of the variants have a tendency toward more aggressive clinical behavior than the classic PTC; hence it is important to be able to recognize them as such.

Cytomorphologic Features

- Smears may show papillary structures, sheets, loosely cohesive groups, or syncytial fragments (Fig. 3.9).
- Cellularity is variable. A large majority of cases is overwhelmingly cellular, whereas cellularity may be scant in tumors with desmoplastic reaction, or those with cystic change.

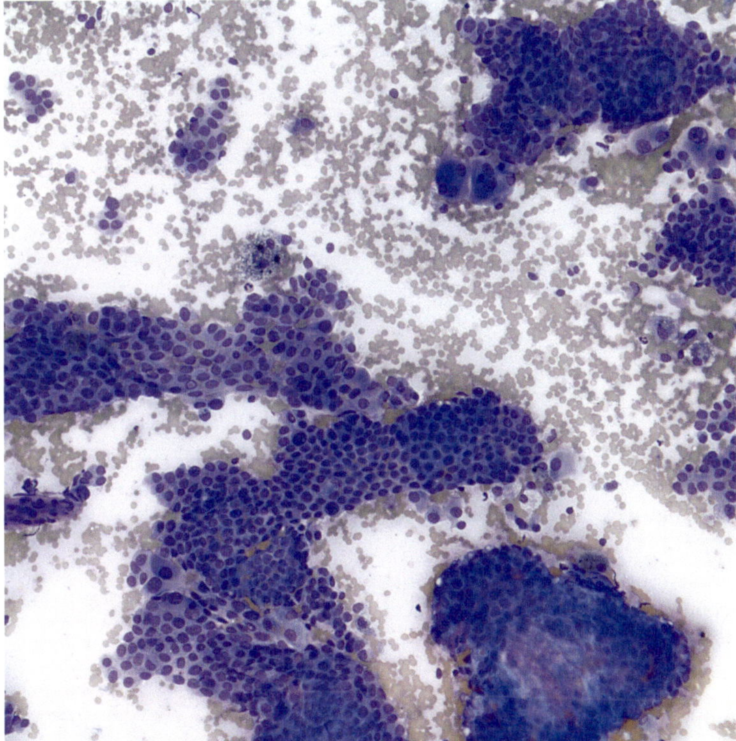

Fig. 3.9 Papillary thyroid carcinoma. Tumor arranged as papillary fragments and syncytial groups (Diff-Quik stain, ×200)

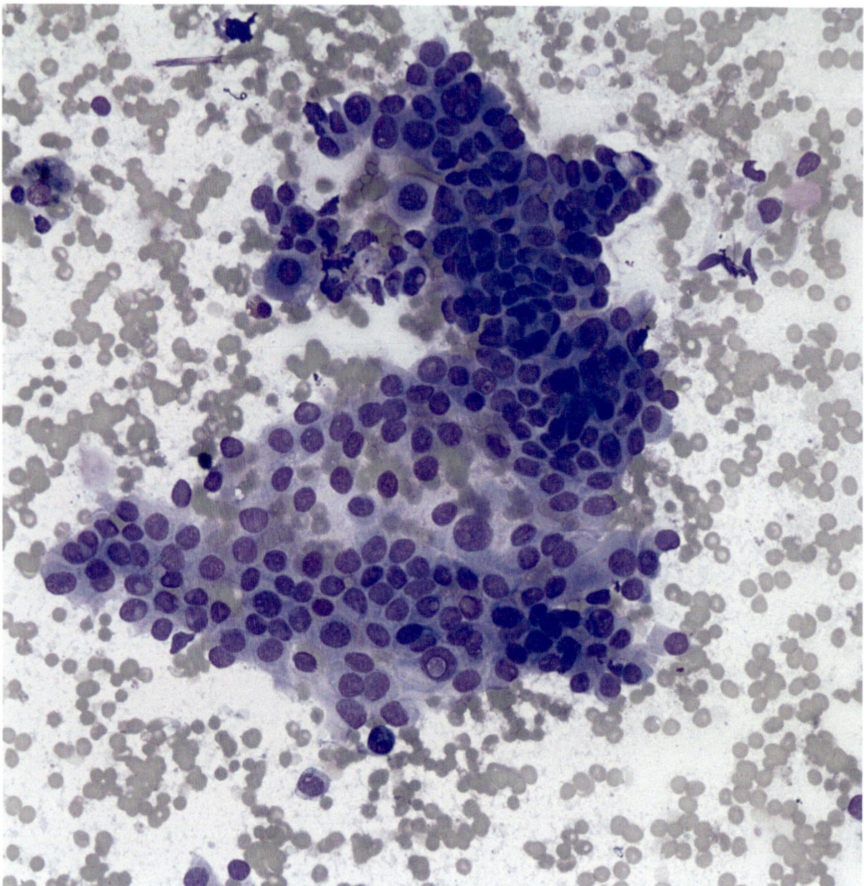

Fig. 3.10 Papillary thyroid carcinoma. Hallmark cytologic features such as nuclear enlargement, nuclear elongation, nuclear grooves, and intranuclear cytoplasmic inclusions (Diff-Quik stain, ×400)

- Nuclear crowding/overlapping.
- The hallmark feature of PTC is the presence of nuclear features such as nuclear enlargement, membrane irregularity, nuclear grooves, nuclear elongation, powdery chromatin, pseudoinclusions, and nucleoli (which may be small or large and may be single or multiple) (Fig. 3.10).
- Cytoplasm is variable – from scant in conventional PTC to abundant, squamoid, vacuolated, or Hürthle-like in other cytomorphologic variants.
- Concentric laminated calcifications also known as psammoma bodies.
- Multinucleated foreign body-type giant cells almost always present with variable number and size of nuclei.

Tips and Pitfalls

- Psammoma bodies must be distinguished from nonspecific, dystrophic calcifications, which are not laminated.
- The presence of conventional PTC nuclear features helps to distinguish oncocytic variant of PTC from Hürthle cell neoplasm. However, the presence of pale chromatin and nuclear grooves is well recognized in Hürthle cells in the absence of PTC [24].
- Tall cell variant of PTC is characterized by neoplastic cells whose height is at least twice their width and the tall cells must comprise at least 30% of the tumor cell population. The tall cells are not as prominent in cytologic preparations as they are on histology. They are frequently seen as large polygonal cells with abundant granular eosinophilic cytoplasm, thereby resembling Hürthle cells [25, 26] (Fig. 3.11).

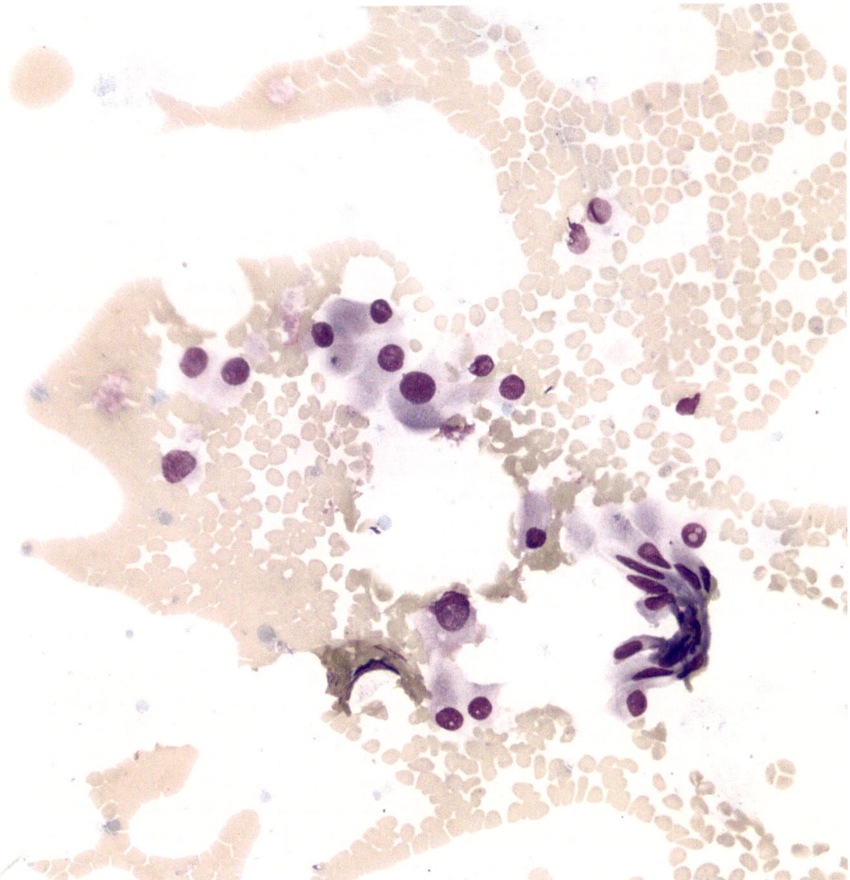

Fig. 3.11 Tall cell variant of papillary thyroid carcinoma. Neoplastic cells whose height is at least twice their width (Diff-Quik stain, ×400)

- The neoplastic cells in columnar variant of PTC are pseudostratified and columnar, but the nuclei do not necessarily demonstrate the typical nuclear features of PTC, and hence the tumor may be confused with metastatic adenocarcinoma to the thyroid.
- Although not entirely specific for the diffuse sclerosing variant of PTC, features such as numerous psammoma bodies, metaplastic squamous epithelium, and marked lymphocytic infiltration are typically seen. The presence of marked lymphocytic infiltrate can obscure the neoplastic follicular cells, mimicking lymphocytic thyroiditis.
- Papillary structures are often not present in solid variant of PTC, and the presence of cohesive syncytial-type tissue fragments, microfollicular/trabecular pattern, or dyshesive single-cell pattern may lead to misdiagnosis of other types of thyroid carcinoma such as poorly differentiated carcinoma, follicular variant of PTC, or medullary carcinoma [27, 28] (Figs. 3.12 and 3.13).

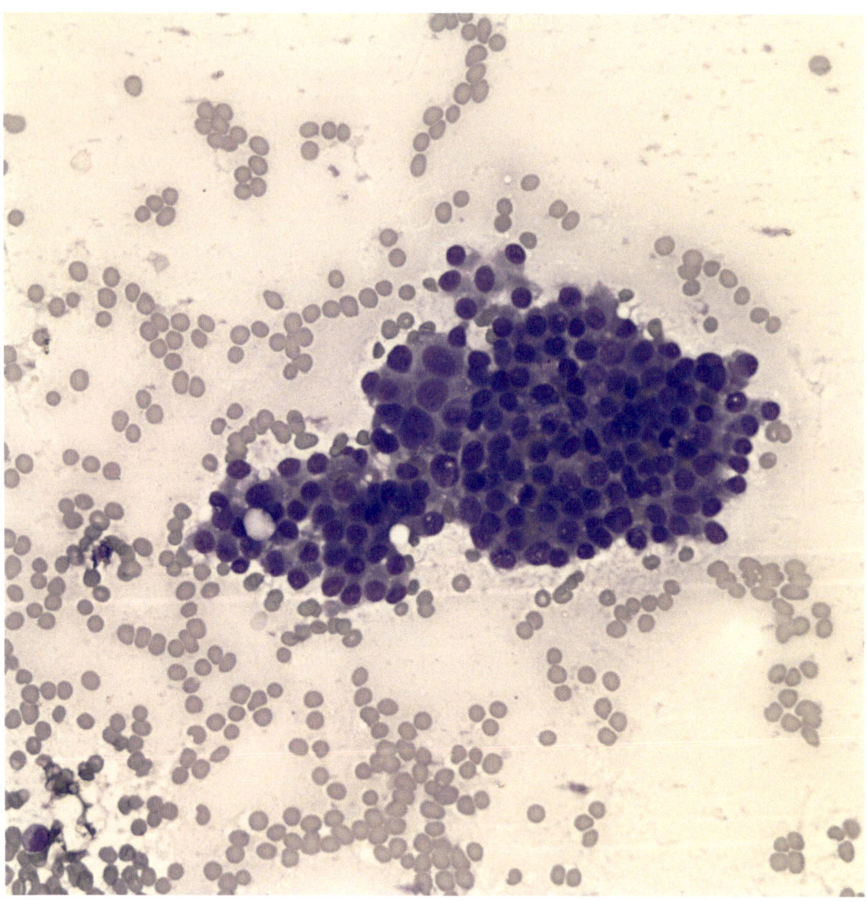

Fig. 3.12 Solid variant of papillary thyroid carcinoma. Tumor arranged as cohesive syncytial-type groups (Diff-Quik stain, ×400)

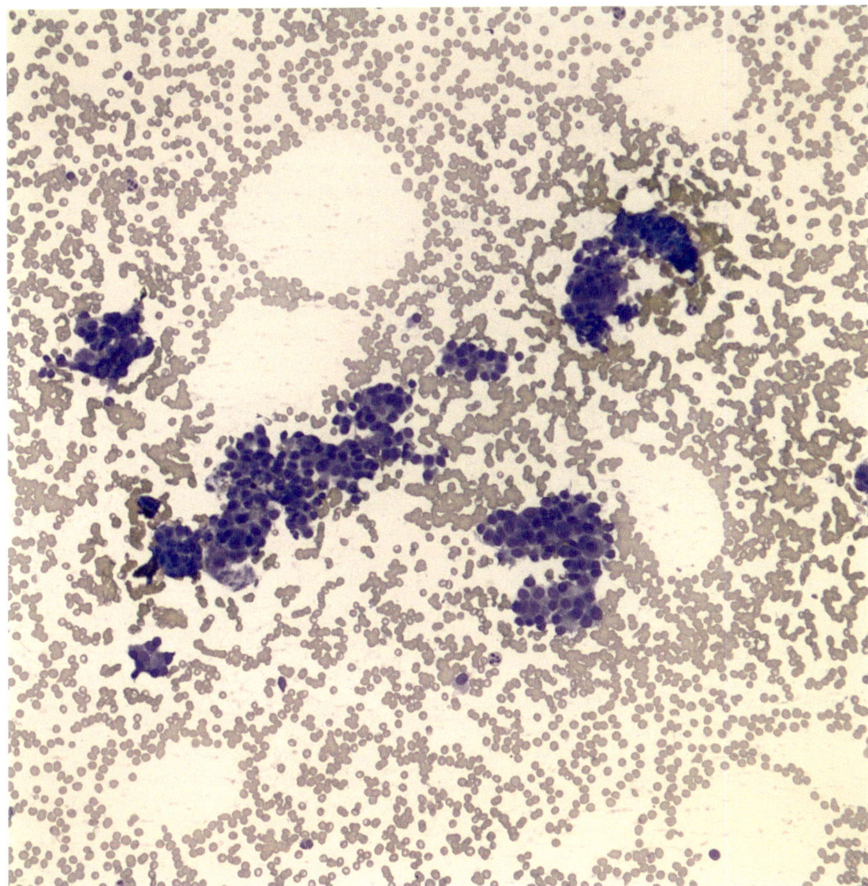

Fig. 3.13 Solid variant of papillary thyroid carcinoma. Tumor arranged in microfollicular and trabecular patterns (Diff-Quik stain, ×200)

Medullary Carcinoma

Diagnostic Consideration

Medullary carcinoma has a wide spectrum of cytomorphologic patterns and hence can mimic a variety of neoplasms. At the time of ROSE, additional pass for cell block material should be obtained if there is a suspicion of medullary carcinoma. This is important because FNA cannot always distinguish medullary carcinoma based on cytology alone, and often, immunohistochemical stain for calcitonin is a useful ancillary study.

Cytomorphologic Features

- Usually highly cellular aspirate, although scant cellularity may be seen with carcinomas containing extensive amyloid deposits and calcification.
- There is a wide spectrum of cytologic features in medullary carcinoma. It is monomorphic if only one cytomorphologic pattern is evident and polymorphic if a combination of different cytomorphologic patterns is seen.
- Tumor cells are predominantly single cells with abundant granular cytoplasm but may also be seen as sheets, loose clusters, syncytia, rosettes, cords, and papillae [29–31] (Figs. 3.14 and 3.15).

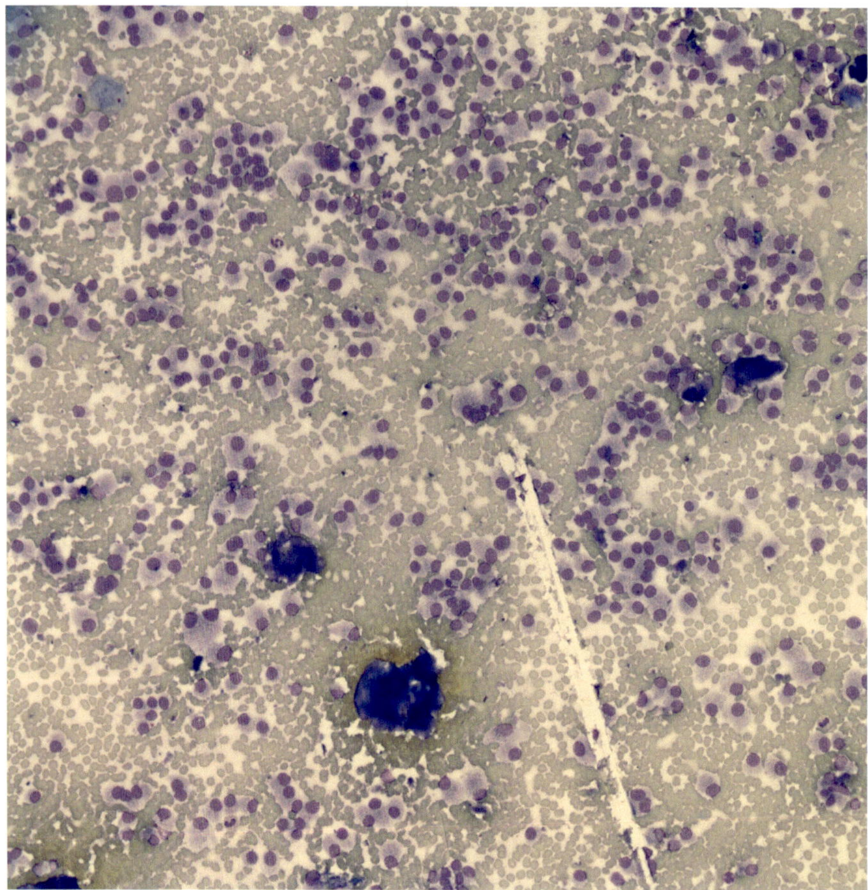

Fig. 3.14 Medullary carcinoma. Single cells with uniform size and shape and abundant granular cytoplasm (Diff-Quik stain, ×200)

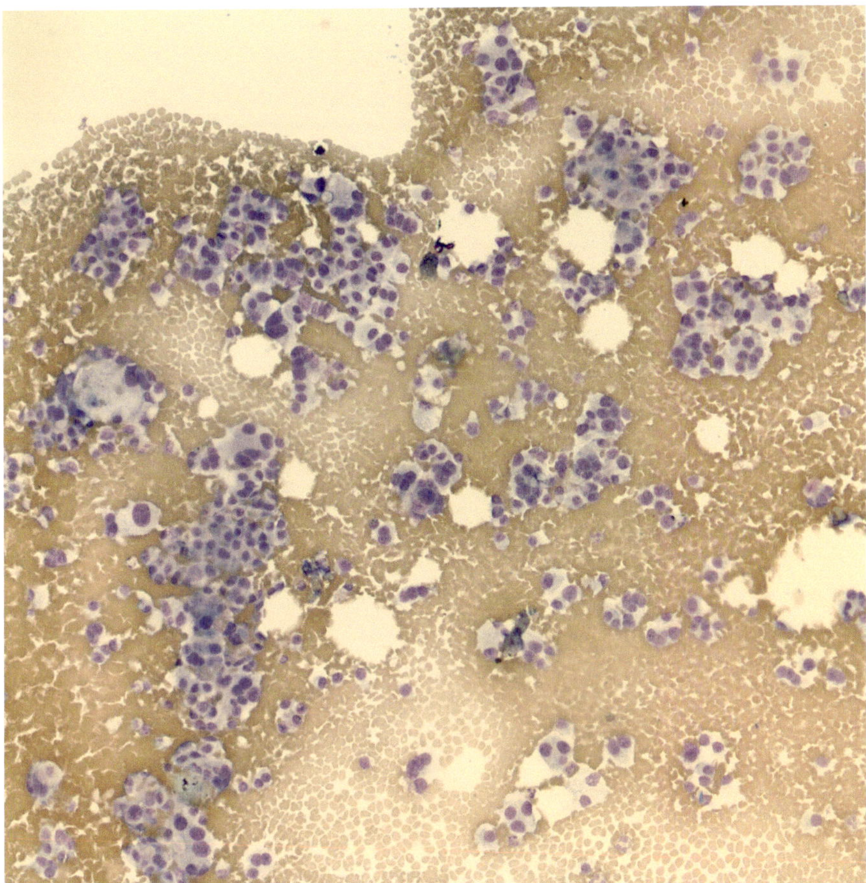

Fig. 3.15 Medullary carcinoma. Loose clusters, rosettes, and cords of tumor cells (Diff-Quik stain, ×200)

- Cells are usually uniform in size and shape but occasionally can present as large, pleomorphic cells. Nuclei are eccentrically placed, giving the cells a plasmacytoid appearance. Binucleation and multinucleation are common. Intranuclear inclusions are frequently seen (Figs. 3.16 and 3.17).

Tips and Pitfalls

- The presence of papillary architecture can mimic papillary carcinoma especially in the presence of intranuclear inclusions and psammoma bodies.

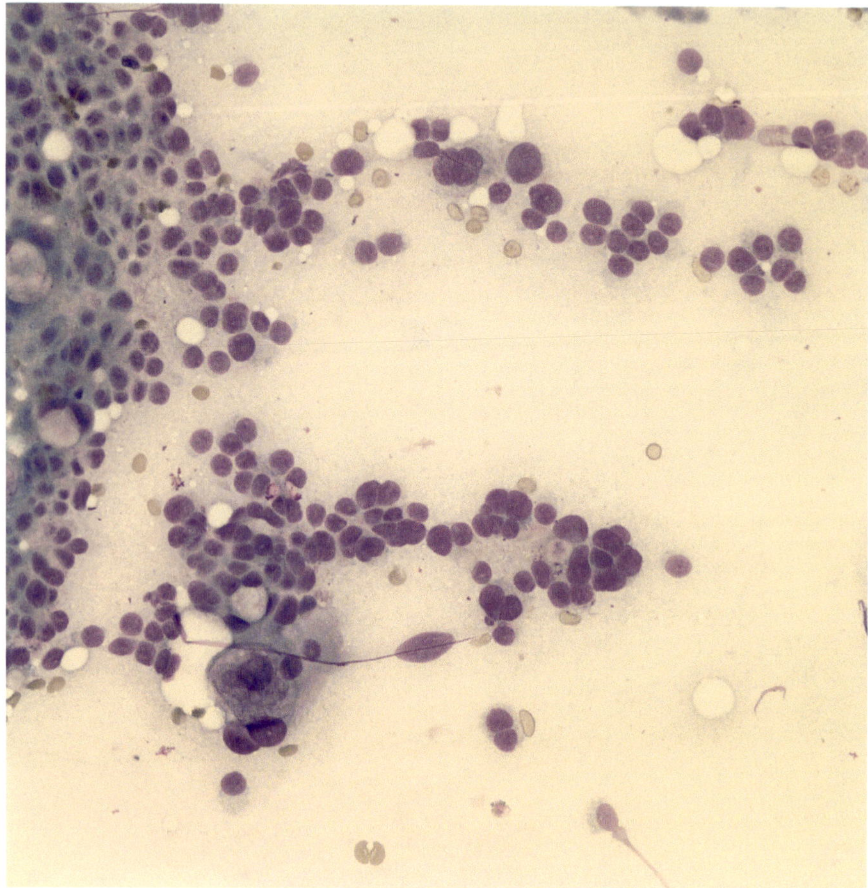

Fig. 3.16 Medullary carcinoma. Large pleomorphic cells (Diff-Quik stain, ×400)

- Tumor cell arrangement as rosettes or microfollicles can mimic a follicular neoplasm or Hürthle cell neoplasm.
- Tumor cell arrangement as cords can mimic poorly differentiated carcinoma, especially the insular type.
- Dispersed single-cell pattern can mimic a lymphoma. When the single cells have prominent plasmacytoid appearance, they can mimic a plasmacytoma.
- Tumors with a predominant spindle cell component can mimic sarcoma, melanoma, or spindle cell carcinoma.
- Amyloid can be confused with thick colloid. If in doubt, additional material should be obtained at the time of ROSE for cell block on which Congo red stain may be performed.

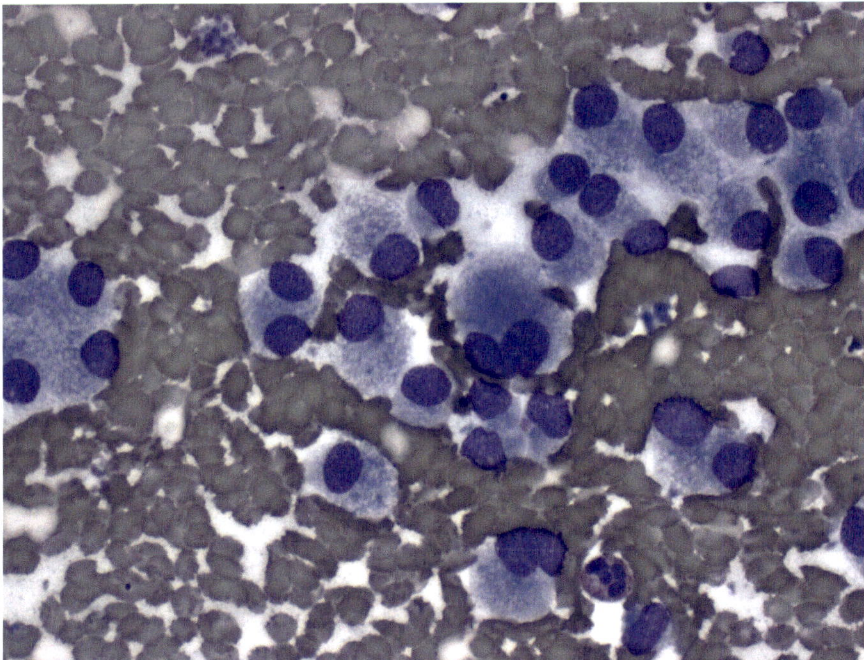

Fig. 3.17 Medullary carcinoma. Single cells with eccentrically placed nuclei. Some of the cells are binucleated (Diff-Quik stain, ×600)

Anaplastic Carcinoma

Diagnostic Consideration

The history is very important in this entity as patients present with rapidly enlarging neck mass which has often metastasized to adjacent structures by the time of diagnosis.

Cytomorphologic Features

- Usually very cellular specimen.
- Noncohesive, large cells with marked nuclear pleomorphism (Figs. 3.18 and 3.19).
- Cells may be epithelioid or spindle-shaped.
- Multinucleated giant cells are usually present.

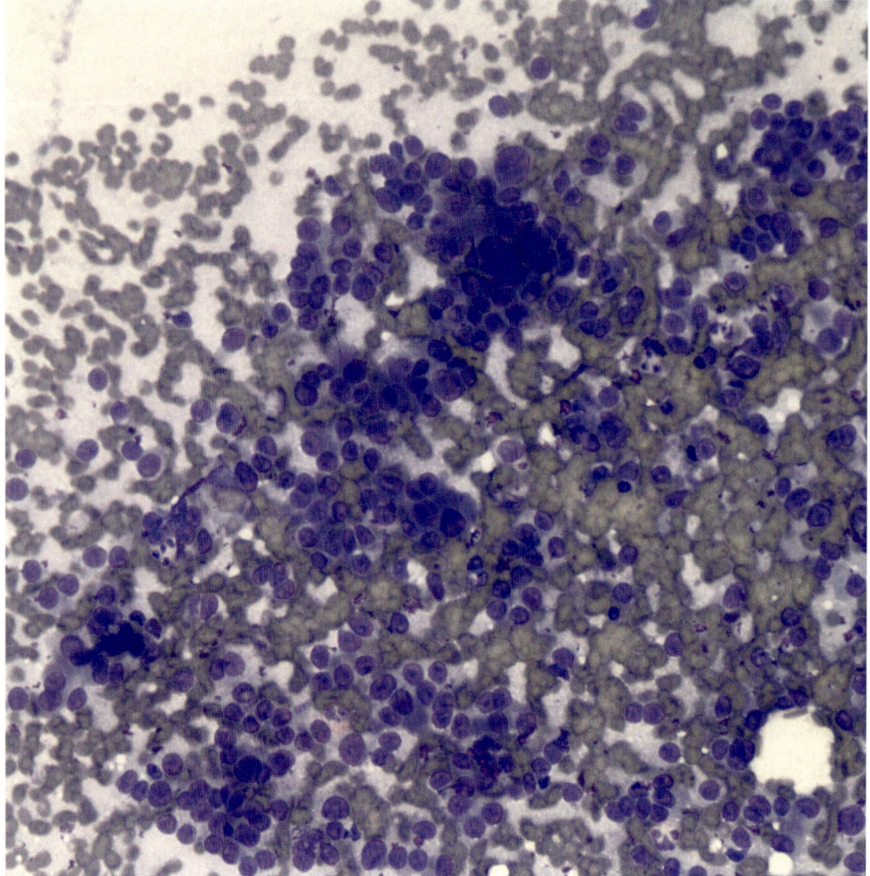

Fig. 3.18 Anaplastic carcinoma. Noncohesive large cells with nuclear pleomorphism (Diff-Quik stain, ×400)

- Extensive necrosis is common, mitoses are numerous, and the Ki67 proliferation index is high [32].
- A good number is associated with a differentiated thyroid carcinoma so marked atypia and pleomorphism may not be prevalent, depending on sampled areas of the tumor.

Tips and Pitfalls

- Anaplastic carcinoma with extensive collagen deposition can mimic Riedel's thyroiditis. The stromal spindle cells from Riedel's thyroiditis are however bland, in comparison to anaplastic carcinoma cells [18].

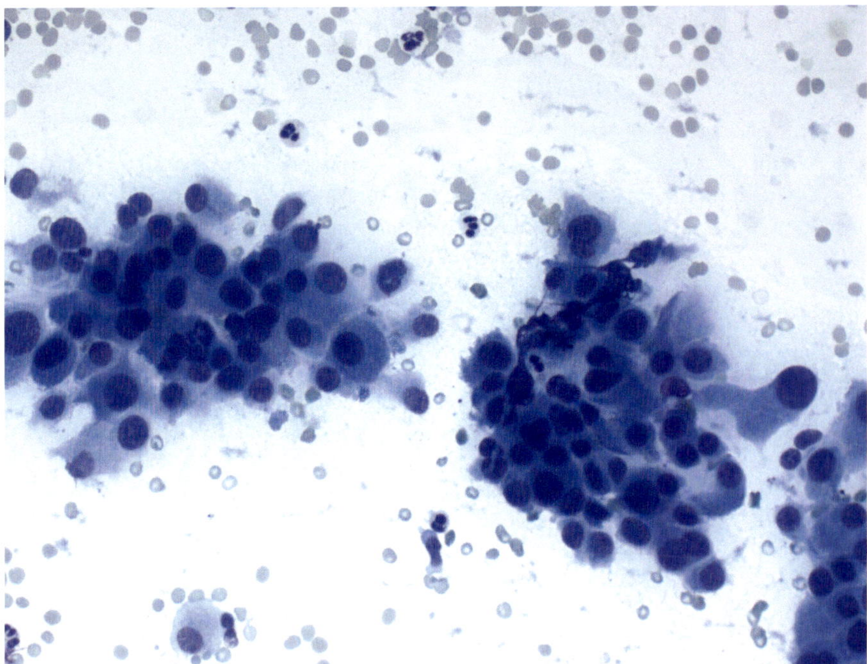

Fig. 3.19 Anaplastic carcinoma. Noncohesive large cells with marked nuclear pleomorphism (Diff-Quik stain, ×400)

- Anaplastic carcinoma cells can be confused with radioactive iodine-induced changes in benign follicular cells after treatment for Graves' disease. These changes include cytomegaly, clumped chromatin, and nucleoli.
- When ossified laryngeal or thyroid cartilage containing hematopoietic tissue is inadvertently sampled, megakaryocytes may mimic anaplastic carcinoma cells. However, megakaryocytes lack the malignant features exhibited by anaplastic carcinoma cells.
- Anaplastic carcinoma cells can mimic poorly differentiated squamous cell carcinoma from direct extension from an adjacent organ in the head and neck. Also, when anaplastic carcinoma has extensive squamous differentiation, it can be mistaken for squamous cell carcinoma [18].
- The medium to large cells of large cell lymphoma, exhibiting high N/C ratios and scant cytoplasm, can sometimes be difficult to differentiate from cells of malignant lymphoma.
- Anaplastic carcinoma can often have a spindle cell pattern, simulating cytologic features of sarcoma.
- Immunohistochemistry can be helpful in the differential diagnosis of anaplastic carcinoma, so additional material should be obtained at the time of ROSE for this purpose.

Metastatic Neoplasms to the Thyroid

Diagnostic Consideration

The possibility of metastasis should always be considered whenever a patient with a history of malignancy elsewhere in the body presents with a thyroid nodule. The thyroid may also be involved by direct extension of malignancies from the head and neck region.

Cytomorphologic Features

- The cytomorphologic pattern of a metastatic tumor depends on the manner of thyroid involvement, the histologic type, and stage of the tumor.
- Cytologic features of metastasis are distinct and different from what is usually seen in primary thyroid tumors. However, there can be an admixture of the tumor with atypical follicular cells [18].

Tips and Pitfalls

- It can be difficult to differentiate between metastatic clear cell renal cell carcinoma and dominant clear cell component within a primary thyroid follicular neoplasm. It may also be difficult to distinguish metastatic clear cell RCC with granular cytoplasm from Hürthle cell neoplasm [18].
- In a patient with a history of breast carcinoma, the presence of single-file pattern of cells and intracytoplasmic lumina is consistent with breast origin [33] (Fig. 3.20).
- Neoplastic cells from metastatic lung adenocarcinoma are usually arranged in three-dimensional clusters and gland-forming clusters. Intranuclear cytoplasmic inclusions may be present and may lead to a misdiagnosis of PTC [34] (Fig. 3.21).
- Benign metaplastic changes seen in the thyroid can mimic squamous cell carcinoma.
- Anaplastic thyroid carcinoma with prominent squamous differentiation can mimic metastatic squamous cell carcinoma.
- In metastatic malignant melanoma, cells may present with clearing of the chromatin, poorly formed nuclear grooves, and intranuclear cytoplasmic inclusions and may lead to a misdiagnosis as PTC [35].
- Whenever metastasis to the thyroid is suspected, especially when there is a history of malignant neoplasms in a different body site, additional material should be obtained at the time of ROSE for immunohistochemical stains and/or molecular studies.

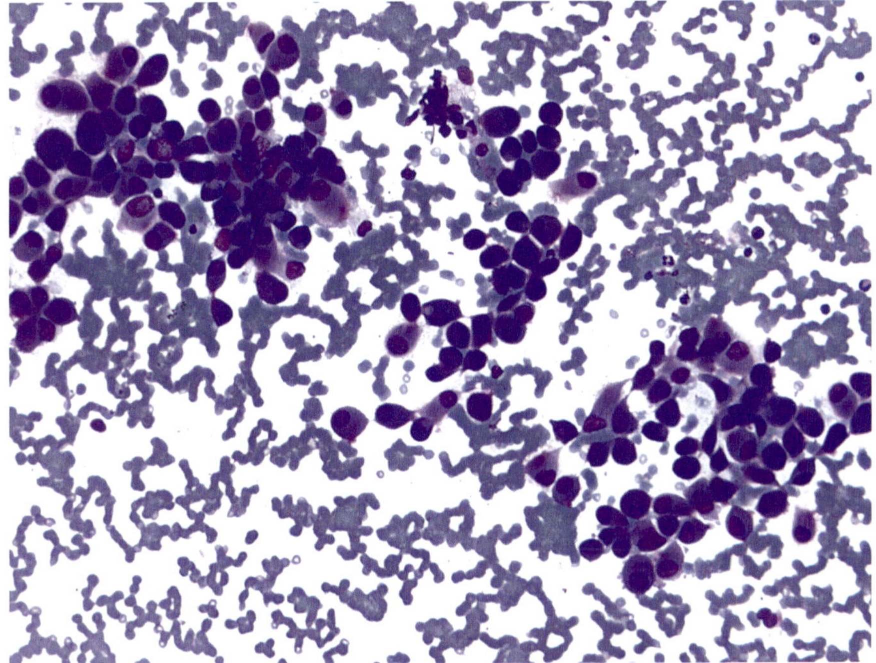

Fig. 3.20 Metastatic breast carcinoma to the thyroid. Loosely cohesive clusters and single tumor cells. The nuclei are eccentrically placed and some of the cells have intracytoplasmic lumina (Diff-Quik stain, ×200)

Parathyroid Tissue Sampling

Diagnostic Consideration

Thyroid tissue has overlapping cytomorphologic features with parathyroid tissue so it may be difficult to distinguish one from the other on FNA [36, 37].

Cytomorphologic Features

- High cellularity.
- Cells are arranged as cohesive sheets, ribbon-like cords, and occasional micro-acini (Fig. 3.22).
- Isolated cells and naked nuclei can be present.
- Round nuclei with stippled chromatin pattern (Fig. 3.23).
- Nucleoli may be absent, small, or prominent.
- Cytoplasm is scant to moderate.

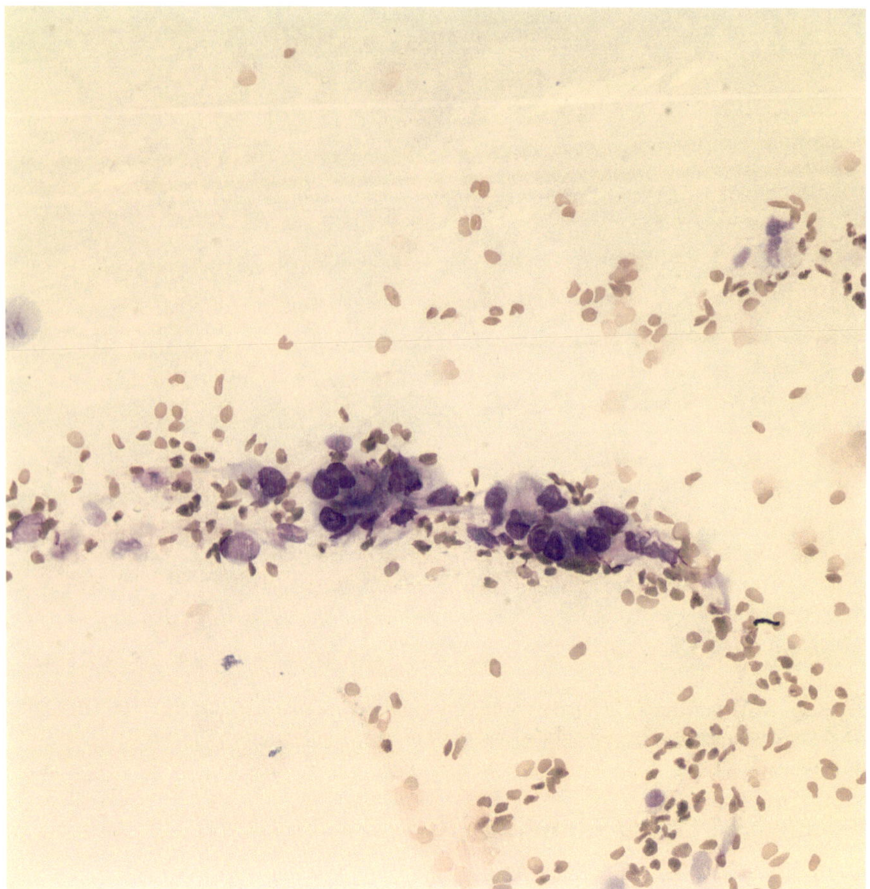

Fig. 3.21 Metastatic lung adenocarcinoma to the thyroid. Gland-forming clusters of tumor cells (Diff-Quik stain, ×400)

Tips and Pitfalls

- Colloid-like material can be produced by hyperplastic parathyroid glands and this can be confused with true colloid [38].
- Parathyroid adenoma smears can show tissue fragments with papillary-like architecture and may be misdiagnosed as papillary carcinoma (Fig. 3.24). Smears with the presence of papillary-like architecture alone without the usual nuclear features of papillary carcinoma should be read with caution [18].
- Parathyroid smears may be interpreted as follicular neoplasm when the cells present as tight, small, three-dimensional clusters in the absence of colloid.

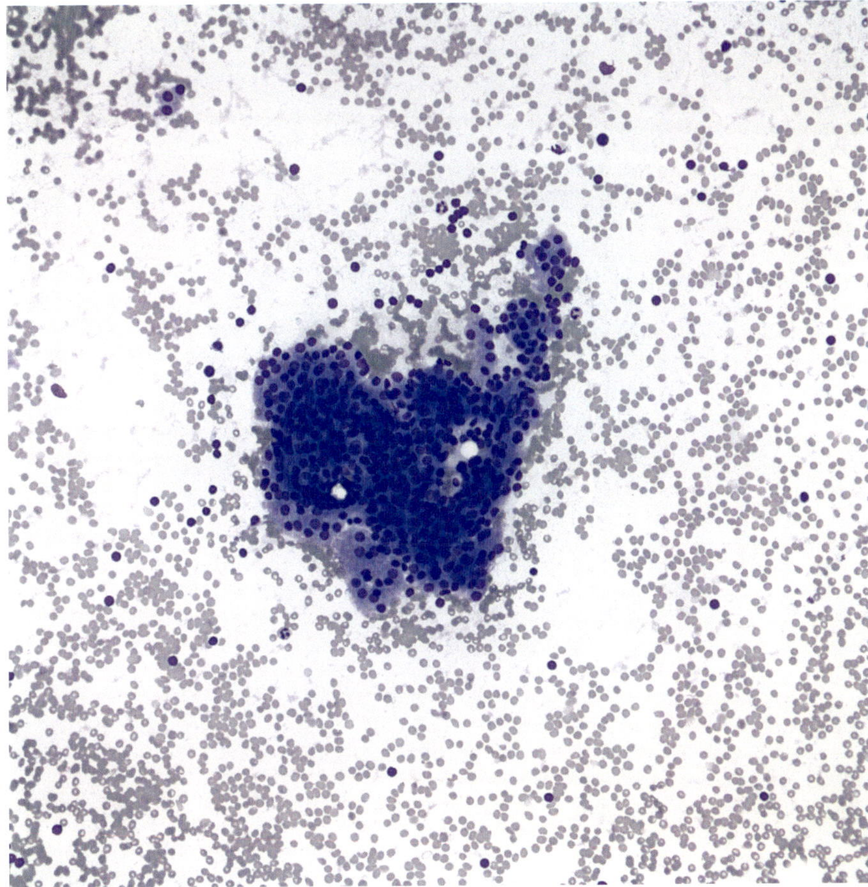

Fig. 3.22 Parathyroid tissue. Cells arranged as cohesive sheets and occasional microacini (Diff-Quik stain, ×400)

- Oncocytic parathyroid adenoma may have follicular structures and can also have colloid-like material in the background, which may lead to a misdiagnosis of Hürthle cell neoplasm. However, Hürthle cell neoplasms of the thyroid have much larger and more prominent nucleoli, and the cells tend to be more discohesive [39, 40].
- When there is a suspicion of parathyroid tissue during ROSE for a thyroid FNA, additional material should be collected for parathyroid hormone (PTH) and/or thyroglobulin immunohistochemical stains. It may also be important to send additional sample for parathyroid assay.

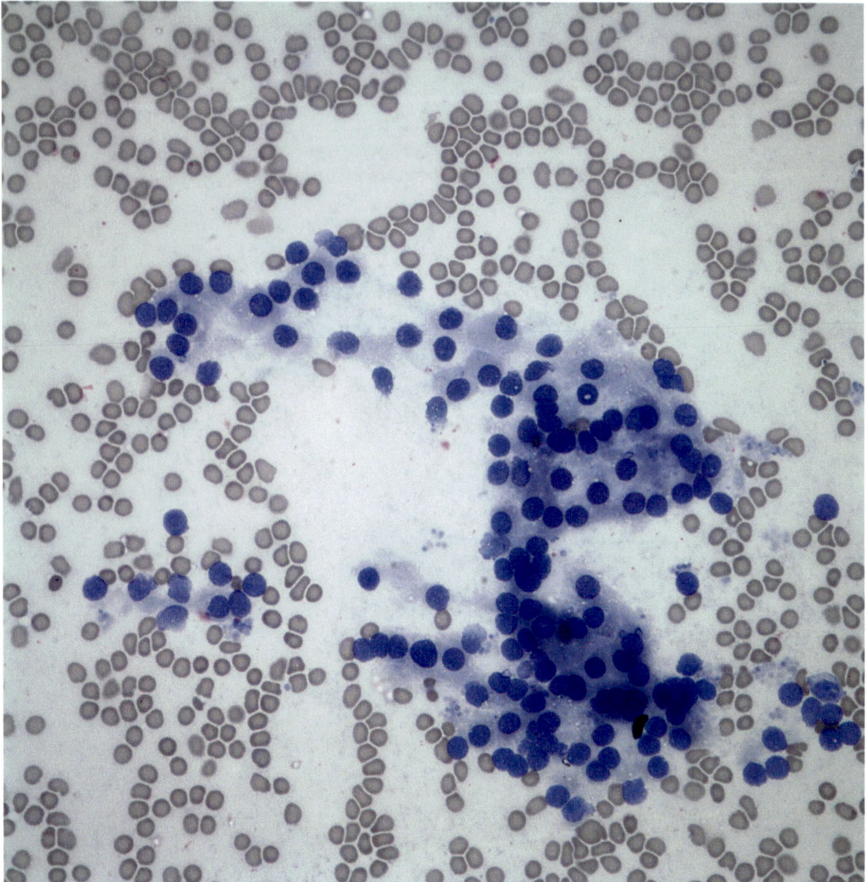

Fig. 3.23 Parathyroid tissue. Cells have round nuclei with stippled chromatin pattern (Diff-Quik stain, ×400)

Ectopic Thyroid Tissue

Diagnostic Consideration

The finding of thyroid tissue in the FNA of a neck mass that is unconnected to the thyroid gland can pose a diagnostic dilemma. The challenge is always to determine whether the aspirate represents a metastatic thyroid malignancy, ectopic thyroid tissue, or benign thyroid inclusion in a lymph node.

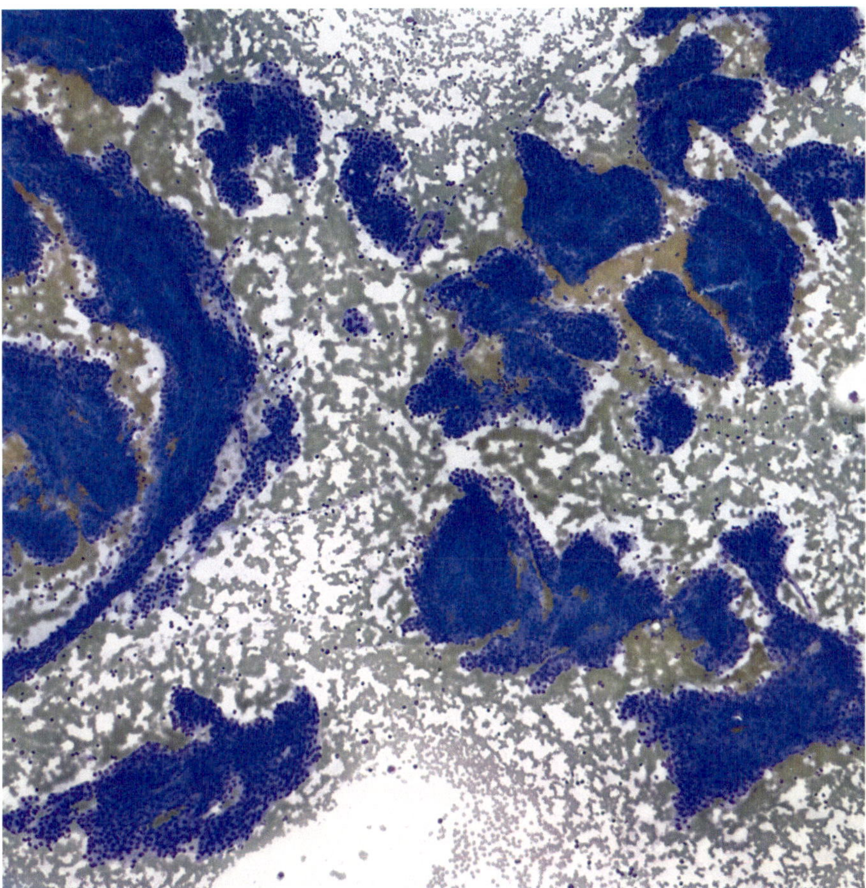

Fig. 3.24 Parathyroid adenoma. Tissue fragments with papillary-like architecture (Diff-Quik stain, ×100)

Cytomorphologic Features

- The cytomorphologic features of ectopic thyroid tissue ranges from normal-appearing follicular cells that are reminiscent of hyperplasia, presence of follicular cells and polymorphous population of lymphocytes in lymphocytic thyroiditis, to rarely, presence of cytologic features of malignancy.
- The presence of a few cytologic features such as unequivocal nuclear features of papillary carcinoma and psammoma bodies is diagnostic of metastases.

Tips and Pitfalls

- Although benign thyroid inclusions may be present in lymph nodes, the presence of thyroid tissue in lateral neck nodes almost always represents nodal metastases from a primary thyroid carcinoma [41, 42].
- The presence of cytologically benign-appearing follicular cells does not necessarily imply a benign process because the pattern of growth of certain thyroid carcinomas may be so well differentiated that they can simulate a nonneoplastic thyroid tissue.
- The presence of cytologic or architectural atypia in follicular cells, even if accompanied by a lymphoid background, does not always indicate metastatic thyroid carcinoma.

Material for Molecular Tests

Molecular testing improves the diagnostic accuracy of FNA for cases in the indeterminate category [43]. It may also provide significant prognostic and therapeutic information preoperatively [44]. The currently available molecular testing can be classified into those involving somatic mutation markers and those involving gene expression classifiers [45]. Several studies have also identified differential expression of several miRNA expressions in thyroid cancers when compared with benign thyroid tissues [45]. More recently, next-generation sequencing has emerged, thus allowing the simultaneous sequencing of large panels of genes [46].

Appropriate and adequate specimen collection at the time of ROSE is key to the success in performance of these tests. It is important to ensure that the specimen/pass evaluated at the time of ROSE is adequately represented in the material sent off for molecular tests.

References

1. Witt BL, Schmidt RL. Rapid onsite evaluation improves the adequacy of fine-needle aspiration for thyroid lesions: a systematic review and meta-analysis. Thyroid. 2013;23:428–35.
2. Redman R, Zalaznick H, Mazzaferri EL, Massoll NA. The impact of assessing specimen adequacy and number of needle passes for fine-needle aspiration biopsy of thyroid nodules. Thyroid. 2006;16:55–60.
3. Yang GC, Liebeskind D, Messina AV. Ultrasound-guided fine-needle aspiration of the thyroid assessed by Ultrafast Papanicolaou stain: data from 1135 biopsies with a two- to six-year follow-up. Thyroid. 2001;11:581–9.
4. Marqusee E, Benson CB, Frates MC, Doubilet PM, Larsen PR, Cibas ES, Mandel SJ. Usefulness of ultrasonography in the management of nodular thyroid disease. Ann Intern Med. 2000;133:696–700.

5. Ghofrani M, Beckman D, Rimm DL. The value of onsite adequacy assessment of thyroid fine-needle aspirations is a function of operator experience. Cancer. 2006;108:110–3.
6. Berner A, Sigstad E, Pradhan M, Grøholt KK, Davidson B. Fine-needle aspiration cytology of the thyroid gland: comparative analysis of experience at three hospitals. Diagn Cytopathol. 2006;34:97–100.
7. Moberly AC, Vural E, Nahas B, Bergeson TR, Kokoska MS. Ultrasound-guided needle aspiration: impact of immediate cytologic review. Laryngoscope. 2010;120:1979–84.
8. Zhu W, Michael CW. How important is on-site adequacy assessment for thyroid FNA? An evaluation of 883 cases. Diagn Cytopathol. 2007;35:183–6.
9. Pitman MB, Abele J, Ali SZ, et al. Techniques for thyroid FNA: a synopsis of the National Cancer Institute thyroid fine-needle aspiration state of the science conference. Diagn Cytopathol. 2008;36:407–24.
10. Cibas ES. Thyroid. In: Cibas ES, Ducatman BS, editors. Cytology: diagnostic principles and clinical correlates. Philadelphia: Saunders Elsevier; 2009. p. 255–84.
11. Goellner JR, Gharib H, Grant CS, Johnson DA. Fine needle aspiration cytology of the thyroid, 1980 to 1986. Acta Cytol. 1987;31:587–90.
12. Grant CS, Hay ID, Gough IR, McCarthy PM, Goellner JR. Long-term follow-up of patients with benign thyroid fine-needle aspiration cytologic diagnoses. Surgery. 1989;106:980–5.
13. Hamburger JI, Husain M. Semiquantitative criteria for fine-needle biopsy diagnosis: reduced false-negative diagnoses. Diagn Cytopathol. 1988;4:14–7.
14. Renshaw AA. Accuracy of thyroid fine-needle aspiration using receiver operator characteristic curves. Am J Clin Pathol. 2001;116:477–82.
15. Jaragh M, Carydis VB, MacMillan C, Freeman J, Colgan TJ. Predictors of malignancy in thyroid fine-needle aspirates "cyst fluid only" cases: can potential clues of malignancy be identified? Cancer. 2009;117:305–10.
16. Baloch Z, LiVolsi V, Asa S, et al. Diagnostic terminology and morphologic criteria for cytologic diagnosis of thyroid lesions: a synopsis of the National Cancer Institute thyroid fine-needle aspiration state of the science conference. Diagn Cytopathol. 2008;36:425–37.
17. Kini SR. Thyroid cytopathology: an atlas and text. Philadelphia: Wolters Kluwer/Lippincott Williams & Wilkins; 2008.
18. Adeniran AJ, Chhieng D. Common diagnostic pitfalls in thyroid cytopathology. New York: Springer; 2016.
19. Kini SR, Miller JM, Hamburger JI, Smith MJ. Cytopathology of papillary carcinoma of the thyroid by fine needle aspiration. Acta Cytol. 1980;24:511–21.
20. Kaur A, Jayaram G. Thyroid tumors: cytomorphology of papillary carcinoma. Diagn Cytopathol. 1991;7:462–8.
21. Renshaw AA. "Histiocytoid" cells in fine-needle aspirations of papillary carcinoma of the thyroid: frequency and significance of an under-recognized cytologic pattern. Cancer. 2002;96:240–3.
22. Louis DN, Vickery AL Jr, Rosai J, Wang CA. Multiple branchial cleft-like cysts in Hashimoto's thyroiditis. Am J Surg Pathol. 1989;13:45–9.
23. DeMay RM. The art and science of cytopathology: superficial aspiration cytology. Chicago: ASCP Press; 2012.
24. Renshaw AA. Fine-needle aspirations of papillary carcinoma with oncocytic features: an expanded cytologic and histologic profile. Cancer Cytopathol. 2011;119:247–53.
25. Lee SH, Jung CK, Bae JS, Jung SL, Choi YJ, Kang CS. Liquid-based cytology improves preoperative diagnostic accuracy of the tall cell variant of papillary thyroid carcinoma. Diagn Cytopathol. 2014;42:11–7.
26. Guan H, Vandenbussche CJ, Erozan YS, et al. Can the tall cell variant of papillary thyroid carcinoma be distinguished from the conventional type in fine needle aspirates? A cytomorphologic study with assessment of diagnostic accuracy. Acta Cytol. 2013;57:534–42.
27. Nikiforov YE, Erickson LA, Nikiforova MN, Caudill CM, Lloyd RV. Solid variant of papillary thyroid carcinoma: incidence, clinical-pathologic characteristics, molecular analysis, and biologic behavior. Am J Surg Pathol. 2001;25:1478–84.

28. Giorgadze TA, Scognamiglio T, Yang GC. Fine-needle aspiration cytology of the solid variant of papillary thyroid carcinoma: a study of 13 cases with clinical, histologic, and ultrasound correlations. Cancer Cytopathol. 2015;123(2):71–81.
29. Papaparaskeva K, Nagel H, Droese M. Cytologic diagnosis of medullary carcinoma of the thyroid gland. Diagn Cytopathol. 2000;22:351–8.
30. Forrest CH, Frost FA, de Boer WB, Spagnolo DV, Whitaker D, Sterrett BF. Medullary carcinoma of the thyroid: accuracy of diagnosis of fine-needle aspiration cytology. Cancer. 1998;84:295–302.
31. Us-Krasovec M, Auersperg M, Bergant D, Golouh R, Kloboves-Prevodnik V. Medullary carcinoma of the thyroid gland: diagnostic cytopathological characteristics. Pathologica. 1998;90:5–13.
32. Lloyd RV, Osamura RY, Kloppel G, Rosai J, editors. World Health Organization classification of tumours. Pathology and genetics of tumours of endocrine organs. Lyon, France: IARC Press; 2017.
33. Schmid KW, Hittmair A, Ofner C, Tötsch M, Ladurner D. Metastatic tumors in fine needle aspiration biopsy of the thyroid. Acta Cytol. 1991;35:722–4.
34. Bellevicine C, Vigliar E, Malapelle U, Carelli E, Fiorelli A, Vicidomini G, Cappabianca S, Santini M, Troncone G. Lung adenocarcinoma and its thyroid metastasis characterized on fine-needle aspirates by cytomorphology, immunocytochemistry, and next-generation sequencing. Diagn Cytopathol. 2015;43:585–9.
35. Miiji LO, Nguyen GK. Metastatic melanoma of the thyroid mimicking a papillary carcinoma in fine-needle aspiration. Diagn Cytopathol. 2005;32:374–6.
36. Dimashkieh H, Krishnamurthy S. Ultrasound guided fine needle aspiration biopsy of parathyroid gland and lesions. Cytojournal. 2006;3:6.
37. Tseleni-Balafouta S, Gakiopoulou H, Kavantzas N, Agrogiannis G, Givalos N, Patsouris E. Parathyroid proliferations: a source of diagnostic pitfalls in FNA of thyroid. Cancer. 2007;111:130–6.
38. Odronic SI, Reynolds JP, Chute DJ. Cytologic features of parathyroid fine-needle aspiration on ThinPrep preparations. Cancer Cytopathol. 2014;122:678–84.
39. Sriphrapradang C, Sornmayura P, Chanplakorn N, Trachoo O, Sae-Chew P, Aroonroch R. Fine-needle aspiration cytology of parathyroid carcinoma mimic Hürthle cell thyroid neoplasm. Case Rep Endocrinol. 2014;2014:680876.
40. Paker I, Yilmazer D, Yandakci K, Arikok AT, Alper M. Intrathyroidal oncocytic parathyroid adenoma: a diagnostic pitfall on fine-needle aspiration. Diagn Cytopathol. 2010;38:833–6.
41. Kozol RA, Geelhoed GW, Flynn SD, Kinder B. Management of ectopic thyroid nodules. Surgery. 1993;114:1103–6. discussion 1106–7.
42. Butler JJ, Tulinius H, Ibanez ML, Ballantyne AJ, Clark RL. Significance of thyroid tissue in lymph nodes associated with carcinoma of the head, neck or lung. Cancer. 1967;20:103–12.
43. Adeniran AJ, Hui P, Chhieng DC, Prasad ML, Schofield K, Theoharis C. BRAF mutation testing of thyroid fine-needle aspiration specimens enhances the predictability of malignancy in thyroid follicular lesions of undetermined significance. Acta Cytol. 2011;55:570–5.
44. Adeniran AJ, Theoharis C, Hui P, Prasad ML, Hammers L, Carling T, Udelsman R, Chhieng DC. Reflex BRAF testing in thyroid fine-needle aspiration biopsy with equivocal and positive interpretation: a prospective study. Thyroid. 2011 Jul;21:717–23.
45. Alexander EK, Schorr M, Klopper J, Kim C, Sipos J, Nabhan F, Parker C, Steward DL, Mandel SJ, Haugen BR. Multicenter clinical experience with the Afirma gene expression classifier. J Clin Endocrinol Metab. 2014;99:119–25.
46. Nikiforov YE, Carty SE, Chiosea SI, Coyne C, Duvvuri U, Ferris RL, Gooding WE, LeBeau SO, Ohori NP, Seethala RR, Tublin ME, Yip L, Nikiforova MN. Highly accurate diagnosis of cancer in thyroid nodules with follicular neoplasm/suspicious for a follicular neoplasm cytology by ThyroSeq v2 next-generation sequencing assay. Thyroid. 2015;25:1217–23.

Chapter 4
Breast

Andrea Hernandez, Tamar C. Brandler, and Joan F. Cangiarella

Introduction

Fine-needle aspiration (FNA) is an accurate and cost-effective method to diagnose breast lesions. A successful FNA necessitates the following conditions: an experienced aspirator, an adequate specimen, good quality smears, and an accurate interpretation from a cytopathologist. Rapid on-site evaluation (ROSE) during aspiration biopsies of the breast has been shown to decrease the number of nondiagnostic samples to less than 1%, with agreement between on-site immediate diagnosis and final diagnosis in 89% of cases [1]. Sakuma et al. reported no false-positive cases after on-site evaluation of 747 breast FNAs when processed with a modified Shorr's stain [2].

Utilizing ROSE allows for proper slide handling and on-site determination of whether additional passes are needed. Based on ROSE findings, immediate triage can ensue with additional sampling of lesions necessitating extra studies (such as flow cytometry or immunohistochemistry). During on-site assessment, quality, color (bloody, clear, green), and consistency (viscous, thin, mucoid) of FNA contents can be evaluated. Additionally, the FNA operator (cytopathologist or radiologist) can provide tactile information regarding the "feel" of the lesion upon needle transversal at the time of ROSE.

A. Hernandez · T. C. Brandler · J. F. Cangiarella (✉)
Department of Pathology, New York University Langone Health, New York, NY, USA
e-mail: Andrea.hernandez@nyulangone.org; Tamar.brandler@nyulangone.org; Joan.cangiarella@nyulangone.org

G. Cai, A. J. Adeniran (eds.), *Rapid On-site Evaluation (ROSE)*,
https://doi.org/10.1007/978-3-030-21799-0_4

Another benefit to ROSE is the interdisciplinary consultation between the cytopathologist and the radiologist in real time. Radiologic features can be reviewed, discussed, and correlated with the cytologic findings. On-site evaluation also allows the cytopathologist to visualize and record a change in lesion size post-aspiration. The greatest advantage of utilizing ROSE is the multidisciplinary approach to patient care and the ability to immediately advise patients on next steps. ROSE eliminates delays in management and determines whether further testing, surgical excision, or clinical monitoring should follow [3].

Specimen Adequacy Assessment

Definitions for adequacy criteria fall under two schools of thought. The first requires the presence of a certain number of ductal epithelial cells, setting the criteria for adequacy to 10 clusters of at least 10 cells, with each cluster on more than one slide, in a background that is neither necrotic nor inflamed [4]. Layfield et al. further determined adequacy to be 4–6 well-visualized epithelial cell groups [4]. The second school of thought does not have a minimum cell requirement, in the context of the right clinical setting. The National Cancer Institute-sponsored conference on breast FNA (1996) determined that there is no specific cellular requirement for specimen adequacy. Instead, adequacy should be based on three components: an appropriately sampled lesion, sufficient quality smears for interpretation, and cytologic findings that are compatible with clinical and radiologic impression [5]. A further recommendation determined that smears should show 6 or more epithelial cell clusters, or the presence of 10 or more intact bipolar cells per ten medium-power fields to minimize false-negative and unsatisfactory rates [4]. It must be recognized that the use of morphology and number of epithelial cells only applies to lesions of epithelial origin. Other breast lesions such as lipomas, fibrous nodules, or intramammary lymph nodes cannot be assessed using these criteria. In a commentary by Stanley et al. [6], Abele notes experience with over 16,000 breast aspiration biopsies and indicates that adequacy should be judged at the clinical level, relying on three elements: clinical and technical assessments at the time of biopsy, a clinically relevant report and the relationship between the referring clinician and the patient [6]. Adequacy relies on the fact that the lesion aspirated correlates with both the physical exam and radiologic impression.

The feel of the lesion ("tactile sensation") as the needle passes through is also important, as dry or gritty sensations may be associated with carcinoma even in the absence of identifiable cells [7]. A well-written report that includes clinical exam findings and the location and characteristics of the biopsied lesion is crucial [6]. Lastly, the limitations of on-site assessment should be acknowledged by both the patient and physician. Patient compliance with required clinical follow-up remains important.

The Use of the Triple Test

The triple test, a combination of the clinical and radiologic findings interpreted in conjunction with the cytologic findings, is critical in the assessment of adequacy for breast FNA [8]. ROSE permits real-time utilization of the triple test for adequacy determination. In combination with the triple test, on-site evaluation allows for greater interpretative accuracy due to cytopathologist review of clinical information, patient exam findings, radiographic/sonographic findings (including awareness of post-aspiration nodule changes), nature/texture of the lesion, and assessment of the aspiration gross and cytologic features. A good example is the FNA of a fibrous breast lesion that may be essentially acellular on ROSE. ROSE may allow, in combination with clinical and radiologic findings and knowledge of the resistance of the lesion to the aspirating needle, the ability to diagnose a less cellular lesion as adequate in the appropriate clinical setting.

Normal Elements in Breast Cytology

The presence of a bimodal population of ductal epithelial cells and myoepithelial cells is a hallmark of benign disease (Fig. 4.1a). Loose dispersed irregular ductal epithelial cells with pleomorphism and a lack of bare oval nuclei is a pattern more commonly seen in carcinoma (Fig. 4.1b).

1. Ductal epithelial cells
   - Cohesive, flat, monolayered, uniform sheets and clusters.
   - Epithelial cells have round to oval nuclei, with smooth nuclear membranes, inconspicuous nucleoli, and fine, evenly distributed chromatin.
   - Epithelial cells have scanty cytoplasm except with apocrine metaplasia where the cytoplasm is abundant and granular.
   - Monolayered sheets of ductal epithelium are also associated with bare oval nuclei.
   - Single, uniform epithelial cells may be seen in ductal hyperplasia.
2. Myoepithelial cells
   - Characteristic feature of benign breast lesions.
   - Appears as bare oval nuclei in the background of smears and among ductal epithelial clusters and sheets.
   - May dominate the smear pattern.
   - Bare oval nuclei have fine chromatin and lack nucleoli.
3. Apocrine metaplastic cells
   - Cohesive sheets of cells with uniform eccentric nuclei.
   - Nuclei are round with bland chromatin and a single prominent nucleolus.
   - Cytoplasm is abundant, amphophilic, and finely granular.
4. Stromal connective tissue fragments
   - Small fragments of collagen may be seen.
   - Adipose tissue fragments are common.

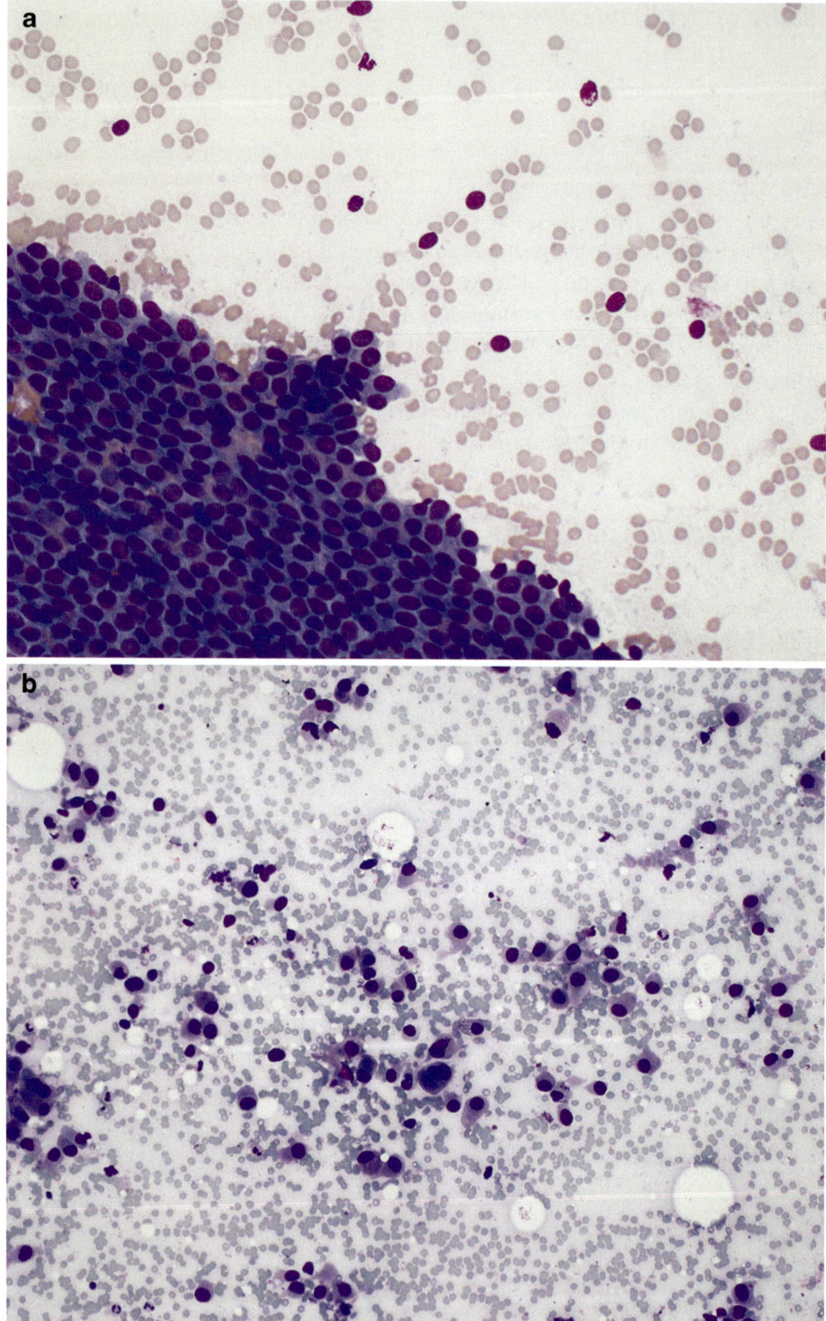

Fig. 4.1 Cytology findings at ROSE in breast FNA. Normal breast cytology shows benign, flat cohesive sheets of ductal epithelial cells and bare oval nuclei (myoepithelial cells) (**a**, Diff-Quik stain, ×400) in contrast to a typical carcinoma that shows numerous single cells with intact cytoplasm and eccentric nuclei (plasmacytoid appearance) (**b**, Diff-Quik stain, ×200)

Cytologic Findings: Acellular or Scant Cellularity

As noted above, cytopathologists who are experienced in the performance of breast FNAs and in physical examination of the breast may prefer not to base adequacy on the number of cells especially if their patient population is comprised of young patients with fibrous or nodular breast lesions where cellularity is limited [9]. FNAs from nonproliferative benign breast nodules are frequently acellular [10]; thus depending on the population referred for aspiration biopsy, the use of cell counts for adequacy would lead to a high unsatisfactory rate. Studies have shown that laboratories receiving a large quantity of breast aspiration biopsies from outside providers should set their own unsatisfactory threshold with the use of clinical and imaging findings rather than cell counting to determine adequacy [11].

Diagnostic Considerations

- Can you determine that the needle is within the mass?
- What was the resistance of the mass upon needle penetration?
- Does this finding correlate with the clinical and radiologic impression?

Differential Diagnoses (Table 4.1)

1. Benign fatty nodule can be considered if nodule is soft on needle penetration and yellow fatty liquid is obtained.
2. Fibrotic lesions in the setting of fibrocystic change, fibrotic or hyalinized fibroadenomas, or physiologic stromal thickening may be acellular; the nodule will be firm on needle penetration.
3. Cystic lesions are almost always benign [12].
   - The fluid should be assessed for viscosity and color, noting the presence of blood.
   - The fluid may be thin, clear or opaque, greenish or brown.

Table 4.1 Key distinguishing cytologic features of acellular or scant smears

	Benign fatty nodule	Benign cyst	Mucocele-like lesion	Cystic carcinoma
Background	Yellow fatty liquid	Clear or opaque, greenish or brown fluid	Viscous mucoid material	Necrosis may be evident
Cytologic features	Fatty fragments, adipocytes	Apocrine cells, foam cells	Muciphages, benign ductal epithelial cells	Atypical epithelial cells

- May be hypocellular or contain foam cells (vacuolated cytoplasm), apocrine metaplastic cells (amphophilic abundant finely granular cytoplasm), and rare clusters or sheets of ductal epithelial cells.
- Clear fluid and the resolution of the mass post-aspiration suggests a benign cyst.

Tips and Pitfalls

- Consider scant cellularity as a false negative from inadequately sampling the lesion.
- The presence of bloody fluid in a presumed cystic aspiration warrants further search for a papillary lesion or malignancy.
- For thick viscous content in a cystic lesion, a mucinous lesion should be considered.
- Apocrine carcinomas may be cystic; therefore careful attention should be given to atypia within apocrine cells [13]. The cell borders in benign apocrine cells are well-defined in contrast to the ragged, indistinct cell borders of apocrine carcinoma [14].

Cytologic Findings: Foam Cells

Cells showing abundant vacuolized cytoplasm, foam cells, are found frequently in benign lesions of the breast and less commonly in malignant tumors. These lesions often impart a wide spectrum of radiologic appearances and at times inconclusive radiologic interpretations. Cytologic on-site assessment is instrumental in elucidating foam cell lesions which are well-known mimickers of malignancy.

Diagnostic Considerations

- What is the macroscopic appearance of the aspirated material? Is it milky; is it oily?
- What is the overall cellularity and background?
- Are the cytoplasmic changes noted in histiocytes or within ductal epithelial cells?
- What is the character of the cytoplasm? Granular? Vacuolated?
- Is there nuclear atypia? Is it minimal or marked?

Differential Diagnoses (Table 4.2, Fig. 4.2a–d)

1. Fat necrosis should be considered in a patient with prior surgical procedure or trauma and an ultrasound appearance of increased echogenicity of subcutaneous tissue or as an anechoic mass with posterior acoustic shadowing [15].
   - Lipid-filled histiocytes with vacuolated cytoplasm are the predominant cell type. Foreign body giant cells surrounding fatty vacuoles also predominate.
   - The background will show degenerated adipocytes (necrosis) and inflammatory cells.

Table 4.2 Key distinguishing cytologic features when foam cells are seen on smears

	Fat necrosis	Lactational changes	Silicone granuloma	Granular cell tumor	Lobular carcinoma
Cellularity	Hypocellular	Moderately to highly cellular	Hypocellular	Moderately cellular	Hypocellular (classic type)
Cytoplasmic quality and content	Foamy, microvacuolated; due to lipid accumulation	Wispy granular or finely vacuolated; containing proteinaceous material	Large vacuoles containing refractile, faintly yellow, translucent, silicone material	Coarsely granular; corresponding to lysosomes	Single punched-out vacuole containing mucin, imparting a signet-ring appearance
Pattern	Abundant histiocytes; multinucleated giant cells engulfing lipid (lipid-laden histiocytes)	Numerous isolated epithelial cells with cytoplasmic characteristics described above; prominent nuclear enlargement with preserved nuclear/cytoplasmic ratio, prominent nucleoli	Abundant histiocytes with cytoplasmic characteristics described above; multinucleated giant cells; asteroid bodies are often seen [17, 20]	Polygonal tumor cells isolated or in aggregates with poorly defined cell borders, round to oval eccentric nuclei with bland chromatin, and an overall low nuclear/cytoplasmic ratio	Small- or intermediate-size uniform, discohesive cells in a loose, single-file arrangement
Background	Dirty; degenerated adipocytes (necrosis), inflammatory cells, calcifications	Many "naked" nuclei and foamy proteinaceous background	Inflammatory cells may be seen	Clean [18] or "sand-like" granules [17]	

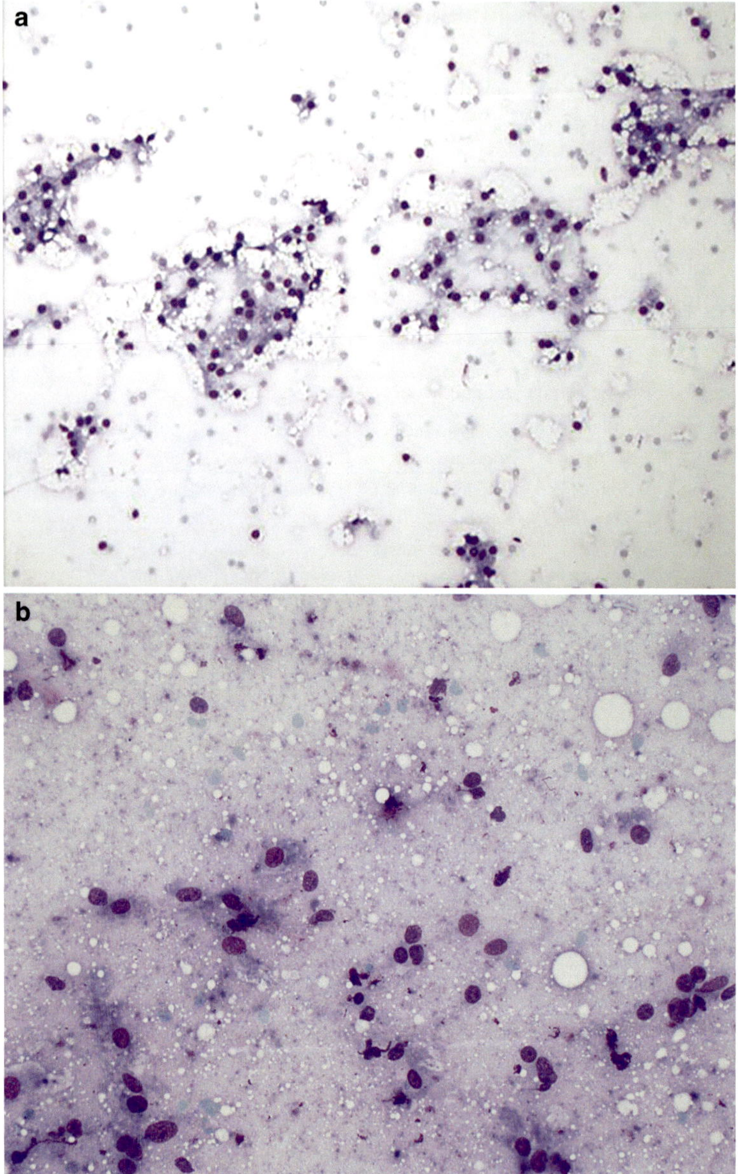

Fig. 4.2 Differential diagnosis of foam cells. Isolated and loose clusters of enlarged ductal cells are seen in this example of lactational change (**a**, Diff-Quik stain, ×200). Granular cell tumor (**b**, Diff-Quik stain, ×400) also displays isolated or "naked" cells, however rarely a loosely cohesive arrangement; when intact, the tumor cells have poorly defined cell borders. The cytoplasm of lactational changes shows the characteristic vacuolated cytoplasm containing proteinaceous material in comparison to the granular cytoplasm of granular cell tumor. Note the prominent nucleoli seen in lactational change, a potential pitfall for malignancy (**c**, ×400). Fat necrosis (**d**, Diff-Quik stain, ×400) shows histiocytes with a foamy, microvacuolated cytoplasm and a "dirty" background with calcific debris. Multinucleated giant cells (**d**), a common feature in fat necrosis, are typically not seen in lactational changes or granular cell tumor

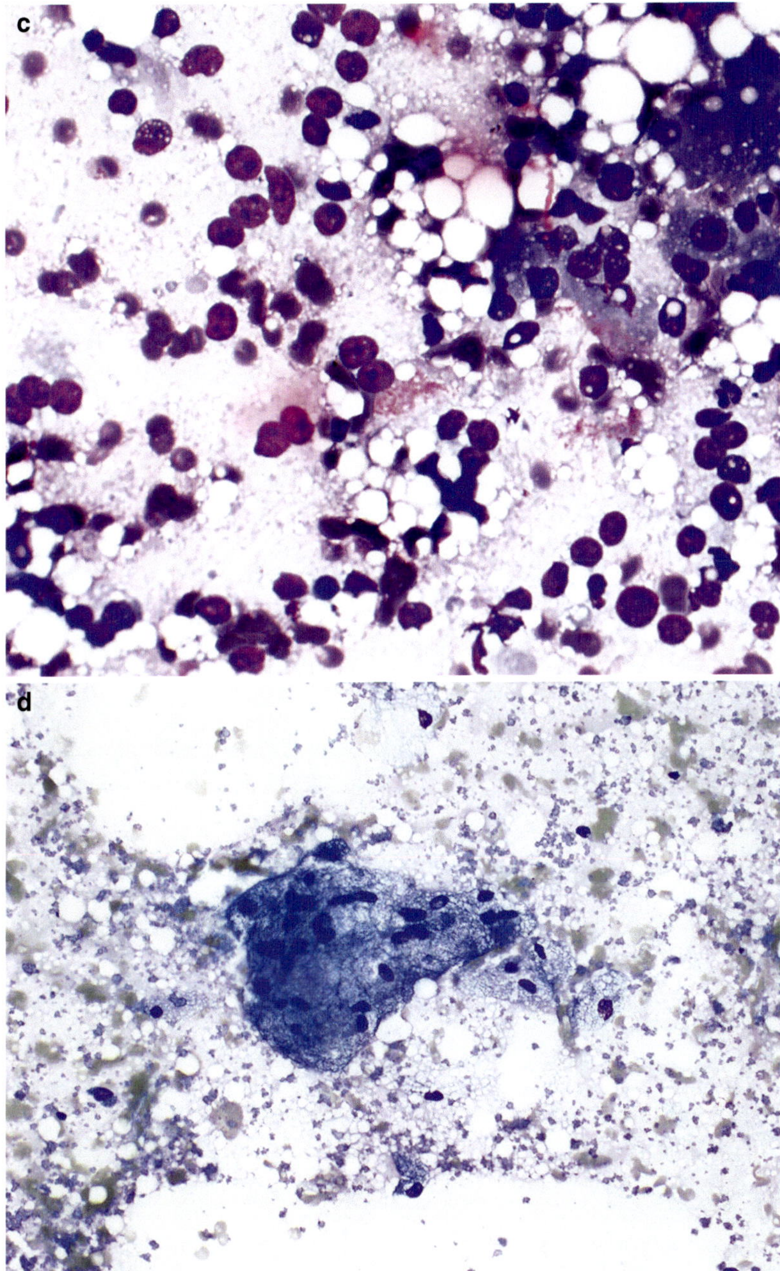

Fig. 4.2 (continued)

2. Lactational changes should be considered in pregnant and newly postpartum women and will show highly cellular smears with a distinctive proteinaceous background.

   - Poorly cohesive but mostly isolated epithelial cells stripped of their cytoplasm, with nuclear enlargement and prominent nucleoli, are seen.
   - The cytoplasm of the epithelial cells is pale, wispy granular, or finely vacuolated. The delicate cytoplasm easily strips away, leading to abundant "naked" nuclei and the characteristic proteinaceous background.
   - Lobular units may be aspirated intact.

3. Granular cell tumor (GCT) is a rare tumor of Schwann cell origin that most commonly occurs in patients of childbearing age and African-American women [16].

   - Ultrasound findings will show a hypoechoic ill-defined, spiculate mass often with posterior shadowing, mimicking carcinoma [16, 17].
   - Polygonal tumor cells, isolated or in aggregates with abundant coarsely granular cytoplasm, round to oval eccentric nuclei with even chromatin, and an overall low nuclear-to-cytoplasmic ratio, are seen.
   - The background will be clean [18] or show "sand-like" granules [17] due to easily stripped away cytoplasm.
   - Necrosis or mitotic activity should raise a concern for malignant GCT [17, 19].

4. Silicone granuloma can show histiocytes with large cytoplasmic vacuoles that contain refractile, faintly yellow translucent crystals which may impart a signet-ring appearance [18].

   - Silicone may be dissolved in processing leaving empty spaces within the vacuoles.
   - Multinucleated giant cells with cytoplasmic vacuolization are common and asteroid bodies have been reported [17, 20].

5. Lobular carcinoma can have variable smear cellularity but is one of the most difficult breast cancers to diagnose by aspiration biopsy [18], often appearing benign on low power.

   - The tumor cells are uniform, small to intermediate size, appearing isolated or in loose, single file arrangements, often with a plasmacytoid appearance.
   - The nuclei are bland with subtle nuclear atypia.
   - Intracytoplasmic single punched-out vacuole with central condensed mucin imparting a signet ring appearance [21] is key to making the correct diagnosis.

Tips and Pitfalls

- Focal, minimal nuclear atypia may be seen in fat necrosis and lactational changes. These entities are commonly associated with *false-positive* interpretations [18, 21]:
  - In fat necrosis, pleomorphic histiocytes and reactive ductal cells may be seen. Background inflammatory cells and abundant foamy histiocytes are helpful clues.
  - In lactational changes, high cellularity and the presence of numerous isolated epithelial cells with prominent nucleoli could also be misinterpreted as malignant. The proteinaceous background and clinical history can be helpful in preventing misinterpretation.
  - Ductal cells encountered in these entities should not display high-grade/marked nuclear atypia including nuclear hyperchromasia, nuclear contour variation, or coarse chromatin; if present, these features should raise concern for carcinoma.
- Granular cell tumor is often misdiagnosed both clinically and radiologically which may lead to anticipated malignant findings during FNA [17, 19]. The absence of bare oval nuclei and the presence of stripped nuclei with minimal nuclear atypia contribute to misinterpretation [19]. A cell block can be useful if considering GCT in the differential diagnosis, as the tumor cells are positive for S100.
- Lobular carcinoma is associated with the highest *false-negative* rate among all breast malignancies [21]. This is due to hypocellular aspirates (predominantly classic type), small tumor cell size, and bland nuclei. The identification of a single file pattern and a mucin containing intracytoplasmic vacuole is helpful.

Cytologic Findings: Squamous Cells

Squamous cells may be seen in a variety of benign and malignant conditions of the breast. Close attention to the cytologic features of the squamous cells and to the background is critical to avoid a false-positive diagnosis [22].

Diagnostic Considerations

- Are the squamous cells nucleated or anucleated? Keratinizing or non-keratinizing?
- Are they atypical?
- Is there an inflammatory background?
- Is there cystic debris or accompanying macrophages?
- Are there other benign or malignant appearing elements?

Differential Diagnoses (Table 4.3, Fig. 4.3a–c)

1. Epidermal inclusion cyst is a rare diagnosis in the breast that shows "cheesy" material upon aspiration, [23] with nucleated and anucleated squames.
2. Subareolar abscess/mastitis presents with pain and redness of the breast in the location of the lesion, primarily in lactating women.
   - Squamous cells are bland and may be anucleated in a background of inflammatory cells, cellular debris, and granulation tissue [24].
3. Primary squamous cell carcinoma is extremely rare.
   - Squamous cells are neoplastic with hyperchromasia and irregular nuclei and keratinization may be present.
4. Metaplastic carcinoma is a rare tumor.
   - Squamous differentiation is often present.
   - The background will show pleomorphic tumor cells with occasional mesenchymal elements (spindle cells, osteoclast-like giant cells, chondromyxoid matrix) [24].

Table 4.3 Key distinguishing cytologic features when squamous cells are seen on smears

	Epidermal inclusion cyst	Subareolar abscess/mastitis	Primary squamous cell carcinoma	Metaplastic carcinoma
Squamous cells: nucleated versus anucleated	Nucleated and anucleated	Nucleated and anucleated	Nucleated	Nucleated
Keratin debris	Present	Present	Present/absent	Present
Necrosis	Absent	Absent	Present	Present
Background	Keratin debris	Inflammation	Keratin debris (+/−)	Non-epithelial components

Fig. 4.3 Differential diagnosis of squamous cells. An epidermal inclusion cyst shows predominantly anucleated squames and keratinaceous debris (**a**, Diff-Quik stain, ×100). A subareolar abscess shows both nucleated and anucleated squamous epithelium and keratinaceous debris but a background of marked acute inflammation, distinguishing this entity from an epidermal inclusion cyst (**b**, Diff-Quik stain, ×200). Metaplastic carcinoma shows abnormal nucleated cells with squamous differentiation with cells that display large nuclei and prominent nucleoli. Some cells display finely vacuolated cytoplasm. This marked nuclear atypia distinguishes squamous cells seen in metaplastic carcinoma from those seen in the aforementioned benign lesions (**c**, Diff-Quik stain, ×200)

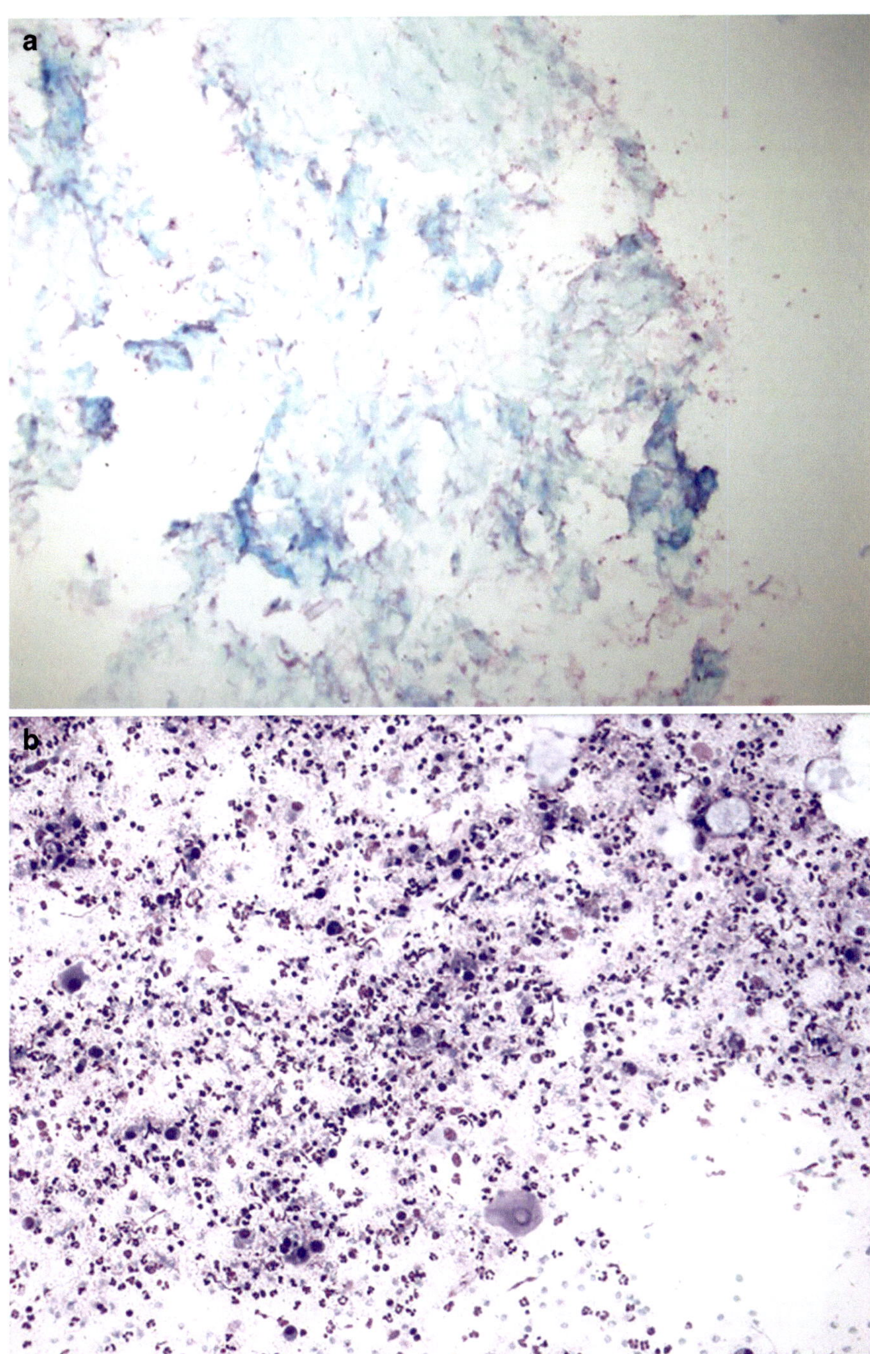
a
b

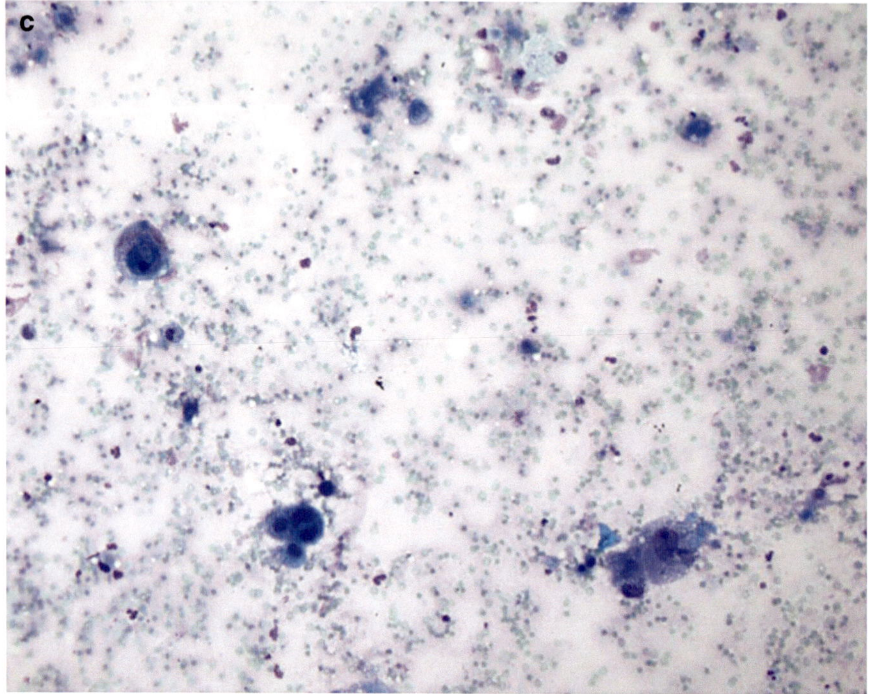

Fig. 4.3 (continued)

Tips and Pitfalls

- Breast abscesses and mastitis may mimic carcinoma.
- Keratin debris may represent benign disease or carcinoma; a search and analysis of well-preserved squames is warranted.
- Spindle cells of metaplastic carcinoma must be distinguished from phyllodes tumor.

Cytologic Findings: Lymphoid Cells

The combination of ultrasound-guided FNA and on-site correlation between radiologist and cytopathologist has been shown to accurately and efficiently determine the axillary lymph node status of women with primary breast cancer. This real-time assessment has increased adequacy rates when compared to ultrasound-guided FNA alone, has allowed for more definitive diagnoses, and, more importantly, has spared many women a more invasive staging procedure [25, 26].

Diagnostic Considerations

- At low magnification, are the cells discohesive or in clusters?
- Is there a mixed lymphoid population? Or is the population monotonous?
- Are there tingible-body macrophages and/or lymphohistiocytic aggregates?
- Are there nonlymphoid cells present?

Differential Diagnoses (Table 4.4)

1. A reactive lymph node appears as a bean-shaped, well-circumscribed round to ovoid nodule with a central lucent hilum on ultrasound.
   - Smears will display a mixed population of small-, intermediate-, and large-size lymphocytes with tingible-body macrophages, germinal centers, and lymphoglandular bodies in the background.
2. Metastatic carcinoma will show a round, hypoechoic lymph node with loss of central hilum and eccentric cortical thickening [27].
   - Epithelial cells may be inconspicuously present within a lymphoid population, or may entirely replace the lymph node with few residual lymphocytes remaining.
   - Appearance of metastatic carcinoma may vary depending on histologic type.

Table 4.4 Key distinguishing cytologic features when lymphoid cells are seen on smears

	Reactive lymph node	Metastatic carcinoma	Non-Hodgkin's lymphoma	Hodgkin's lymphoma
Lymphoid population	Heterogeneous lymphocytes of varying shape and size	Heterogeneous lymphocytes of varying shape and size, presence of lymphocytes depends on extent of metastasis	Monotonous lymphocytes, may be uniformly small or large	Heterogeneous lymphocytes of varying shape and size; Reed-Sternberg cells
Background	Tingible-body macrophages, germinal centers, lymphoglandular bodies, crush artifact	Intermediate or large cells, may be present inconspicuously singly or in clusters with prominent nucleoli (ductal) or intracytoplasmic mucin vacuole (lobular)	Lymphoglandular bodies, crush artifact	Necrosis, inflammatory cells (neutrophils, eosinophils, plasma cells)

  - Ductal carcinoma will typically appear as large cells, when compared to adjacent lymphocytes or red blood cells, and found singly or in clusters, with prominent nucleoli and irregular nuclear contours.
  - Lobular carcinoma can be very challenging to identify, due to a discohesive or single-cell infiltrative pattern [28], which can resemble discohesive lymphocytes at low power. Higher magnification will show tumor cells with a plasmacytoid appearance and subtle nuclear atypia. The presence of a mucin-containing intracytoplasmic punched-out vacuole is helpful for the diagnosis.

3. Lymphoma identified in an axillary lymph node is unusual and usually an unexpected finding in women with breast cancer. Primary breast lymphoma is rare and usually occurs secondary to systemic disease.

   - Smears of non-Hodgkin's lymphoma will show a discohesive, atypical lymphoid population. The lymphocytes will appear monotonous with variable degree of atypia, often with irregular nuclear contours and prominent nucleoli.
   - Hodgkin's lymphoma is an exception, as it is associated with a polymorphous background of lymphocytes and mixed inflammatory infiltrate including eosinophils and plasma cells. Reed-Sternberg cells appear as large, binucleated cells with prominent nucleoli.

Tips and Pitfalls

- Lymphocytes may cluster together, a feature which at low magnification can be mistaken for metastatic carcinoma.
- Dedicated needle passes should be performed to collect a sufficient sample for flow cytometry in the following cases:
  - Atypical lymphoid proliferation is observed.
  - Heterogeneous population is lacking.
  - Clinical or radiologic suspicion exists.
- A diagnosis of Hodgkin's and large cell lymphoma can be made on cytomorphology alone [17]. Flow cytometry to establish clonality or to exclude non-Hodgkin's lymphoma may be useful.

Cytologic Findings: Papillary Structures

A papillary pattern can be seen in a variety of breast lesions. Distinguishing true papillae (true fibrovascular cores with endothelial cells lined by epithelium) from "pseudopapillary" (epithelial projections that lack fibrovascular cores) arrangements is helpful during ROSE for proper triaging of these lesions. The presence of papillary structures in breast FNA can be challenging as there is significant overlap with other nonpapillary breast lesions [29]. Papillary (true fibrovascular cores lined by epithelium) or "pseudopapillary" (epithelial projections that lack fibrovascular cores) patterns can be seen in papillomas, papillary carcinomas, micropapillary ductal carcinoma in situ, fibroadenomas, fibrocystic change, and other low-grade in situ and invasive ductal carcinomas [30]. Distinguishing benign papillomas from carcinomas can be problematic but equally as challenging is differentiating papillomas from fibroadenomas or fibrocystic change [31]. Papillary lesions may present as palpable masses, nipple discharge, or solid lesions or complex intracystic lesions on ultrasound [29].

Diagnostic Considerations

- Are the arrangements truly papillary? Can you identify fibrovascular cores?
- What cells are seen in the background? Columnar cells? Histiocytes?
- Do the cells appear atypical?
- Do you see stroma in the background?

Differential Diagnoses (Table 4.5, Fig. 4.4a–c)

1. Papillary neoplasms are hypercellular with three-dimensional cohesive clusters of ductal epithelial cells with fibrovascular cores. In papillomas, myoepithelial cells are seen within the three-dimensional epithelial cell clusters but are scanty. Apocrine cells and columnar-shaped cells can be seen in a bloody or cystic background containing hemosiderin-laden macrophages [30].
2. Fibroadenomas show pseudopapillary cell clusters that appear more two dimensional than three dimensional and lack true fibrovascular cores. Clusters of epithelial cells should overlap and fold at their edges in contrast to three-dimensional bulbous edges in papillary neoplasms. Myoepithelial cells are seen in the background and in association with epithelial cell clusters.
3. Papillary carcinomas have increased nuclear hyperchromasia and stratification of nuclei.
4. Ductal carcinomas may have pseudopapillary groups of malignant ductal epithelial cells but typically lack fibrovascular cores. Discohesive tumor cells with intact cytoplasm and atypical nuclear features are noted. Less evidence of a cystic background and lesser numbers of macrophages are seen [30].

Table 4.5 Key distinguishing cytologic features when papillary structures are seen on smears

	Papilloma	Fibrocystic change	Fibroadenoma	Papillary carcinoma	Ductal carcinoma
Cellularity	Moderate to markedly cellular smears	Variably cellular smears	Moderately cellular smears	Moderately to highly cellular smears	Moderately to highly cellular smears
Architecture	Three-dimensional clusters with fibrovascular cores lined by endothelial cells Dyshesive columnar-shaped cells commonly seen in background, palisaded rows of columnar cells	Two-dimensional clusters of ductal epithelial cells lacking fibrovascular cores	Staghorn epithelial clusters, two-dimensional rather than three, lacking fibrovascular cores	Columnar cells seen in higher numbers than in papillomas	Atypical ductal epithelial cells in pseudopapillary arrangements lacking fibrovascular cores
Stroma	Scanty, sclerosed acellular stroma		Fibromyxoid stromal tissue fragments that may be cellular		Fragments of stroma may be associated with atypical cells (desmoplastic stroma)
Background	Paucity of myoepithelial cells Apocrine cells usually present Hemorrhagic or cystic background Numerous foamy or hemosiderin-laden macrophages Psammomatous calcifications can be seen	Hemorrhagic or cystic background Prominent apocrine metaplastic cells Scattered bare oval nuclei	Numerous "naked" bare oval nuclei in background Macrophages, but in lesser amounts than seen in papillomas	Paucity of myoepithelial cells Necrotic background may be seen Hemorrhagic or cystic background Psammomatous calcifications can be seen	Single atypical epithelial cells
Cytomorphology of epithelial cells	Atypia can be present; can be severe in infarction		Epithelial sheets with flat edges and blunt edges Columnar cells in small numbers at edges of clusters	Atypia is variable Hyperchromatic, elongated nuclei	Atypical epithelial cells with intact cytoplasm and moderate to severe nuclear abnormalities

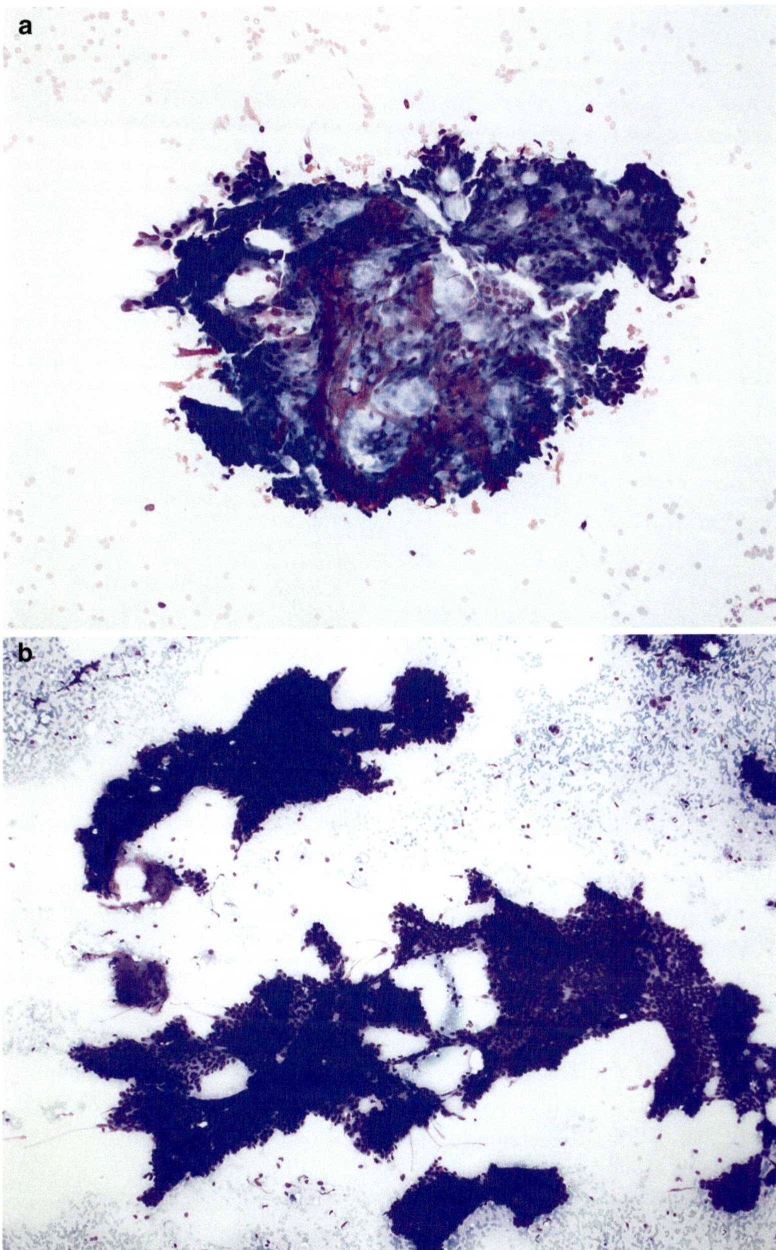

Fig. 4.4 Differential diagnosis of papillary arrangements. A papilloma shows papillary arrangements of ductal epithelial cells with fibrovascular cores and columnar cell appearance (**a**, Diff-Quik stain, ×100). While fibroadenoma can show ductal epithelial cells in "pseudopapillary" arrangements, they lack true fibrovascular cores. Myoepithelial cells also appear more prominent in the background and isolated stromal fragments are noted (**b**, Diff-Quik stain, ×100). Papillary carcinomas may be more cellular but may be difficult to distinguish from papilloma on cytology; it is important to look for increased columnar or single plasmacytoid cells as compared to a simple papilloma (**c**, Diff-Quik stain, ×200)

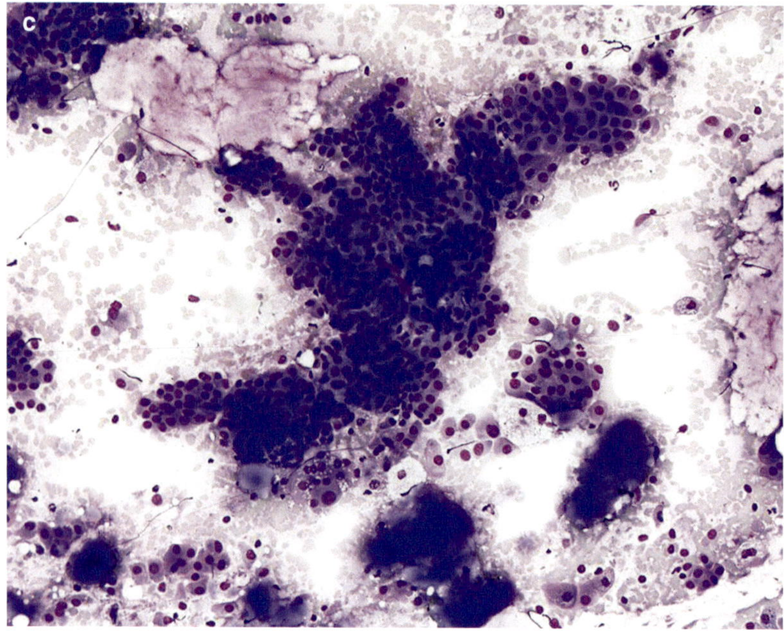

Fig. 4.4 (continued)

Tips and Pitfalls

- Diagnosis of papillary lesions on FNA is difficult due to the overlap of cytologic findings with other benign breast lesions and with carcinomas.
- The cytologic features of benign papillary lesions overlap with other benign breast lesions that show a "pseudopapillary" pattern. In 1 study of 70 cases reported as papillary on fine-needle aspiration biopsy, more than 50% were not true papillary lesions with one-quarter diagnosed as fibroadenoma or fibrocystic change [32].
- Distinguishing benign from malignant papillary lesions is difficult unless obvious features of malignancy are seen [33]; thus most lesions are diagnosed as papillary neoplasms with a recommendation for excision. It is important to recognize that cellular dispersion in papillomas can mimic malignancy to avoid a false-positive diagnosis.
- Marked cellularity, single ductal epithelial cells with marked atypia, the lack of bland columnar cells, and a background with foam cells and apocrine metaplasia favor a papillary carcinoma [31].
- Atypical epithelial cells with high nuclear-to-cytoplasmic ratios and coarse granular chromatin and necrosis should not be equated with malignancy as these cytologic findings can be seen in infarcted intraductal papillomas [34].
- Core biopsy in the diagnosis of papillary lesions does not add additional information as fragmentation of cores, presence of focal atypia due to sampling, and

overlap of histologic features of benign and malignant papillary lesions require surgical excision for definitive diagnosis in many cases [32]. Therefore, when these features are present during ROSE, additional sampling can be avoided and surgical excision can be promptly scheduled.

Cytologic Findings: Single Epithelial Cells

Single cells on breast smears often connote a cancerous diagnosis. However, the features of the single cells must be examined before jumping to a positive diagnosis. Single myoepithelial cells appear in benign fibrocystic breasts and abundantly in benign fibroadenomas as bare oval nuclei. Single columnar cells often appear in cases of papillary lesions, as the cells fall off the tips of the papillae. Large single cells with eccentric nuclei and prominent nucleoli are a suspicious finding and an examination for carcinoma must ensue.

Diagnostic Considerations

- Do the cells have cytoplasm, or are they stripped nuclei?
- If they have cytoplasm, is it eccentric?
- Are the cells large or small?
- Are the cells columnar? Or spindled?
- Are the single cells atypical or bland?
- What type of epithelial or stromal groups (if any) occur on the slide?

Differential Diagnoses (Table 4.6)

1. Benign entities can be considered if stripped nuclei represent myoepithelial cells such as in fibroadenomas. Remaining slide elements will contribute to the diagnosis (i.e., stromal fragments and staghorn epithelial sheets).
2. Smearing artifact may lead to the presence of single bland epithelial cells; these cells will be small and similar in appearance to benign epithelium.
3. Atypical epithelial proliferations can show rare large single cells with eccentric nuclei and prominent nucleoli in a predominantly benign appearing background.
4. Papillary lesions may have large groups of ductal epithelial cells with elongated or columnar-shaped single cells in the background.
   - Fibrovascular cores may indicate a papillary lesion.
5. In situ/invasive carcinomas should be considered if large pleomorphic single cells with eccentric nuclei and prominent nucleoli are present.
   - Single cells are often abundant, occasionally appearing adjacent to three-dimensional groups of enlarged ductal epithelial cells.

Table 4.6 Key distinguishing cytologic features when single cells are seen on smears

	Benign entities	Smearing artefact	Atypical epithelial cells	Papillary lesions	In situ/ invasive carcinoma
Cellularity	Low to moderate	Variably cellular smears	Moderately cellular smears	Moderately to highly cellular smears	Moderately to highly cellular smears
Single cells: stripped versus intact	Most commonly stripped nuclei-myoepithelial cells	Cells may be both with and without cytoplasm	With cytoplasm	With cytoplasm	With cytoplasm
Size or shape/ cytomorphology	Small myoepithelial cells scattered throughout the background and within sheets of ductal epithelium	Small, bland epithelial and myoepithelial cells may be present	Cells may appear larger with eccentric nuclei and conspicuous nucleoli	Elongated or columnar-shaped single cells, falling off the tips of papillae	Large pleomorphic single cells with eccentric nuclei and prominent nucleoli

Tips and Pitfalls

- The differential diagnosis of elongated single cells is papillary versus mesenchymal lesions.
- Stripped nuclei indicative of myoepithelial cells do not always imply benign lesions.
  - Stripped nuclei accompanied by large pleomorphic single cells may suggest an in situ malignancy.
  - Myoepithelial cells may be aspirated by the needle as it passes through benign breast tissue before sampling a malignant lesion.
- When atypical single cells with eccentric and enlarged nuclei are noted and are not definitive for malignancy, a core biopsy should be considered.
- In cases with a definitive diagnosis of malignancy, a core biopsy should be considered for biomarker assessment.

Cytologic Findings: Mucin

Colloid or mucinous carcinoma is the most commonly recognized mucinous lesion of the breast. However, the presence of mucin is not specific for colloid carcinoma as benign breast lesions may also yield abundant extracellular mucinous material. Most mucinous lesions can be accurately distinguished and classified by FNA, with findings similar to those noted on core biopsy [32, 35, 36].

Diagnostic Considerations

- What is the overall cellularity?
- What is the character of the mucin? Are there coursing thin-walled vessels within the mucin?
- What is the arrangement/pattern of the epithelial ductal cells?
- Are there epithelial cells embedded within the mucin?
- Are there background oval bare nuclei (myoepithelial cells)?

Differential Diagnoses (Table 4.7, Fig. 4.5a–c)

1. Colloid carcinoma should be considered in an older patient with well-defined, round, isoechoic, or hypoechoic mass or a mass that feels soft to the needle.
    - Smears show moderate or high cellularity with abundant background mucin (metachromatic on modified Giemsa stain and purple-blue on Papanicolaou stain) with branching capillaries ("chicken wire blood vessels") coursing through mucin.

Table 4.7 Key distinguishing cytologic features when mucin is seen on smears

	Mucocele-like lesion	Fibrocystic change with mucin	Myxoid fibroadenoma	Colloid carcinoma
Cellularity	Hypocellular	Hypocellular to highly cellular	Highly cellular	Moderately to highly cellular
Quality and content of mucinous material	Thin and wispy or thick and colloid-like [39]; may be acellular or contain macrophages or benign ductal cells	Thin and wispy or thick and colloid-like [39]; may be acellular or contain macrophages, apocrine cells, or benign ductal cells	Slightly fibrillary or strandy due to degeneration of myxoid stromal fragments [37]; contain myoepithelial cells	Thin and wispy or thick and colloid-like [39] with coursing thin-walled vessels
Pattern	Cohesive, monolayered clusters of benign ductal cells	Flat sheets and clusters of benign ductal cells	Staghorn epithelial sheets admixed with or separate from myxoid stromal fragments (+/− vasculature)	Floating epithelial cells in mucin in three-dimensional clusters, ball-like aggregates or sheets with overlapping and crowding, discohesive or as dissociated single cells
Atypia	None	None	None to minimal	Minimal to moderate
Background	Macrophages	Bare oval nuclei; macrophages or apocrine cells	Numerous bare oval nuclei	No oval bare nuclei; no stromal fragments

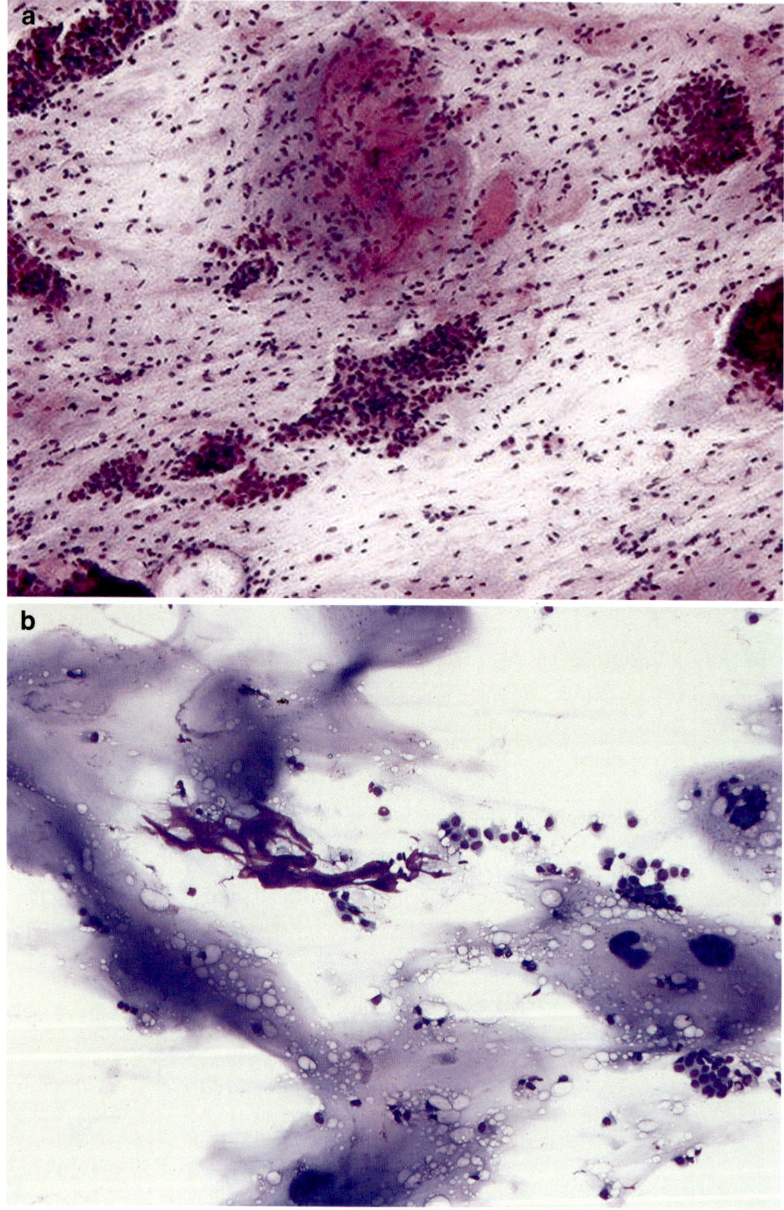

Fig. 4.5 Differential diagnosis of mucinous lesions. Background mucin or mucin-like material characterizes these three lesions. Branching groups of benign ductal cells, abundant bare oval nuclei, and fibromyxoid stromal fragments are seen in this example of myxoid fibroadenoma (**a**, Diff-Quik stain, ×200). Myoepithelial cells are not seen in colloid carcinoma (**b**, Diff-Quik stain, ×100). A variable ductal cell arrangement is characteristic of colloid carcinoma as these tumors most commonly display three-dimensional ball-like aggregates or dispersed single cells in comparison to myxoid FA or fibrocystic change (**c**, Diff-Quik stain, ×200) which show branching clusters or flat sheets. Vasculature may be seen in the stromal fragments of myxoid FA, not to be confused with the coursing thin-walled vessels seen embedded in the background mucin of colloid carcinoma (**b**)

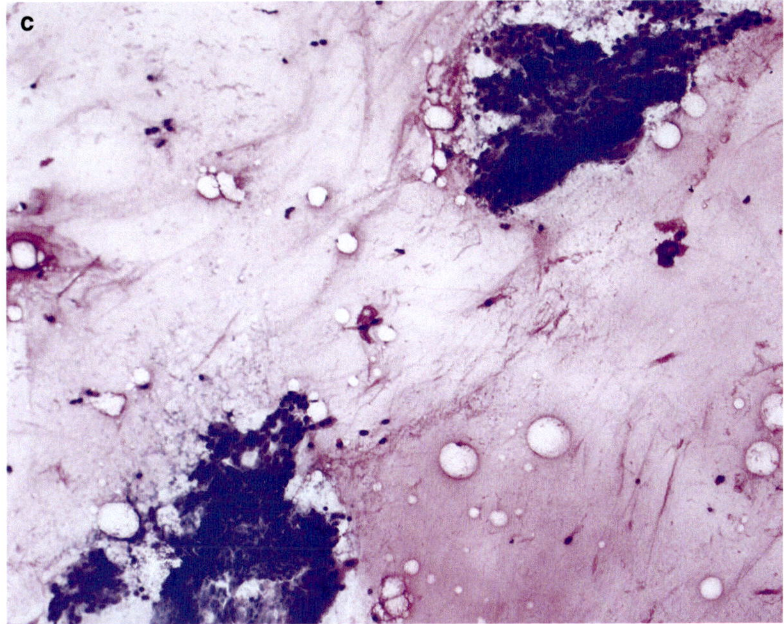

Fig. 4.5 (continued)

- There are three-dimensional clusters, cohesive sheets, and single intact cells floating within the mucin.
- Cells have bland cytologic features with round, uniform nuclei, fine nuclear chromatin without nucleoli, and absent myoepithelial cells.

2. Myxoid fibroadenoma (FA) is noted in younger patients and can be highly cellular.

   - Epithelial ductal cells are arranged in large, flat staghorn sheets with numerous oval bare nuclei in the background. Dissociated single epithelial cells, with no or minimal atypia may be seen.
   - Fibromyxoid stromal fragments (+/− coursing vessels) appear metachromatic on modified Giemsa stain and may be fibrillary but should not be mistaken for extracellular mucin [37].

3. Fibrocystic change (FCC) may also show extracellular mucin that originates from distended ducts and microcysts [38].

   - Cellularity can be variable with features of FCC including a mixed population of cohesive epithelial ductal cells and myoepithelial cells, apocrine metaplastic cells, and macrophages.

4. Mucocele-like lesion (MLL) is uncommon with mucin-filled cysts that rupture and extravasate mucin into the adjacent breast tissue.

- Represents spectrum of lesions ranging from benign and atypical to malignant etiology, with reported association with ADH, DCIS, and invasive ductal carcinoma [21, 39, 40].
- Circumscribed and often palpable [40] with radiologic calcifications on mammogram; on ultrasound they tend to be noted as oval clustered small cystic hypoechoic lesions, suggestive of complex cysts [17, 41].
- In benign MLL, smears will show abundant mucin and low cellularity, cohesive, monolayered clusters of benign ductal cells with absence of nuclear atypia; rarely single intact epithelial cells may be seen.
- Not infrequently detached epithelial lining and histiocytes/muciphages forming clusters may float in the extravasated mucin, features which may be misleading.
- Malignant MLL show cytologic features which may be indistinguishable from colloid carcinoma.

Tips and Pitfalls

- The most helpful cytomorphologic findings distinguishing myxoid FA, FCC, and MLL from colloid carcinoma include the presence of myoepithelial cells in the background and in association with epithelial groups, the absence of crowding or overlapping of ductal cells in three-dimensional clusters, and the absence or rarity of dissociated single atypical epithelial cells and thin-walled vasculature floating within mucin [39].
- Acellular or paucicellular mucin-rich aspirates that may be a MLL warrant surgical excision due to the association with DCIS or carcinoma at excision as there are no definitive clinical or radiologic features that can distinguish a benign mucocele [32].
- In the presence of marked/high-grade nuclear atypia, consider a mixed tumor, as the distinction between pure mucinous carcinoma and a mixed mucinous and ductal carcinoma is not possible by FNA [18]. Descriptive terminology such as "adenocarcinoma with prominent mucinous features" is preferred for reporting.

Cytologic Findings: Stroma

Breast FNA smears with a significant spindle cell or mesenchymal component are uncommon and represent a diverse group of lesions [42]. Fibroadenomas are common, with the presence of stroma observed in more than half of cases [43]. Compared to phyllodes tumors, the stroma is less cellular and less atypical [44].

Diagnostic Considerations

- What is the content of the fragment?
- What is the cellularity level of the fragment?
- What is the location of the fragment with respect to the epithelial cells (if epithelial cells are present)?
- Are there few or many stromal fragments?
- What is the overall cellularity and background seen on the slide?

Differential Diagnoses (Table 4.8, Fig. 4.6a–c)

1. Fibroadenoma should be considered in young patients with a solid, homogeneous, mobile breast lesion with smooth or lobulated borders [45].
    - Stromal fragments are of low to moderate cellularity and are separate from, or at the periphery of, large branching sheets of epithelial cells.
    - The background displays numerous bare oval nuclei.

Table 4.8 Key distinguishing cytologic features when stroma is seen on smears

	Fibroadenoma	Phyllodes	Papillary lesion	Spindle cell/ mesenchymal lesion	Sarcoma
Cellularity of stromal fragment	Low	Moderate to high	Moderate	Low to high	High
Stromal quality	Fibromyxoid	Fibrous	Fibrovascular	Fibrous, myxoid, collagenous, chondroid	Variable
Architecture	Stroma at periphery of epithelial sheets	Increased number of large stromal fragments [21]	Papillary fragments with fibrovascular cores	Scant stromal fragments	Highly cellular stromal fragments with atypical to pleomorphic spindled nuclei
Background	Bare oval nuclei	Spindled stromal cells [21]	High cellularity, columnar epithelium, bare oval to elongated nuclei, macrophages	Scant cellularity	Atypical spindle cells, blood (in angiosarcoma), other mesenchymal elements (depending on sarcoma type)
Cytomorphology of epithelial cells	Bland to atypical	Bland to atypical	Low to high Atypia	N/A	N/A

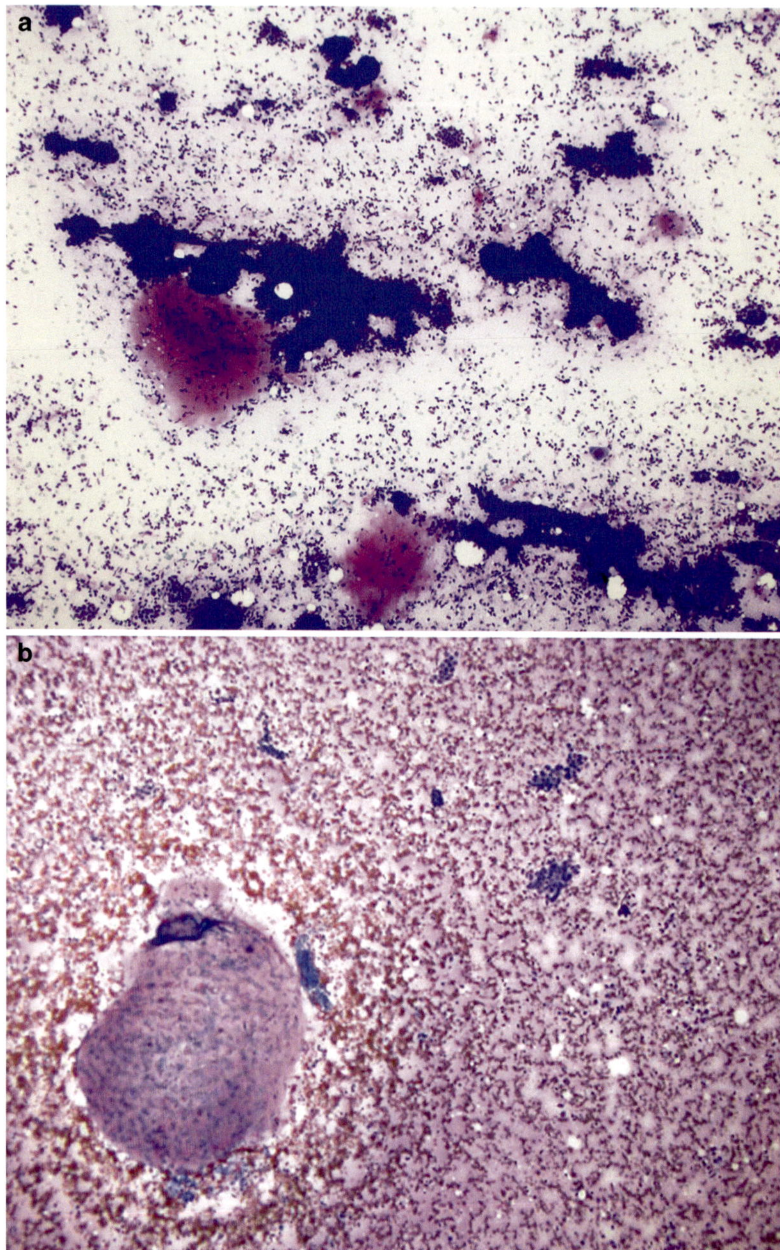

Fig. 4.6 Differential diagnosis of stroma. Fibroadenoma showing characteristic stromal fragments and large branching, staghorn sheets of epithelial cells in a background of numerous bare oval nuclei; of note, the stroma in a fibroadenoma is typically of low cellularity and often appears fibromyxoid (**a**, Diff-Quik stain, ×100), whereas the stromal fragments of phyllodes tumor show increased cellularity (**b**, Diff-Quik stain, ×100). Sarcoma shows significant atypia with spindle-shaped cells appearing as very large single cells, some with enlarged nuclei with irregular nuclear borders, as distinguished from both fibroadenoma and phyllodes which have benign cells in the background (epithelium and myoepithelium) (**c**, Diff-Quik stain, ×400)

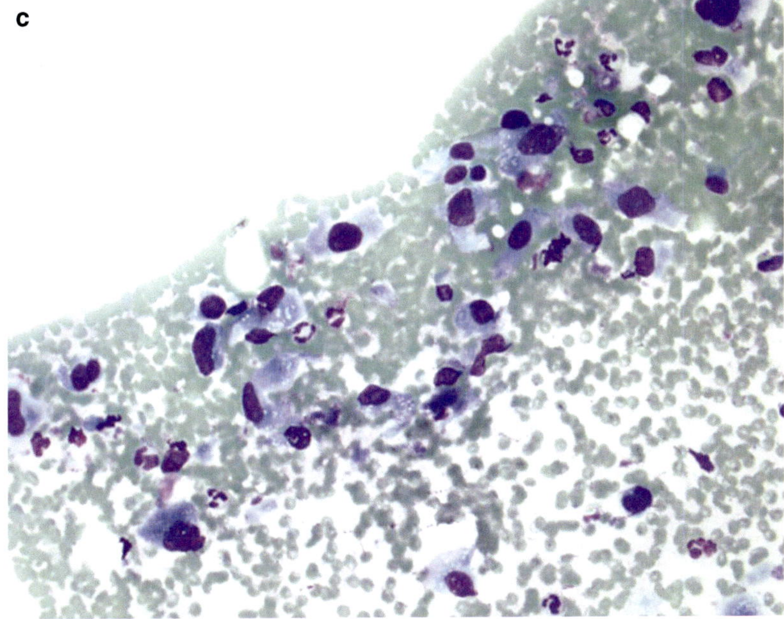

Fig. 4.6 (continued)

2. Phyllodes tumor occurs in the second or fifth decade and clinically and radiologically presents as a rapid growth of a well-circumscribed lesion with lobulated borders [45].
   - Stromal fragments are of moderate to high cellularity, are large and numerous, and may display atypia of both stromal and epithelial cell components.
3. Papillary lesions present as retroareolar breast lesions with abnormal breast discharge [45].
   - Stromal fragments are of low to moderate cellularity and contain fibrovascular cores that are centrally placed in the large epithelial fragments.
   - The background is highly cellular with scattered single columnar cells together with or lacking bare oval nuclei, macrophages, and cyst fluid.
   - Three-dimensional papillary epithelial cell clusters and cell balls are noted [46].
4. Spindle cell/mesenchymal lesions can present with a stellate mass that clinically and radiologically mimics carcinoma.
   - Stromal fragments may be scanty but may also predominate the smear.
   - The background may display other elements:
     - Mesenchymal, i.e., lipomatous elements in spindle cell lipoma
     - Inflammatory, i.e., inflammatory cells in nodular fasciitis [46]

5. Sarcomas are uncommon lesions in the breast.
   - Stromal fragments are of high cellularity with large pleomorphic cells and mitotic figures.
   - The background lacks epithelial elements and may show abundant blood, i.e., angiosarcoma.

Tips and Pitfalls

- Cases with branching epithelial sheets, a background of bare oval nuclei, and stromal fragments both in the periphery and in the center of epithelial sheets should be scrutinized for the presence of fibrovascular cores, to avoid missing a papillary lesion.
- If a papillary lesion is diagnosed during ROSE, surgical planning can begin immediately.
- Sarcomatoid carcinoma must remain in the differential diagnosis for an atypical spindle cell lesion.
- In cases with scant cellularity and rare stromal fragments, adequacy must be determined based on the clinical and radiologic findings with awareness that the lesion may represent a stromal or fibrotic lesion that is difficult to aspirate.

References

1. Nasuti JF, Gupta PK, Baloch ZW. Diagnostic value and cost-effectiveness of on-site evaluation of fine-needle aspiration specimens: review of 5,688 cases. Diagn Cytopathol. 2002;27(1):1–4.
2. Sakuma T, Mimura A, Tanigawa N, Takamizu R, Morishima H, Matsunami N. Rapid on-site cytologic examination of 1500 breast lesions using the modified Shorr's stain. Breast Cancer (Tokyo, Japan). 2015;22(3):280–6.
3. Kocjan G, Bourgain C, Fassina A, Hagmar B, Herbert A, Kapila K, et al. The role of breast FNAC in diagnosis and clinical management: a survey of current practice. Cytopathology. 2008;19(5):271–8.
4. Layfield LJ, Mooney EE, Glasgow B, Hirschowitz S, Coogan A. What constitutes an adequate smear in fine-needle aspiration cytology of the breast? Cancer. 1997;81(1):16–21.
5. The uniform approach to breast fine-needle aspiration biopsy. Am J Surg. 1997;174(4):371–85.
6. Stanley MW, Abele J, Kline T, Silverman JF, Skoog L. What constitutes adequate sampling of palpable breast lesions that appear benign by clinical and mammographic criteria? Diagn Cytopathol. 1995;13(5):473–82.
7. Roberts JC, Rainsbury RM. 'Tactile sensation': a new clinical sign during fine needle aspiration of breast lumps. Ann R Coll Surg Engl. 1994;76(2):136–8.
8. Hermansen C, Skovgaard Poulsen H, Jensen J, Langfeldt B, Steenskov V, Frederiksen P, et al. Diagnostic reliability of combined physical examination, mammography, and fine-needle puncture ("triple-test") in breast tumors. A prospective study. Cancer. 1987;60(8):1866–71.
9. Abati A, Simsir A. Breast fine needle aspiration biopsy: prevailing recommendations and contemporary practices. Clin Lab Med. 2005;25(4):631–54, v.

10. Abele J, Stanley MW, Rollins SD, Miller TR. What constitutes an adequate smear in fine-needle aspiration cytology of the breast? Cancer. 1998;84(1):57–61.
11. Howell LP, Gandour-Edwards R, Folkins K, Davis R, Yasmeen S, Afify A. Adequacy evaluation of fine-needle aspiration biopsy in the breast health clinic setting. Cancer. 2004;102(5):295–301.
12. Smith DN, Kaelin CM, Korbin CD, Ko W, Meyer JE, Carter GR. Impalpable breast cysts: utility of cytologic examination of fluid obtained with radiologically guided aspiration. Radiology. 1997;204(1):149–51.
13. Onoue S, Katoh T, Chigira H, Matsuo K, Suzuki M, Shibata Y, et al. A case of apocrine carcinoma of the breast presenting as two cysts. Breast Cancer (Tokyo, Japan). 1997;4(3):193–6.
14. Agarwal C, Pujani M, Sharma N, Rana D, Prajapati D. Apocrine carcinoma of breast: a rare entity posing cytological challenge. Diagn Cytopathol. 2017;45(12):1156–8.
15. Kerridge WD, Kryvenko ON, Thompson A, Shah BA. Fat necrosis of the breast: a pictorial review of the mammographic, ultrasound, CT, and MRI findings with Histopathologic correlation. Radiol Res Pract. 2015;2015:613139.
16. Irshad A, Pope TL, Ackerman SJ, Panzegrau B. Characterization of sonographic and mammographic features of granular cell tumors of the breast and estimation of their incidence. J Ultrasound Med. 2008;27(3):467–75.
17. Cangiarella J, Simsir A, Tabbara SO, editors. Breast cytohistology. Cambridge: Cambridge University Press; 2013. (Cytohistology of Small Tissue Samples).
18. Barbara S, Ducatman HW. Breast. In: Cibas ES, editor. Cytology: diagnostic principles and clinical correlates. 4th ed. Philadelphia: Saunders Elsevier; 2014. p. 233–65.
19. Pieterse AS, Mahar A, Orell S. Granular cell tumour: a pitfall in FNA cytology of breast lesions. Pathology. 2004;36(1):58–62.
20. Malzone MG, Campanile AC, Gioioso A, Fucito A, D'Aiuto G, Botti G, et al. Silicone lymphadenopathy: presentation of a further case containing asteroid bodies on fine-needle cytology sample. Diagn Cytopathol. 2015;43(1):57–9.
21. Cangiarella J, Simsir A. Breast. In: Svante R, Orell GS, editors. Orell and Sterrett's fine needle aspiration cytology. 5th ed. Edinburgh: Churchill Livingstone; 2012. p. 156–209.
22. Ng WK, Kong JH. Significance of squamous cells in fine needle aspiration cytology of the breast. A review of cases in a seven-year period. Acta Cytol. 2003;47(1):27–35.
23. DeMay R. Practical principles of cytopathology. 1st ed. Chicago: American Society for Clinical Pathology; 2007. p. 420.
24. Schmitt F, Gerhard R, Stanley DE, Domanski HA. Breast. In: Domanski HA, editor. Atlas of fine needle aspiration cytology. 2014th ed. London: Springer; 2013.
25. Fung AD, Collins JA, Campassi C, Ioffe OB, Staats PN. Performance characteristics of ultrasound-guided fine-needle aspiration of axillary lymph nodes for metastatic breast cancer employing rapid on-site evaluation of adequacy: analysis of 136 cases and review of the literature. Cancer Cytopathol. 2014;122(4):282–91.
26. O'Leary DP, O'Brien O, Relihan N, McCarthy J, Ryan M, Barry J, et al. Rapid on-site evaluation of axillary fine-needle aspiration cytology in breast cancer. Br J Surg. 2012;99(6):807–12.
27. Alvarez S, Anorbe E, Alcorta P, Lopez F, Alonso I, Cortes J. Role of sonography in the diagnosis of axillary lymph node metastases in breast cancer: a systematic review. AJR Am J Roentgenol. 2006;186(5):1342–8.
28. Topps A, Clay V, Absar M, Howe M, Lim Y, Johnson R, et al. The sensitivity of pre-operative axillary staging in breast cancer: comparison of invasive lobular and ductal carcinoma. Eur J Surg Oncol. 2014;40(7):813–7.
29. Prathiba D, Rao S, Kshitija K, Joseph LD. Papillary lesions of breast – an introspect of cytomorphological features. J Cytol. 2010;27(1):12–5.
30. Nayar R, De Frias DV, Bourtsos EP, Sutton V, Bedrossian C. Cytologic differential diagnosis of papillary pattern in breast aspirates: correlation with histology. Ann Diagn Pathol. 2001;5(1):34–42.

31. Simsir A, Waisman J, Thorner K, Cangiarella J. Mammary lesions diagnosed as "papillary" by aspiration biopsy: 70 cases with follow-up. Cancer. 2003;99(3):156–65.
32. Simsir A, Cangiarella J. Challenging breast lesions: pitfalls and limitations of fine-needle aspiration and the role of core biopsy in specific lesions. Diagn Cytopathol. 2012;40(3):262–72.
33. Jeffrey PB, Ljung BM. Benign and malignant papillary lesions of the breast. A cytomorphologic study. Am J Clin Pathol. 1994;101(4):500–7.
34. Kobayashi TK, Ueda M, Nishino T, Watanabe S, Yakushiji M. Spontaneous infarction of an intraductal papilloma of the breast: cytological presentation on fine needle aspiration. Cytopathology. 1992;3(6):379–84.
35. Dawson AE, Mulford DK. Fine needle aspiration of mucinous (colloid) breast carcinoma. Nuclear grading and mammographic and cytologic findings. Acta Cytol. 1998;42(3):668–72.
36. Renshaw AA. Can mucinous lesions of the breast be reliably diagnosed by core needle biopsy? Am J Clin Pathol. 2002;118(1):82–4.
37. Ly A, Kong CS. Fine needle aspiration cytology. In: Kristen A, Atkins CK, editors. Practical breast pathology: a diagnostic approach E-book: a volume in the pattern recognition series. 1st ed. Philadelphia: Saunders; 2012. p. 254–77.
38. Simsir A, Tsang P, Greenebaum E. Additional mimics of mucinous mammary carcinoma: fibroepithelial lesions. Am J Clin Pathol. 1998;109(2):169–72.
39. Ventura K, Cangiarella J, Lee I, Moreira A, Waisman J, Simsir A. Aspiration biopsy of mammary lesions with abundant extracellular mucinous material. Review of 43 cases with surgical follow-up. Am J Clin Pathol. 2003;120(2):194–202.
40. Wong NL, Wan SK. Comparative cytology of mucocelelike lesion and mucinous carcinoma of the breast in fine needle aspiration. Acta Cytol. 2000;44(5):765–70.
41. Begum SM, Jara-Lazaro AR, Thike AA, Tse GM, Wong JS, Ho JT, et al. Mucin extravasation in breast core biopsies–clinical significance and outcome correlation. Histopathology. 2009;55(5):609–17.
42. Chhieng DC, Cangiarella JF, Waisman J, Fernandez G, Cohen JM. Fine-needle aspiration cytology of spindle cell lesions of the breast. Cancer. 1999;87(6):359–71.
43. Dejmek A, Lindholm K. Frequency of cytologic features in fine needle aspirates from histologically and cytologically diagnosed fibroadenomas. Acta Cytol. 1991;35(6):695–9.
44. Maritz RM, Michelow PM. Cytological criteria to distinguish Phyllodes tumour of the breast from Fibroadenoma. Acta Cytol. 2017;61(6):418–24.
45. Sencha AN, Evseeva EV, Mogutov MS, Patrunov Y. Breast ultrasound. 2013th ed. Berlin: Springer; 2013. p. 258.
46. Masood S, Rosa M. Cytopathology of the breast. In: Gattuso P, Reddy VB, Masood S, editors. Differential diagnosis in cytopathology. 1st ed. Cambridge: Cambridge University Press; 2009. p. 760.

Chapter 5
Salivary Gland

Adebowale J. Adeniran

Introduction

Fine needle aspiration (FNA) biopsy is the procedure of choice in the preoperative evaluation of salivary gland lesions. The procedure is easily accessible, minimally invasive, safe, and cost-effective [1–5]. Coupled with the high sensitivity, specificity, and diagnostic accuracy, it helps in the risk stratification of patients and has been shown to decrease the number of surgeries when included into the initial assessment [6]. The procedure is also preferred because alternative procedures such as incisional biopsy are associated with an increased risk of infection and potential contamination of surgical planes. Inadequate sampling is an important limitation of salivary gland FNA [7–9]. The advent of rapid on-site evaluation at the time of the procedure has greatly enhanced the assessment of adequacy of FNA specimens especially in the areas of increased diagnostic yield and optimal preparation of specimens [1, 10].

Because the normal parotid gland contains numerous intraparotid and periparotid lymph nodes [11], primary lymphomas and metastatic tumors mimicking salivary gland neoplasms are commonly seen, and ROSE is also essential to determine the cell of origin of tumor, to determine whether the tumor is primary or secondary, and to determine whether or not additional passes are needed for ancillary studies like flow cytometry (in the case of lymphoid lesions) and cell block material (in the case of diagnostically challenging lesions and metastatic tumors).

A. J. Adeniran (✉)
Department of Pathology, Yale University School of Medicine, New Haven, CT, USA
e-mail: adebowale.adeniran@yale.edu

G. Cai, A. J. Adeniran (eds.), *Rapid On-site Evaluation (ROSE)*,
https://doi.org/10.1007/978-3-030-21799-0_5

Diagnostic Consideration

Specimen Adequacy Assessment

There are no established criteria for assessing specimen adequacy. However, the presence of normal salivary gland elements on the smear in a patient with a radiologically confirmed mass lesion should be treated as nondiagnostic. It should be noted though that an aspirate containing exclusively both ducts and acini may represent sialosis, a salivary gland swelling without evidence of neoplasia, infection, or inflammation [12]. Cystic lesions are also notorious for nondiagnostic yield, so when a cystic salivary gland lesion is aspirated, any residual mass lesion should be resampled after the fluid has been aspirated [13, 14]. Recommendations for optimal specimen preparation include the use of air-dried and alcohol-fixed slides, prepared for Romanowsky and Papanicolaou staining, respectively, with supplemental combinations of liquid-based or cytospin preparations, cell blocks, and RPMI for flow cytometric evaluation where appropriate and possibly sterile material for microbiology. For cyst-fluid-only specimens, only one or two smears are recommended with the remainder being processed as either cytospin or liquid-based preparations.

Normal Salivary Gland Tissue

Aspirates of normal salivary gland tissue usually have low cellularity and they are composed of acinar cells, ductal cells, and admixed adipose tissue (Fig. 5.1) [12, 15]. Occasionally naked acinar nuclei and myoepithelial cells are present. Acinar cells form cohesive, spherical groups composed of polyhedral cells with vacuolated or granular cytoplasm and small, uniform nuclei. The ductal cells form either flat honeycomb sheets of small, uniform cuboidal cells with centrally located round nuclei or tight tubular structures composed of similar cells.

Nonneoplastic Conditions

Acute Sialadenitis

Aspirates from acute sialadenitis are usually hypocellular and consist of abundant neutrophils, necrotic debris, and fibrin [16]. As the infection progresses, lymphocytes, histiocytes, plasma cells, and granulation tissue are seen in varying proportions. Fragments of ductal and acinar cells with reactive and regenerative atypia may also be present.

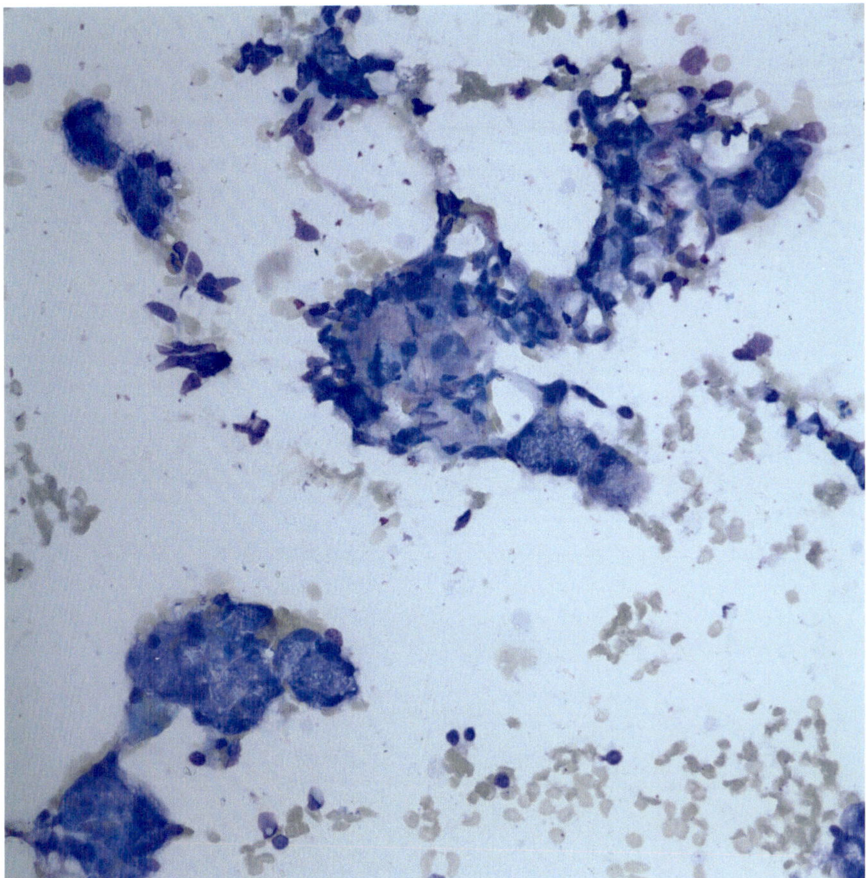

Fig. 5.1 Normal acinar cells and admixed adipose tissue (Diff-Quik stain, ×400)

Chronic Sialadenitis

Aspirates from chronic sialadenitis are sparsely cellular. They contain lymphocytes, plasma cells, and fibrous tissue, in a mucoid background, admixed with blood and proteinaceous debris (Fig. 5.2). There is paucity of acinar cells.

Granulomatous Sialadenitis

Aspirates show aggregates of epithelioid histiocytes and sometimes multinucleated forms in a background of granular, necrotic debris and inflammation. Epithelioid histiocytes have elongated, bland nuclei, with folded nuclear membranes, fine

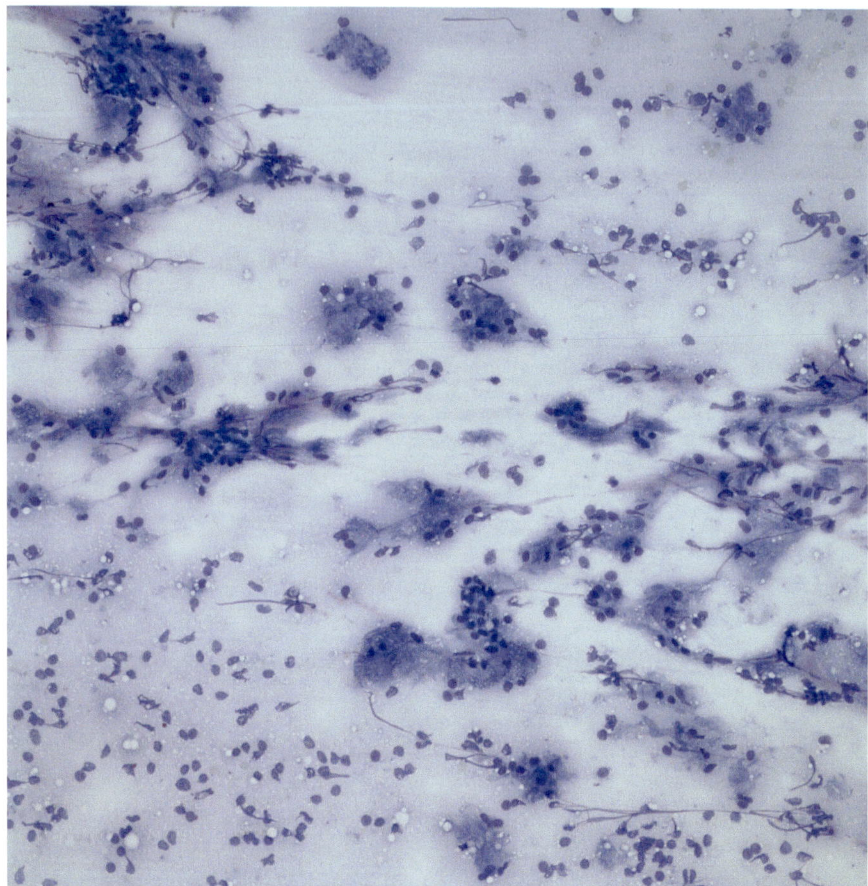

Fig. 5.2 Chronic sialadenitis. Acinar cells and numerous lymphocytes in a mucoid background (Diff-Quik stain, ×200)

chromatin, and small, inconspicuous nucleoli. The cytoplasm is abundant and eosinophilic [17, 18]. Asteroid bodies, Schaumann bodies, and calcium oxalate crystals can be present in sarcoidosis [14].

Tips and Pitfalls

- If the aspirate is grossly recognizable as pus, or an infectious etiology is suspected, material should be collected and sent for microbiologic studies at the time of ROSE.
- If there is significant epithelial atypia or suspicion of a neoplastic process, repeat FNA after the infection has resolved should be recommended.

- In chronic sialadenitis, the presence of atypical metaplastic squamous cells in a background of mucus can mimic mucoepidermoid carcinoma [19].
- The presence of psammoma bodies has been described in chronic sialadenitis [20] and should not be interpreted as a feature of malignancy.
- Special stains and culture for organisms in cases of granulomatous sialadenitis are important and additional material should be collected for this purpose at the time of ROSE.

Cystic Lesions

Mucocele

Mucoceles are pseudocysts because they lack an epithelial lining. Aspirates are sparsely cellular and composed of histiocytes, some with intracellular mucin, granular debris, extracellular mucin, amylase crystalloids, and inflammatory cells [14].

Retention Cyst

The diagnosis of benign retention cyst on FNA is usually based on the presence of fluid (clear, turbid, or viscous), containing neutrophils, foamy macrophages, and amorphous cell debris. Cholesterol crystals, acinar and ductal cells, as well as metaplastic squamous cells can also be seen [21].

Benign Lymphoepithelial Cyst

These cysts have been observed in increasing frequency in patients with acquired immunodeficiency syndrome (AIDS). The cysts are lined by squamous epithelium and surrounded by dense lymphoid tissue with reactive lymphoid follicles [22]. Aspirates contain an abundant, heterogeneous population of reactive lymphocytes and macrophages in clear cyst fluid. There may be a few clusters of squamous or sometimes columnar or cuboidal epithelial cells [23].

Tips and Pitfalls

- The presence of muciphages and extracellular mucin alone has a wide differential diagnosis, which includes mucocele, mucus retention cyst, and chronic sialadenitis with mucus metaplasia. Furthermore, low-grade mucoepidermoid

carcinoma is also to be considered. It is a prudent practice to regard the diagnosis as atypical and add a comment to describe the differential diagnosis. A residual mass after cyst aspiration, however, is highly suspicious for mucoepidermoid carcinoma.
- Distinction of benign lymphoepithelial cyst from Warthin tumor may be difficult because the oncocytes of a Warthin tumor can show extensive squamous metaplasia.
- In benign squamous-lined cysts, cystic squamous cell carcinoma cannot be entirely excluded and must be considered. It is important to add a comment to the diagnosis to reflect this.

Benign Neoplasms

Pleomorphic Adenoma

The proportions of the cellular constituents are extremely variable from one tumor to another and within an individual tumor. Hence it is important to obtain multiple passes from different areas of the tumor [14].

A. Cytomorphologic features

- Aspirates have a thick, gelatinous consistency and cellularity is variable.
- Smears consist of epithelial cells, myoepithelial cells, and chondromyxoid matrix.
- Uniform, medium-sized epithelial cells are present in cohesive groups, usu ally in a honeycomb pattern, often forming ducts or small sheets. Individual cells may also be present. The epithelial cells are typically intermixed with the chondromyxoid stroma (Fig. 5.3) [24, 25].
- Myoepithelial cells are usually present as single cells, within matrix material (Fig. 5.4), in loose clusters, or in larger, haphazardly arranged clusters, and they have a variety of appearances: spindle-shaped, epithelioid, clear cell, and plasmacytoid.
- The presence of chondromyxoid fibrillary matrix is the most characteristic finding. When seen at ROSE, it is magenta-colored and metachromatic on Romanowsky-type stain.
- Tyrosine crystalloids may be present, although these are nonspecific.

B. Tips and pitfalls

- When there is paucity or absence of matrix and predominance of epithelial elements (Fig. 5.5), there may be a misdiagnosis as monomorphic adenoma, basal cell adenoma, or carcinoma, while predominance of myoepithelial cells may lead to a misdiagnosis of myoepithelioma [25–27]. In this context,

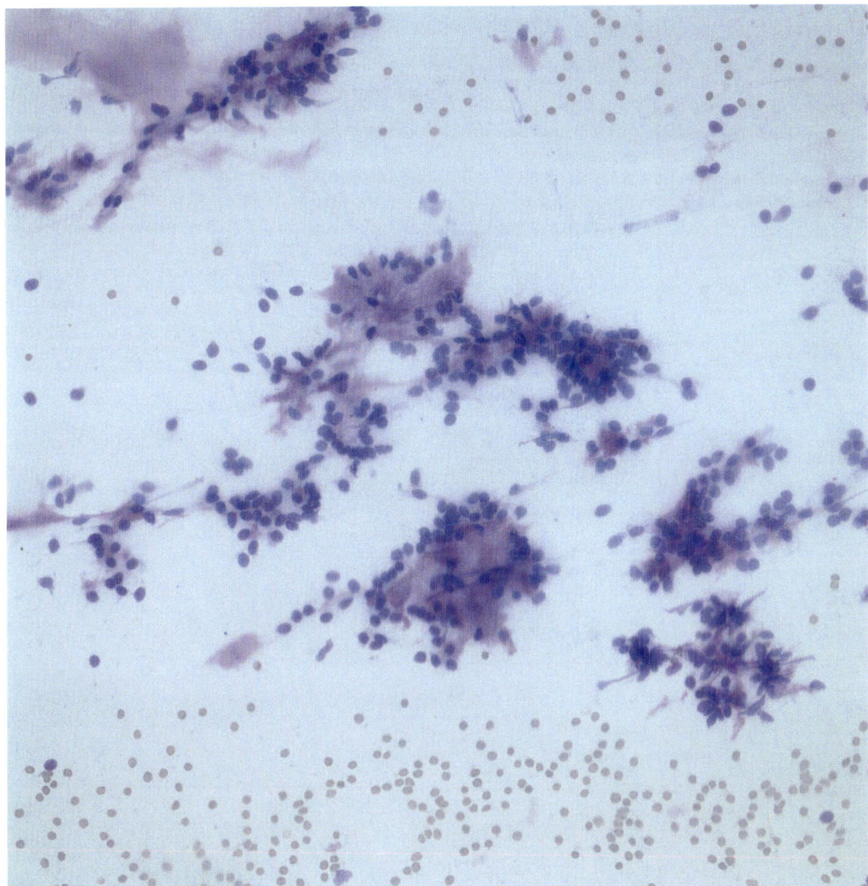

Fig. 5.3 Pleomorphic adenoma. Epithelial cells in cohesive groups, intermixed with chondromyxoid stroma (Diff-Quik stain, ×200)

rather than making a definitive diagnosis of pleomorphic adenoma, it may be expedient to give a list of differential diagnoses.

- Aspirates from pleomorphic adenoma may contain homogeneous globules surrounded by monomorphous epithelial cells (cylindromatous areas) thereby mimicking adenoid cystic carcinoma and making distinction between the 2 entities difficult [21, 28, 29]. Multiple sampling from different areas of the tumor will most likely reduce this diagnostic error.
- When tumors are dominated by a mature chondroid substance, they may be difficult to tell apart from a true chondroid neoplasm.
- Severe cytologic atypia usually raises the possibility of carcinoma ex pleomorphic adenoma. [28] Atypical cells in pleomorphic adenoma can be seen frequently. The smears may contain single cells of stromal type

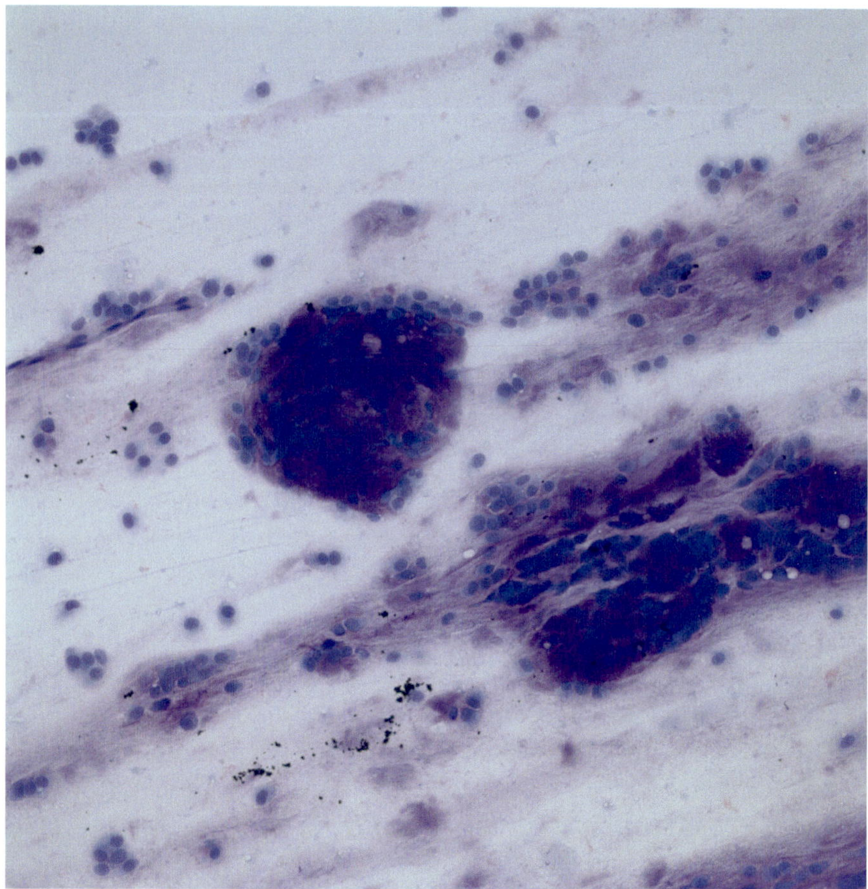

Fig. 5.4 Pleomorphic adenoma. Myoepithelial cells present as single cells and loose clusters within matrix material (Diff-Quik stain, ×200)

that have very large, irregular, often multiple or multilobate, bizarre nuclei [21]. When there is no accompanying necrosis or abundant mitoses, the diagnosis of pleomorphic adenoma with atypia is justified, with a comment that the finding could be indicative of early malignant change [14].

- Extensive squamous or mucinous metaplasia in pleomorphic adenoma may lead to an erroneous diagnosis of squamous cell carcinoma or low-grade mucoepidermoid carcinoma [30, 31].

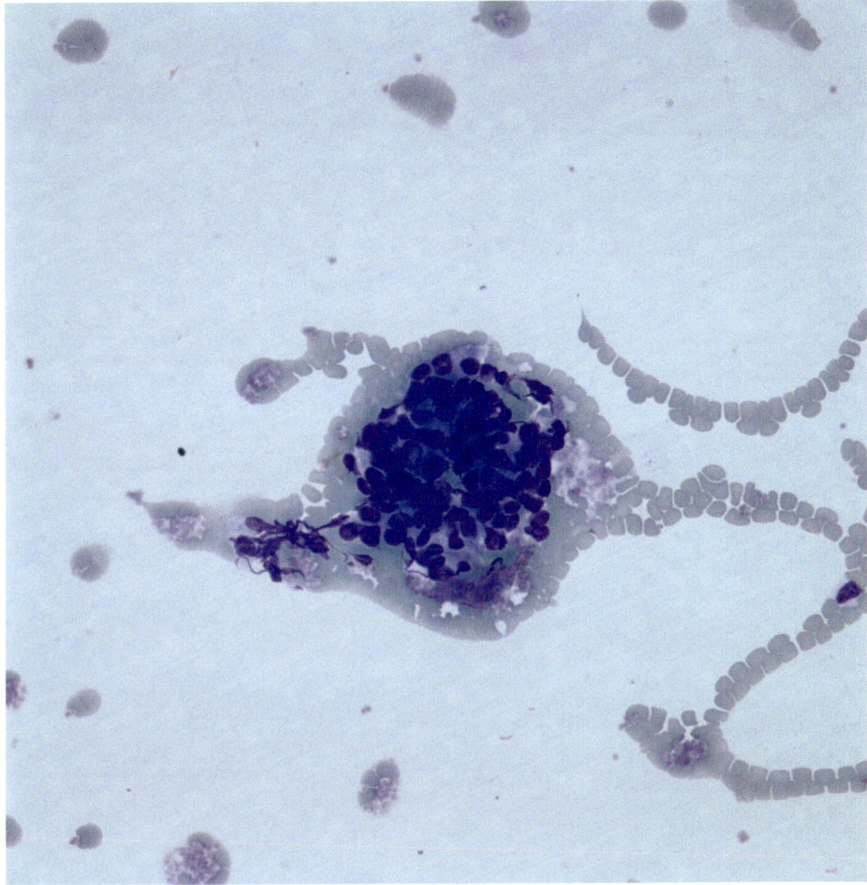

Fig. 5.5 Pleomorphic adenoma. Predominance of epithelial cells and absence of matrix (Diff-Quik stain, ×400)

Warthin Tumor

Warthin tumor has a cystic appearance and the aspirate contains distinctive, thick, brown-green, granular fluid grossly resembling motor engine oil.

A. Cytomorphologic features

- Variable cellularity, ranging from barely optimum cellularity to occasional hypercellularity.

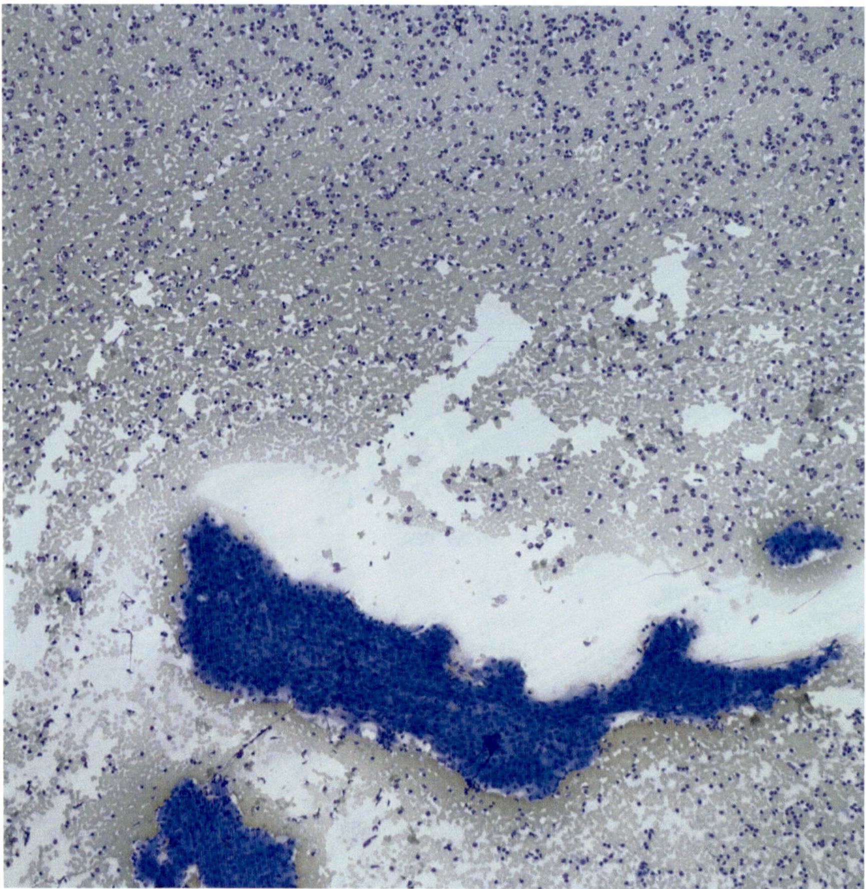

Fig. 5.6 Warthin tumor. Epithelial fragments in a background of abundant lymphocytes (Diff-Quik stain, ×100)

- Admixture of epithelial fragments, occasional single epithelial cells, and abundant lymphocytes in a granular cystic background [32] (Fig. 5.6).
- Epithelial cells are oncocytic in appearance, and they are arranged in cohesive, monolayered sheets, with large nuclei, prominent nucleoli, and moderately abundant granular cytoplasm (Fig. 5.7).
- Background of lymphocytes, in single dispersed cells and as crushed lymphoid tangles.

B. Tips and pitfalls

- When the epithelial component predominates, smears may show large sheets of oncocytic cells, with relatively few lymphocytes, and this may be misinterpreted as oncocytoma.
- Degenerated oncocytes in the presence of abundant mucoid material may lead to an erroneous diagnosis of mucoepidermoid carcinoma [32].

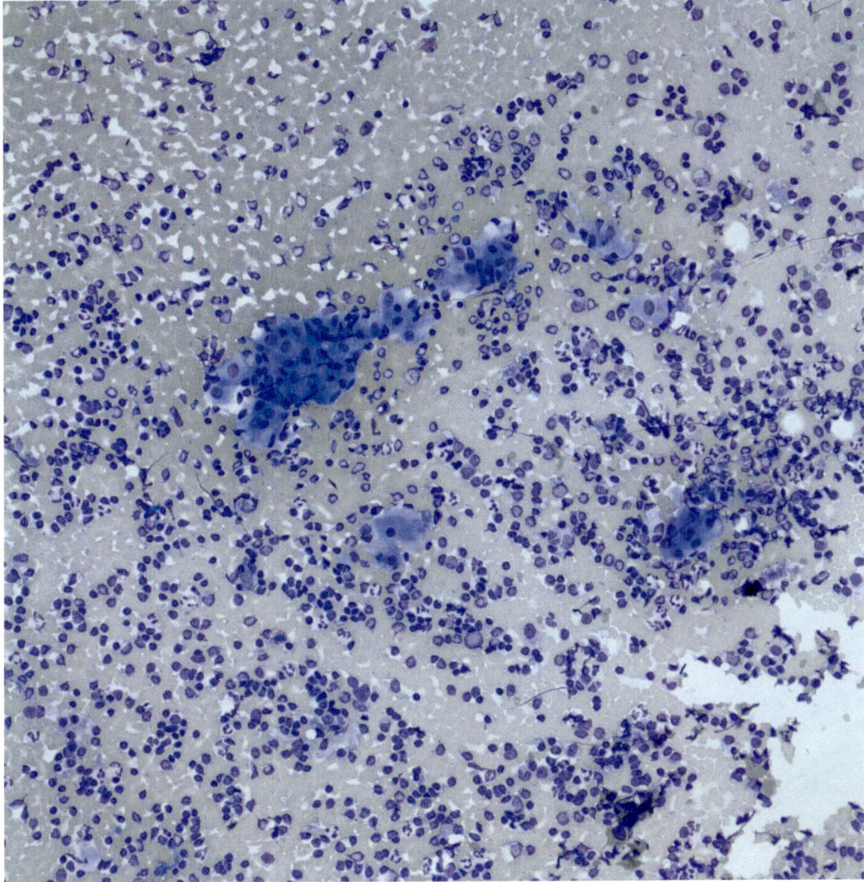

Fig. 5.7 Warthin tumor. Oncocytic cells with moderately abundant granular cytoplasm in a background of abundant lymphocytes (Diff-Quik stain, ×200)

- In cases associated with marked inflammation, squamous metaplasia may be present, suggesting a diagnosis of squamous cell carcinoma with extensive background necrosis [33].

Malignant Neoplasms

Mucoepidermoid Carcinoma

Mucoepidermoid carcinoma (MEC) has extreme cytomorphologic heterogeneity thus making a definitive FNA diagnosis of this neoplasm very challenging. Cytologic features differ between low-grade and high-grade mucoepidermoid carcinoma. The

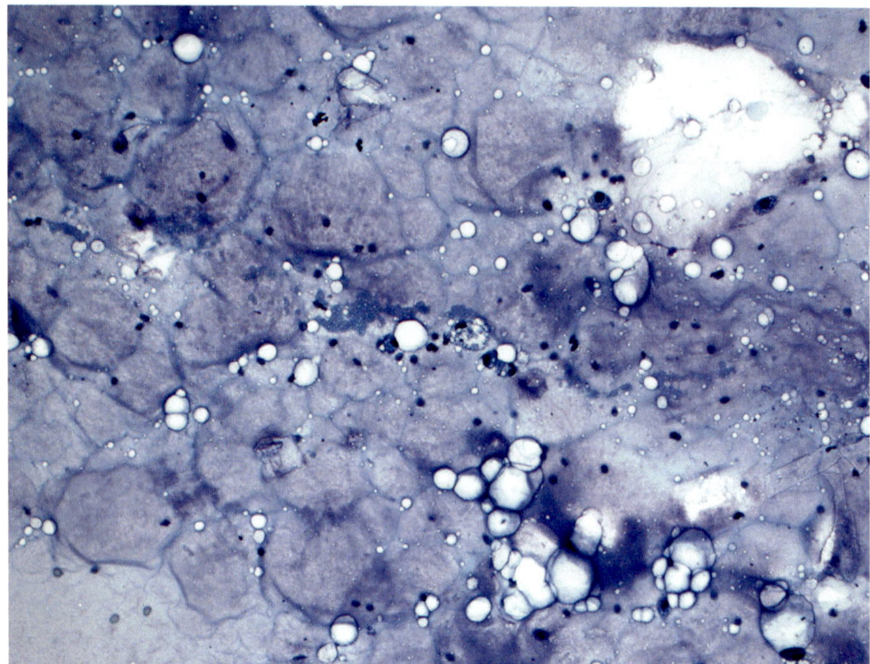

Fig. 5.8 Low-grade mucoepidermoid carcinoma. Mucin-secreting cells in a background of muciphages and mucous (Diff-Quik stain, ×200)

diagnostic difficulty is more common in low-grade tumors that usually present as cystic lesions.

A. Cytomorphologic features

- Variable cellularity.
- The diagnostic feature of MEC is the combination of mucous cells, epidermoid (squamoid) cells, and intermediate cells, with clear cells often present as well.
- Low-grade tumors are usually cystic with predominantly mucin-secreting cells and intermediate cells with round to oval nuclei; moderate amount of dense cytoplasm, in a dirty background of muciphages, mucous and nuclear debris (Fig. 5.8) [21, 34].
- Intermediate-grade tumors show a greater proportion of intermediate cells and squamous cells with mild to moderate atypia [35].
- High-grade tumors show obviously malignant poorly cohesive clusters and singly scattered squamous epithelial cells with moderate to abundant eosinophilic cytoplasm, pleomorphic hyperchromatic nuclei, and a few intermediate cells in a necrotic background. Mucin-secreting cells may be difficult to find [36] (Fig. 5.9).

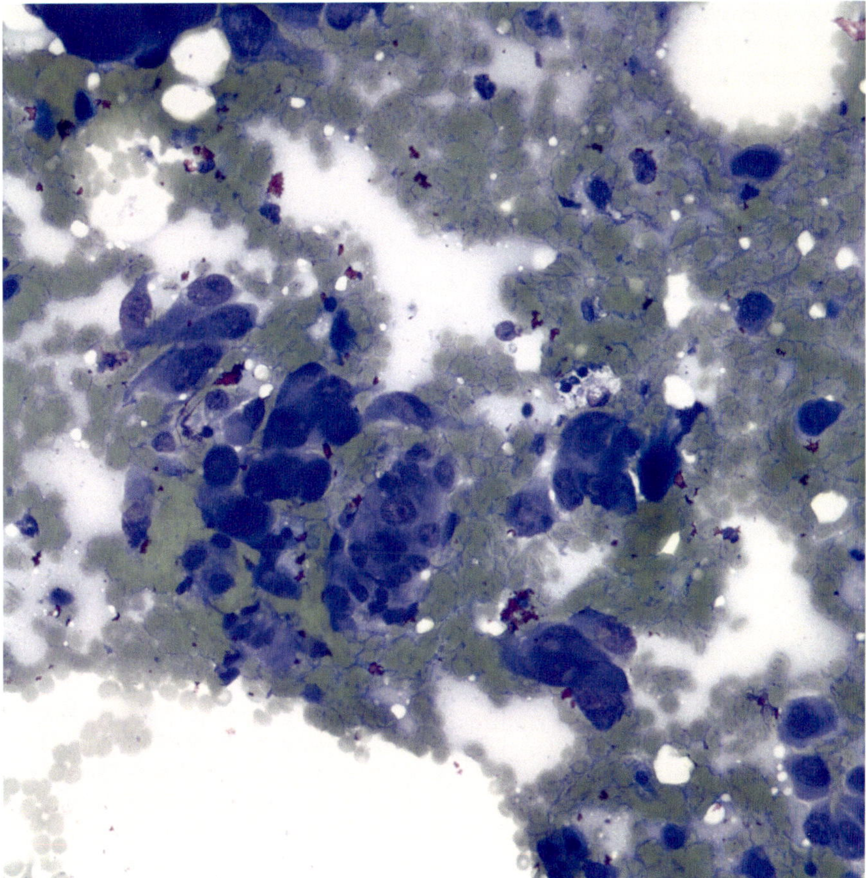

Fig. 5.9 High-grade mucoepidermoid carcinoma. Malignant poorly cohesive clusters and singly scattered epithelial cells with moderate eosinophilic cytoplasm and pleomorphic nuclei (Diff-Quik stain, X200)

B. Tips and pitfalls

- MEC may be misdiagnosed as mucous cyst if there is paucicellular smear either from sampling error or cyst-fluid-diluting tumor cells and presence of mucous cells in a mucinous background [34, 36].
- A partially solid and cystic tumor may be misdiagnosed as being entirely cystic if the solid component is not sampled [34, 37, 38]. Due to this pitfall, cases diagnosed as mucinous cystic lesion should be reported with the caveat that low-grade MEC cannot be excluded.
- In high-grade tumors with malignant squamous epithelial cells, the paucity or absence of intermediate and mucin-secreting cells can lead to a misdiagnosis as metastatic squamous cell carcinoma.

- Underdiagnosis as pleomorphic adenoma is a recognized pitfall as intermediate cells and stromal cells can be interpreted as benign epithelial cells and myoepithelial cells of pleomorphic adenoma, respectively. Furthermore, thick extracellular mucin can be perceived as pale chondromyxoid matrix. The presence of squamous metaplasia can also lead to the misdiagnosis of MEC as pleomorphic adenoma [39].
- Ancillary studies such as reverse transcription polymerase chain reaction (RT-PCR) and fluorescence in situ hybridization (FISH) have been found to be useful in the diagnosis of morphologically ambiguous cases of MEC and to determine biologic behavior of tumors [34]; hence material should be collected for ancillary studies at the time of ROSE.

Adenoid Cystic Carcinoma

There are three variants of adenoid cystic carcinoma, and they are often present in combination – tubular, cribriform, and solid. It is important to recognize the solid pattern because of its more aggressive clinical course.

A. Cytomorphologic features

- The cells are variably sized, often large, basaloid, with scant cytoplasm, and hyperchromatic often angulated nuclei (Fig. 5.10) [25, 40].
- Abundant acellular matrix that is arranged in discrete globules and cylinders with sharp borders (Fig. 5.11).
- Globules are intensely metachromatic with a Romanowsky-type stain.
- Basaloid cells predominate and there is scant matrix in solid variant of adenoid cystic carcinoma.

B. Tips and pitfalls

- When basaloid cells predominate and there is scant matrix, it is often impossible to distinguish solid variant of adenoid cystic carcinoma from basal cell adenoma.
- The hyaline matrix material is similar to the fibromyxoid stroma of pleomorphic adenoma. The hyaline stroma material in adenoid cystic carcinoma is, however, more homogeneous than that in pleomorphic adenoma (Fig. 5.12). It can appear glassy, granular, or laminated, but not fibrillar like the stroma material characteristic of pleomorphic adenoma. Also, the matrix of adenoid cystic carcinoma has sharp edges, with a characteristic "cookie cutter" appearance. Moreover, the neoplastic cells of adenoid cystic carcinoma surround the matrix material but are not embedded in it [14], resulting in discreet islands of variably sized globules and fingerlike projections of matrix-like material.

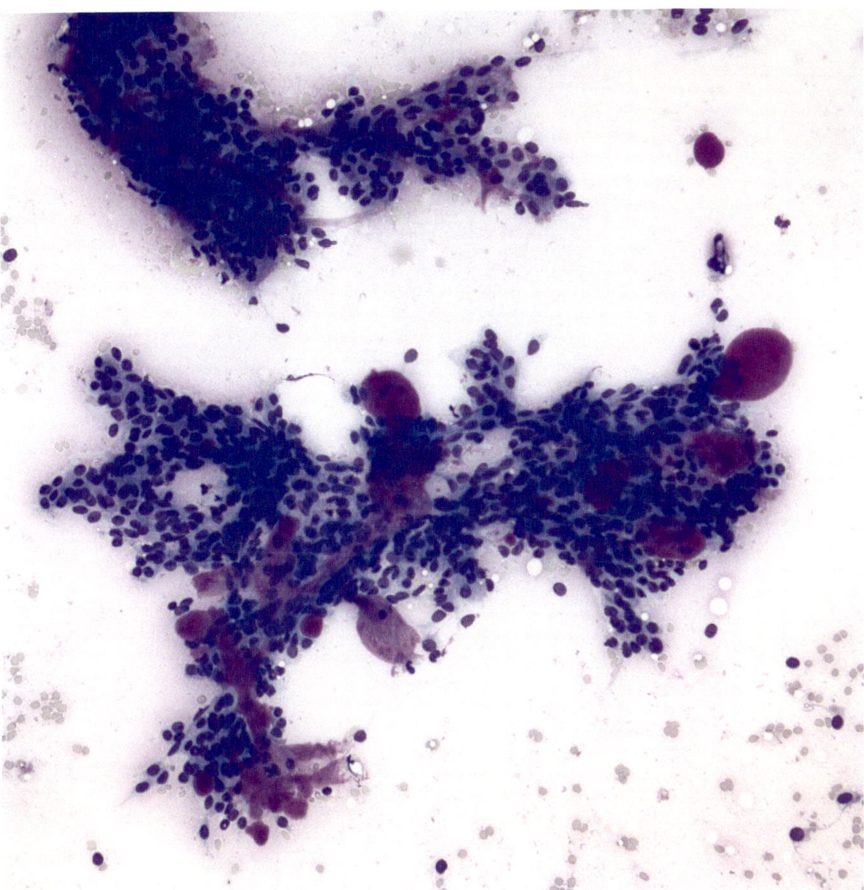

Fig. 5.10 Adenoid cystic carcinoma. Variably sized basaloid cells with scant cytoplasm (Diff-Quik stain, ×200)

- Polymorphous low-grade adenocarcinoma can have stromal spheres, but unlike adenoid cystic carcinoma, the nuclei are not hyperchromatic.
- Adenoid cystic carcinoma has so much in common cytomorphologically with benign dermal eccrine cylindroma; that distinction between both can only be made by tumor location [41].
- Immunohistochemistry for MYB overexpression and fluorescence in situ hybridization (FISH) for the MYB gene rearrangement are useful for diagnosis; hence, additional material should be collected for these ancillary studies at the time of ROSE [42, 43].

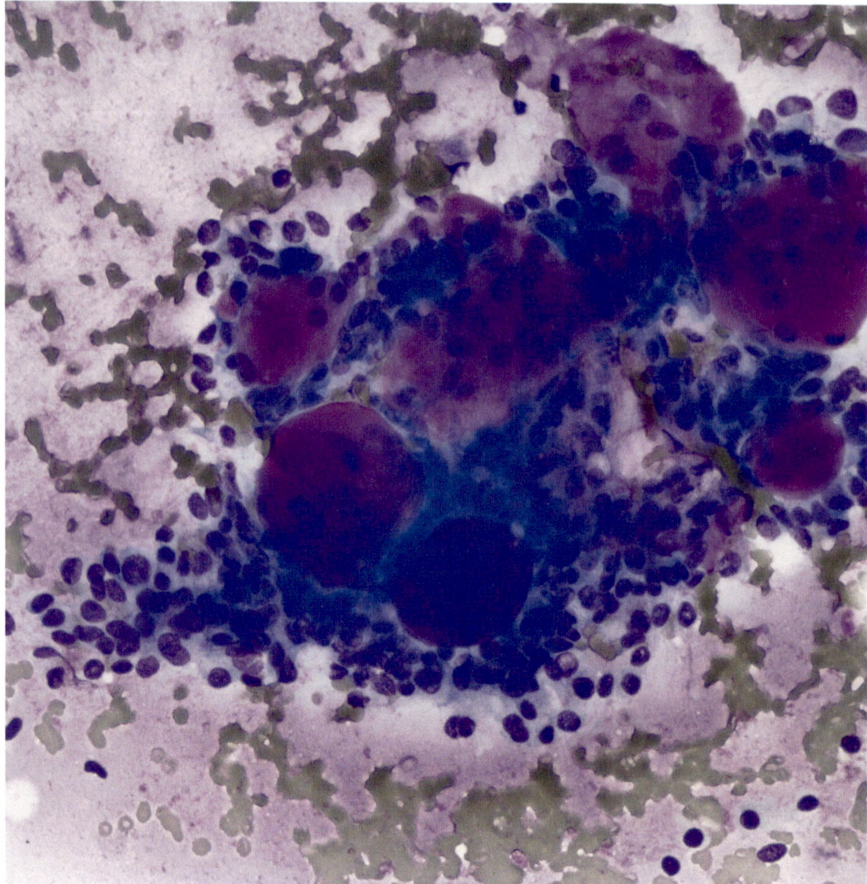

Fig. 5.11 Adenoid cystic carcinoma. Abundant acellular matrix that is arranged in discrete globules and cylinders with sharp borders (Diff-Quik stain, ×400)

Acinic Cell Carcinoma

Acinic cell carcinoma is usually a low-grade malignancy, which usually resembles normal salivary gland, but is more cellular, and the acinic structures are more disorganized and discohesive.

A. Cytomorphologic features

- Cellular aspirate containing cells that are arranged in irregular clusters forming linear, acinar, and glandular structures, accompanied by a visible network of capillaries (Fig. 5.13).
- Cohesive clusters of large, polygonal serous cells with variation in size and shape [44]. They have eccentric, small nuclei, sometimes with visible nucleoli and with delicate, vacuolated, basophilic cytoplasm (Fig. 5.14).

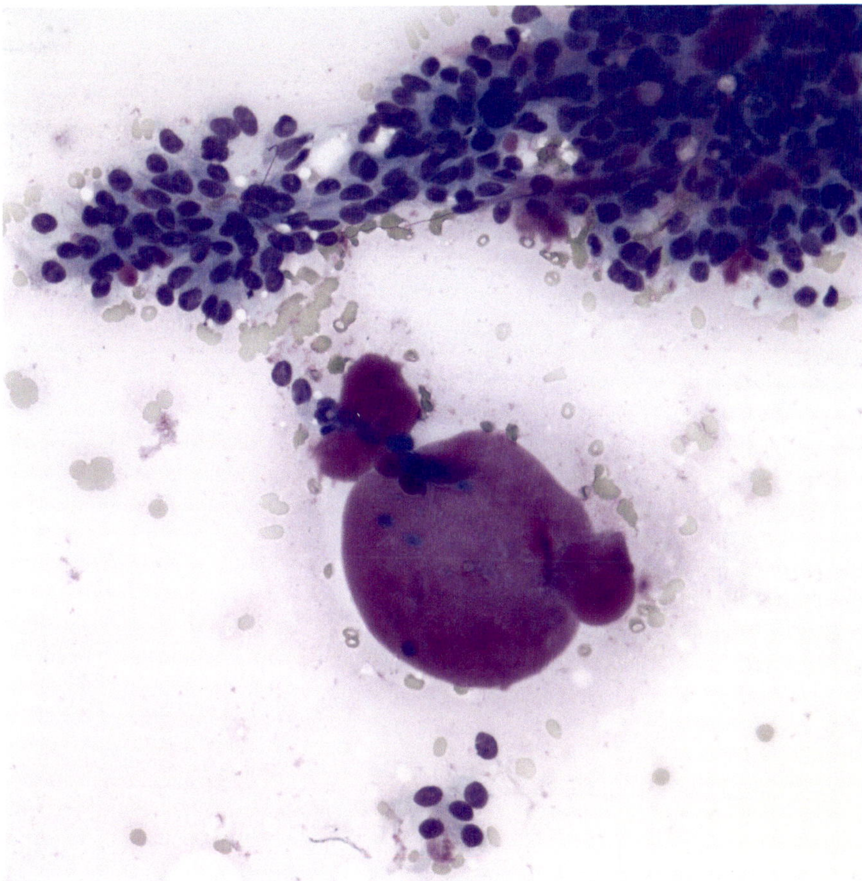

Fig. 5.12 Adenoid cystic carcinoma. The hyaline stroma is homogeneous in appearance (Diff-Quik stain, ×400)

- The cytoplasm may contain occasional coarse zymogen granules that are metachromatic with Romanowsky stains. The cytoplasmic granules are PAS-positive and diastase-resistant.

B. Tips and pitfalls

- A variant of acinic cell carcinoma with psammoma bodies may yield calcific material between acinar cells, leading to a false-negative diagnosis of sialolithiasis [20, 45].
- A predominant papillary architecture may be present and this may cause confusion with metastatic adenocarcinoma.
- Lymphoid cells are present in approximately one third of acinic cell carcinoma, with a predominant lymphoid pattern in 10% of them. The dense lymphoid cells intermixed with acinar cells can mimic chronic sialadenitis [46].

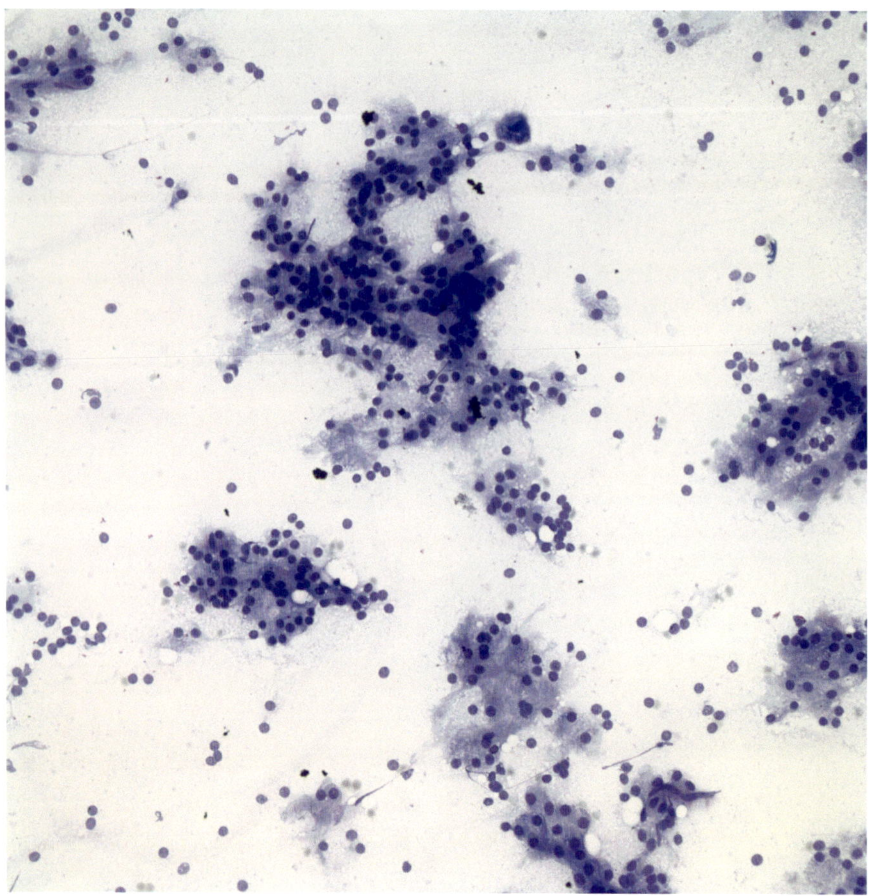

Fig. 5.13 Acinic cell carcinoma. Cellular aspirate with cells arranged in irregular clusters, forming acinar structures (Diff-Quik stain, ×200)

- Vacuolated cells of acinic cell carcinoma resemble the sebaceous cells of sebaceous carcinoma, but sebaceous cells contain lipid and are PAS-positive and diastase-sensitive.
- When high-grade transformation occurs in acinic cell carcinoma, the cells demonstrate more marked nuclear atypia and less acinar differentiation, and they are difficult to distinguish from high-grade carcinomas [47].

Polymorphous Low-Grade Adenocarcinoma

Polymorphous low-grade adenocarcinoma (PLGA) is a low-grade adenocarcinoma involving predominantly minor salivary glands. Tumors are characterized by architectural diversity and cytologic uniformity. A variety of growth patterns can be seen and these include papillary, cribriform, tubular, solid, and fascicular [48].

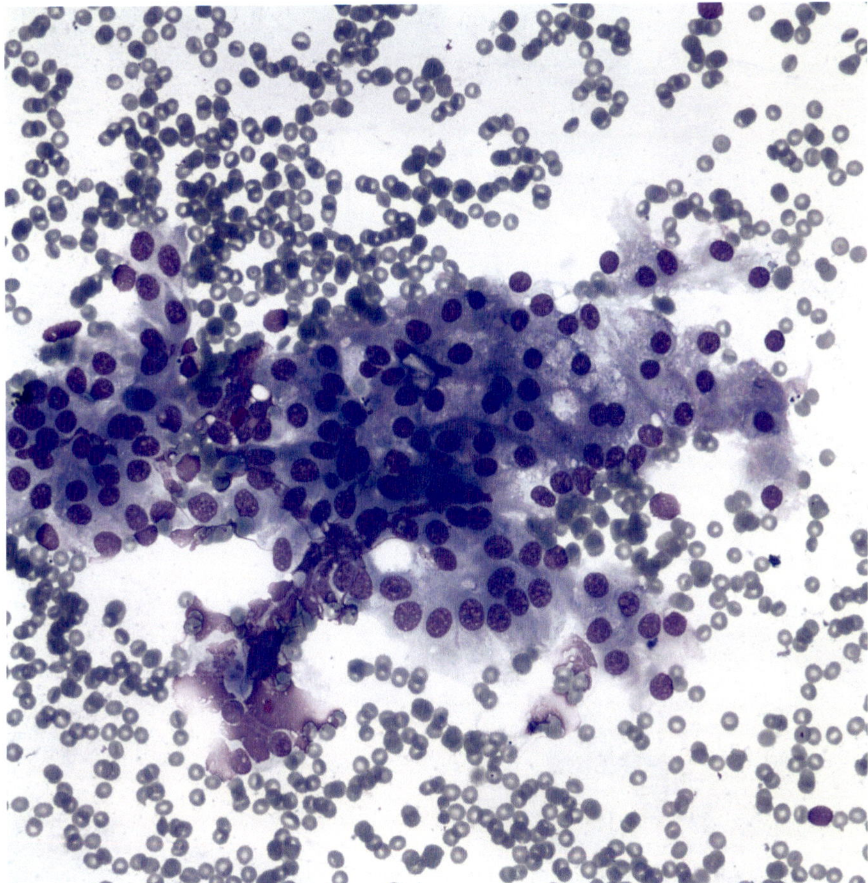

Fig. 5.14 Acinic cell carcinoma. Large polygonal cells with eccentric nuclei and delicate, vacuolated, basophilic cytoplasm (Diff-Quik stain, ×400)

A. Cytomorphologic features

- Hypercellular smears, consisting mainly of branching papillary clusters and sheets of bland uniform cells (Fig. 5.15).
- The nuclei are round to oval, spindled with fine chromatin and inconspicuous nucleoli, with a moderate amount of eosinophilic cytoplasm [48].
- Intranuclear inclusions frequently seen.
- Abundant hyaline globules within gland-like spaces in the clusters of cells.
- Dispersed myxohyaline matrix with bare nuclei in the background.

B. Tips and pitfalls

- The biphasic combination of epithelial cells and matrix can lead to a misdiagnosis of pleomorphic adenoma. The usually more abundant matrix in pleomorphic adenoma frequently has a more fibrillary appearance. The spindled myoepithelial cells are admixed with the matrix, a feature not seen in

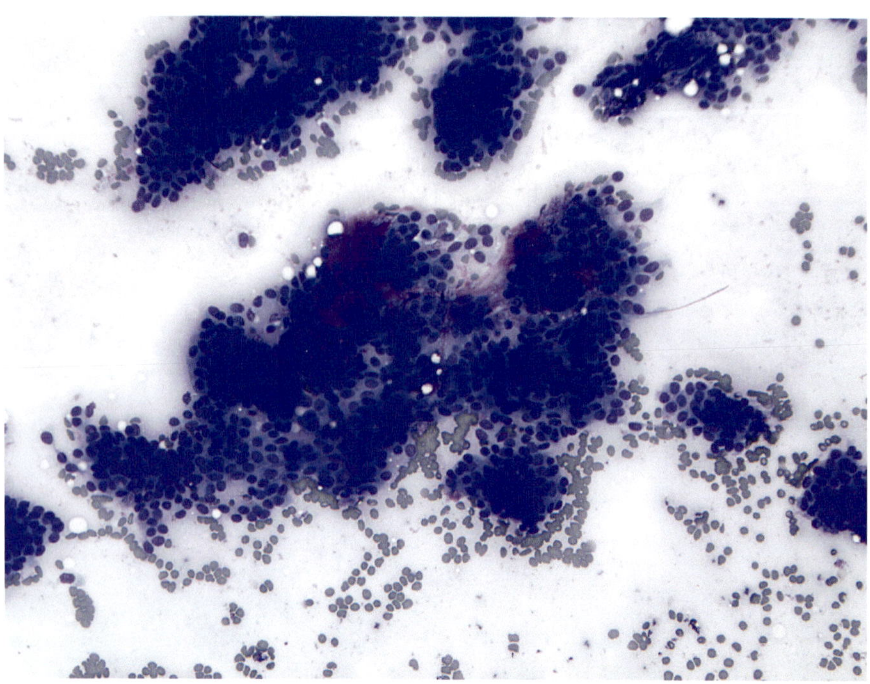

Fig. 5.15 Polymorphous low-grade adenocarcinoma. Cellular aspirate with bland papillary clusters and sheets of bland uniform cells. The nuclei are round to oval. Hyaline globules are seen within gland-like spaces in cell clusters (Diff-Quik stain, ×200)

PLGA. Also, the presence of pseudopapillary formations are not typically seen in pleomorphic adenoma [48].

- The presence of abundant hyaline globules within gland-like spaces in the clusters of cells is similar to the globules of adenoid cystic carcinoma. Adenoid cystic carcinoma can be distinguished by its characteristic hyperchromatic basaloid cells with scant cytoplasm and without spindling, in contrast to the cuboidal oval to round cells of PLGA, which have dispersed chromatin and moderate amount of cytoplasm [25].
- When epithelial-myoepithelial carcinoma is monomorphous and mostly composed of myoepithelial cells, it may be difficult to differentiate from PLGA. Epithelial-myoepithelial carcinoma exhibits isolated cells and clusters of oval cells, frequently arranged in pseudopapillary fragments with stromal cores, but rarely with hyaline globules [25].

Salivary Duct Carcinoma

Salivary duct carcinoma is an uncommon but distinctive type of salivary gland tumor that resembles a high-grade, comedo-type ductal carcinoma of the breast, but a low-grade variant reminiscent of low-grade ductal carcinoma in situ of the breast has also been described [49, 50].

A. Cytomorphologic features

- Moderate cellularity with large, anaplastic tumor cells arranged in cohesive clusters, sheets, or papillary fragments [25]
- Prominent background necrosis

B. Tips and pitfalls

- Similar high-grade appearance may be seen in other high-grade primary tumors of the salivary gland and in metastatic carcinomas.
- Cases with bland nuclear features in conjunction with a stromal component may lead to a misdiagnosis as pleomorphic adenoma.
- Salivary duct carcinoma is usually immunoreactive for Her2 and androgen receptor; hence additional material should be obtained for these ancillary studies at the time of ROSE [51, 52].

Squamous Cell Carcinoma

Squamous cell carcinoma is a rare primary malignancy in the salivary gland. Metastasis to the gland or intraparenchymal lymph node is far more common [14]. Diagnosis is established if an adequate aspirate of salivary gland tumor contains only cells of squamous carcinoma without admixture of mucous or glandular epithelium.

A. Cytomorphologic features

- Cytologically tumor has the classic features of squamous carcinoma, usually keratinizing type (although some may be nonkeratinizing).
- Nuclei are hyperchromatic with coarse chromatin (Fig. 5.16).
- Cytoplasm is dense and has discrete cell boundaries.
- Pearls, bizarre-shaped cells, and dyskeratotic cells are characteristic [15, 25, 53, 54].

B. Tips and pitfalls

- It is often impossible to distinguish high-grade nonkeratinizing squamous cell carcinoma from other high-grade salivary gland tumors, especially mucoepidermoid carcinoma. The presence of intracytoplasmic mucin suggests mucoepidermoid carcinoma [14].
- Metastatic squamous cell carcinoma from other sites or direct extension from the head and neck area must be excluded. In reporting squamous cell carcinoma of the salivary gland, a comment must be added that clinical-radiologic correlation is recommended to exclude a metastasis.

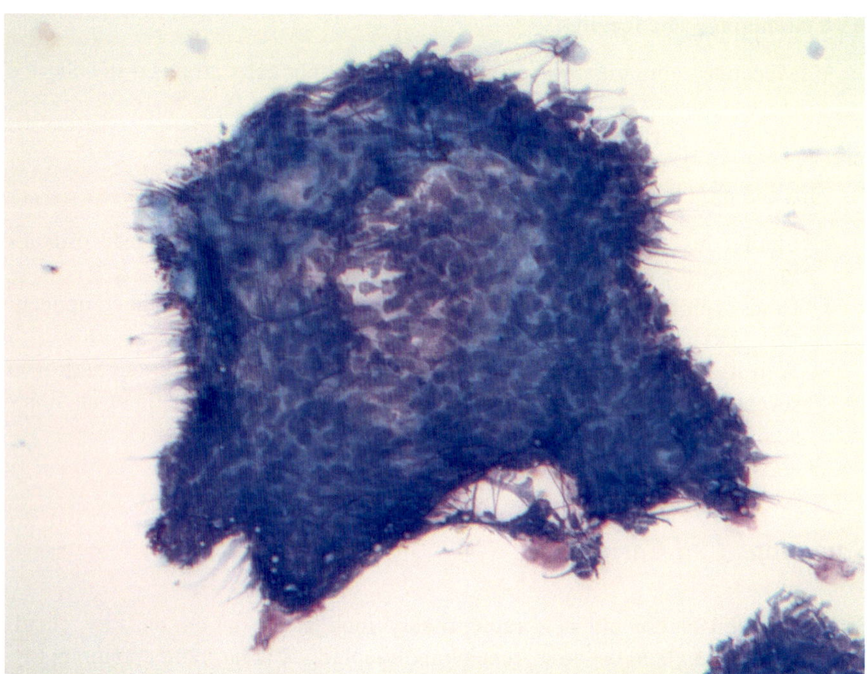

Fig. 5.16 Squamous cell carcinoma, nonkeratinizing type. Hyperchromatic nuclei and coarse chromatin (Diff-Quik stain, ×200)

Malignant Lymphoma

The lymphoid tissue of the salivary glands is a component of the mucosa-associated lymphoid tissue (MALT). Lymphoma can arise de novo or in association with pre-existing lymphoid lesions, especially lymphoepithelial sialadenitis or Sjogren syndrome. The most common types of lymphoma in the salivary gland are (1) marginal zone B-cell lymphoma (MALT lymphoma, which typically arises in patients with lymphoepithelial sialadenitis), (2) follicular lymphoma, and (3) diffuse large B-cell lymphoma (DLBCL), an aggressive form of lymphoma that diffusely involves the parenchyma of salivary gland tissue [55]. Follicular lymphomas mainly involve periparotid lymph nodes rather than the salivary gland itself [14].

A. Cytomorphologic features

- Aspirates of MALT contain monomorphous population of small- to intermediate-sized lymphoid cells with a moderate amount of pale cytoplasm, round-to-irregular nuclei, condensed chromatin, and small nucleoli, admixed with scattered immunoblasts [56].
- Tingible body macrophages are usually scant to absent.
- DLBCL aspirate shows malignant population of large, centroblastic, and/or immunoblastic cells with prominent central, large nucleoli in a large, round,

vesicular nucleus. The cytoplasm is abundant and plasmacytoid, or clear to pale [56]. Pleomorphic, multilobated cells may be present, as well as signet ring cell type or spindle cells [57, 58].

B. Tips and pitfalls

- Lymphoid cells in MALT lymphoma may have plasmacytoid features. Mature plasma cells may even be present. Differentiation from lymphoplasmacytic lymphoma may be difficult because both types of lymphoma may have marked plasmacytoid differentiation [56].
- DLBCL cells are often seen in large aggregates and this may lead to misdiagnosis as an epithelial neoplasm, most notably carcinoma and melanoma.
- Additional material should be obtained at the time of ROSE for immunohistochemical stains.
- Flow cytometry is an important ancillary study and additional material should be obtained at the time of ROSE in RPMI solution for flow cytometry.

Metastatic Tumors

Because the normal parotid gland contains numerous intraparotid and periparotid lymph nodes [11], primary lymphomas and metastatic tumors mimicking salivary gland neoplasms are commonly seen. Metastatic squamous cell carcinoma and malignant melanoma account for the vast majority of metastatic tumors to the salivary gland.

A. Cytomorphologic features

- The cytomorphologic pattern of a metastatic tumor depends on the manner of involvement and type of the salivary gland involved, the histologic type, and the stage of the tumor.
- Cytologic features of metastasis are distinct and different from what is usually seen in primary salivary gland tumors. However, there can be an admixture of the tumor with atypical salivary gland tissue (e.g., from prior radiation).

B. Tips and pitfalls

- In patients with salivary gland tumors and known past or present history of malignant tumor at another site, the possibility of metastasis must always be considered.
- Several primary salivary gland carcinomas like primary squamous cell carcinoma, salivary duct carcinoma, acinic cell carcinoma, and neuroendocrine carcinoma may have cytomorphologic features in common with their extrasalivary counterparts, and diagnosis may be challenging, especially when the primary tumor is unknown [59].
- Immunohistochemistry may be crucial for a definitive diagnosis; hence additional material should be obtained for this purpose at the time of ROSE whenever metastatic tumor is suspected.

References

1. Wangsiricharoen S, Lekawanvijit S, Rangdaeng S. Agreement between rapid on-site evaluation and the final cytological diagnosis of salivary gland specimens. Cytopathology. 2017;28:321–8.
2. Colella G, Cannavale R, Flamminio F, Foschini MP. Fine-needle aspiration cytology of salivary gland lesions: a systematic review. J Oral Maxillofac Surg. 2010;6(8):2146–53.
3. Consamus EN, Smith D, Oviedo SP, Mody DR, Takei H. Diagnostic accuracy of fine-needle aspiration cytology of salivary gland lesions: a 6-year retrospective review. J Am Soc Cytopathol. 2015;4:63–73.
4. Rossi ED, Wong LQ, Bizzarro T, et al. The impact of FNAC in the management of salivary gland lesions: institutional experiences leading to a risk-based classification scheme. Cancer Cytopathol. 2016;124:38 8–396.
5. Seethala RR, LiVolsi VA, Baloch ZW. Relative accuracy of fine-needle aspiration and frozen section in the diagnosis of lesions of the parotid gland. Head Neck. 2005;27:217–23.
6. Layfield LJ, Gopez E, Hirschowitz S. Cost efficiency analysis for fine needle aspiration in the workup of parotid and submandibular gland nodules. Diagn Cytopathol. 2006;34:734–8.
7. Mohammed Nur M, Murphy M. Adequacy and accuracy of salivary gland fine needle aspiration cytology. Ir J Med Sci. 2016;185:711–6.
8. Mallon DH, Kostalas M, MacPherson FJ, et al. The diagnostic value of fine needle aspiration in parotid lumps. Ann R Coll Surg Engl. 2013;95:258–62.
9. Griffith CC, Pai RK, Schneider F, et al. Salivary gland tumor fine-needle aspiration cytology: a proposal for a risk stratification classification. Am J Clin Pathol. 2015;143:839–53.
10. Shield PW, Cosier J, Ellerby G, Gartrell M, Papadimos D. Rapid on-site evaluation of fine needle aspiration specimens by cytology scientists: a review of 3032 specimens. Cytopathology. 2014;25:322–9.
11. McKean ME, Lee K, McGregor IA. The distribution of lymph nodes in and around the parotid gland: an anatomical study. Br J Plast Surg. 1985;38:1–5.
12. Henry-Stanley MJ, Beneke J, Bardales RH, Stanley MW. Fine-needle aspiration of normal tissue from enlarged salivary glands: sialosis or missed target? Diagn Cytopathol. 1995;13:300–3.
13. Geisinger KR, Weidner N. Aspiration cytology of salivary glands. Semin Diagn Pathol. 1986;3:219–26.
14. Krane JF, Faquin WC. Salivary gland. In: Cibas ES, Ducatman BS, editors. Cytology: diagnostic principles and clinical correlates. Philadelphia: Saunders Elsevier; 2014. p. 299–332.
15. Layfield LJ, Glasgow BJ. Diagnosis of salivary gland tumors by fine-needle aspiration cytology: a review of clinical utility and pitfalls. Diagn Cytopathol. 1991;7:267–72.
16. Droese M. Cytological diagnosis of sialadenosis, sialadenitis, and parotid cysts by fine-needle aspiration biopsy. Adv Otorhinolaryngol. 1981;26:49–96.
17. Mair S, Leiman G, Levinsohn D. Fine needle aspiration cytology of parotid sarcoidosis. Acta Cytol. 1989;33:169–72.
18. Tambouret R, Geisinger KR, Powers CN, Khurana KK, Silverman JF, Bardales R, Pitman MB. The clinical application and cost analysis of fine-needle aspiration biopsy in the diagnosis of mass lesions in sarcoidosis. Chest. 2000;117:1004–11.
19. Stanley MW, Bardales RH, Beneke J, Korourian S, Stern SJ. Sialolithiasis. Differential diagnostic problems in fine-needle aspiration cytology. Am J Clin Pathol. 1996;106:229–33.
20. Frierson HF Jr, Fechner RE. Chronic sialadenitis with psammoma bodies mimicking neoplasia in a fine-needle aspiration specimen from the submandibular gland. Am J Clin Pathol. 1991;95:884–8.
21. Boccato P, Altavilla G, Blandamura S. Fine needle aspiration biopsy of salivary gland lesions. A reappraisal of pitfalls and problems. Acta Cytol. 1998;42:888–98.
22. Weidner N, Geisinger KR, Sterling RT, Miller TR, Yen TS. Benign lymphoepithelial cysts of the parotid gland. A histologic, cytologic, and ultrastructural study. Am J Clin Pathol. 1986;85:395–401.

23. Elliott JN, Oertel YC. Lymphoepithelial cysts of the salivary glands. Histologic and cytologic features. Am J Clin Pathol. 1990;93:39–43.
24. Kapadia SB, Dusenbery D, Dekker A. Fine needle aspiration of pleomorphic adenoma and adenoid cystic carcinoma of salivary gland origin. Acta Cytol. 1997;41:487–92.
25. Klijanienko J, Vielh P. Fine-needle sampling of salivary gland lesions. I. Cytology and histology correlation of 412 cases of pleomorphic adenoma. Diagn Cytopathol. 1996;14:195–200.
26. Elsheikh TM, Bernacki EG. Fine needle aspiration cytology of cellular pleomorphic adenoma. Acta Cytol. 1996;40:1165–75.
27. Handa U, Dhingra N, Chopra R, Mohan H. Pleomorphic adenoma: Cytologic variations and potential diagnostic pitfalls. Diagn Cytopathol. 2009;37:11–5.
28. Viguer JM, Vicandi B, Jiménez-Heffernan JA, López-Ferrer P, Limeres MA. Fine needle aspiration cytology of pleomorphic adenoma. An analysis of 212 cases. Acta Cytol. 1997;41:786–94.
29. Lee SS, Cho KJ, Jang JJ, Ham EK. Differential diagnosis of adenoid cystic carcinoma from pleomorphic adenoma of the salivary gland on fine needle aspiration cytology. Acta Cytol. 1996;40:1246–52.
30. Jacobs JC. Low grade mucoepidermoid carcinoma ex pleomorphic adenoma. A diagnostic problem in fine needle aspiration biopsy. Acta Cytol. 1994;38:93–7.
31. Pitman MB. Mucoepidermoid carcinoma ex pleomorphic adenoma of the parotid gland. Acta Cytol. 1995;39:604–6.
32. Parwani AV, Ali SZ. Diagnostic accuracy and pitfalls in fine-needle aspiration interpretation of Warthin tumor. Cancer. 2003;99:166–71.
33. Mooney EE, Dodd LG, Layfield LJ. Squamous cells in fine-needle aspiration biopsies of salivary gland lesions: potential pitfalls in cytologic diagnosis. Diagn Cytopathol. 1996;15:447–52.
34. Joseph TP, Joseph CP, Jayalakshmy PS, Poothiode U. Diagnostic challenges in cytology of mucoepidermoid carcinoma: report of 6 cases with histopathological correlation. J Cytol. 2015;32:21–4.
35. Auclair PL, Ellis GL. Mucoepidermoid carcinoma. In: Ellis GL, Auclair PL, Gnepp DR, editors. Surgical pathology of the salivary glands. Philadelphia: WB Saunders; 1991. p. 279–86.
36. Vasudevan G, Bishnu A, Singh BMK, Singh VK. Mucoepidermoid carcinoma of salivary gland: limitations and pitfalls on FNA. J Clin Diagn Res. 2017;11:ER04–6.
37. Edwards PC, Wasserman P. Evaluation of cystic salivary gland lesions by fine needle aspiration: an analysis of 21 cases. Acta Cytol. 2005;49:489–94.
38. Frable MA, Frable WJ. Fine-needle aspiration biopsy of salivary glands. Laryngoscope. 1991;101:245-9.
39. Kocjan G, Nayagam M, Harris M. Fine needle aspiration cytology of salivary gland lesions: advantages and pitfalls. Cytopathology. 1990;1:269–75.
40. Nagel H, Hotze HJ, Laskawi R, Chilla R, Droese M. Cytologic diagnosis of adenoid cystic carcinoma of salivary glands. Diagn Cytopathol. 1999;20:358–66.
41. Bondeson L, Lindholm K, Thorstenson S. Benign dermal eccrine cylindroma. A pitfall in the cytologic diagnosis of adenoid cystic carcinoma. Acta Cytol. 1983;27:326–8.
42. Brill LB 2nd, Kanner WA, Fehr A, Andrén Y, Moskaluk CA, Löning T, Stenman G, Frierson HF Jr. Analysis of MYB expression and MYB-NFIB gene fusions in adenoid cystic carcinoma and other salivary neoplasms. Mod Pathol. 2011;24:1169–76.
43. West RB, Kong C, Clarke N, Gilks T, Lipsick JS, Cao H, Kwok S, Montgomery KD, Varma S, Le QT. MYB expression and translocation in adenoid cystic carcinomas and other salivary gland tumors with clinicopathologic correlation. Am J Surg Pathol. 2011;35:92–9.
44. Palma O, Torri AM, de Cristofaro JA, Fiaccavento S. Fine needle aspiration cytology in two cases of well-differentiated acinic-cell carcinoma of the parotid gland. Discussion of diagnostic criteria. Acta Cytol. 1985;29:516–21.
45. Whitlatch SP. Psammoma bodies in fine-needle aspiration biopsies of acinic cell tumor. Diagn Cytopathol. 1986;2:268–9.
46. Daneshbod Y, Daneshbod K, Khademi B. Diagnostic difficulties in the interpretation of fine needle aspirate samples in salivary lesions: diagnostic pitfalls revisited. Acta Cytol. 2009;53:53–70.

47. Johnykutty S, Miller CH, Hoda RS, Giampoli EJ. Fine-needle aspiration of dedifferentiated acinic cell carcinoma: report of a case with cyto-histological correlation. Diagn Cytopathol. 2009;37:763–8.
48. Gibbons D, Saboorian MH, Vuitch F, Gokaslan ST, Ashfaq R. Fine-needle aspiration findings in patients with polymorphous low grade adenocarcinoma of the salivary glands. Cancer. 1999;87:31–6.
49. Khurana KK, Pitman MB, Powers CN, Korourian S, Bardales RH, Stanley MW. Diagnostic pitfalls of aspiration cytology of salivary duct carcinoma. Cancer. 1997;81:373–8.
50. Delgado R, Klimstra D, Albores-Saavedra J. Low grade salivary duct carcinoma. A distinctive variant with a low grade histology and a predominant intraductal growth pattern. Cancer. 1996;78:958–67.
51. Glisson B, Colevas AD, Haddad R, Krane J, El-Naggar A, Kies M, Costello R, Summey C, Arquette M, Langer C, Amrein PC, Posner M. HER2 expression in salivary gland carcinomas: dependence on histological subtype. Clin Cancer Res. 2004;10:944–6.
52. Jaspers HC, Verbist BM, Schoffelen R, Mattijssen V, Slootweg PJ, van der Graaf WT, van Herpen CM. Androgen receptor-positive salivary duct carcinoma: a disease entity with promising new treatment options. J Clin Oncol. 2011;29:e473–6.
53. Jayaram N, Ashim D, Rajwanshi A, Radhika S, Banerjee CK. The value of fine-needle aspiration biopsy in the cytodiagnosis of salivary gland lesions. Diagn Cytopathol. 1989;5:349–54.
54. Orell SR. Diagnostic difficulties in the interpretation of fine needle aspirates of salivary gland lesions: the problem revisited. Cytopathology. 1995;6:285–300.
55. Harris NL. Lymphoid proliferations of the salivary glands. Am J Clin Pathol. 1999;111:S94–103.
56. Young NA, Al-Saleem T. Diagnosis of lymphoma by fine-needle aspiration cytology using the revised European-American classification of lymphoid neoplasms. Cancer. 1999;87:325–45.
57. Weiss L, Arber D, Chang K. Lymph nodes and spleen. In: Silverberg S, DeLellis R, Frable W, editors. Principles and practice of surgical pathology and cytopathology, vol. 1. 3rd ed. New York: Churchill Livingstone; 1997. p. 675–772.
58. Dardick I, Srinivasan R, Al-Jabi M. Signet-ring cell variant of large cell lymphoma. Ultrastruct Pathol. 1983;5:195–200.
59. Lussier C, Klijanienko J, Vielh P. Fine-needle aspiration of metastatic nonlymphomatous tumors to the major salivary glands: a clinicopathologic study of 40 cases cytologically diagnosed and histologically correlated. Cancer. 2000;90:350–6.

Chapter 6
Lymph Node

Guoping Cai

Introduction

The etiologies of lymph node enlargement are diverse and include reactive, infectious, and neoplastic processes [1–3]. Whether enlarged lymph nodes are subject for biopsy depends upon clinical presentation and suspicion. For example, an enlarged mobile tender cervical lymph node in a patient with a known history of recent oral or upper respiratory tract infection is more likely a reactive process, and a close clinical follow-up is sufficient. Enlarged firm and/or fused cervical lymph nodes in a patient with history of head and neck squamous cell carcinoma is highly suspicious for metastatic disease; biopsy of the enlarged lymph nodes is warranted. Enlarged lymph nodes, especially in deep-seated regions, without reasonable explanation may also need further evaluation.

Lymph nodes can be evaluated by fine needle aspiration (FNA) biopsy by palpation or under ultrasound guidance if superficially located or under the guidance of other imaging techniques if deep seated [4]. FNA biopsy has relatively high sensitivity and diagnostic accuracy, which can help confirm a clinical impression of reactive process, identify an infectious etiology, and diagnose a suspected malignancy [1–5]. If malignancy is identified, further classification of the tumor can be achieved by cytomorphologic analysis and pertinent ancillary studies [5–10]. Implementation of rapid on-site evaluation (ROSE) can further improve the diagnostic performance of FNA by ensuring adequate sampling and appropriate specimen triage for ancillary studies that are crucial for rendering a definite diagnosis [11–14].

G. Cai (✉)
Department of Pathology, Yale University School of Medicine, New Haven, CT, USA
e-mail: guoping.cai@yale.edu

G. Cai, A. J. Adeniran (eds.), *Rapid On-site Evaluation (ROSE)*,
https://doi.org/10.1007/978-3-030-21799-0_6

Diagnostic Considerations

Specimen Adequacy Assessment

Adequacy of lymph node sampling should be assessed by cytological findings as well as correlation with clinical impression. The specimens are generally considered as adequate if (a) malignancy, primary or metastatic, is identified or (b) necrosis or granulomatous inflammation with or without infectious agents is present. There are however no established criteria regarding the required cellularity when the results suggest a benign/reactive process although certain cellularity has been suggested for specific site lymph node sampling [15]. It is recommended that multiple passes should be performed before a negative diagnosis is considered.

The cellularity of lymph node sampling can be influenced by several factors, including the location of lymph node, the nature of lesions, and biopsy techniques. Inguinal lymph nodes are known to be fibrotic, pelvic lymph nodes often have fat replacement, and mediastinal lymph nodes may have abundant anthracotic pigment-containing histiocytes. The lymph nodes involved by lymphomas such as Hodgkin lymphoma and diffuse large B-cell lymphoma may sometimes be fibrotic, which leads to low cellularity by FNA biopsy.

Normal Elements Lymph Node Cytology

Aspiration of a benign or reactive lymph node yields a polymorphous population of lymphocytes ranging from small, intermediate, and occasionally large in size. The lymphocytes can be recognized by the following features: (a) disperse single cells, (b) lymphoglandular bodies from fractioned cytoplasm seen in the background, and (c) nuclear streaming, a smearing artifact created due to fragility of lymphocytes (Figs. 6.1 and 6.2). However, lymphocytes can sometimes present as clusters, which may represent lymphohistiocytic aggregates from germinal centers (Fig. 6.3).

In addition to lymphoid cells, histiocytes are often present. The numbers of histiocytes may vary depending on the location and underlying etiologies of lymph node enlargement. Abundant anthracotic pigment-containing histiocytes can be seen in mediastinal lymph node sampling. Other inflammatory cells such as eosinophils and mast cells, endothelial cells, capillaries, as well as scant fibrous tissue, probably from lymph node capsule, can be seen.

Approach for Reactive/Infectious Lymphadenopathy

- Clinical and imaging findings are very helpful.
- Specimens should be triaged according to the findings during on-site evaluation.

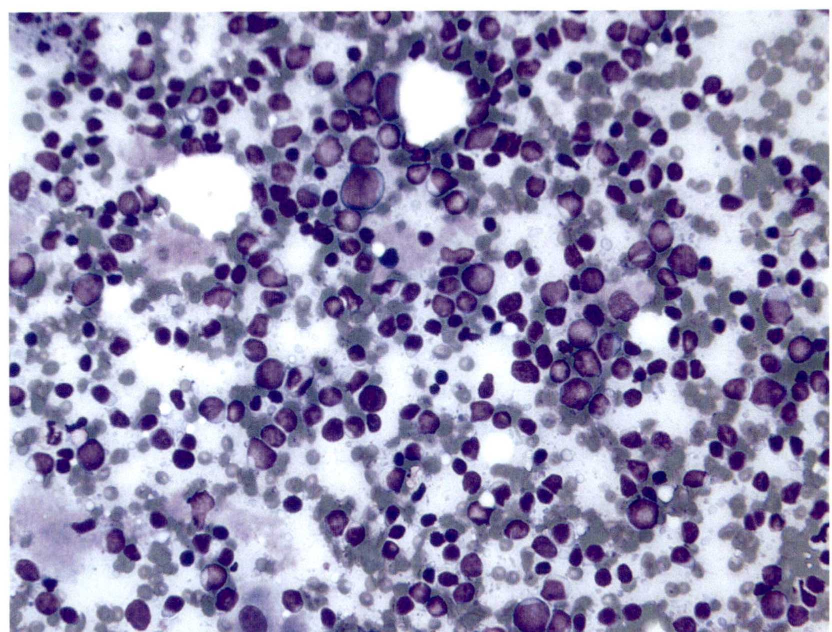

Fig. 6.1 Lymph node sampling. Dispersed polymorphous lymphocytes with background lymphoglandular bodies (Diff-Quik stain, ×400)

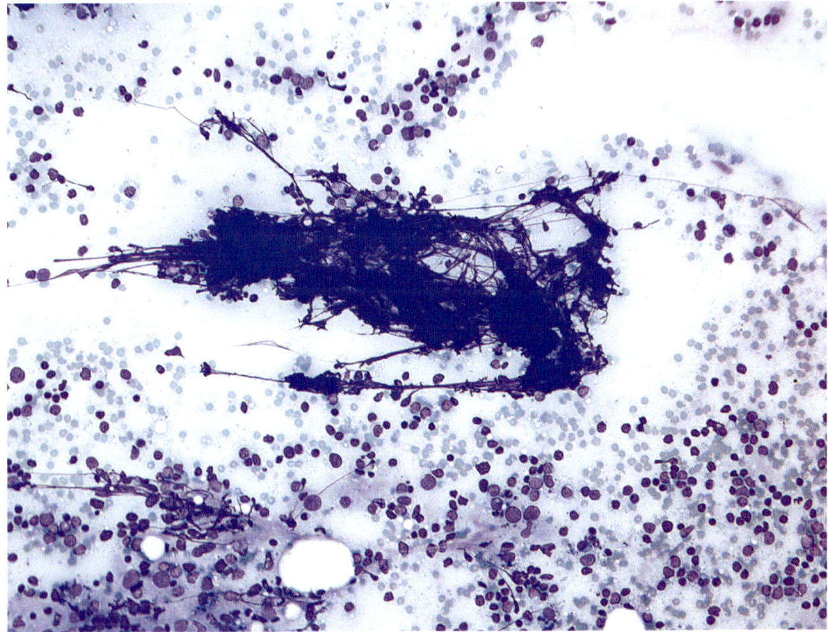

Fig. 6.2 Lymph node sampling. Dispersed polymorphous lymphocytes with nuclear streaming artifact (Diff-Quik stain, ×200)

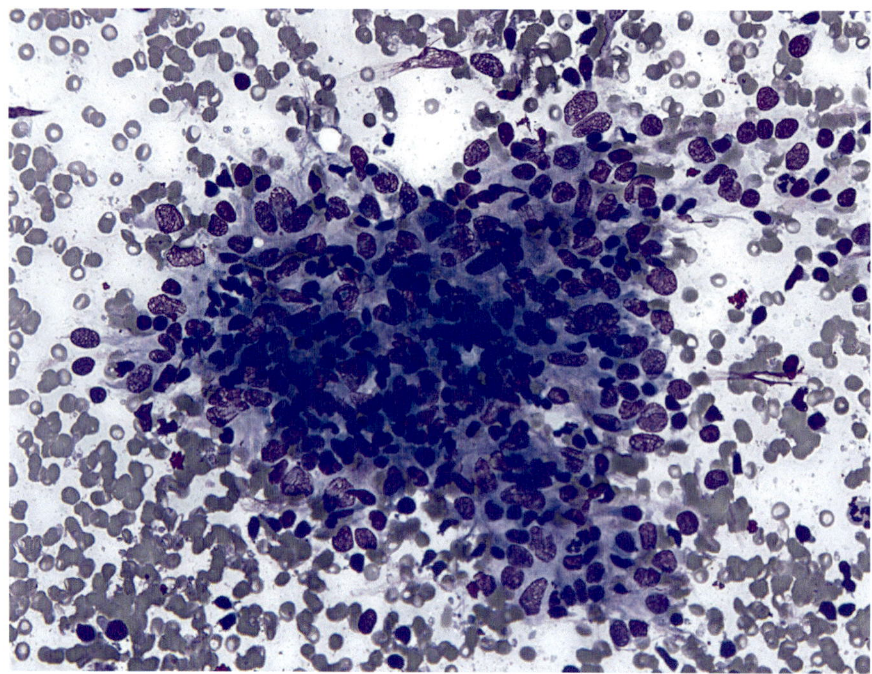

Fig. 6.3 Lymph node sampling. Lymphohistiocytic aggregate (Diff-Quik stain, ×400)

- If an infectious etiology is suspected, specimen should be submitted for microbiology culture study.
- Additional specimen should be saved for special stains for identification of microorganisms.

Approach for Lymphoproliferative Disorders

- When lymphoid cells show a monotonous appearance or display significant cytological atypia, a lymphoproliferative disorder should be considered.
- If a lymphoproliferative disorder is suspected, specimen should be submitted for flow cytometry analysis which is less needed for Hodgkin lymphoma.
- In elderly patients with an unknown etiology of lymphadenopathy, flow cytometry analysis is recommended to rule out a lymphoproliferative disorder even if a polymorphous population of lymphocytes is present.
- If lymph node sampling yields a low cellularity specimen, core needle may be indicated if the procedure is clinically deemed to be safe [1, 16].
- Excisional biopsy may be needed for an inconclusive diagnosis after FNA and/or core needle biopsy.
- For a primary diagnosis, multimodal approaches are recommended, including cytomorphology, flow cytometry, immunocytochemical analysis, and molecular cytogenetic testing.

- For a diagnosis of recurrent disease, documentation of similar immunophenotypic features may be sufficient. However, cytomorphologic evaluation is important to rule out a progression or transformation from a low-grade to high-grade lymphoproliferative disorder.

Approach for Metastatic Tumors

- In patients with known history of or by imaging studies highly suspicious for carcinomas such as lung cancers, lymph node sampling is part of tumor staging workup [17, 18].
- Knowledge of patient's prior history of malignancy is important and can serve as the diagnostic clues; however, metastasis can be seen as a primary presentation in some cases.
- In case suspicious for a metastatic disease, specimen should be saved for preparation of a cell block.
- Immunocytochemical studies are essential for diagnosis of metastatic tumor and identification of tumor origin.

Nonneoplastic Lymphadenopathy

Reactive Lymphadenopathy

Lymph node enlargement could be the result of a nonspecific response to infectious or noninfectious conditions such as viral infection, tissue injury, and systemic nonneoplastic diseases.

1. Cytomorphologic features [2, 3] (Fig. 6.4)
    - Polymorphous population of lymphocytes.
    - Increased numbers of large lymphocytes including centroblasts and immunoblasts.
    - Tingible body macrophages (histiocytes containing cellular debris).
    - Lymphohistiocytic aggregates.
    - Capillary vasculatures with plump endothelial cells; plump endothelial cells can also be seen individually.
2. Tips and pitfalls
    - Reactive lymphadenopathy can, at least in most cases, trace back to a possible etiology.
    - Due to the presence of a polymorphous population of lymphocytes, reactive lymphoid hyperplasia should be differentiated from Hodgkin lymphoma as well as some non-Hodgkin lymphomas.

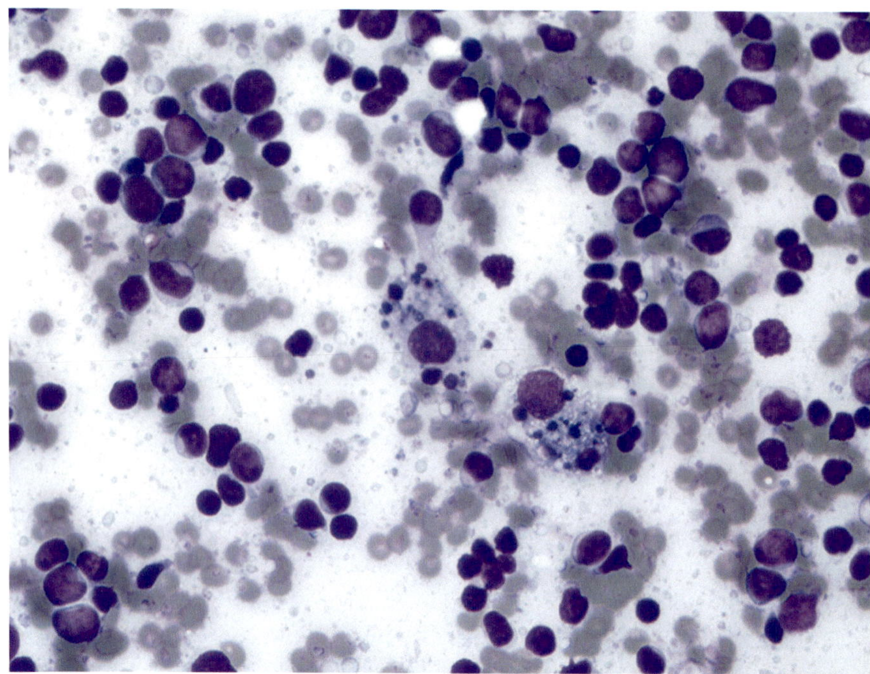

Fig. 6.4 Reactive lymph node. Dispersed polymorphous lymphocytes with a few tingible body macrophages (Diff-Quik stain, ×400)

- Centroblasts and immunoblasts seen in reactive lymphadenopathy are large, but still they are significantly smaller than Hodgkin cells and lack typical cytomorphology such as binucleated Reed-Sternberg cells.
- Non-Hodgkin lymphomas such as diffuse large B-cell lymphoma and anaplastic large cell lymphoma have significant cytological atypia, helping differentiate from a reactive process.
- However, some lymphomas such as follicular lymphoma can have overlapping cytomorphologic features with that seen in reactive lymphadenopathy. Sampling for flow cytometry to rule out a lymphoproliferative disorder is recommended if there is an uncertainty about clinical presentation.

Infectious Lymphadenopathy

Lymph nodes can be enlarged due to infection by specific agents such as bacteria, mycobacteria, or fungal organisms.

1. Cytomorphologic features [2, 3]

   - Mixed inflammatory cells, from neutrophils predominant to lymphocytes/histiocytes predominant.

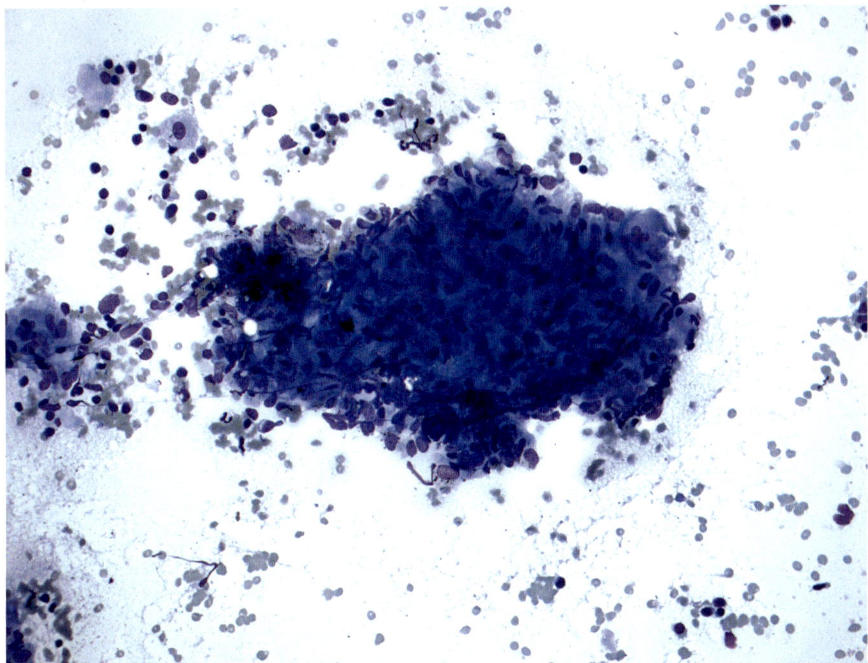

Fig. 6.5 Non-necrotizing granuloma. A cluster of epithelioid histiocytes and intermixed small lymphocytes (Diff-Quik stain, ×200)

- Granulomatous inflammation is commonly seen, characterized by clusters of epithelioid histiocytes mixed with scant lymphocytes with or without multinucleated histiocytes/giant cells (Fig. 6.5).
- Necrosis is often present with or without granulomatous inflammation (Fig. 6.6).
- Infectious microorganisms may be stained or visible as negative images on Diff-Quik stain.

2. Tips and pitfalls

- It is important to triage specimen to include microbiology culture studies in cases suspicious for infectious lymphadenopathy.
- Identification of specific agents may need specific stains such as Gram, acid-fast, and GMS stain. The final classification of microorganisms should be correlated with culture study results.
- The presence of necrosis, even if abundant, does not rule out malignancy. Metastatic squamous cell carcinoma in a lymph node can mimic an infectious etiology.
- Granulomatous inflammation can coexist with a malignant process including metastatic tumors or lymphoproliferative disorders.

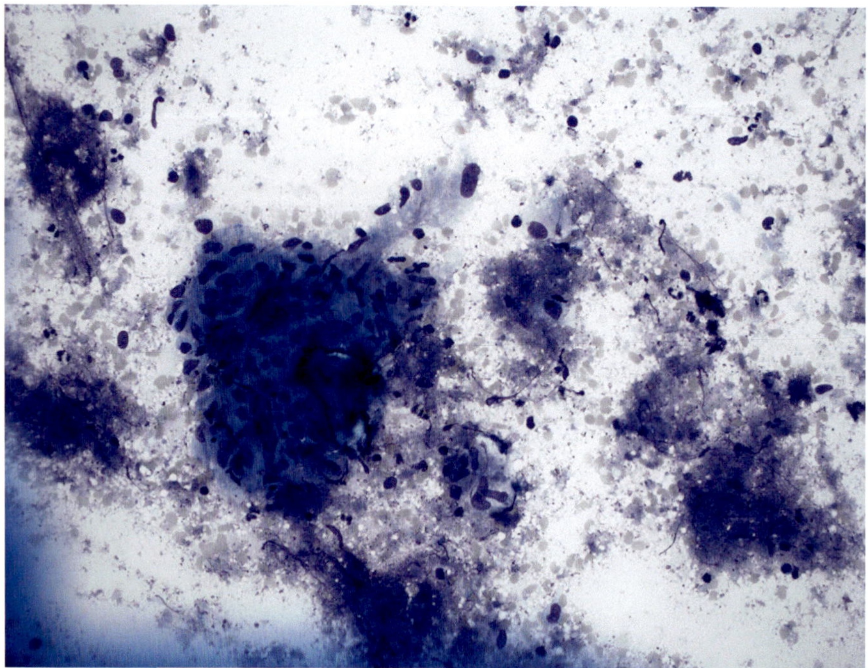

Fig. 6.6 Necrotizing granuloma. A cluster of epithelioid histiocytes and intermixed small lymphocytes with necrotic debris (Diff-Quik stain, ×200)

Hodgkin Lymphoma

Hodgkin lymphoma is one of the common lymphoproliferative disorders frequently present as lymphadenopathy, often as enlarged and/or fused lymph nodes in cervical and deep-seated regions. Hodgkin lymphomas are classified as classical Hodgkin lymphoma and nodular lymphocyte predominant Hodgkin lymphoma, differing in their morphologic and more obviously immunophenotypic features [19]. Based on histomorphology, classical Hodgkin lymphoma can be further classified into nodular sclerosing, lymphocyte-rich, mixed cellularity, and lymphocyte-depleted forms. FNA biopsy can diagnose Hodgkin lymphoma and may be able to separate classical from nodular lymphocyte predominant Hodgkin lymphomas with the aid of immunocytochemical studies [20–23]. It is however very difficult to further classify classical Hodgkin lymphomas on cytological material.

Classical Hodgkin Lymphoma

It is the most common form, accounting for about 90% of all Hodgkin lymphomas. The patients with classical Hodgkin lymphoma are often very young or elderly individuals, with a characteristic bimodal age distribution.

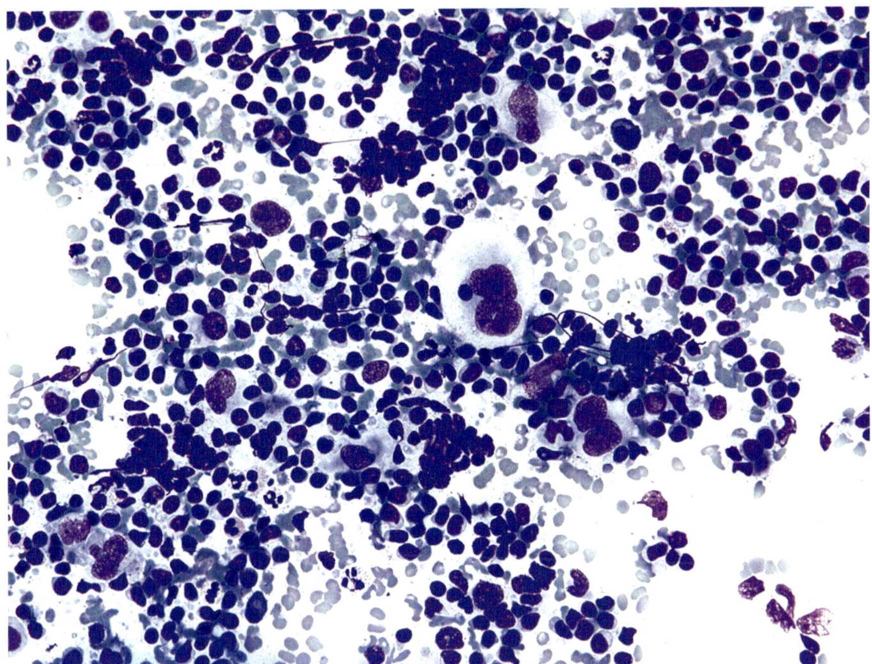

Fig. 6.7 Hodgkin lymphoma. A few large mononuclear and binucleated cells with prominent nucleolus in a background of small lymphocytes and occasional eosinophils and plasma cells (Diff-Quik stain, ×200)

1. Cytomorphologic features [2, 3, 20–22] (Figs. 6.7 and 6.8)

   - Scattered large cells, mononuclear or binucleated, with large prominent nucleolus (Reed-Sternberg cells, classical or mononuclear forms)
   - Predominant small lymphocytes in the background
   - Variable numbers of eosinophils, plasma cells, and histiocytes
   - Lymphohistiocytic aggregates and tingible body macrophages often absent

2. Tips and pitfalls

   - Hodgkin lymphoma should be differentiated from reactive lymphoid hyperplasia, anaplastic large cell lymphoma, T-cell-rich large B-cell lymphoma, metastatic poorly differentiated carcinoma or sarcoma, and particularly metastatic melanoma.
   - In cases suspicious for Hodgkin lymphoma during on-site evaluation, additional specimen should be saved for cell block for immunocytochemical studies, which are often required for diagnosis and differential diagnosis.
   - The neoplastic cells in Hodgkin lymphoma most likely stain positive for CD30 and PAX5 but less likely for CD20. CD45 is negative. Hodgkin lymphoma is often EBV associated, which can be documented by EBER in situ hybridization study.

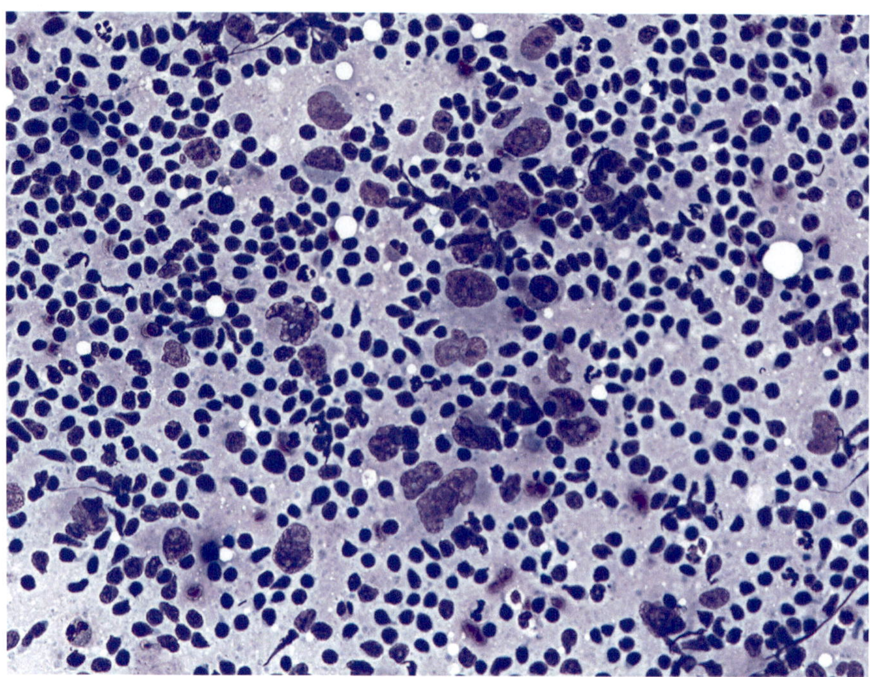

Fig. 6.8 Hodgkin lymphoma. Scattered large mononuclear and rare binucleated cells with prominent nucleolus in a background of small lymphocytes and occasional histiocytes, eosinophils, and plasma cells (Diff-Quik stain, ×200)

- In cases unsure for Hodgkin or non-Hodgkin lymphomas during on-site evaluation, specimen may be submitted for flow cytometry study. An increased CD4/CD8 ratio, although not specific, is a common finding in Hodgkin lymphoma [24].
- In difficult cases, core needle or excisional biopsy may be needed to render a definite diagnosis.

Nodular Lymphocyte Predominant Hodgkin Lymphoma

This type of Hodgkin lymphoma is far more less likely seen, accounting for about 10% of all Hodgkin lymphomas. It affects predominant male patients between 30 and 50 years of age and involves cervical, axillary, and inguinal lymph nodes. Mediastinal involvement is rare.

1. Cytomorphologic features [2, 3, 19, 23]

   - Scattered large cells, often folded mononuclear or binucleated, with smaller nucleolus (popcorn cells).

- Predominant small lymphocytes in the background.
- Eosinophils, plasma cells, and histiocytes are minimal.
- Lymphohistiocytic aggregates and tingible body macrophages often absent.

2. Tips and pitfalls

- Hodgkin lymphoma should be differentiated from reactive lymphoid hyperplasia, anaplastic large cell lymphoma, T-cell-rich large B-cell lymphoma, and metastatic poorly differentiated carcinoma, sarcoma, or melanoma.
- In cases suspicious for Hodgkin lymphoma during on-site evaluation, additional specimen should be saved for cell block for immunocytochemical studies, which are often required for diagnosis and differential diagnosis.
- The neoplastic cells in this Hodgkin lymphoma are often positive for CD45, CD20, and PAX5, while negative for CD30 contrasting to the classical form. EBV infection is uncommonly seen.
- In difficult cases, core needle or excisional biopsy may be needed to render a definite diagnosis.

Non-Hodgkin B-Cell Lymphomas

Non-Hodgkin B-cell lymphomas (NHLs) comprise a long list of entities which have diverse clinical, morphologic, and cytogenetic features [19]. The goal of FNA biopsy is not aimed to resolve diagnostic issues for all entities but rather to focus on the most common types of B-cell NHLs, which together account for more than 80% of cases. In the remaining cases, the efforts are primarily to confirm or suggest the possibility of a neoplastic lymphoid proliferation by documenting the monoclonality through flow cytometry (light chain kappa or lambda restriction) or molecular approach (heavy chain immunoglobulin rearrangement) [5, 6, 9, 25]. It is therefore crucial to secure specimen for flow cytometry analysis. Additional samples are also recommended for potential immunocytochemical and molecular studies. FNA biopsy can be used to establish a new diagnosis or to document a recurrent or persistent disease. Morphologic transformation or progression of lymphoma should also be evaluated [26].

Small Cell Lymphomas

Included in this group are the lymphomas with similar cytomorphologic features of small lymphocytes predominance, including grade 1 or 2 follicular lymphoma (FL), mantle cell lymphoma (MCL), marginal zone lymphoma (MZL), and chronic lymphocytic leukemia/small lymphocytic lymphoma (CLL/SLL). These lymphomas most likely occur in patients with age of 60 years old or above and often have an indolent clinical course except for mantle cell lymphoma.

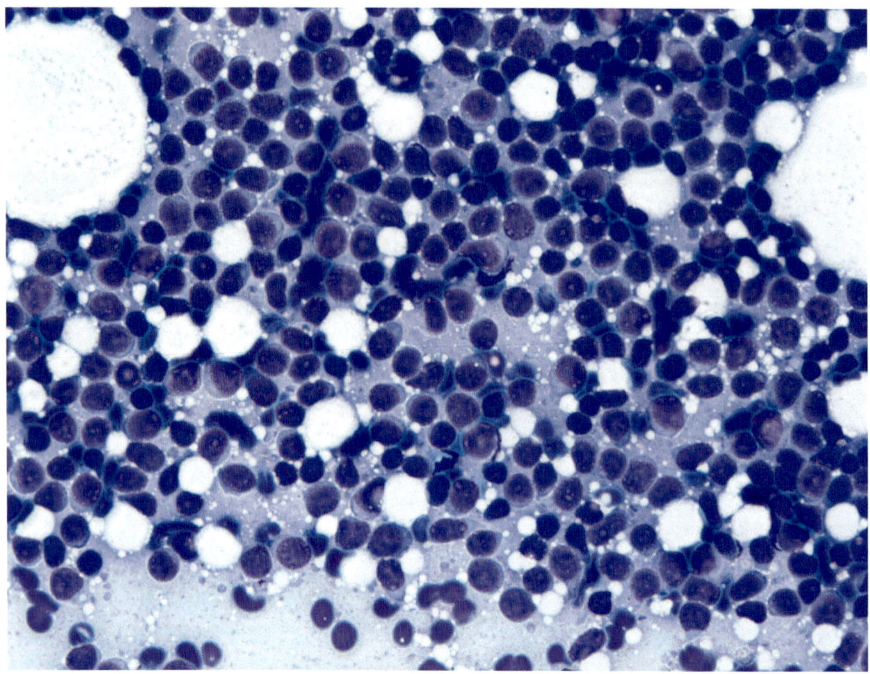

Fig. 6.9 Chronic lymphocytic leukemia/small lymphocytic lymphoma. Monotonous small lymphocyte with scant cytoplasm and round nuclei with smooth nuclear contours and inconspicuous nucleolus (Diff-Quik stain, ×400)

1. Cytomorphologic features [2, 3, 27–30]
   - Predominant small lymphocytes.
   - Tingible body macrophages often absent.
   - Monotonous appearance in CLL/SLL and MCL while scattered intermediate-sized cells seen in FL and MZL.
   - CLL/SLL: small lymphocytes with scant cytoplasm, smooth nuclear contours, clumped chromatin (soccer ball appearance), and small nucleoli (Fig. 6.9).
   - MCL: small lymphocytes with scant cytoplasm, irregular nuclear contours, fine chromatin, and small nucleoli (Fig. 6.10).
   - FL: predominant small cleaved lymphocytes and scattered intermediate-sized lymphocytes with cleaved or noncleaved nuclei seen in low-grade tumors (Fig. 6.11).
   - MZL: mixed small- and intermediate-sized lymphocytes with moderate amount of cytoplasm and eccentrically placed round nuclei (monocytoid cells) (Fig. 6.12).
2. Tips and pitfalls
   - The primary differential diagnosis is reactive lymphoid hyperplasia. Polymorphous lymphoid population and tingible body macrophages favor a reactive process. Flow cytometry study is often required.
   - Combination of cytomorphologic, immunophenotypic, and cytogenetic features may be required to classify this group of lymphomas (Table 6.1).

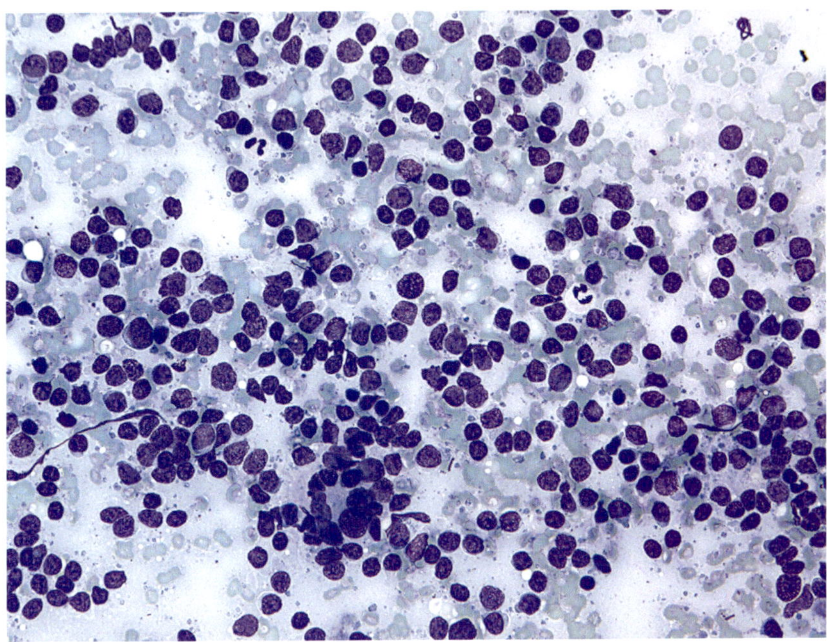

Fig. 6.10 Mantle cell lymphoma. Monotonous small lymphocyte with scant cytoplasm and round to oval nuclei with irregular nuclear contours (Diff-Quik stain, ×400)

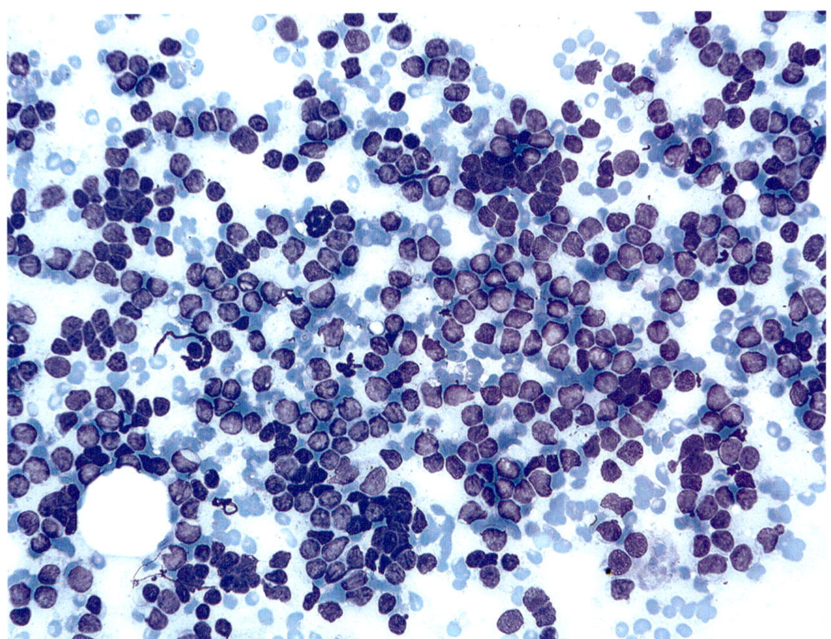

Fig. 6.11 G1/2 Follicular lymphoma. Monotonous small lymphocyte with scant cytoplasm and cleaved round nuclei (Diff-Quik stain, ×400)

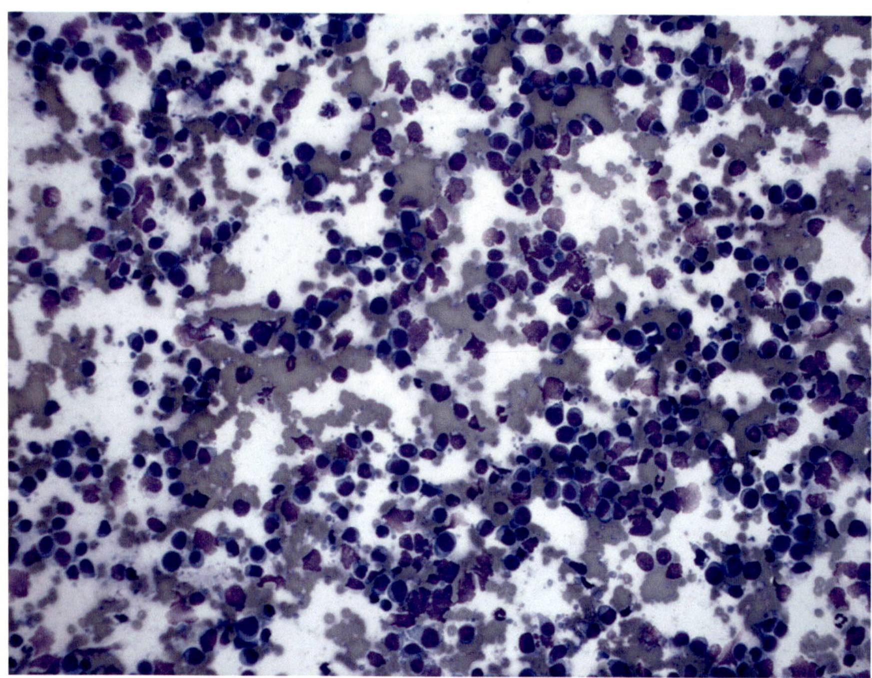

Fig. 6.12 Marginal zone lymphoma. Monotonous small lymphocyte with scant cytoplasm and eccentrically located round nuclei with smooth nuclear contours (Diff-Quik stain, ×200)

Table 6.1 Cytomorphologic, immunophenotypic, and cytogenetic features of small cell lymphomas

	CLL/SLL	FL (G1/G2)	MCL	MZL
Cytomorphology	Monomorphic small lymphocytes with smooth nuclear contours and clumped chromatin	Predominant small cleaved lymphocytes and scattered cleaved or noncleaved intermediate lymphocytes	Monomorphic small lymphocytes with irregular nuclear contours and fine chromatin	Mixed small and intermediate lymphocytes with eccentrically placed nuclei
Immunophenotype	CD10−, CD5+, CD23+, cyclin D1−	CD10+, CD5−, CD23−/+, cyclin D1−	CD10−, CD5+, CD23−, cyclin D1+	CD10−, CD5−, CD23−, cyclin D1−
Cytogenetics	Trisomy 12[a]	t (14:18)	t (11:14)	Trisomy 3[b]

CLL/SLL chronic lymphocytic leukemia/small lymphocytic lymphoma, *FL* grade 1 or 2 follicular lymphoma, *MCL* mantle cell lymphoma, *MZL* marginal zone lymphoma
[a]Trisomy 12 is seen in about 30% of CLL/SLL cases
[b]Trisomy 3 is commonly seen in extranodal MZL

Intermediate-Sized Cell Lymphomas

This group of lymphomas are aggressive tumors, the most common types of which are Burkitt lymphoma and B-/T-lymphoblastic lymphoma. Blastoid variant of mantle cell lymphoma is also included.

1. Cytomorphologic features [2, 3, 31–33]

   - Relatively uniform intermediate-sized lymphocytes.
   - Mitoses and apoptotic bodies.
   - Tingible body macrophages.
   - Burkitt lymphoma: uniform intermediate lymphocytes with scant deep blue cytoplasm, prominent cytoplasmic fine vacuoles, round nuclei, and conspicuous nucleoli (Fig. 6.13).
   - Lymphoblastic lymphoma: uniform intermediate lymphocytes with scant cytoplasm, round nuclei, fine chromatin, and inconspicuous nucleoli (Fig. 6.14).
   - Blastoid mantle cell lymphoma: uniform intermediate lymphocytes with scant cytoplasm, round nuclei, fine chromatin, and conspicuous nucleoli.

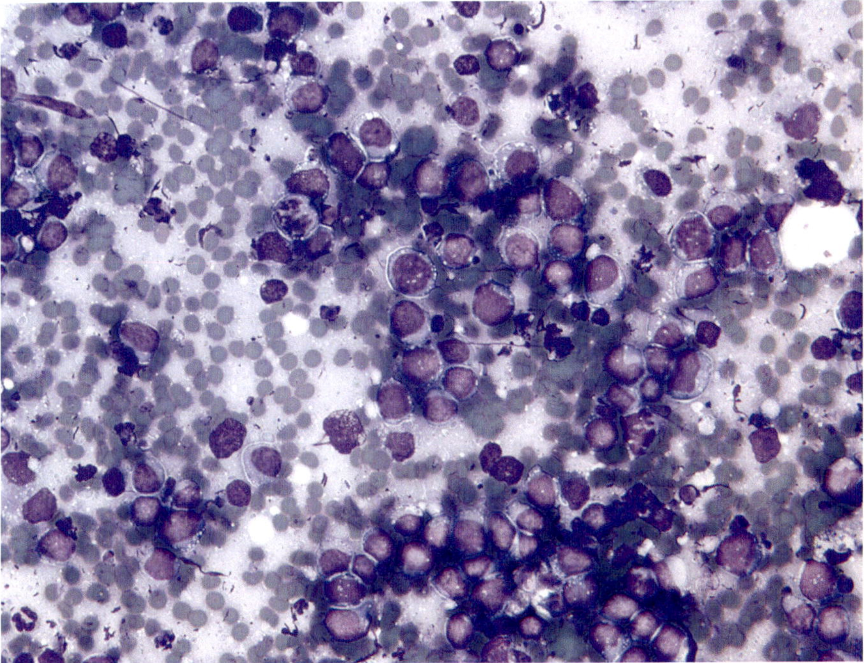

Fig. 6.13 Burkitt lymphoma. Relatively monotonous intermediate-sized lymphocyte with scant cytoplasm, fine cytoplasmic vacules and round nuclei with irregular nuclear contours, fine chromatin, and inconspicuous nucleolus (Diff-Quik stain, ×400)

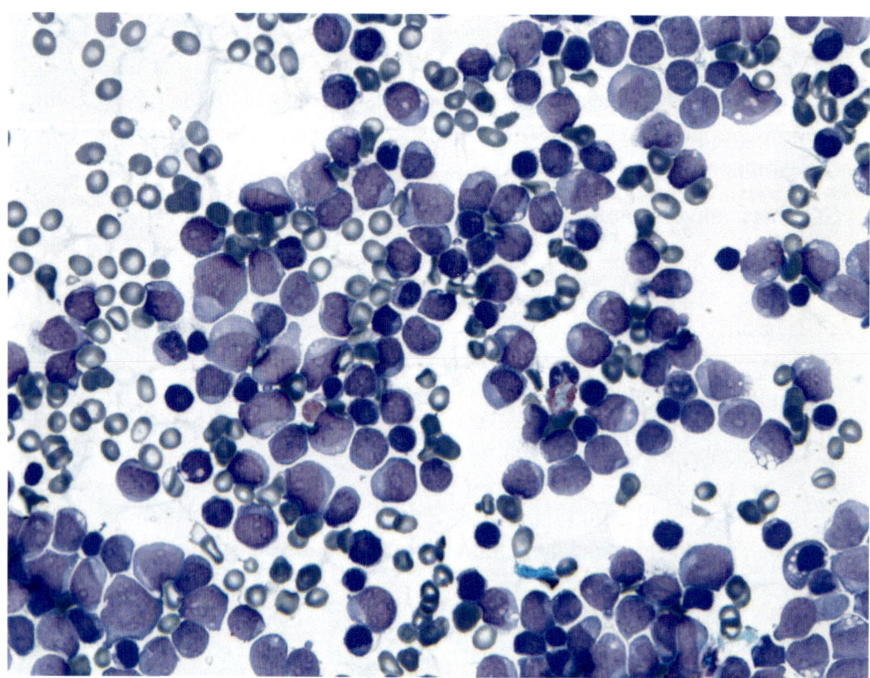

Fig. 6.14 Lymphoblastic lymphoma. Monotonous intermediate-sized lymphocyte with scant cytoplasm and round nuclei with smooth nuclear contours (Diff-Quik stain, ×400)

2. Tips and pitfalls

- The lymphomas in this group should be differentiated from non-lymphoid tumors such as poorly differentiated carcinoma and melanoma. Immunocytochemical studies are essential for a correct diagnosis.
- Plasmablastic lymphoma and myeloma may share similar cytomorphologic features.
- In addition to cytomorphology, immunophenotypic and cytogenetic features are helpful for differential diagnosis between Burkitt lymphoma and lymphoblastic lymphoma. Burkitt lymphoma is positive for c-myc, is always EBV-associated, and has characteristic t (8:14) with a near 100% of Ki-67 index. The tumor cells of lymphoblastic lymphoma are positive for TdT.

Large Cell Lymphomas

Diffuse large B-cell lymphoma (DLBCL) is the most common type of large cell lymphomas and should be further classified as follicular center origin versus non-follicular center origin due to their difference in prognosis. Grade 3 follicular

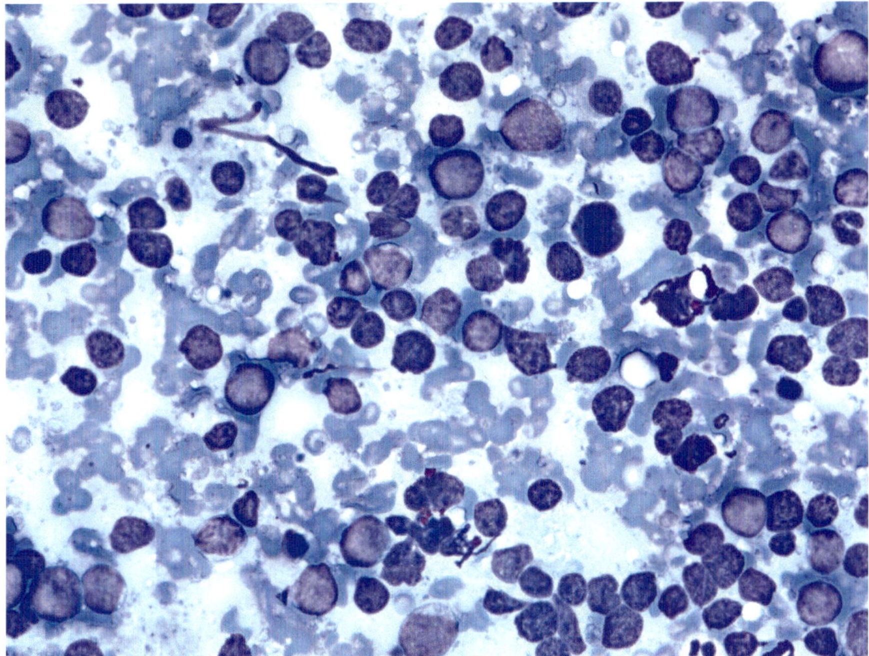

Fig. 6.15 Diffuse large B-cell lymphoma. Polymorphic large lymphocyte with scant cytoplasm, irregular nuclear contours, and conspicuous nucleolus (Diff-Quik stain, ×400)

lymphoma (FL) may share similar morphology. Both DLBCL and FL are seen in elderly patients; however, primary mediastinal large B-cell lymphoma, a variant of DLBCL, occurs primarily in young adults.

1. Cytomorphologic features [2, 3, 31] (Figs. 6.15 and 6.16)

   - Polymorphous population of lymphocytes.
   - Variable number large atypical lymphocytes mixed with background small lymphocytes.
   - Large atypical cells with nuclear pleomorphism, irregular nuclear contours, and conspicuous nucleoli.

2. Tips and pitfalls

   - This group of lymphomas should be differentiated from other high-grade lymphomas as well as non-hematopoietic malignancy. Flow cytometry and/or immunocytochemistry would be helpful for their differential diagnosis.
   - Grade 3 follicular lymphoma (FL) may be difficult to distinguish from DLBCLs of follicular center origin. In this setting, a diagnostic term of high-grade large B-cell lymphoma is acceptable for clinical management (Fig. 6.17).

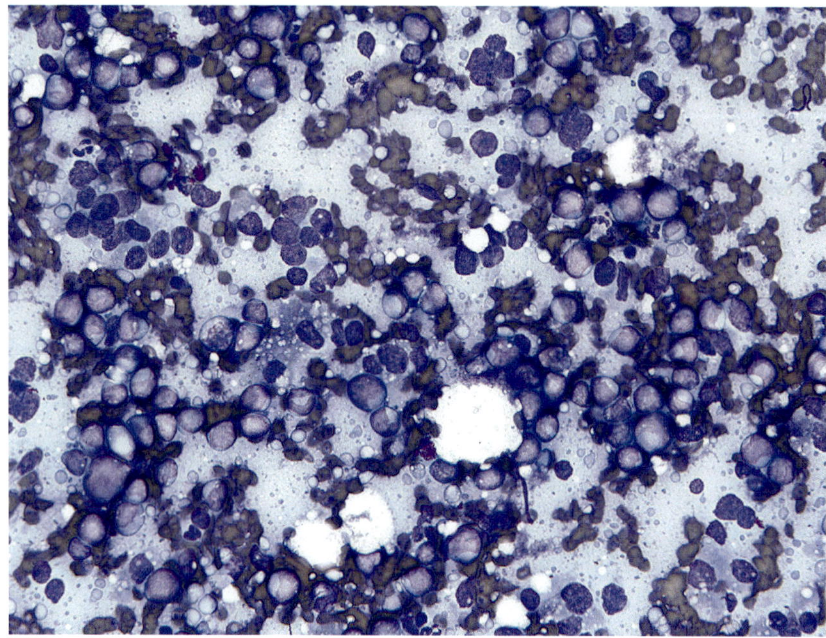

Fig. 6.16 G3 follicular lymphoma. Polymorphous population of small, intermediate, and large lymphocyte with scant cytoplasm, cleaved nuclei, and conspicuous nucleolus (Diff-Quik stain, ×400)

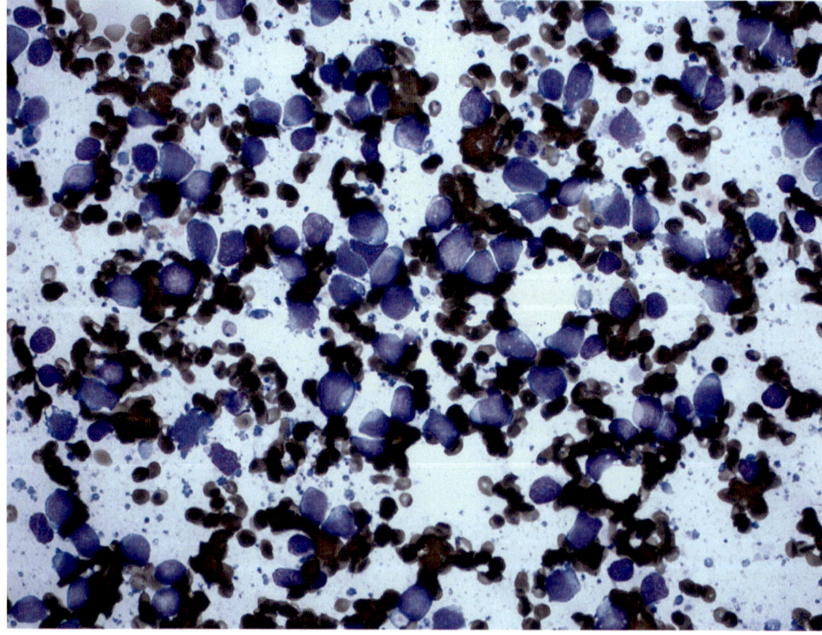

Fig. 6.17 High-grade large B-cell lymphoma (progressed or transformed from G1/2 tumor follicular lymphoma). Polymorphic intermediate and large lymphocyte with scant cytoplasm, irregular nuclear contours, and conspicuous nucleolus (Diff-Quik stain, ×400)

Lymphomas with Plasmacytoid Morphology

Hematopoietic neoplasms with plasmacytoid morphology include plasma cell neoplasm (PCN) and lymphoplasmacytic lymphoma (LPL), both occurring primarily in elderly patients. They share plasmacytoid cell morphology and CD138 positivity. Plasma cell neoplasms can be further classified as plasmacytoma as a solitary lesion and multiple myeloma as multiple simultaneous lesions.

1. Cytomorphologic features [2, 3]
   - Relative uniform cell population.
   - Many cells with eccentrically placed nuclei (plasmacytoid appearance).
   - PCN: almost exclusive plasma cells with paranuclear hofs, occasional binucleation, and multinucleation (Fig. 6.18).
   - LPL: mixed small lymphocytes, plasma cells, and plasmacytoid cells.
2. Tips and pitfalls
   - The tumors in this group should be differentiated from other tumors with plasmacytoid appearance including marginal zone lymphoma (monocytoid appearance) [34], metastatic melanoma, metastatic well-differentiated neuroendocrine tumor, and metastatic lobular breast carcinoma.

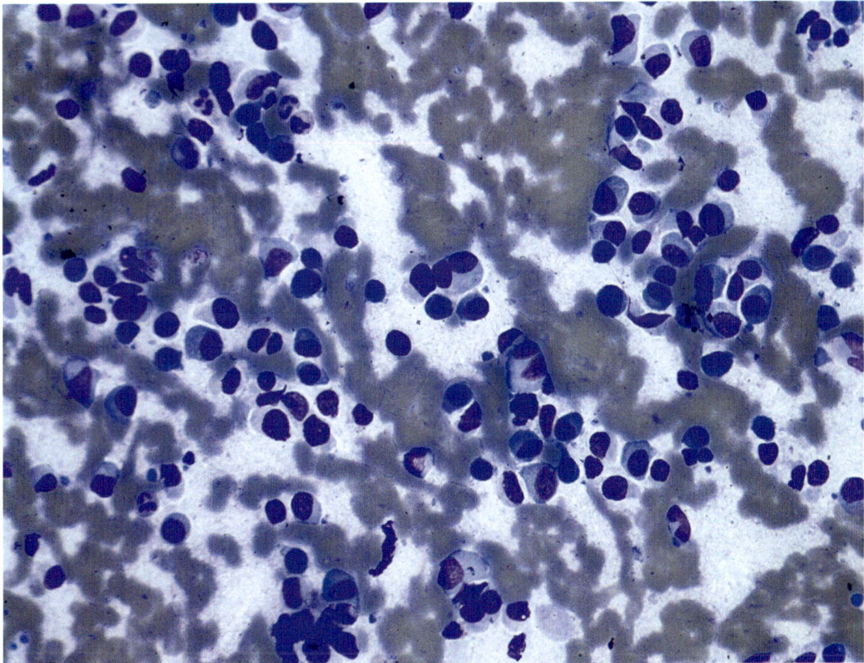

Fig. 6.18 Plasma cell neoplasm. Relatively uninform cells with moderate amount of cytoplasm and eccentrically located nuclei. Perinuclear hofs and occasional binucleation are seen (Diff-Quik stain, ×400)

- PCN and LPL both express CD138 but differ in their cell components and other immunophenotypic features. PCN often does not usually express B-cell marker such as CD19/CD20 and is also negative for CD45, while LPL usually expresses CD45 and CD19/CD20.
- Flow cytometry analysis has a limited role in diagnosing PCN but is helpful for its differential diagnosis. Flow cytometry with cytoplasmic light chain analysis may also help establish clonality of PCN.

Non-Hodgkin T-Cell Lymphomas

T-cell non-Hodgkin lymphomas are relatively uncommon, accounting for about 10% of non-Hodgkin lymphomas (NHL). As compared to B-cell NHLs, T-cell lymphomas often display significant cytological atypia. Diagnosis of T-cell lymphomas can be established by cytomorphologic atypia, aberrant T-cell antigen expression, and T-cell receptor gene rearrangement [19]. The commonly seen T-cell lymphomas involving lymph nodes include peripheral T-cell lymphoma (PTCL) and anaplastic large cell lymphoma (ALCL).

Peripheral T-Cell Lymphoma

PTCL is a heterogenous group of mature T-cell lymphoma and the most common type of T-cell lymphoma, which primarily affects adult patients and has an aggressive clinical course.

1. Cytomorphologic features [2, 3] (Fig. 6.19)

   - Polymorphous population of lymphocytes or monotonous large lymphocytes.
   - Large lymphocytes have irregular hyperchromatic nuclei with prominent nucleoli.
   - Background small lymphocytes, eosinophils, plasma cells, and histiocytes, sometimes epithelioid histiocytes.
   - Rare Reed-Sternberg-like cells may be present.

2. Tips and pitfalls

   - PTCL may share similar morphologic features with Hodgkin lymphoma, anaplastic large cell lymphoma, and high-grade B-cell non-Hodgkin lymphomas such as diffuse large B-cell lymphoma.
   - PTCL often shows loss of some T-cell-associated antigens and sometimes aberrant CD4/CD8 expression such as double negative CD4/CD8 and double positive CD4/CD8.

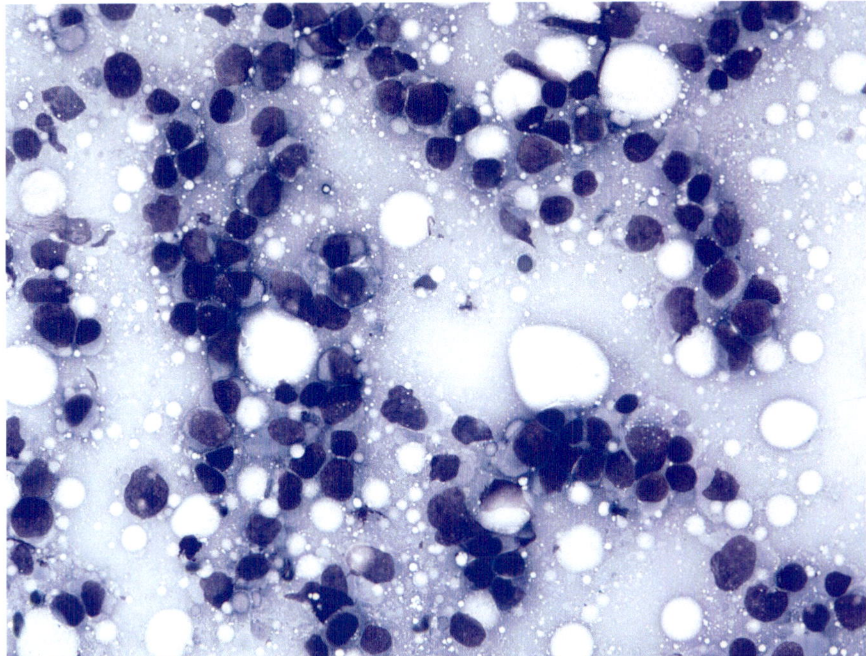

Fig. 6.19 Peripheral T-cell lymphoma. Polymorphic intermediate and large lymphocyte with scant cytoplasm, irregular nuclear contours, and conspicuous nucleolus (Diff-Quik stain, ×400)

Anaplastic Large Cell Lymphoma

ALCL is a T-cell lymphoma which has characteristic morphologic features. According to the most recent WHO classification, ALCL are divided into ALK-positive and ALK-negative ALCL. ALK-positive ALCL primarily affects patients in their first three decades of life, while ALK-negative counterpart can occur in patients of any age. The latter has a poorer prognosis as compared to ALK-positive tumor.

1. Cytomorphologic features [2, 3, 35] (Figs. 6.20 and 6.21)
    - Pleomorphic population of lymphocytes.
    - Large atypical lymphoid cells with abundant cytoplasm and large irregular nuclei, horseshoe- or donut-shaped, with prominent nucleoli.
    - Rare Reed-Sternberg-like cells may be present.
    - Scattered histiocytes and neutrophils.
    - Small cell variant has been described.
2. Tips and pitfalls
    - ALCL should be distinguished from Hodgkin lymphoma, peripheral T-cell lymphoma, high-grade B-cell lymphomas, and metastatic tumors.

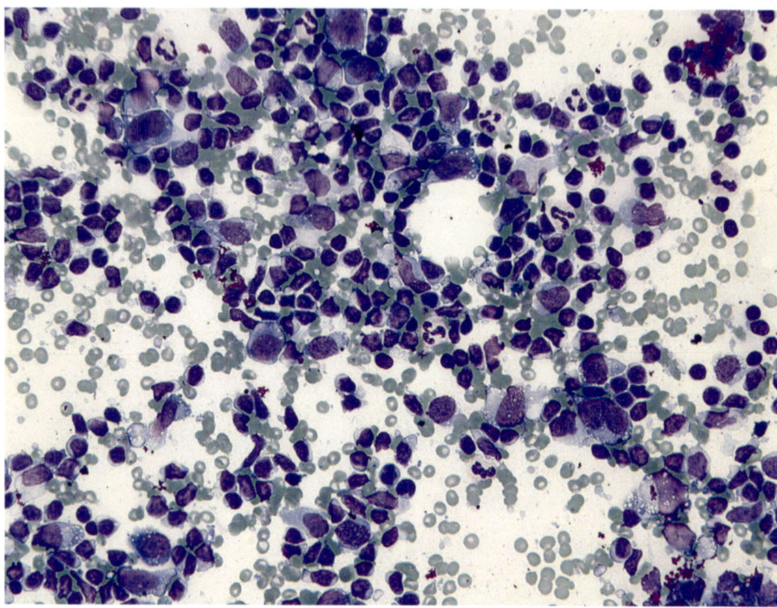

Fig. 6.20 Anaplastic large cell lymphoma. Mixed small, intermediate, and large lymphocyte with irregular nuclear contours. The large lymphocytes have moderate amount of cytoplasm and conspicuous nucleolus. Occasional large bilobed atypical cells are seen (Diff-Quik stain, ×400)

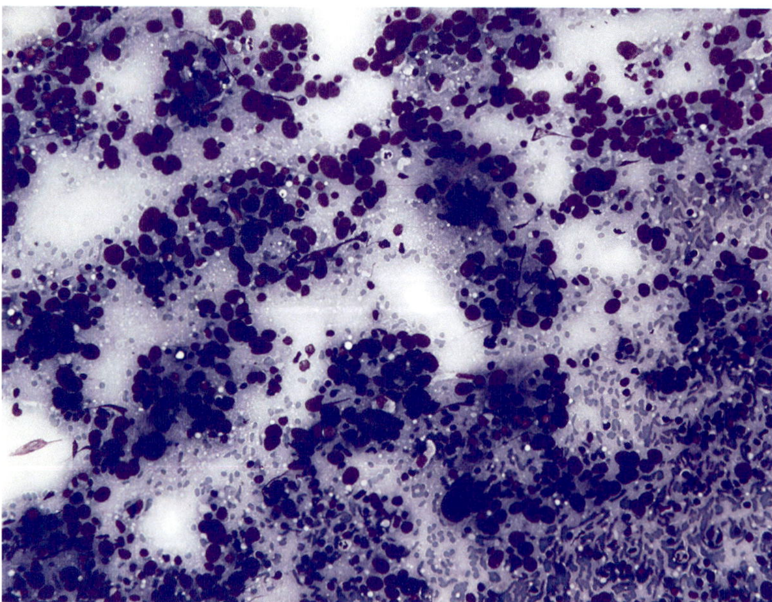

Fig. 6.21 Anaplastic large cell lymphoma. Large atypical lymphocyte with irregular nuclear contours and conspicuous nucleolus. Scattered small lymphocytes and occasional large bilobed multinucleated atypical cells are seen (Diff-Quik stain, ×400)

- ALCL can be ALK positive or negative by immunostaining.
- There is a small portion of ALCL cases showing lymphohistiocytic, small cell and Hodgkin-like pattern.

Other Hematopoietic Neoplasms

Other hematopoietic tumors, either myeloid or histiocytic origin, can involve lymph nodes although uncommon.

Myeloid Sarcoma

Myeloid sarcoma is defined as a tumor mass consisting of myeloid blasts, with or without maturation, occurring at an anatomic site other than the bone marrow.

1. Cytomorphologic features [2, 3, 36]
   - Relatively monomorphic population.
   - In most cases, tumor cells display myelomonocytic or pure monoblastic morphology.
   - Myelomonocytic morphology: moderate amount of cytoplasm, folded nuclei, inconspicuous nucleolus.
   - Monoblastic morphology: scant cytoplasm, round nuclei, and prominent nucleolus.
2. Tips and pitfalls
   - The major differential of myeloma sarcoma is with malignant lymphomas. Immunophenotypic analysis is required to establish a diagnosis of myeloid sarcoma, expressing myeloperoxidase (MPO) and CD33 and also often immature markers such as CD34 and CD117.
   - Myeloid sarcoma should also be differentiated from extramedullary hematopoiesis. The later comprises of the cells of three lineages.

Histiocytic/Dendritic Cell Neoplasms

Tumors of histiocytic and dendritic cell origin are rare and account for less than 1% of lymphoid lesions. The tumors include histiocytic sarcoma, Langerhans cell histiocytosis, and interdigitating/follicular dendritic cell sarcoma.

1. Cytomorphologic features [2, 3, 37]
   - Histiocytic sarcoma: polymorphous population of atypical cells with irregular nuclei.

- Langerhans cell histiocytosis: cells with abundant cytoplasm and indented or grooved nuclei in a background of mixed eosinophils, lymphocytes, and neutrophils.
- Dendritic cell sarcoma: epithelioid or spindle-shaped cells.

2. Tips and pitfalls

- Differential diagnosis may include lymphoid tumors as well as reactive process.
- Immunophenotypic analysis is crucial for diagnosis. Histiocytic sarcoma is positive for CD68, Langerhans cell histiocytosis is positive for S100 and CD1a, and dendritic cell sarcoma is either positive for S100 (interdigitating) or CD21 and CD35 (follicular).

Metastatic Tumors

Secondary involvement by metastatic tumors, mostly carcinomas, is one of the major causes for lymphadenopathy. Most metastatic tumors can be recognized by their distinct morphologic features, but some may impose a diagnostic challenge due to overlapping morphology with lymphomas or reactive lymphadenopathy.

Metastatic Melanoma

1. Cytomorphologic features [38, 39] (Fig. 6.22)

- Dispersed single cells.
- Eccentrically placed nuclei with prominent nucleolus.
- Occasional binucleation, intranuclear inclusions, and melanin pigments.
- Spindle cell variant seen in a small number of cases.

2. Tips and pitfalls

- Presence of single dispersed cells in a background of lymphocytes may mimic lymphomas.
- Intranuclear inclusions and melanin pigments, if present, help in the differential diagnosis. Positivity of melanocytic markers such as SOX10, Melan A, HMB45, and S100 is diagnostic of metastatic melanoma.
- Patient's history is also helpful.

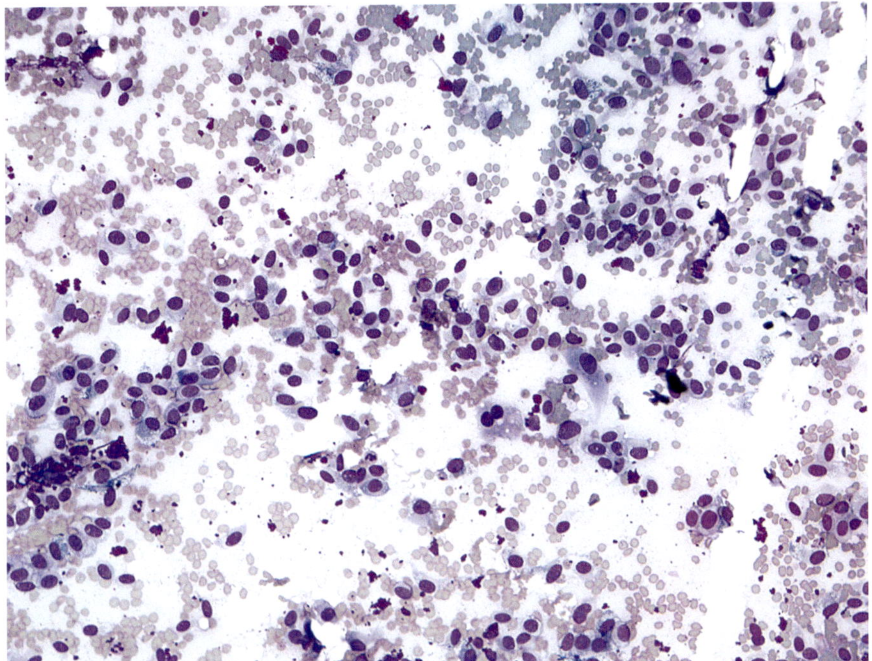

Fig. 6.22 Metastatic melanoma. Dispersed relative uniform cells with oval nuclei and occasional intracytoplasmic melanin pigments (Diff-Quik stain, ×200)

Metastatic Breast Carcinoma

1. Cytomorphologic features [40, 41] (Fig. 6.23)
   - Dispersed single or loose groups of epithelioid cells, predominantly single cells in lobular carcinoma.
   - Epithelioid cells have round to oval nuclei.
   - Variable polymorphous population of lymphocytes in the background.
2. Tips and pitfalls
   - Intermixed dispersed single cells or dyscohesive groups of epithelioid cells with lymphocytes seen in metastatic carcinoma may mimic lymphoproliferative disorder.
   - Immunocytochemical study may be needed in difficult cases. Metastatic breast carcinomas are cytokeratin and GATA3 positive.

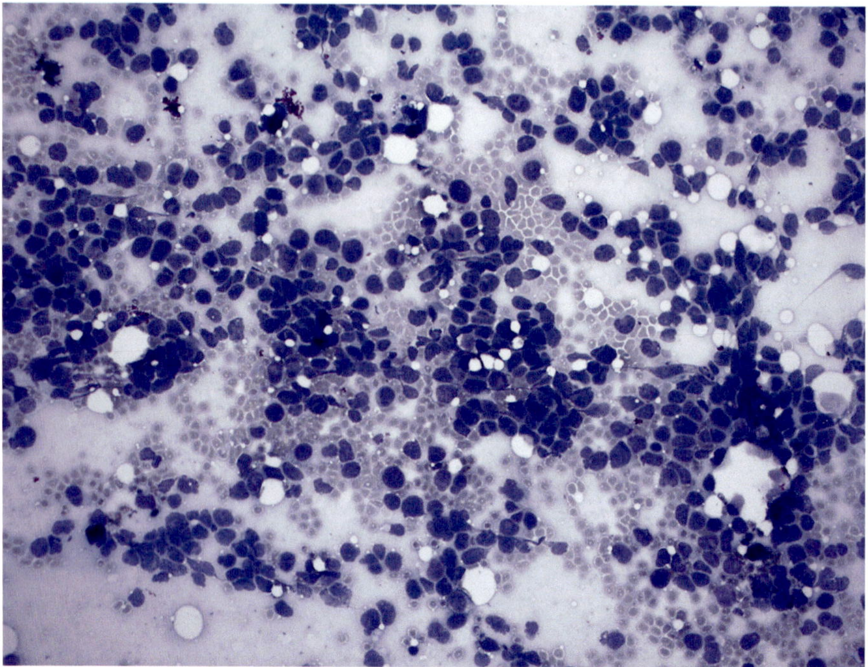

Fig. 6.23 Metastatic breast carcinoma. Single and loose cohesive groups of relative uniform cells with scant cytoplasm and irregular nuclear contours (Diff-Quik stain, ×200)

Metastatic Small Cell Carcinoma

1. Cytomorphologic features [42, 43] (Fig. 6.24)
   - Dispersed single or loosely cohesive groups of intermediate-sized tumor cells with high nuclear-to-cytoplasmic ratios and focal nuclear molding.
   - Nuclear streaming artifacts often present.
   - Necrosis and apoptotic bodies often present.
2. Tips and pitfalls
   - Small cell carcinoma and lymphomas share some cytomorphologic features including dyscohesive tumor cells and nuclear streaming artifacts. However, necrosis and nuclear molding are uncommon for lymphomas.
   - Immunocytochemical studies with neuroendocrine markers are diagnostic of small cell carcinoma.
   - During the on-site evaluation, it is advised to save specimen for flow cytometry analysis and immunochemistry if there is an uncertainty whether the lesion represents small cell carcinoma or lymphoma.

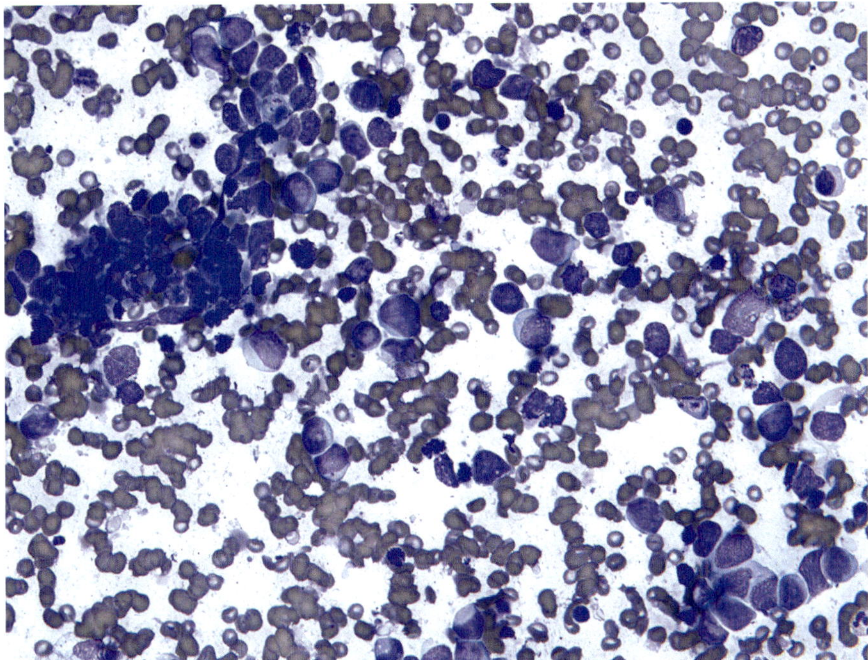

Fig. 6.24 Metastatic small cell carcinoma. Single and loose cohesive groups of relative uniform cells with scant cytoplasm and irregular nuclear contours. Focal nuclear molding and nuclear streaming artifact are present (Diff-Quik stain, ×200)

Metastatic Germ Cell Tumor (Seminoma/Germinoma)

1. Cytomorphologic features [44, 45] (Fig. 6.25)
    - A mixture of dyscohesive neoplastic cells and lymphocytes.
    - Neoplastic cells have round nuclei with conspicuous nucleolus.
    - Tigroid background often seen.
2. Tips and pitfalls
    - Seminoma/germinoma share some cytomorphologic features with lymphomas. However, lymphomas less likely have a tigroid background, which if present help the diagnosis of seminoma/germinoma.
    - Diagnosis of seminoma/germinoma can be supported by positive SALL4 and OCT4 immunostains.

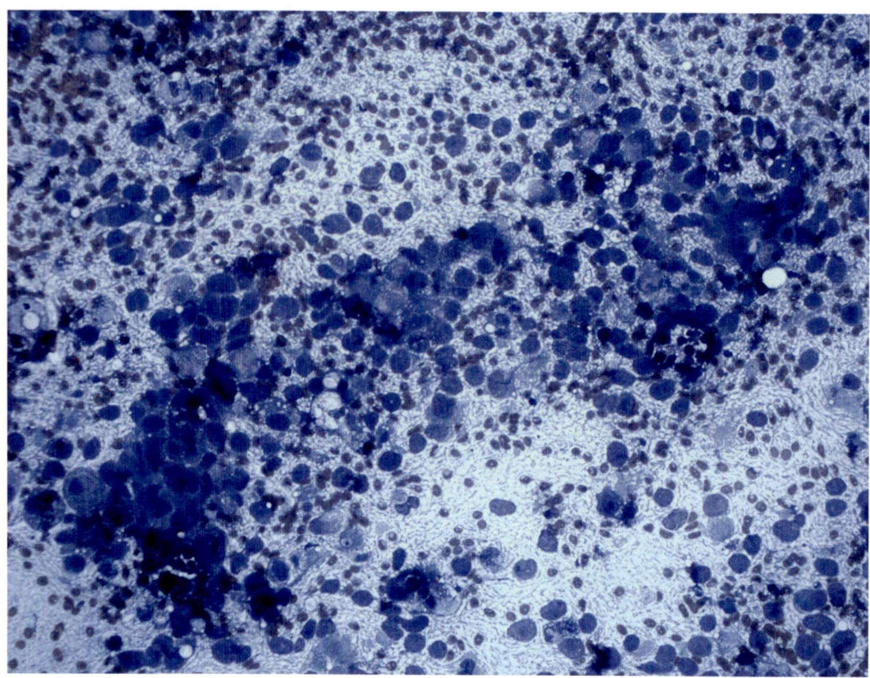

Fig. 6.25 Metastatic germ cell tumor. Single and loose cohesive groups of relative uniform cells with scant cytoplasm, fine cytoplasmic vacuoles, and round nuclei in a tigroid background (Diff-Quik stain, ×200)

Metastatic Squamous Cell Carcinoma

1. Cytomorphologic features (Fig. 6.26)
   - In most cases, squamous cell carcinoma can be easily distinguished from lymphomas.
   - However, extensive necrosis can be seen in some metastatic squamous cell carcinoma, which can mimic infectious/necrotic lymphadenopathy or squamous epithelium-lined cystic lesions.
2. Tips and pitfalls
   - In metastatic squamous cell carcinoma with extensive necrosis, tumor cells are necrotic but may still have maintained the outlines as atypical ghost cells.
   - Careful search for viable non-keratinizing atypical cells with high nuclear-to-cytoplasmic ratios is important for a diagnosis of malignancy.
   - Papanicolaou stain is helpful to highlight abnormal keratinization.

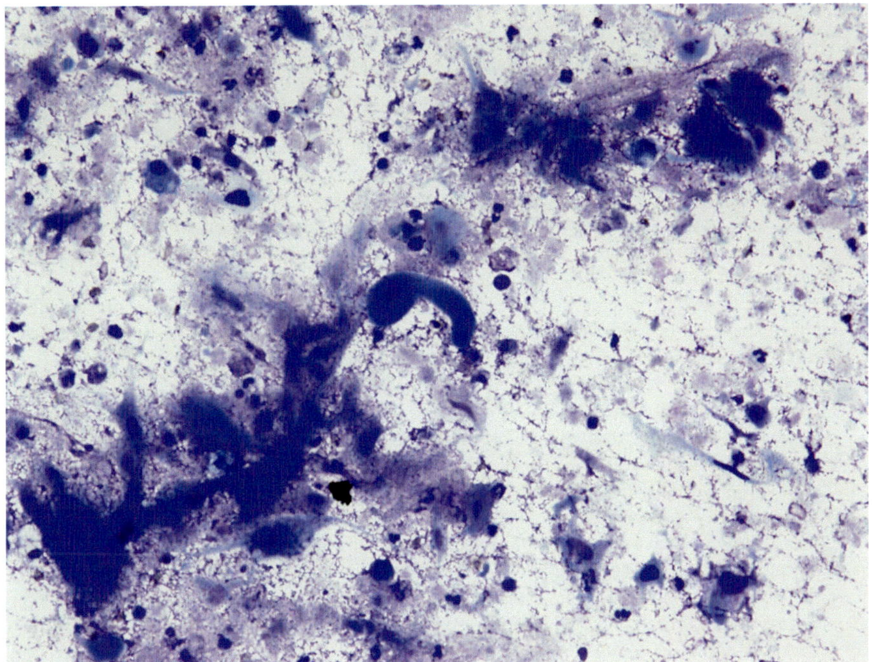

Fig. 6.26 Metastatic squamous cell carcinoma. Scattered polymorphic cells with dense cytoplasm and hyperchromatic nuclei in a necrotic background (Diff-Quik stain, ×400)

References

1. Metzgeroth G, Schneider S, Walz C, Reiter S, Hofmann WK, Marx A, Hastka J. Fine needle aspiration and core needle biopsy in the diagnosis of lymphadenopathy of unknown aetiology. Ann Hematol. 2012;91(9):1477–84.
2. Wieczorek TJ, Wakely PE Jr. In: Cibas ES, Ducatman BS, editors. Cytology. Diagnostic principles and clinical correlates. 4th ed. Edinburg: Saunders/Elsevier; 2014. p. 333–71.
3. Young NA, Dulaimi E, Al-Saleem T. In: Bibbo M, Wilbur DC, editors. Comprehensive cytopathology. 4th ed. New York: Elsevier; 2015. p. 545–80.
4. Nunez AL, Jhala NC, Carroll AJ, Mikhail FM, Reddy VV, Xian RR, Jhala DN. Endoscopic ultrasound and endobronchial ultrasound-guided fine-needle aspiration of deep-seated lymphadenopathy: analysis of 1338 cases. Cytojournal. 2012;9:14.
5. Wakely PE Jr. Fine-needle aspiration cytopathology in diagnosis and classification of malignant lymphoma: accurate and reliable? Diagn Cytopathol. 2000;22(2):120–5.
6. Caraway NP. Evolving role of FNA biopsy in diagnosing lymphoma: past, present, and future. Cancer Cytopathol. 2015;123(7):389–93.
7. Demurtas A, Accinelli G, Pacchioni D, Godio L, Novero D, Bussolati G, Palestro G, Papotti M, Stacchini A. Utility of flow cytometry immunophenotyping in fine-needle aspirate cytologic diagnosis of non-Hodgkin lymphoma: a series of 252 cases and review of the literature. Appl Immunohistochem Mol Morphol. 2010;18(4):311–22.

8. da Cunha Santos G, Ko HM, Geddie WR, Boerner SL, Lai SW, Have C, Kamel-Reid S, Bailey D. Targeted use of fluorescence in situ hybridization (FISH) in cytospin preparations: results of 298 fine needle aspirates of B-cell non-Hodgkin lymphoma. Cancer Cytopathol. 2010;118(5):250–8.
9. Ensani F, Mehravaran S, Irvanlou G, Aghaipoor M, Vaeli S, Hajati E, Khorgami Z, Nasiri S. Fine-needle aspiration cytology and flow cytometric immunophenotyping in diagnosis and classification of non-Hodgkin lymphoma in comparison to histopathology. Diagn Cytopathol. 2012;40(4):305–10.
10. Loya A, Nadeem M, Yusuf MA. Use of ancillary techniques in improving the yield of samples obtained at endoscopic ultrasound-guided fine needle aspiration of thoracic and abdominal lymph nodes. Acta Cytol. 2014;58(2):192–7.
11. Mehmood S, Jahan A, Loya A, Yusuf MA. Onsite cytopathology evaluation and ancillary studies beneficial in EUS-FNA of pancreatic, mediastinal, intra-abdominal, and submucosal lesions. Diagn Cytopathol. 2015;43(4):278–86.
12. Fung AD, Collins JA, Campassi C, Ioffe OB, Staats PN. Performance characteristics of ultrasound-guided fine-needle aspiration of axillary lymph nodes for metastatic breast cancer employing rapid on-site evaluation of adequacy: analysis of 136 cases and review of the literature. Cancer Cytopathol. 2014;122(4):282–91.
13. Cleveland P, Gill KR, Coe SG, Woodward TA, Raimondo M, Jamil L, Gross SA, Heckman MG, Crook JE, Wallace MB. An evaluation of risk factors for inadequate cytology in EUS-guided FNA of pancreatic tumors and lymph nodes. Gastrointest Endosc. 2010;71(7):1194–9.
14. da Cunha Santos G, Boerner SL, Geddie WR. Maximizing the yield of lymph node cytology: lessons learned from rapid onsite evaluation of image- and endoscopic-guided biopsies of hilar and mediastinal lymph nodes. Cancer Cytopathol. 2011;119(6):361–6.
15. Jeffus SK, Joiner AK, Siegel ER, Massoll NA, Meena N, Chen C, Post SR, Bartter T. Rapid on-site evaluation of EBUS-TBNA specimens of lymph nodes: comparative analysis and recommendations for standardization. Cancer Cytopathol. 2015;123(6):362–72.
16. Amador-Ortiz C, Chen L, Hassan A, Frater JL, Burack R, Nguyen TT, Kreisel F. Combined core needle biopsy and fine-needle aspiration with ancillary studies correlate highly with traditional techniques in the diagnosis of nodal-based lymphoma. Am J Clin Pathol. 2011;135(4):516–24.
17. Annema JT, van Meerbeeck JP, Rintoul RC, Dooms C, Deschepper E, Dekkers OM, De Leyn P, Braun J, Carroll NR, Pract M, de Ryck F, Vansteenkiste J, Vermassen F, Versteegh MI, Veseliç M, Nicholson AG, Rabe KF, Tournoy KG. Mediastinoscopy vs endosonography for mediastinal nodal staging of lung cancer: a randomized trial. JAMA. 2010;304(20):2245–52.
18. Lilo MT, Allison DB, Younes BK, Cui M, Askin FB, Gabrielson E, Li QK. The critical role of EBUS-TBNA cytology in the staging of mediastinal lymph nodes in lung cancer patients: a correlation study with positron emission tomography findings. Cancer Cytopathol. 2017;125(9):717–25.
19. Stein H, Pileri SA, Weiss LM, Poppema S, Gascoyne RD, Jaffe ES. In: WHO classification of tumours haematopoietic and lymphoid tissues. 4th Ed. (Swerdlow SH, Campo E, Harris NL, Jaffe ES, Pileri SA, Stein H and Thiele J, eds). Lyon: IARC Press. 2017: 423-442.
20. Chhieng DC, Cangiarella JF, Symmans WF, Cohen JM. Fine-needle aspiration cytology of Hodgkin disease: a study of 89 cases with emphasis on false-negative cases. Cancer. 2001;93(1):52–9.
21. Jiménez-Heffernan JA, Vicandi B, López-Ferrer P, Hardisson D, Viguer JM. Value of fine needle aspiration cytology in the initial diagnosis of Hodgkin's disease. Analysis of 188 cases with an emphasis on diagnostic pitfalls. Acta Cytol. 2001;45(3):300–6.
22. Das DK, Francis IM, Sharma PN, Sathar SA, John B, George SS, Mallik MK, Sheikh ZA, Haji BE, Pathan SK, Madda JP, Mirza K, Ahmed MS, Junaid TA. Hodgkin's lymphoma: diagnostic difficulties in fine-needle aspiration cytology. Diagn Cytopathol. 2009;37(8):564–73.
23. Subhawong AP, Ali SZ, Tatsas AD. Nodular lymphocyte-predominant Hodgkin lymphoma: cytopathologic correlates on fine-needle aspiration. Cancer Cytopathol. 2012;120(4):254–60.

24. Hernandez O, Oweity T, Ibrahim S. Is an increase in CD4/CD8 T-cell ratio in lymph node fine needle aspiration helpful for diagnosing Hodgkin lymphoma? A study of 85 lymph node FNAs with increased CD4/CD8 ratio. Cytojournal. 2005;2:14.
25. Monaco SE, Teot LA, Felgar RE, Surti U, Cai G. Fluorescence in situ hybridization studies on direct smears: an approach to enhance the fine-needle aspiration biopsy diagnosis of B-cell non-Hodgkin lymphomas. Cancer. 2009;117(5):338–48.
26. Catrina Reading F, Schlette EJ, Stewart JM, Keating MJ, Katz RL, Caraway NP. Fine-needle aspiration biopsy findings in patients with small lymphocytic lymphoma transformed to hodgkin lymphoma. Am J Clin Pathol. 2007;128(4):571–8.
27. Dong HY, Harris NL, Preffer FI, Pitman MB. Fine-needle aspiration biopsy in the diagnosis and classification of primary and recurrent lymphoma: a retrospective analysis of the utility of cytomorphology and flow cytometry. Mod Pathol. 2001;14(5):472–81.
28. Murphy BA, Meda BA, Buss DH, Geisinger KR. Marginal zone and mantle cell lymphomas: assessment of cytomorphology in subtyping small B-cell lymphomas. Diagn Cytopathol. 2003;28(3):126–30.
29. Bangerter M, Brudler O, Heinrich B, Griesshamnuer M. Fine needle aspiration cytology and flow cytometry in the diagnosis and subclassification of non-Hodgkin's lymphoma based on the World Health Organization classification. Acta Cytol. 2007;51(3):390–8.
30. Schmid S, Tinguely M, Cione P, Moch H, Bode B. Flow cytometry as an accurate tool to complement fine needle aspiration cytology in the diagnosis of low grade malignant lymphomas. Cytopathology. 2011;22(6):397–406.
31. Meda BA, Buss DH, Woodruff RD, Cappellari JO, Rainer RO, Powell BL, Geisinger KR. Diagnosis and subclassification of primary and recurrent lymphoma. The usefulness and limitations of combined fine-needle aspiration cytomorphology and flow cytometry. Am J Clin Pathol. 2000;113(5):688–99.
32. Silowash R, Pantanowitz L, Craig FE, Simons JP, Monaco SE. Utilization of flow cytometry in pediatric fine-needle aspiration biopsy specimens. Acta Cytol. 2016;60(4):344–53.
33. Patel RA, Sheehan AM, Finch CJ, Lopez-Terrada D, Hernandez VS, Curry CV. Fine-needle aspiration cytology of T-lymphoblastic lymphoma associated FGFR1 rearrangement myeloproliferative neoplasm. Diagn Cytopathol. 2014;42(1):45–8.
34. Nasu A, Igawa T, Sato H, Yanai H, Yoshino T, Sato Y. Extranodal marginal zone B-cell lymphoma of mucosa-associated lymphoid tissue with plasma cell differentiation: periodic acid-schiff reaction-positive Dutcher body is a diagnostic clue to distinguish it from plasmacytoma. Diagn Cytopathol. 2017;45(6):547–51.
35. Kim SE, Kim SH, Lim BJ, Hong SW, Yang WI. Fine needle aspiration cytology of small cell variant of anaplastic large cell lymphoma. A case report. Acta Cytol. 2004;48(2):254–8.
36. Suh YK, Shin HJ. Fine-needle aspiration biopsy of granulocytic sarcoma: a clinicopathologic study of 27 cases. Cancer. 2000;90(6):364–72.
37. Hang JF, Siddiqui MT, Ali SZ. Fine needle aspiration of Langerhans cell histiocytosis: a cytopathologic study of 37 cases. Acta Cytol. 2017;61(2):96–102.
38. Galli F, Petraitiene V, Muthu SK, James S, Koppana VR, Arya A. Challenges in the differential diagnosis of interdigitating dendritic cell sarcoma of intraparotid lymph node vs. metastatic malignant melanoma with unknown primary site. Int J Surg Pathol. 2015;23(3):248–52.
39. Piao Y, Guo M, Gong Y. Diagnostic challenges of metastatic spindle cell melanoma on fine-needle aspiration specimens. Cancer. 2008;114(2):94–101.
40. Alkuwari E, Auger M. Accuracy of fine-needle aspiration cytology of axillary lymph nodes in breast cancer patients: a study of 115 cases with cytologic-histologic correlation. Cancer. 2008;114(2):89–93.
41. Boughey JC, Middleton LP, Harker L, Garrett B, Fornage B, Hunt KK, Babiera GV, Dempsey P, Bedrosian I. Utility of ultrasound and fine-needle aspiration biopsy of the axilla in the assessment of invasive lobular carcinoma of the breast. Am J Surg. 2007;194(4):450–5.

42. Afify A, Das S, Mingyi C. Two smalls in one: coincident small cell carcinoma and small lymphocytic lymphoma in a lymph node diagnosed by fine-needle aspiration biopsy. Cytojournal. 2012;9:5.
43. Kang HK, Um SW, Jeong BH, Lee KJ, Kim H, Kwon OJ, Han J. The utility of endobronchial ultrasound-guided transbronchial needle aspiration in patients with small-cell lung cancer. Intern Med. 2016;55(9):1061–6.
44. Yang X, Cole A, Cajigas A, Khader S. Fine needle aspiration of a metastatic germ cell tumor to supraclavicular lymph node. Lab Med. 2014;45(2):151–5.
45. Ustün M, Heilo A, Fosså S, Aass N, Berner A. Ultrasound-guided fine needle cytology of retroperitoneal masses in patients with malignant germ cell tumours: diagnosis and therapeutic impact. Eur Urol. 2002;42(3):221–8.

Part III
Image-Guided Biopsies of Deep-Seated Organs

Chapter 7
Liver

Guoping Cai

Introduction

Fine needle aspiration (FNA) biopsy has been widely used to evaluate focal hepatic lesions, most of which are solid and could represent primary hepatic or metastatic diseases. While metastatic tumors are often multifocal, primary liver lesions could present as a solitary or multifocal lesion. Cystic hepatic lesions are seldom biopsied by FNA due to a low diagnostic yield. However, FNA biopsy may be used to reduce the risk of rupture when cystic lesions are large or used to rule out a malignancy when in appropriate clinical setting.

FNA have high sensitivity and specificity in diagnosing space-occupying hepatic lesions [1–9]. The reported sensitivity and specificity range from 85% to 95% and 98–100%, respectively [2, 5, 9]. FNA is safe procedure with very low complication rates [5–7, 9]. In addition to cytomorphology, ancillary studies performed on cell block sections play an important role to substantialize the diagnostic yield of FNA biopsy, to confirm malignancy, and if appropriate to elucidate tumor origin [10–13]. It is crucial to secure sufficient material during on-site evaluation. Rapid on-site evaluation (ROSE) allows adequate sampling and appropriate specimen triage and further improves diagnostic yield of FNA biopsy [14, 15].

FNA biopsy offers excellent diagnostic results for metastatic tumors. Primary hepatic tumors, especially those well-differentiated hepatocellular carcinomas or cholangiocarcinoma, may impose diagnostic challenges on FNA [3, 10, 12, 13]. Follow-up with core needle biopsy may help with diagnosis in difficult cases [16–20].

G. Cai (✉)
Department of Pathology, Yale University School of Medicine, New Haven, CT, USA
e-mail: guoping.cai@yale.edu

G. Cai, A. J. Adeniran (eds.), *Rapid On-site Evaluation (ROSE)*,
https://doi.org/10.1007/978-3-030-21799-0_7

Diagnostic Considerations

Specimen Adequacy Assessment

There are no established numeric criteria in terms of adequate assessment. The ultimate reference would be whether the findings of FNA biopsy can fully explain the lesion revealed on imaging studies. A diagnosis of malignancy is apparently considered adequate. When a malignancy is rendered, additional work-up should be followed to further classify tumors and, if metastatic, to elucidate tumor origin. It could be difficult to distinguish a reactive process for a benign tumor and further classify benign tumors on FNA alone. For a cystic lesion, the biopsy may show only cyst contents. Correlation with imaging findings is always required to ensure adequate sampling.

Normal Elements and Contaminants in Liver Cytology

1. Hepatocytes (Figs. 7.1, 7.2, and 7.3)
   - Polygonal cells in small groups or cohesive clusters.
   - Abundant granular cytoplasm.

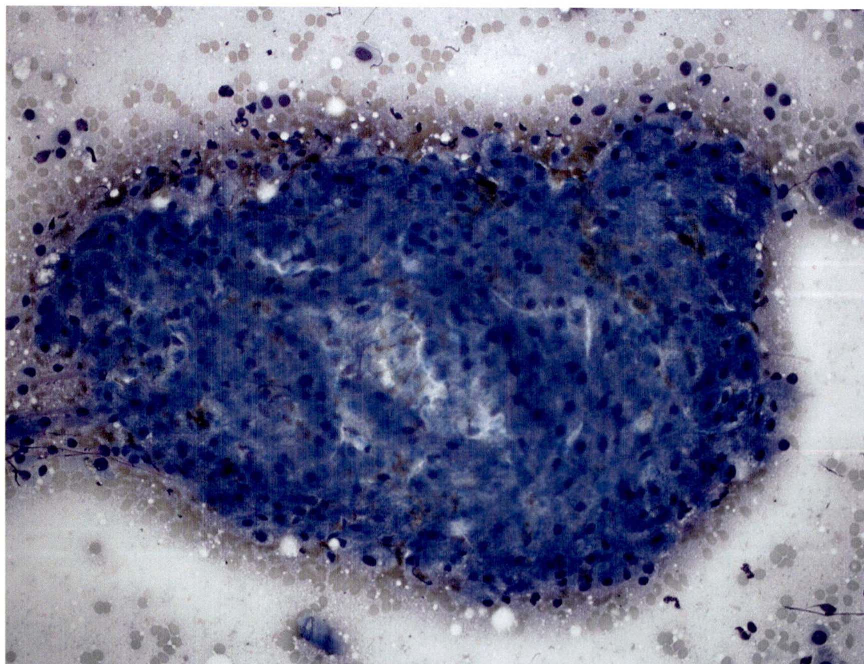

Fig. 7.1 Normal hepatocytes. A cohesive cluster of uniform hepatocytes (Diff-Quik stain, ×200)

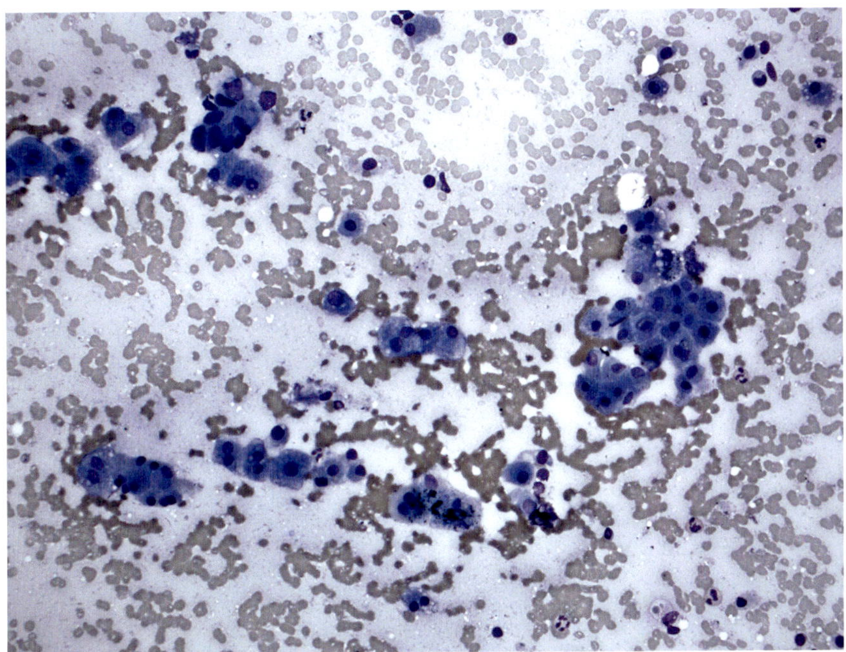

Fig. 7.2 Normal hepatocytes. Single and small groups of uniform hepatocytes with small round nuclei, abundant granular cytoplasm, and occasional cytoplasmic bile pigments (Diff-Quik stain, ×200)

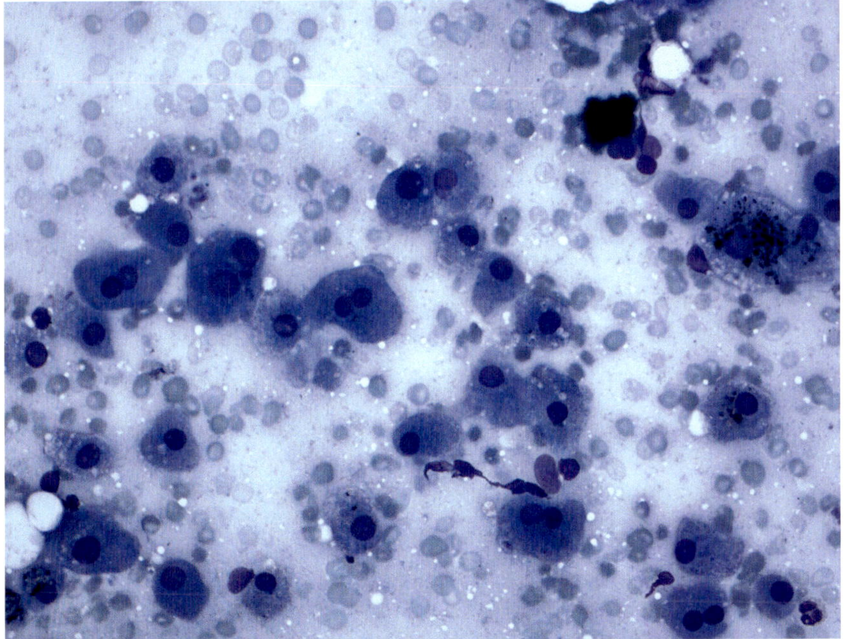

Fig. 7.3 Normal hepatocytes. Single and small groups of hepatocytes with small round nuclei, abundant granular cytoplasm, and occasional binucleation and cytoplasmic bile pigments (Diff-Quik stain, ×400)

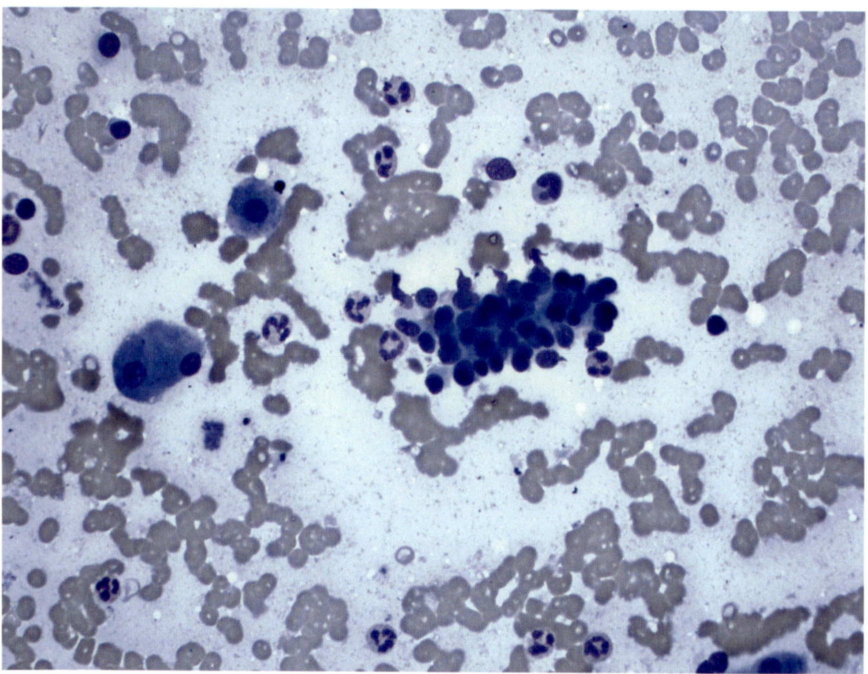

Fig. 7.4 Normal bile ductal epithelial cells. A single group of uniform epithelial cells with small uniform round nuclei and vacuolated cytoplasm. A few normal hepatocytes also seen (Diff-Quik stain, ×400)

- Round nuclei with conspicuous nucleolus.
- Cytoplasmic vacuoles/fat droplets may be present.
- Cytoplasmic bile pigments may be present.

2. Bile duct epithelial cells (Fig. 7.4)

   - Small uniform cuboidal cells arranged in small groups and flat sheets.
   - Round nuclei with smooth nuclear contours, evenly distributed chromatin, and small nucleolus.
   - Moderate amount of vacuolated cytoplasm.

3. Mesothelial cells (Fig. 7.5)

   - Most commonly seen in transabdominal biopsy specimens.
   - Uniform polygonal cells with distinct cell borders arranged in flat sheets.
   - Round to oval nuclei with clearing chromatin, nuclear grooves, and small nucleolus.
   - Moderate to abundant dense cytoplasm.

4. Gastrointestinal epithelial cells

   - Seen in endoscopy-guided biopsy specimens, transgastric or transduodenal.

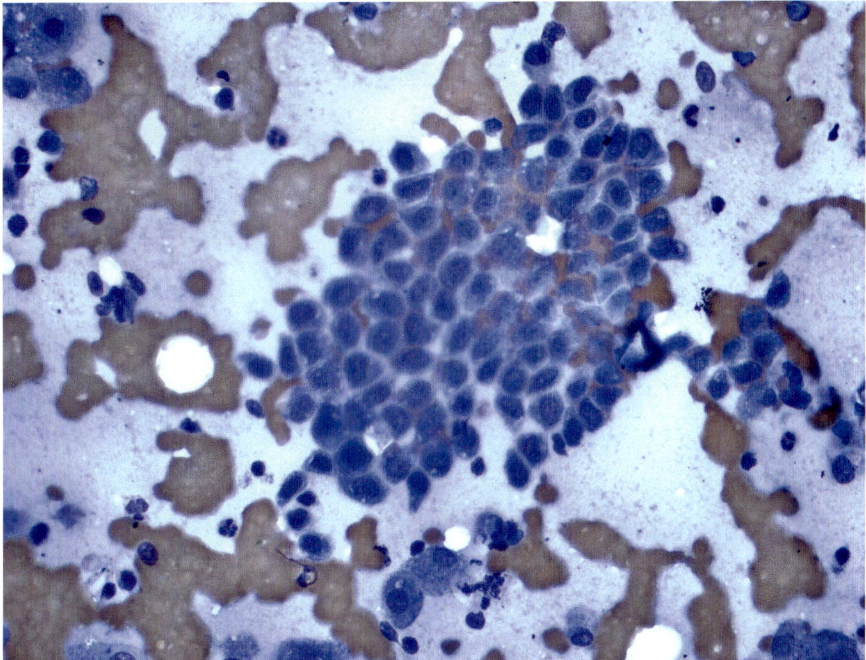

Fig. 7.5 Mesothelial cells. A sheet of benign-appearing mesothelial cells with dense cytoplasm, distinct cell borders, and oval nuclei. A few normal hepatocytes also seen (Diff-Quik stain, ×400)

- Duodenal epithelium: Cohesive sheets or clusters of uniform columnar epithelial cells intermixed with mucin-containing goblet cells.
- Gastric epithelium: Small groups, sheets, and clusters of a variety of epithelial cells; epithelial cells may include foveolar epithelial cells, chief cells, and parietal cells (Fig. 7.6).

Tips

- FNA biopsy of the liver can be performed under the guidance of abdominal ultrasound, computed tomography, or endoscopic ultrasound. The biopsies under the guidance of these imaging techniques shows similar diagnostic yields [2, 4, 6, 7]. Choice of imaging techniques may be dependent on the location of lesions and expertise available.
- Endoscopic ultrasound may be best used for the lesions located in the left lobe of the liver and is preferred when endoscopic ultrasound is also used for evaluation of primary lesions in the pancreas, biliary tract, duodenum, and stomach.
- It is always important to know the clinical aspect of lesion being biopsied including clinical differential diagnosis and travel history if an infectious etiology is suspected.

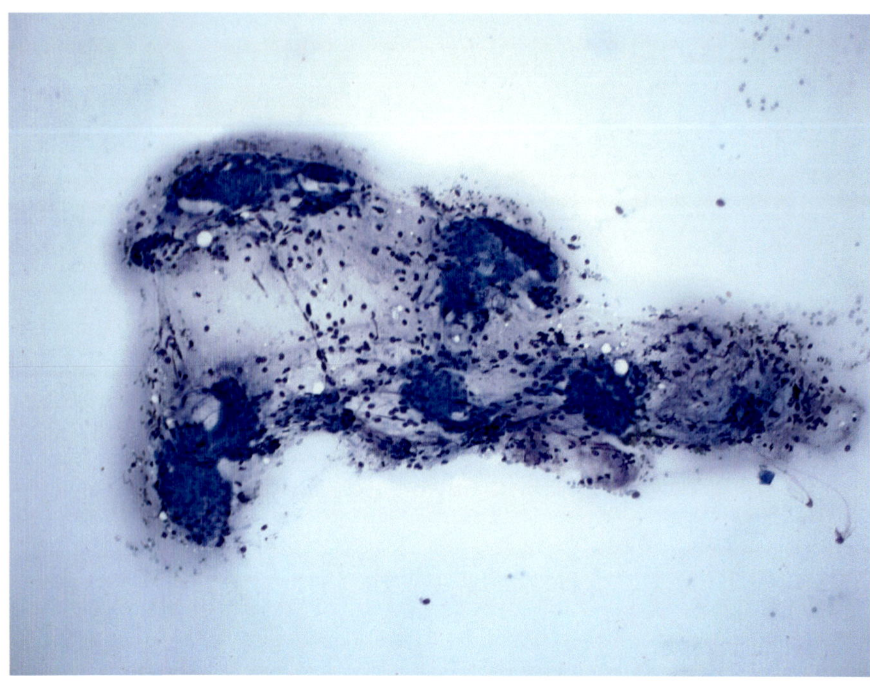

Fig. 7.6 Gastric epithelial cells. Small groups and clusters of uniform epithelial cells with small round nuclei and vacuolated cytoplasm (Diff-Quik stain, ×100)

- Knowledge of background liver diseases such as cirrhosis needs to be kept in mind, especially in rendering diagnosis of hepatocellular carcinoma.
- Based on on-site findings, it is crucial to appropriately triage specimen. Specimen needs to be submitted for culture study if infection is suspected. In cases suspected for metastatic tumors, specimen should be saved for preparation of a cell block, on which immunophenotypic analysis can be performed.
- On-site evaluation has a minimal value for evaluation of simple cystic lesions.
- In cases suspected for a well-differentiated hepatocellular carcinoma or cholangiocarcinoma, core needle biopsy may be suggested if clinically indicated.

Cystic Lesions of the Liver

Hepatic cysts are rare as compared to solid mass-forming lesions and affect about 5% of the general population. The differential diagnosis is broad and includes nonneoplastic diseases (i.e., congenital, acquired, infectious, noninfectious cysts) and, in rare cases, cystic neoplasms. FNA may be helpful in diagnosis, but findings are often nonspecific with specimens containing predominantly fluid, histiocytes, and acellular debris.

Developmental/Congenital Cyst

This is the most common hepatic cyst, accounting for more than 90% of hepatic cysts. It occurs in adults of 20–50 years with a female predominance. Unilocular; single or multiple. Usually small but may become symptomatic when larger. May be seen in polycystic liver disease.

1. Cytomorphologic features
    - Scattered histiocytes.
    - Cyst lining cells may be present.
    - Most cyst lining cells are bile duct-type glandular cells.
    - Metaplastic squamous cells may be seen.
2. Tips and pitfalls
    - The primary goal of the biopsy is to rule out a malignancy.
    - Differential diagnosis includes pseudocyst and parasitic cyst.

Hydatid Cyst

Hydatid cyst is commonly seen in Mediterranean, African, and Oceania countries and it primarily affects immigrant population in the USA. Majority of patients develop unilocular cyst; predominantly in the right hepatic lobe. May have calcifications in the cyst wall.

1. Cytomorphologic features [21, 22]
    - Cellular debris.
    - Fragments of laminated membranes.
    - Scolices and hooklets may be present.
2. Tips and pitfalls
    - Biopsy carries a risk of anaphylactic shock.
    - Differential diagnosis may include other parasitic cystic lesions.

Abscess

Liver abscess is often caused by infectious agents such as bacteria and amoeba. Patients have associated clinical symptoms.

1. Cytomorphologic features
    - Abundant neutrophils.
    - Scattered histiocytes and lymphocytes.
    - Necrotic debris.

2. Tips and pitfalls

   - It is not challenging for diagnosis in patient with clinical symptoms and typical FNA findings.
   - The caveat is to rule out a malignancy since malignancy can be associated with inflammation and necrosis.
   - Part of specimen should be sent for culture study for identification of infectious agents.

Hepatocellular Lesions

Hepatic lesions of hepatocellular origin are the most commonly encountered diseases subjected to FNA biopsy. These lesions range from nonneoplastic changes to malignant neoplasms. FNA biopsy is able, at least in most cases, to differentiate a nonneoplastic or benign lesion from malignant. However, further classification of benign lesions may be difficult based on cytomorphological analysis alone. Core needle biopsy may be needed for classification of benign lesions as well as diagnosis of well-differentiated hepatocellular carcinoma.

Regenerative Nodule

Regenerative nodules, variable in size, are the common findings in cirrhotic liver. Since cirrhosis is a risk factor for development of hepatocellular carcinoma, the possibility of hepatocellular carcinoma should be ruled out if a nodule, usually greater than 1 cm, is found in the background of cirrhosis. FNA biopsy could help, at least in most cases, the distinction of these two entities.

1. Cytomorphologic features (Figs. 7.7 and 7.8) [3, 23–25]

   - Moderate to high cellularity.
   - Normal-appearing hepatocytes in small groups and clusters.
   - Hepatocytes may have intracytoplasmic fat droplets and/or bile pigments.
   - Hepatocytes may show focal reactive atypia such as variation in nuclear size, prominent nucleolus, and binucleation.

2. Tips and pitfalls

   - Differential diagnosis may include hepatic adenoma and well-differentiated hepatocellular carcinoma.
   - Hepatic adenoma has more uniform benign-appearing hepatocytes.
   - Well-differentiated hepatocellular carcinoma is accompanied with prominent vasculatures, the feature demonstrated as endothelial wrapping and capillary traversing.

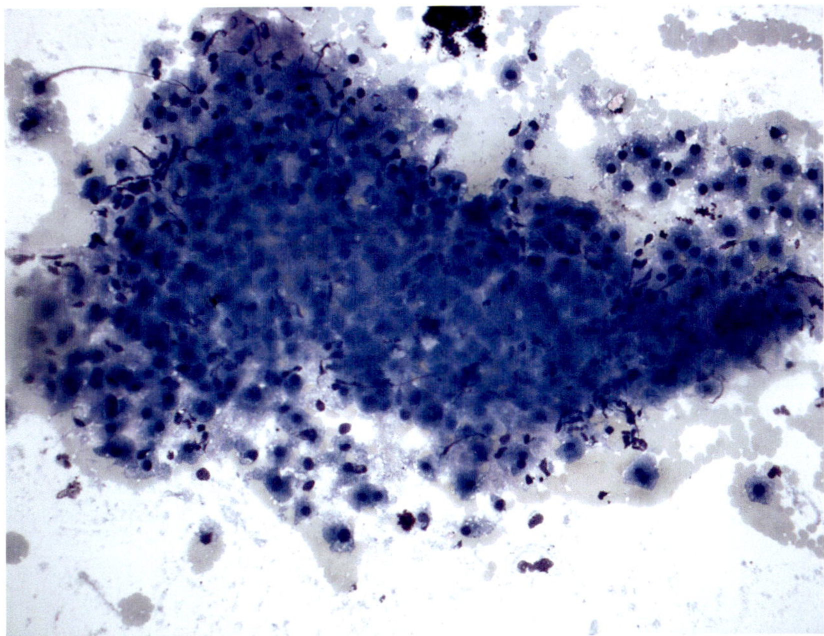

Fig. 7.7 Regenerative nodule. A cohesive cluster of hepatocytes with small round nuclei, abundant granular cytoplasm, and cytoplasmic fat droplets intermixed with a few lymphocytes (Diff-Quik stain, ×200)

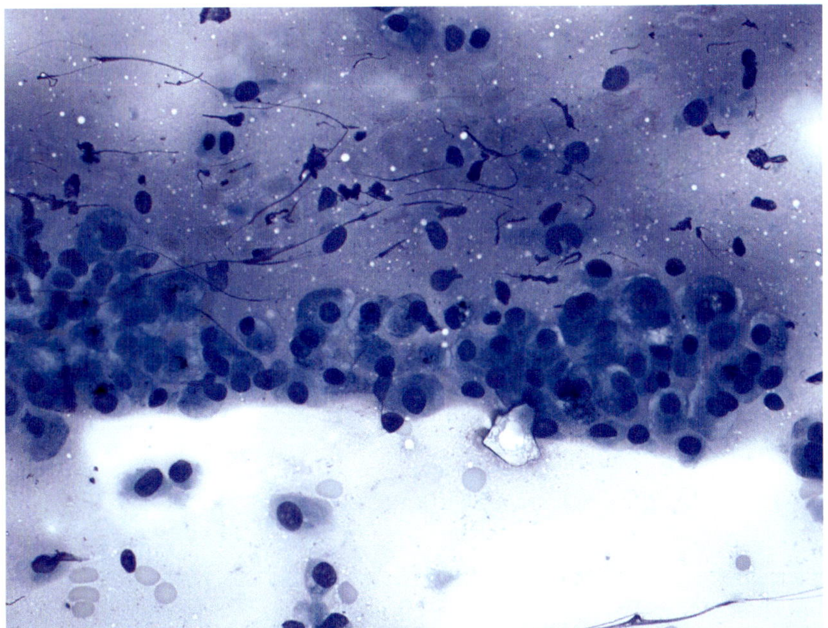

Fig. 7.8 Regenerative nodule. Single and loose groups of hepatocytes with variable-sized round nuclei, abundant granular cytoplasm, and occasional binucleation and cytoplasmic bile pigments intermixed with a few lymphocytes (Diff-Quik stain, ×400)

Focal Nodular Hyperplasia

Focal nodular hyperplasia is a benign lesion and often present as a solitary mass characterized by proliferation of hepatocytes and bile ducts with a central scar. It occurs most commonly in women of young ages.

1. Cytomorphologic features [3, 26, 27]
   - Moderate cellularity.
   - Benign-appearing hepatocytes as well as benign-appearing bile ductal cells.
   - Minimal cytological atypia.
   - Variable amount of bile ductal cells.
2. Tips and pitfalls
   - Cytologically it is difficult to distinguish from normal liver sampling.
   - In cases with a low number of bile ductal cells, differential diagnosis may include regenerative nodule and hepatic adenoma.

Hepatic Adenoma

Hepatic adenoma is a benign neoplasm. It occurs predominantly in women under the age of 30 who have history of long-term use of oral contraceptives.

1. Cytomorphologic features [3, 12, 28]
   - Moderate to high cellularity.
   - Benign-appearing uniform hepatocytes.
   - Minimal cytological atypia.
   - Bile ductal cells absent.
2. Tips and pitfalls
   - Differential diagnosis includes normal liver sampling and regenerative nodule.
   - Patient's clinical and imaging information is important for the differential diagnosis.

Well-Differentiated Hepatocellular Carcinoma

Hepatocellular carcinoma is the most common primary hepatic malignant neoplasm. It occurs mostly in patients with cirrhosis. There are wide ranges of tumor differentiation. FNA biopsy has a relatively high diagnostic accuracy for hepatocellular carcinoma.

1. Cytomorphologic features (Figs. 7.9 and 7.10) [1, 3, 10, 12, 23–25, 29, 30]

   - High cellularity.
   - Single, small groups, sheets, and clusters of relative uniform hepatocytes.
   - Hepatocytes show mild cytological atypia including increased nuclear-to-cytoplasmic ratios, nuclear enlargement, prominent nucleolus, and occasional intranuclear inclusions.
   - Hepatocytes may contain cytoplasmic bile pigments.
   - Spindle-shaped endothelial cells surround groups of hepatocytes (endothelial wrapping).
   - Groups of hepatocytes with embedded capillary vasculatures (capillary traversing).
   - Increased naked nuclei.

2. Tips and pitfalls

   - Differential diagnosis includes cirrhosis/regenerative nodule and hepatic adenoma.
   - Vascular proliferation is the key feature seen in hepatocellular carcinoma manifested by endothelial wrapping and capillary traversing on FNA cytology specimens.
   - In difficult cases, core needle biopsy may help settle diagnostic challenge.

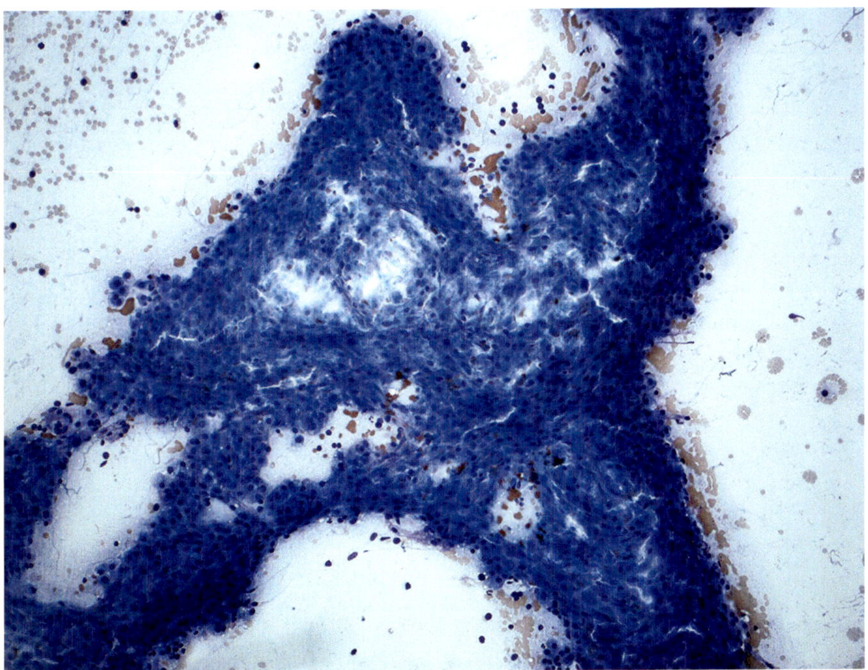

Fig. 7.9 Well-differentiated hepatocellular carcinoma. A large cohesive cluster of relatively uniform hepatocytes with round nuclei and granular cytoplasm. Capillary vasculatures with spindle nuclei seen within the cluster (Diff-Quik stain, ×100)

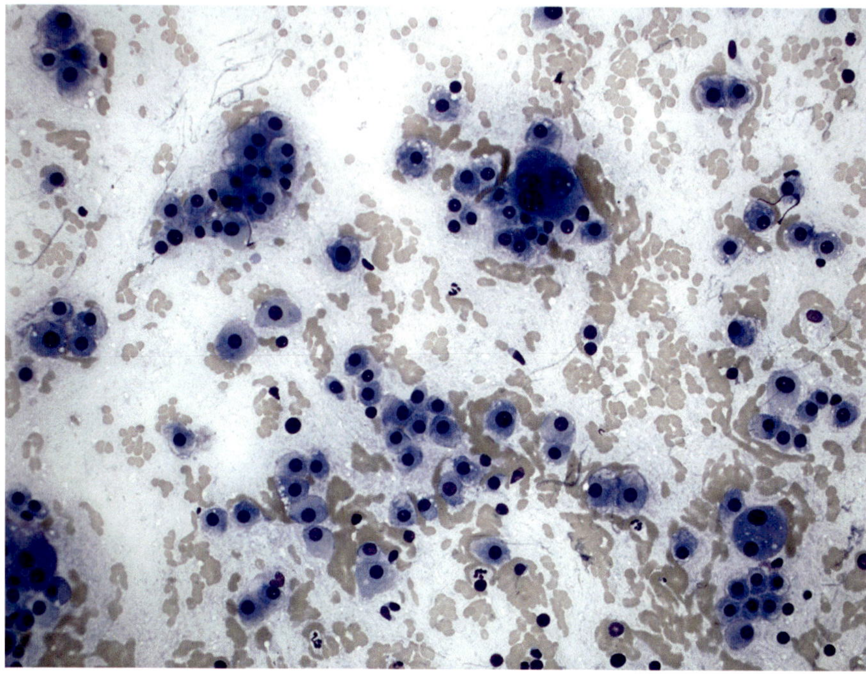

Fig. 7.10 Well-differentiated hepatocellular carcinoma. Single and small groups of hepatocytes with variable-sized round nuclei, abundant granular cytoplasm, and occasional cytoplasmic fat droplets (Diff-Quik stain, ×200)

Moderate to Poorly Differentiated Hepatocellular Carcinoma

1. Cytomorphologic features (Figs. 7.11, 7.12 and 7.13) [1, 3, 12, 29, 31]
    - High cellularity.
    - Abundant single hepatocytes besides those in small groups, cords, sheets, and clusters.
    - Pleomorphic nuclei with prominent nucleolus, occasional multinucleation, and atypical mitoses.
    - Many naked nuclei.
    - Endothelial wrapping and capillary traversing may be seen.
    - Fatty changes may be seen in some cells.
    - Morphologic variants of hepatocellular carcinoma have been described including clear cell and spindle cell variants.
2. Tips and pitfalls
    - Diagnostic challenge is that poorly differentiated hepatocellular carcinoma may have subtle or even lose morphologic characteristics of hepatocytic phenotype and then must be differentiated from poorly differentiated cholangiocarcinoma and metastatic carcinoma.

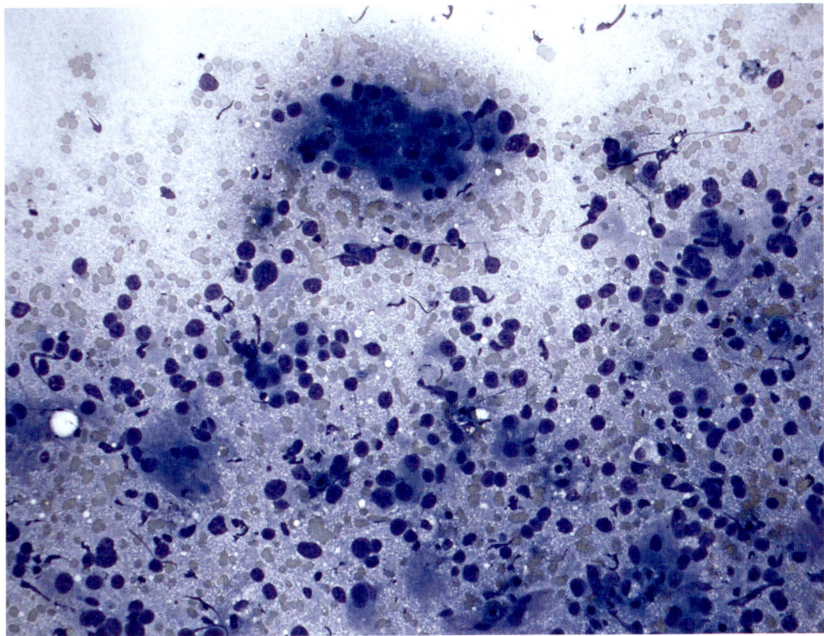

Fig. 7.11 Moderately differentiated hepatocellular carcinoma. Single and small groups of hepatocytes with variable-sized round nuclei, abundant granular cytoplasm, and conspicuous nucleolus. Fat droplets seen in cytoplasm as well as background (Diff-Quik stain, ×200)

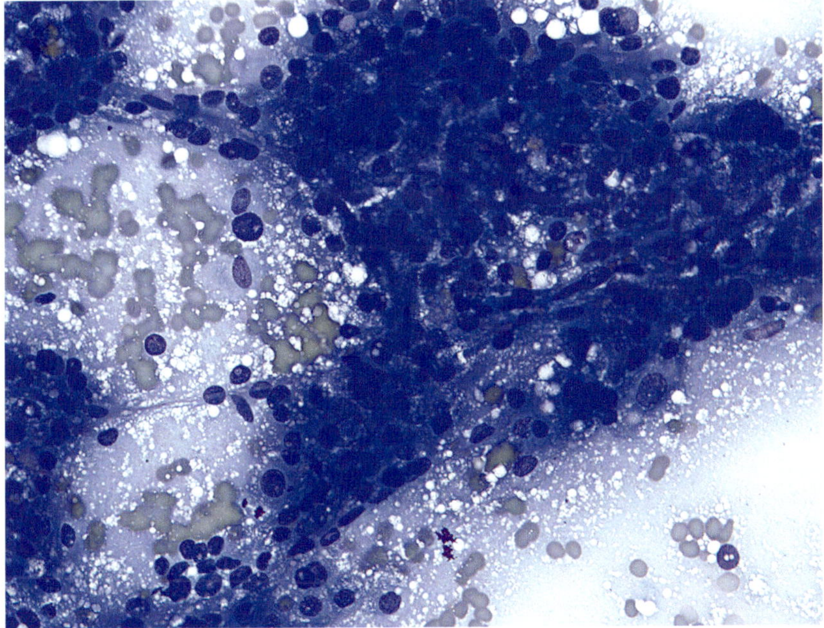

Fig. 7.12 Moderately differentiated hepatocellular carcinoma. Clusters of hepatocytes with traversing capillary vasculatures. Hepatocytes showing variable-sized round nuclei, abundant granular cytoplasm, and conspicuous nucleolus. Fat droplets seen in cytoplasm as well as background (Diff-Quik stain, ×400)

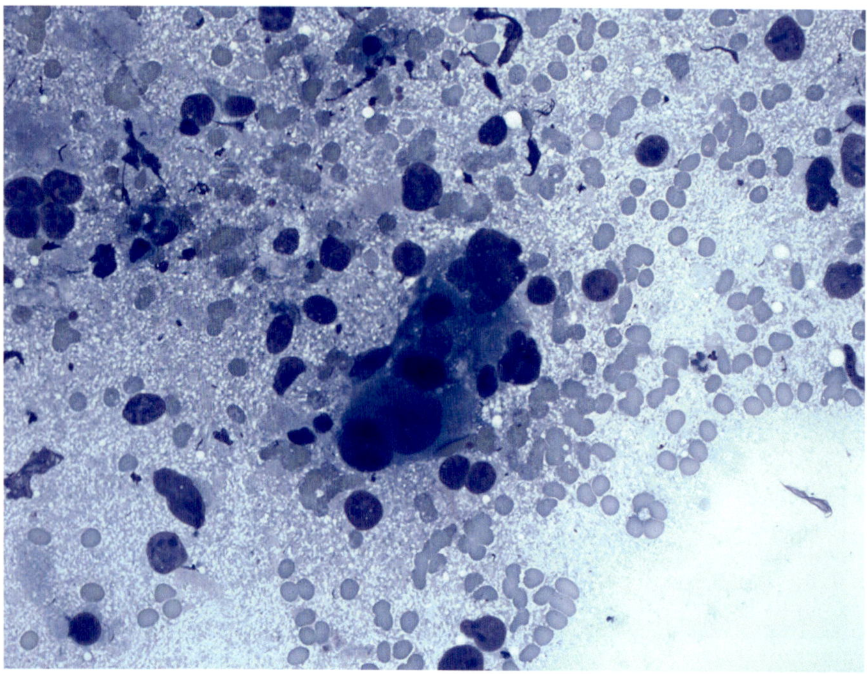

Fig. 7.13 Poorly differentiated hepatocellular carcinoma. Single and small groups of hepatocytes with pleomorphic nuclei, abundant granular cytoplasm, and prominent nucleolus. Fat droplets seen in cytoplasm as well as background (Diff-Quik stain, ×400)

- Immunophenotypic analysis with hepatocytic markers such as HepPar1 and arginase as well as glypican 3 may help establish diagnosis of poorly differentiated hepatocellular carcinoma.

Fibrolamellar Hepatocellular Carcinoma

Fibrolamellar hepatocellular carcinoma is an uncommon malignant tumor with distinct clinical and histopathologic features. It occurs almost exclusively in young patients with ages under 35. The tumor is not associated with cirrhosis.

1. Cytomorphologic features [32, 33]

   - High cellularity.
   - Single and loose clusters of large pleomorphic cells.
   - Abundant granular cytoplasm with possible intracytoplasmic hyaline globules.

- Large vesicular nuclei with large prominent nucleolus.
- Scant fibrous tissue may be seen separating clusters of hepatocytes.

2. Tips and pitfalls

- Although tumor cells are large, nuclear-to-cytoplasmic ratios are low in fibrolamellar hepatocellular carcinoma.
- Patient's unique demographic and clinical information is helpful for diagnosis.
- Tumor cells stains positive for hepatocyte markers but also stain positive for CK7.

Hepatoblastoma

Hepatoblastoma is a rare malignant tumor which occurs mostly in children under age of 5. It is characterized by variable combination of several epithelial and mesenchymal elements.

1. Cytomorphologic features [34–36]

- Moderate to high cellularity.
- Epithelial and mesenchymal elements in varying proportions and at variable stages of differentiation.
- Epithelial elements: wide-range morphologies of hepatocyte-like cells, large anaplastic cells, and undifferentiated small cells.
- Variable amounts of mesenchymal elements: fibrous, calcified stroma, and osteoid-like tissue.

2. Tips and pitfalls

- Difficult to diagnose by FNA; extensive sampling is needed.
- Differential diagnosis includes the tumors that may occur in young patients, including infantile hemangioendothelioma, mesenchymal hamartoma, and angiomyolipoma.

Bile Duct Lesions

Bile duct lesions are much less common and include reactive bile ductile proliferation, bile duct adenoma, and intrahepatic cholangiocarcinoma. It is important to separate cholangiocarcinoma from other lesions. Core needle biopsy may be required for diagnosis of well-differentiated cholangiocarcinoma.

Reactive Bile Ductile Proliferation

Reactive bile ductal proliferation is often associated with cirrhosis, biliary tract disorders, and focal nodular hyperplasia and present as multiple irregular nodules.

1. Cytomorphologic features

   - Low to moderate cellularity.
   - Small uniform epithelial cells arranged in small acinar groups or flat sheets.
   - Vacuolated cytoplasm and round nuclei with smooth nuclear contours and evenly distributed chromatin.
   - Mild cytological atypia including nuclear enlargement or conspicuous nucleolus may be seen; bile pigments may be seen.
   - Variable number of benign-appearing hepatocytes may be present.

2. Tips and pitfalls

   - Differential diagnosis includes bile duct adenoma/hamartoma and cholangiocarcinoma.
   - It is difficult to distinguish reactive bile ductile proliferation from bile duct adenoma or hamartoma based on the cytomorphology alone. Clinical and imaging findings may be helpful.
   - It is important to exclude cholangiocarcinoma which shows more cytological atypia. In difficult cases, follow-up with core needle biopsy should be considered.

Bile Duct Adenoma/Hamartoma

Bile duct adenoma is typically a single small subcapsular nodule, while bile duct hamartoma has multiple nodules, also known as von Meyenburg complex. They share the same histopathologic feature, i.e., proliferating bile ducts embedded in fibrous tissue.

1. Cytomorphologic features

   - Hypocellular specimen.
   - Small uniform epithelial cells arranged in small acinar groups or flat sheets.
   - Vacuolated cytoplasm and round nuclei with smooth nuclear contours and evenly distributed chromatin.
   - Hepatocytes often absent.

2. Tips and pitfalls

   - Diagnostic clue is a single population of bland bile ductal cells.
   - Differential diagnosis includes reactive bile duct proliferation and more importantly cholangiocarcinoma.

Cholangiocarcinoma

Cholangiocarcinoma is less common than hepatocellular carcinoma but is the second most common primary malignant tumor of the liver. It can arise in the intrahepatic or extrahepatic bile duct and is often not associated with cirrhosis. Dependent on the location, tumor can be sampled via bile duct brushing/biopsy or be evaluated by FNA [37, 38].

1. Cytomorphologic features (Figs. 7.14, 7.15, and 7.16) [4, 8, 39, 40]
   - Moderate to hypercellular specimen.
   - Single, loose groups and clusters of cuboidal or low columnar tumor cells.
   - Scant to moderate amount of vacuolated cytoplasm.
   - Enlarged nuclei with variation in size and nuclear overlapping.
   - Coarse chromatin and conspicuous nucleolus.
2. Tips and pitfalls
   - Differential diagnosis includes hepatocellular carcinoma and metastatic adenocarcinoma.
   - Cholangiocarcinoma may have some overlapping cytomorphologic features with hepatocellular carcinoma, especially clear cell hepatocellular carcinoma.

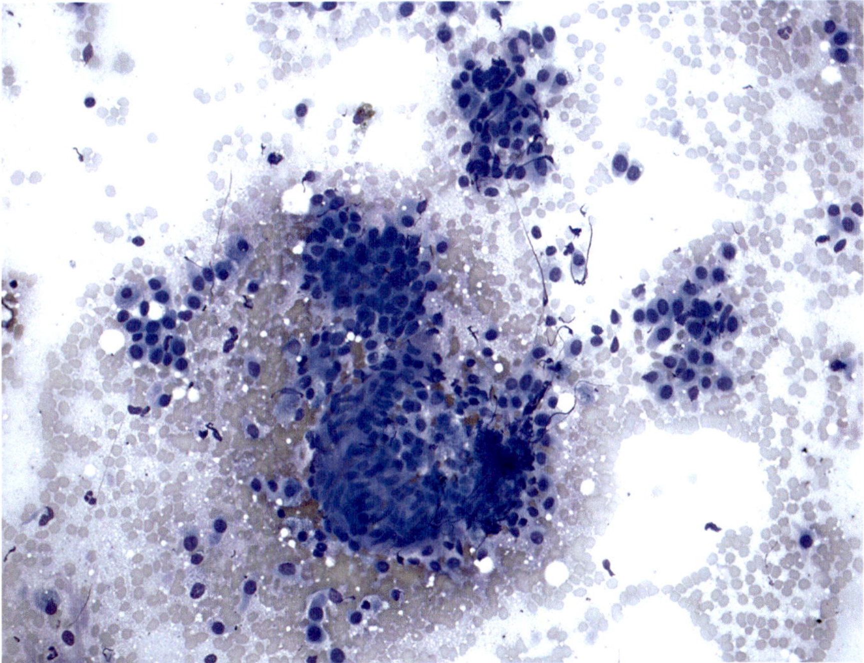

Fig. 7.14 Well-differentiated cholangiocarcinoma. Single and small groups of epithelial cells with enlarged round nuclei and vacuolated cytoplasm (Diff-Quik stain, ×200)

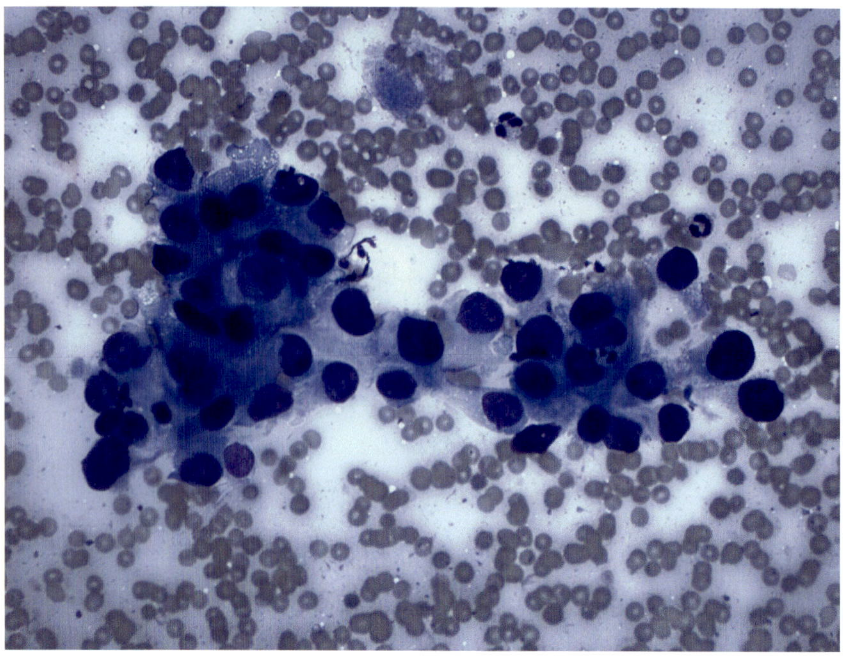

Fig. 7.15 Well-differentiated cholangiocarcinoma. Single groups of epithelial cells with enlarged round to oval nuclei, vacuolated cytoplasm, and conspicuous nucleolus (Diff-Quik stain, ×400)

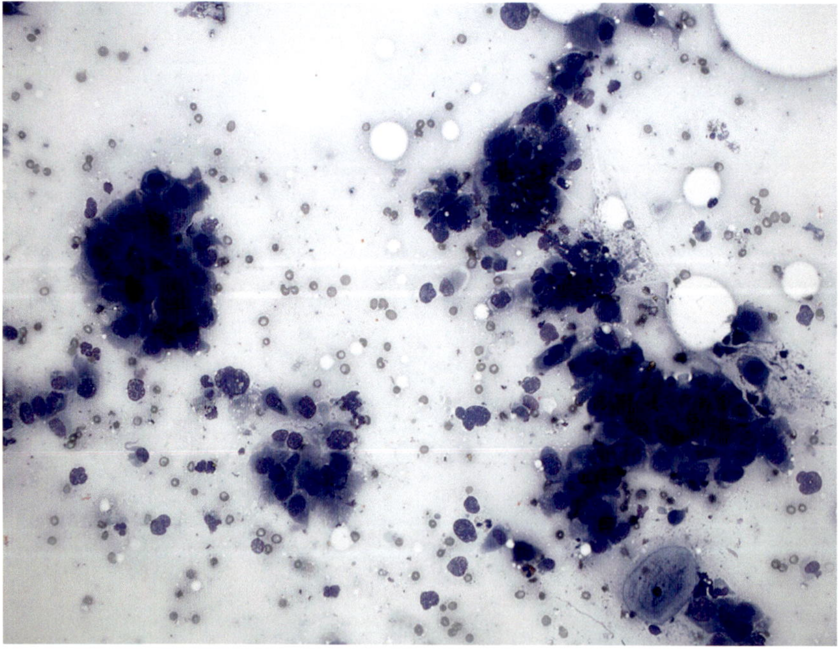

Fig. 7.16 Poorly differentiated cholangiocarcinoma. Single and small clusters of epithelial cells with enlarged pleomorphic nuclei, vacuolated cytoplasm, and conspicuous nucleolus (Diff-Quik stain, ×200)

However, cholangiocarcinoma does not have sinusoidal capillary vasculatures and bile pigments. Immunocytochemical analysis offers a discriminatory profile that helps separate these two entities.
- Morphologically, it is almost impossible to differentiate cholangiocarcinoma from metastatic adenocarcinomas, particularly of breast and pancreas origin. Clinical history, imaging findings, and immunophenotyping are often needed.

Combined Hepatocellular Carcinoma and Cholangiocarcinoma

Combined hepatocellular carcinoma and cholangiocarcinoma is a rare occurrence.

1. Cytomorphologic features
   - Hypercellular specimen.
   - Duo populations of tumor cells in variable proportions.
   - Hepatocellular carcinoma component: polygonal cells with granular cytoplasm, round nuclei, prominent nucleolus, and sometimes bile pigments.
   - Cholangiocarcinoma component: cuboidal or low columnar cells with vacuolated cytoplasm, round or oval nuclei, and small conspicuous nucleolus.
2. Tips and pitfalls
   - Differential diagnosis may include cholangiocarcinoma, hepatocellular carcinoma, as well as metastatic carcinoma.
   - Morphological demonstration of duo tumor cell population with confirmatory immunocytochemical analysis may be required for a diagnosis.

Vascular Lesions

Vascular tumors are commonly seen in the liver, ranging from benign hemangioma to malignant angiosarcoma. Most of hepatic vascular tumors are benign with hemangioma being the most common benign tumor found in the liver. FNA biopsy of hepatic vascular tumors most likely yields low cellularity specimen with bloody background. Clinical correlation and correlation with imaging findings are critically important for diagnosing this category of tumors.

Hemangioma

Hemangioma is the tumor with dilated vascular spaces lined by benign endothelial cells. It has characteristic imaging findings and is infrequently subjected to FNA biopsy. Rather, FNA is often used to rule out malignancy in cases with atypical findings on imaging.

1. Cytomorphologic features [4, 13]

   - Very low cellularity.
   - Isolated or small clusters of spindle cells with bland cytomorphology.
   - Bloody background.
   - Benign hepatocytes may be present.

2. Tips and pitfalls

   - Bloody specimen with rare bland spindle cells is a common finding.
   - Spindle cells may be not present in some cases; and thus, confirming biopsy needle location may help ease the concern for inadequate sampling.
   - Correlation with imaging findings is required.

Angiosarcoma

Angiosarcoma is an uncommon malignant tumor in the liver, accounting for less than 1% of primary hepatic malignancies.

1. Cytomorphologic features [41] (Fig. 7.17)

   - Single and clusters of spindle cells or epithelioid cells.
   - Pleomorphic nuclei with prominent nucleoli.

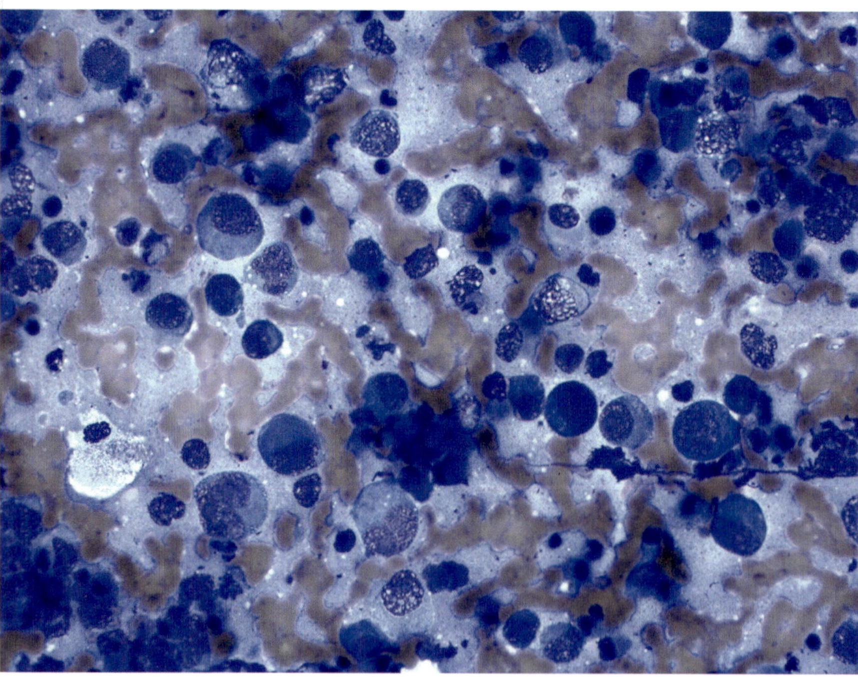

Fig. 7.17 Epithelioid angiosarcoma. Single and loose cohesive groups of large pleomorphic cells with high nuclear-to-cytoplasmic ratios, eccentrically located nuclei, and occasional mitoses (Diff-Quik stain, ×400)

- Vacuolated cytoplasm may contain red blood cells or neutrophils.
- Frequent mitoses including atypical mitoses.
- Necrosis may be present.

2. Tips and pitfalls

- Differential diagnosis may include poorly differentiated primary or metastatic tumors.
- Cytomorphologic features are not entirely specific; and confirmatory immunostains with ERG, CD31, and CD34 are diagnostic.

Epithelioid Hemangioendothelioma

Epithelioid hemangioendothelioma is an uncommon vascular tumor with a less aggressive clinical course as compared to angiosarcoma.

1. Cytomorphologic features [42]

- Moderate to high cellularity.
- Dispersed single or clusters of epithelioid cells with folded nuclei and conspicuous nucleoli.
- Spindle tumor cells may be present.
- Occasional cytoplasmic vacuoles.
- Mitoses are rare and necrosis is absent.

2. Tips and pitfalls

- Epithelioid hemangioendothelioma should be distinguished from angiosarcoma, which is largely based on cytomorphological analysis.
- Due to its epithelioid cell morphology, the differential diagnosis should include cholangiocarcinoma, hepatocellular carcinoma, metastatic carcinoma, and melanoma.
- The diagnosis requires confirmatory ERG, CD31, and CD34 immunostains but with a low Ki-67 index.

Angiomyolipoma

Although uncommon, liver is the most common site outside the kidney to have angiomyolipoma. The presence of fat component in angiomyolipoma allows an accurate diagnosis by imaging studies.

1. Cytomorphologic features [43]

- Moderate cellularity.
- Mixed fat, epithelioid cells/spindle cells (myoid cells), and vascular tissue in variable proportions.
- Epithelioid variant shows predominant epithelioid cells.
- Extramedullary hematopoiesis may be seen in some cases.

2. Tips and pitfalls

    - Although angiomyolipoma has a triad of fat, vessel, and myoid elements, only the myoid component is specific for the diagnosis. Myoid element can be confirmed by melanocytic markers such as Melan A and HMB45 as well as smooth muscle marker SMA.
    - Angiomyolipoma should be differentiated from myelolipoma and nodular hematopoiesis.
    - Differential diagnosis for epithelioid angiomyolipoma may include hepatocellular carcinoma, cholangiocarcinoma, and metastatic tumor.

Metastatic Tumors

Metastatic tumors are more commonly seen than primary neoplasms in the liver. The liver has a unique duo blood supply system through the hepatic artery and portal vein; thus, metastatic tumors can originate from organs of the portal systems such as the gastrointestinal tract and pancreaticobiliary as well as from the organs such as the lung, breast, and skin through the systemic circulation [11, 12, 17, 44]. Most metastatic tumors have cytomorphologic features which can help differential diagnosis from primary hepatic tumors, mainly hepatocellular carcinoma and intrahepatic cholangiocarcinoma. However, there are cytomorphologic features that are shared by primary and some metastatic tumors. For example, metastatic well-differentiated pancreatic ductal adenocarcinoma or extrahepatic cholangiocarcinoma can have similar features as primary intrahepatic cholangiocarcinoma. In addition to cytomorphology, clinical history, imaging findings, and immunophenotypic analysis are often required to render a diagnosis of metastatic tumor.

Metastatic Colorectal Adenocarcinoma

This is one of the most common metastatic tumors seen in the liver. Most patients have a documented history of colorectal adenocarcinoma.

1. Cytomorphologic features (Figs. 7.18 and 7.19)

    - Clusters of tumor cells in a necrotic background.
    - Tumor cells are columnar in shape and have vacuolated cytoplasm and oval hyperchromatic nuclei, arranged in sheets or acinar pattern.
    - Single tumor cells may be seen.

2. Tips and pitfalls

    - History of colorectal adenocarcinoma with classic cytomorphologic features is often sufficient for a diagnosis.
    - In some cases, immunostains may be needed for differential diagnosis. The tumor cells are typically positive for CK20 and CDX2 while negative for CK7.

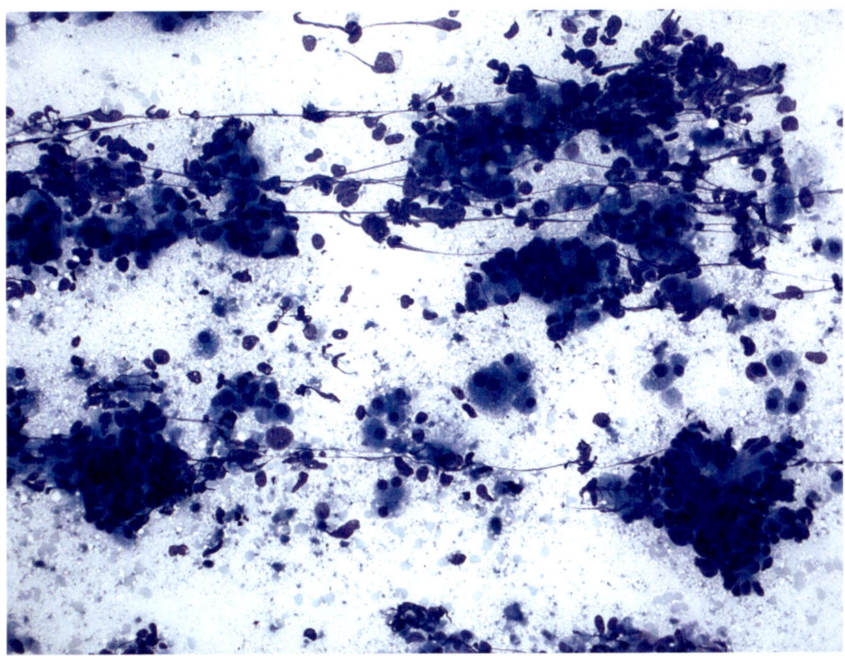

Fig. 7.18 Metastatic colonic adenocarcinoma. Single and small groups of epithelial cells with oval to columnar nuclei and vacuolated cytoplasm in a necrotic background. Scattered reactive hepatocytes also seen (Diff-Quik stain, ×200)

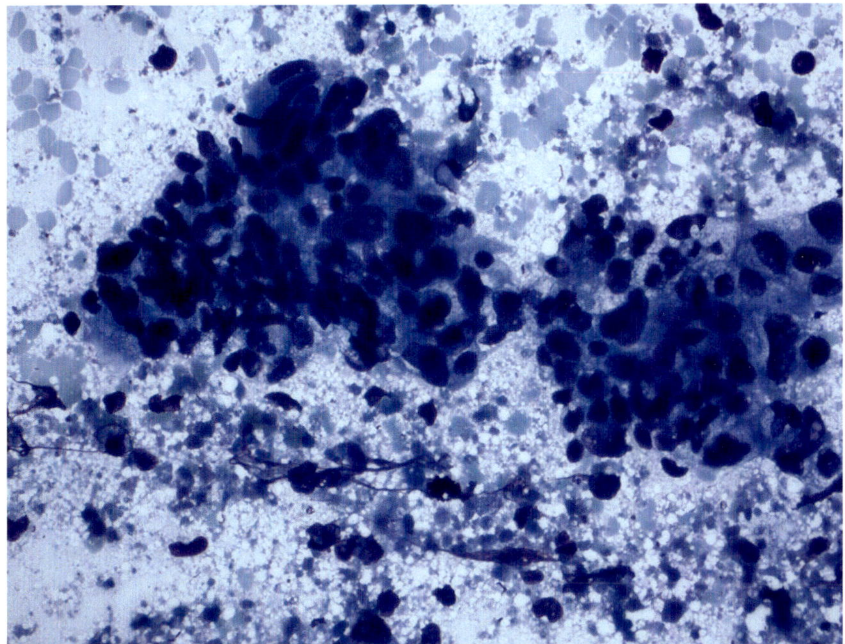

Fig. 7.19 Metastatic colonic adenocarcinoma. Small groups of epithelial cells with oval to columnar nuclei and vacuolated cytoplasm in a necrotic background (Diff-Quik stain, ×400)

Metastatic Pancreatic Adenocarcinoma

Liver is the common primary site for pancreatic adenocarcinoma to metastasize to. Metastasis can be documented during initial evaluation of pancreatic tumors or after patients receive treatments.

1. Cytomorphologic features (Fig. 7.20)
   - Clusters of tumor cells with scattered single cells.
   - Variable cytological atypia.
   - Tumor cells have vacuolated cytoplasm, irregular nuclear contours, and conspicuous nucleolus.
   - Necrosis may be present.
2. Tips and pitfalls
   - Morphological comparison with primary pancreatic tumor is the key to establish a diagnosis of metastatic disease.
   - Differential diagnosis should include cholangiocarcinoma and metastatic adenocarcinoma from other primaries.
   - Immunostains may be helpful for exclusion of other primary sites such as lung and breast.

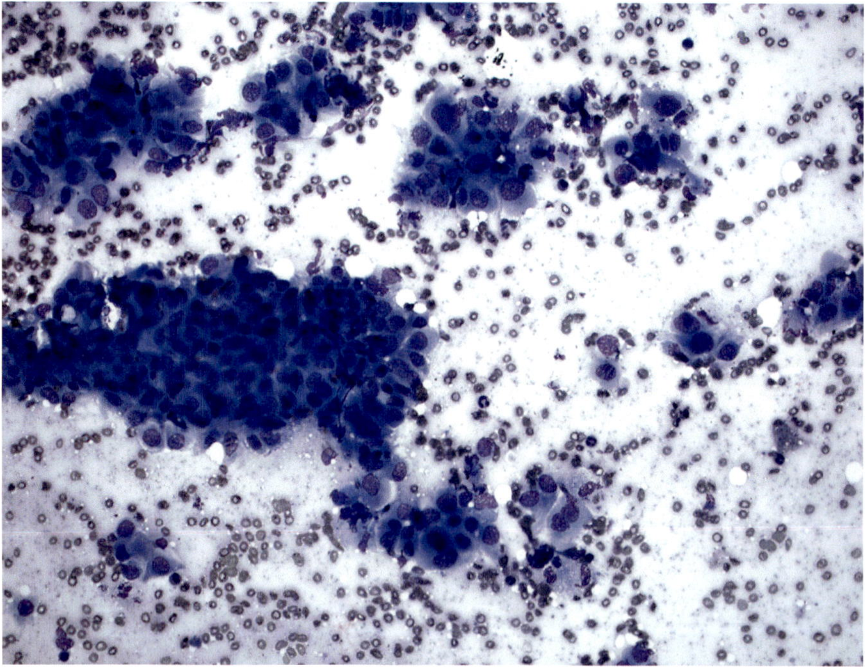

Fig. 7.20 Metastatic pancreatic adenocarcinoma. Single and small groups of epithelial cells with round to oval nuclei, variation in nuclear size, vacuolated cytoplasm, and conspicuous nucleolus (Diff-Quik stain, ×200)

Metastatic Lung Carcinoma

Most patients have a recent diagnosis of lung carcinoma, including adenocarcinoma, squamous cell carcinoma, and small cell carcinoma.

1. Cytomorphologic features
   - Adenocarcinoma: single and loose cohesive clusters of tumor cells with vacuolated cytoplasm, pleomorphic nuclei, irregular nuclear contours, and conspicuous nucleolus (Fig. 7.21).
   - Squamous cell carcinoma: loose groups or sheets of tumor cells with dense cytoplasm, pleomorphic hyperchromatic nuclei, and inconspicuous nucleolus. Necrosis is often present (Fig. 7.22).
   - Small cell carcinoma: single and dyscohesive clusters of intermediate-sized tumor cells with scant cytoplasm, nuclear molding, and inconspicuous nucleolus. Necrosis and apoptosis are often seen.
2. Tips and pitfalls
   - Patient's history plays an important role for metastatic work-up.
   - The markers such as TTF-1 and Napsin A are helpful for elucidation of lung origin of metastatic adenocarcinoma.

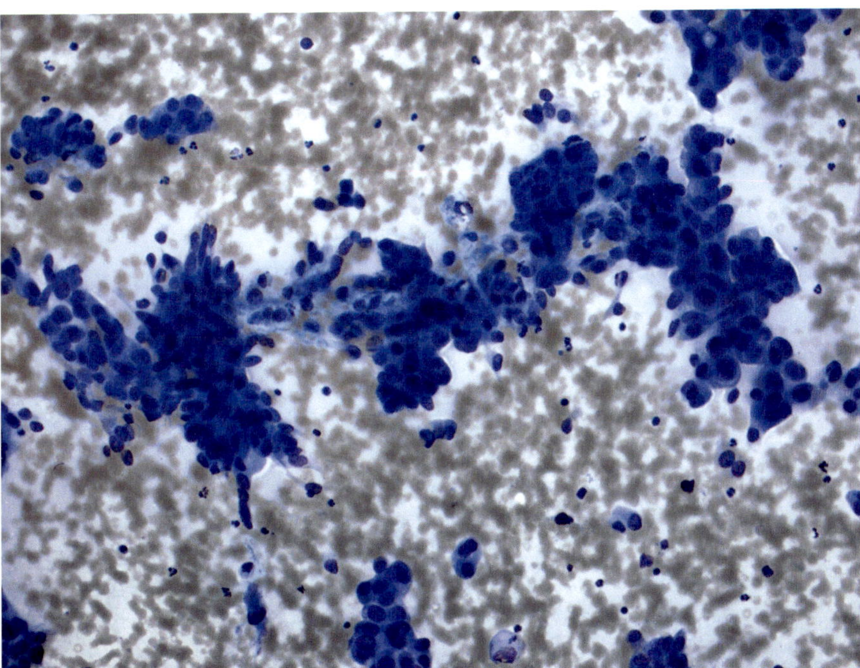

Fig. 7.21 Metastatic lung adenocarcinoma. Single and small groups of epithelial cells with round to oval nuclei, variation in nuclear size, vacuolated cytoplasm, and conspicuous nucleolus (Diff-Quik stain, ×200)

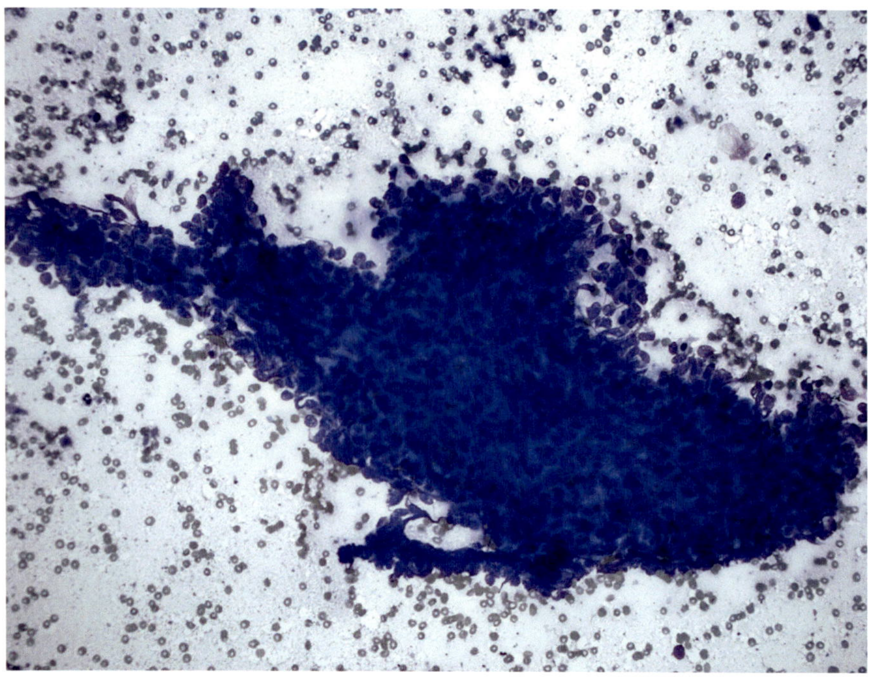

Fig. 7.22 Metastatic lung squamous cell carcinoma. A single cluster of epithelial cells with high nuclear-to-cytoplasmic ratios, oval nuclei, and dense cytoplasm (Diff-Quik stain, ×200)

- In cases of metastatic small cell carcinoma, TTF-1 is not a reliable marker for lung primary since TTF-1 positivity has been seen in small cell carcinomas of non-lung origin.

Metastatic Breast Carcinoma

Breast carcinoma is the most common type of cancers seen in women. Ductal carcinoma is far more common than lobular carcinoma. Metastatic breast carcinoma can occur many years after initial diagnosis and treatment.

1. Cytomorphologic features (Fig. 7.23)

   - Ductal carcinoma: clusters of relatively uniform tumor cells with moderate amount of cytoplasm, eccentrically located nuclei, and conspicuous nucleolus.
   - Lobular carcinoma: single and loose groups of relatively uniform tumor cells with electrically located nuclei and occasional cytoplasmic vacuoles.

2. Tips and pitfalls

   - Tumor cells with relatively bland cytomorphology raises the possibility of metastatic breast carcinoma.
   - The differential diagnosis may include cholangiocarcinoma and metastatic well-differentiated pancreatic ductal adenocarcinoma.

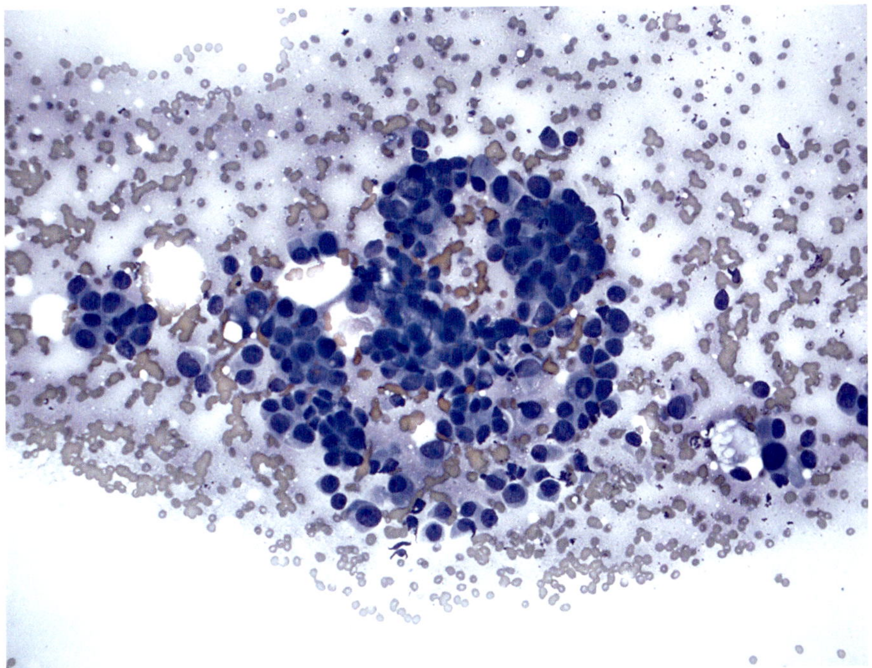

Fig. 7.23 Metastatic breast adenocarcinoma. Single and small groups of epithelial cells with eccentrically located round to oval nuclei, variation in nuclear size, vacuolated cytoplasm, and conspicuous nucleolus (Diff-Quik stain, ×200)

- Additional material should be requested for preparation of cell block, on which breast origin markers such as GATA3, mammaglobin, and GCDFP15 as well as ER, PR, and HER2 tests can be performed.

Metastatic Neuroendocrine Neoplasm

Neuroendocrine tumors metastatic to the liver mostly originate from the pancreas and gastrointestinal tract, most of which are well differentiated.

1. Cytomorphologic features (Fig. 7.24)
   - Loosely cohesive groups of relatively uniform tumor cells.
   - Tumor cells have moderate amount of cytoplasm and eccentrically located oval nuclei with inconspicuous nucleolus.
   - Occasional binucleation.
2. Tips and pitfalls
   - Documented history and morphological comparison are the most important elements.
   - Immunophenotypic analysis help confirm neuroendocrine differentiation but add little for identification of possible primary sites.

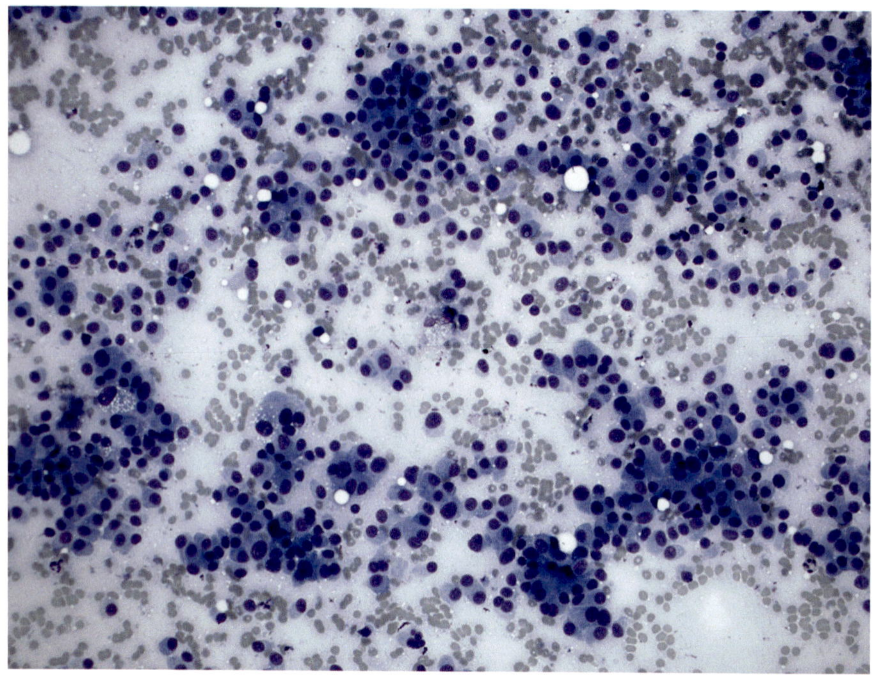

Fig. 7.24 Metastatic well-differentiated neuroendocrine tumor. Single and small groups of epithelioid cells with eccentrically located round to oval nuclei, dense cytoplasm with occasional cytoplasmic vacuoles, and inconspicuous nucleolus (Diff-Quik stain, ×200)

Metastatic Sarcoma

Metastatic sarcoma to the liver is a rare occurrence.

1. Cytomorphologic features (Fig. 7.25)

   - Single or loose groups of tumor cells.
   - Often spindle cells, but could be epithelioid.
   - Variable cytological atypia.
   - Matrix may be present in the background or intermixed with tumor cells.

2. Tips and pitfalls

   - Patients often have history of sarcoma.
   - Comparison with histological or cytological specimen of the original tumor is the key to render a correct diagnosis.

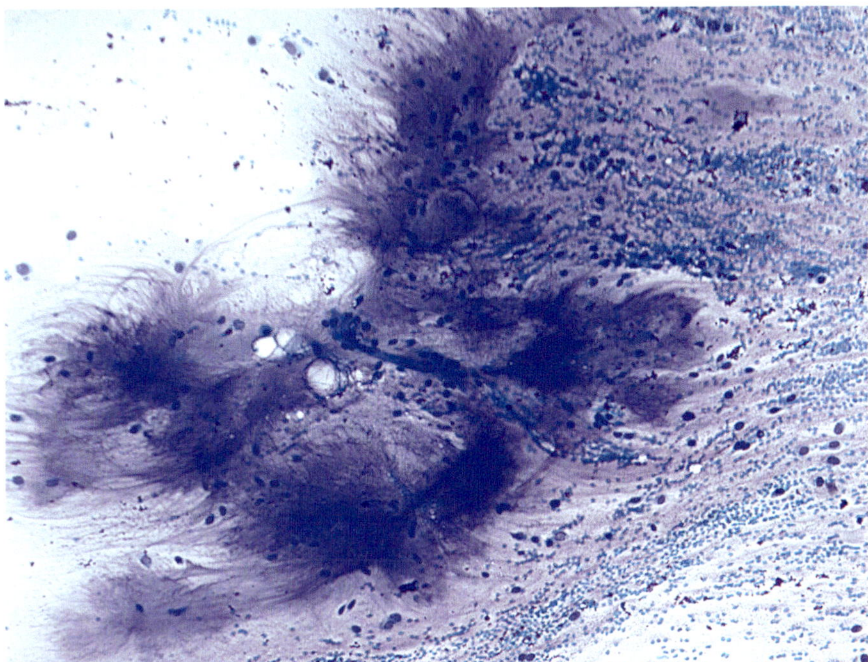

Fig. 7.25 Metastatic myxoid liposarcoma. Abundant myxoid material, scattered epithelioid cells with scant cytoplasm intermixed with occasional lipoblasts, and capillary vasculature (Diff-Quik stain, ×100)

Metastatic Melanoma

Patients vary in ages and often have documented history of melanoma.

1. Cytomorphologic features (Fig. 7.26)

   - Melanoma is a great mimic for many tumors due to its diverse morphologic features.
   - Dispersed single cells and loosely cohesive groups.
   - Epithelioid cells or spindle cells.
   - Classical morphology includes large tumor cells with eccentrically located nuclei, prominent nucleoli, and occasional intranuclear inclusions and binucleation.
   - Melanin pigments may be present.

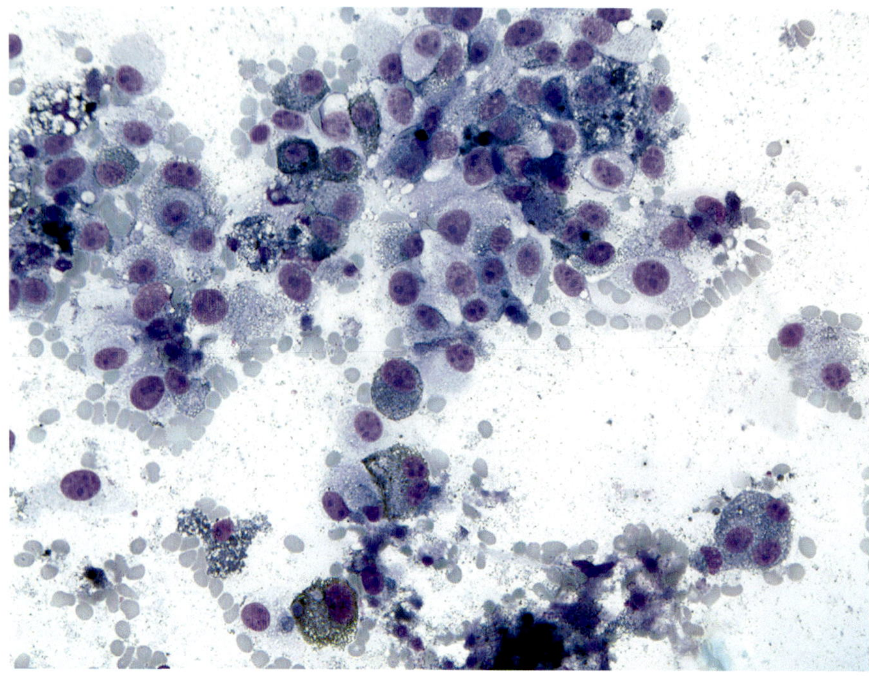

Fig. 7.26 Metastatic melanoma. Single and small groups of epithelioid cells with oval nuclei and prominent nucleolus and abundant cytoplasmic melanin pigments (Diff-Quik stain, ×200)

2. Tips and pitfalls

   - Metastatic melanoma should always be included in the differential diagnosis for metastatic tumor work-up, especially in patients with history of melanoma.
   - No single morphologic feature can reliably rule in or rule out metastatic melanoma.
   - Immunocytochemical analysis with melanocytic markers such as SOX10, Melan A, and HMB45 is often required for rendering a diagnosis. S100 may need to be included in the panel when dealing spindle cell melanoma.

References

1. Bottles K, Cohen MB. An approach to fine needle aspiration biopsy diagnosis of hepatic masses. Diagn Cytopathol. 1991;7(2):204–10.
2. Edoute Y, Tibon-Fisher O, Ben-Haim SA, Malberger E. Imaging-guided and nonimaging-guided fine needle aspiration of liver lesions: experience with 406 patients. J Surg Oncol. 1991;48(4):246–51.
3. Dodd LG, Mooney EE, Layfield LJ, Nelson RC. Fine-needle aspiration of the liver and pancreas: a cytology primer for radiologists. Radiology. 1997;203(1):1–9.

4. Hertz G, Reddy VB, Green L, Spitz D, Massarani-Wafai R, Selvaggi SM, Kluskens L, Gattuso P. Fine-needle aspiration biopsy of the liver: a multicenter study of 602 radiologically guided FNA. Diagn Cytopathol. 2000;23(5):326–8.
5. Guo Z, Kurtycz DF, Salem R, De Las Casas LE, Caya JG, Hoerl HD. Radiologically guided percutaneous fine-needle aspiration biopsy of the liver: retrospective study of 119 cases evaluating diagnostic effectiveness and clinical complications. Diagn Cytopathol. 2002;26(5): 283–9.
6. tenBerge J, Hoffman BJ, Hawes RH, Van Enckevort C, Giovannini M, Erickson RA, Catalano MF, Fogel R, Mallery S, Faigel DO, Ferrari AP, Waxman I, Palazzo L, Ben-Menachem T, Jowell PS, McGrath KM, Kowalski TE, Nguyen CC, Wassef WY, Yamao K, Chak A, Greenwald BD, Woodward TA, Vilmann P, Sabbagh L, Wallace MB. EUS-guided fine needle aspiration of the liver: indications, yield, and safety based on an international survey of 167 cases. Gastrointest Endosc. 2002;55(7):859–62.
7. DeWitt J, LeBlanc J, McHenry L, Ciaccia D, Imperiale T, Chappo J, Cramer H, McGreevy K, Chriswell M, Sherman S. Endoscopic ultrasound-guided fine needle aspiration cytology of solid liver lesions: a large single-center experience. Am J Gastroenterol. 2003;98(9): 1976–81.
8. Crowe DR, Eloubeidi MA, Chhieng DC, Jhala NC, Jhala D, Eltoum IA. Fine-needle aspiration biopsy of hepatic lesions: computerized tomographic-guided versus endoscopic ultrasound-guided FNA. Cancer. 2006;108(3):180–5.
9. Eloubeidi MA, Tamhane A. Prospective assessment of diagnostic utility and complications of endoscopic ultrasound-guided fine needle aspiration. Results from a newly developed academic endoscopic ultrasound program. Dig Dis. 2008;26(4):356–63.
10. Kuo FY, Chen WJ, Lu SN, Wang JH, Eng HL. Fine needle aspiration cytodiagnosis of liver tumors. Acta Cytol. 2004;48(2):142–8.
11. Khurana U, Handa U, Mohan H, Sachdev A. Evaluation of aspiration cytology of the liver space occupying lesions by simultaneous examination of smears and cell blocks. Diagn Cytopathol. 2009;37(8):557–63.
12. Wee A. Fine needle aspiration biopsy of hepatocellular carcinoma and hepatocellular nodular lesions: role, controversies and approach to diagnosis. Cytopathology. 2011;22(5): 287–305.
13. Soudah B, Schirakowski A, Gebel M, Potthoff A, Braubach P, Schlue J, Krech T, Dämmrich ME, Kreipe HH, Abbas M. Overview and evaluation of the value of fine needle aspiration cytology in determining the histogenesis of liver nodules: 14 years of experience at Hannover Medical School. Oncol Rep. 2015;33(1):81–7.
14. Mohanty SK, Pradhan D, Sharma S, Sharma A, Patnaik N, Feuerman M, Bonasara R, Boyd A, Friedel D, Stavropoulos S, Gupta M. Endoscopic ultrasound guided fine-needle aspiration: what variables influence diagnostic yield? Diagn Cytopathol. 2018;46(4): 293–8.
15. Eloubeidi MA, Tamhane A, Jhala N, Chhieng D, Jhala D, Crowe DR, Eltoum IA. Agreement between rapid onsite and final cytologic interpretations of EUS-guided FNA specimens: implications for the endosonographer and patient management. Am J Gastroenterol. 2006;101(12):2841–7.
16. Kaçar Özkara S, Ozöver Tuneli I. Fine needle aspiration cytopathology of liver masses: 101 cases with cyto−/histopathological analysis. Acta Cytol. 2013;57(4):332–6.
17. McGahan JP, Bishop J, Webb J, Howell L, Torok N, Lamba R, Corwin MT. Role of FNA and core biopsy of primary and metastatic liver disease. Int J Hepatol. 2013;2013:174103.
18. Lee YN, Moon JH, Kim HK, Choi HJ, Choi MH, Kim DC, Lee TH, Lee TH, Cha SW, Kim SG, Kim YS. Usefulness of endoscopic ultrasound-guided sampling using core biopsy needle as a percutaneous biopsy rescue for diagnosis of solid liver mass: combined histological-cytological analysis. J Gastroenterol Hepatol. 2015;30(7):1161–6.
19. Pineda JJ, Diehl DL, Miao CL, Johal AS, Khara HS, Bhanushali A, Chen EZ. EUS-guided liver biopsy provides diagnostic samples comparable with those via the percutaneous or transjugular route. Gastrointest Endosc. 2016;83(2):360–5.

20. Schulman AR, Thompson CC, Odze R, Chan WW, Ryou M. Optimizing EUS-guided liver biopsy sampling: comprehensive assessment of needle types and tissue acquisition techniques. Gastrointest Endosc. 2017;85(2):419–26.
21. Das DK, Bhambhani S, Pant CS. Ultrasound guided fine-needle aspiration cytology: diagnosis of hydatid disease of the abdomen and thorax. Diagn Cytopathol. 1995;12(2):173–6.
22. Babu KS, Goel D, Prayaga A, Rao IS, Kumar A. Intraabdominal hydatid cyst: a case report. Acta Cytol. 2008;52(4):464–6.
23. Das DK. Cytodiagnosis of hepatocellular carcinoma in fine-needle aspirates of the liver: its differentiation from reactive hepatocytes and metastatic adenocarcinoma. Diagn Cytopathol. 1999;21(6):370–7.
24. Longchampt E, Patriarche C, Fabre M. Accuracy of cytology vs. microbiopsy for the diagnosis of well-differentiated hepatocellular carcinoma and macroregenerative nodule. Definition of standardized criteria from a study of 100 cases. Acta Cytol. 2000;44(4):515–23.
25. Hill KA, Nayar R, DeFrias DV. Cytohistologic correlation of cirrhosis and hepatocellular carcinoma. Pitfall in diagnosis? Acta Cytol. 2004;48(2):127–32.
26. Ruschenburg I, Droese M. Fine needle aspiration cytology of focal nodular hyperplasia of the liver. Acta Cytol. 1989;33(6):857–60.
27. Laiq Z, Bishop JA, Ali SZ. Liver lesions in children and adolescents: cytopathologic analysis and clinical correlates in 44 cases. Diagn Cytopathol. 2012;40(7):586–91.
28. Yang GC, Yang GY, Tao LC. Distinguishing well-differentiated hepatocellular carcinoma from benign liver by the physical features of fine-needle aspirates. Mod Pathol. 2004;17(7):798–802.
29. Kung IT, Chan SK, Fung KH. Fine-needle aspiration in hepatocellular carcinoma. Combined cytologic and histologic approach. Cancer. 1991;67(3):673–80.
30. Pitman MB, Szyfelbein WM. Significance of endothelium in the fine-needle aspiration biopsy diagnosis of hepatocellular carcinoma. Diagn Cytopathol. 1995;12(3):208–14.
31. Balani S, Malik R, Malik R, Kapoor N. Cytomorphological variables of hepatic malignancies in fine needle aspiration smears with special reference to grading of hepatocellular carcinoma. J Cytol. 2013;30(2):116–20.
32. Pérez-Guillermo M, Masgrau NA, García-Solano J, Sola-Pérez J, de Agustín y de Agustín P. Cytologic aspect of fibrolamellar hepatocellular carcinoma in fine-needle aspirates. Diagn Cytopathol. 1999;21(3):180–7.
33. Crowe A, Knight CS, Jhala D, Bynon SJ, Jhala NC. Diagnosis of metastatic fibrolamellar hepatocellular carcinoma by endoscopic ultrasound-guided fine needle aspiration. Cytojournal. 2011;8:2.
34. Ersöz C, Zorludemir U, Tanyeli A, Gümürdülü D, Celiktaş M. Fine needle aspiration cytology of hepatoblastoma. A report of two cases. Acta Cytol. 1998;42(3):799–802.
35. Parikh B, Jojo A, Shah B, Bansal R, Trivedi P, Shah MJ. Fine needle aspiration cytology of hepatoblastoma: a study of 20 cases. Indian J Pathol Microbiol. 2005;48(3):331–6.
36. Vlajnic T, Brisse HJ, Aerts I, Fréneaux P, Cellier C, Fabre M, Klijanienko J. Fine needle aspiration in the diagnosis and classification of hepatoblastoma: analysis of 21 new cases. Diagn Cytopathol. 2017;45(2):91–100.
37. Weilert F, Bhat YM, Binmoeller KF, Kane S, Jaffee IM, Shaw RE, Cameron R, Hashimoto Y, Shah JN. EUS-FNA is superior to ERCP-based tissue sampling in suspected malignant biliary obstruction: results of a prospective, single-blind, comparative study. Gastrointest Endosc. 2014 Jul;80(1):97–104.
38. Brandi G, Venturi M, Pantaleo MA, Ercolani G, GICO. Cholangiocarcinoma: Current opinion on clinical practice diagnostic and therapeutic algorithms: a review of the literature and a long-standing experience of a referral center. Dig Liver Dis. 2016;48(3):231–41.
39. Fritscher-Ravens A, Broering DC, Sriram PV, Topalidis T, Jaeckle S, Thonke F, Soehendra N. EUS-guided fine-needle aspiration cytodiagnosis of hilar cholangiocarcinoma: a case series. Gastrointest Endosc. 2000;52(4):534–40.

40. Chaudhary HB, Bhanot P, Logroño R. Phenotypic diversity of intrahepatic and extrahepatic cholangiocarcinoma on aspiration cytology and core needle biopsy: case series and review of the literature. Cancer. 2005;105(4):220–8.
41. Geller RL, Hookim K, Sullivan HC, Stuart LN, Edgar MA, Reid MD. Cytologic features of angiosarcoma: a review of 26 cases diagnosed on FNA. Cancer Cytopathol. 2016;124(9):659–68.
42. Jurczyk M, Zhu B, Laskin W, Lin X. Pitfalls in the diagnosis of hepatic epithelioid hemangioendothelioma by FNA and needle core biopsy. Diagn Cytopathol. 2014;42(6):516–20.
43. Zhou H, Guo M, Gong Y. Challenge of FNA diagnosis of angiomyolipoma: a study of 33 cases. Cancer Cytopathol. 2017;125(4):257–66.
44. Saeed OAM, Cramer H, Wang X, Wu HH. Fine needle aspiration cytology of hepatic metastases of neuroendocrine tumors: a 20-year retrospective, single institutional study. Diagn Cytopathol. 2018;46(1):35–9.

Chapter 8
Kidney and Adrenal Gland

Adebowale J. Adeniran

Kidney

Introduction

In the past, clinical management of patients was based on characteristic radiologic features; hence there was no clear role for fine needle aspiration (FNA) of renal tumors [1]. The great majority of renal lesions are radiologically benign cysts, which require no treatment. All solid renal cortical lesions, except metastases, were subject to surgical resection. More recently, FNA has been of increasing value. It is helpful in preventing unnecessary surgeries in patients with benign lesions such as oncocytoma, in patients with malignant lesions who are otherwise nonsurgical candidates, in patients with radiologically indeterminate cysts, and in other patients for whom partial nephrectomy rather than radical nephrectomy may be a preferred alternative treatment, especially in patients with tumors such as papillary renal cell carcinoma (papillary RCC), chromophobe RCC, and mucinous tubular and spindle cell carcinoma, which have a good prognosis [1–4]. Current management of small renal masses involves ablating the masses using cryotherapy, radiofrequency, or ethanol injections. FNA is done in this category of patients to confirm malignancy before the ablation procedure [5]. Advances in neoadjuvant targeted therapies for RCC have made the knowledge of the histological subtype critical for tailoring clinical trials and follow-up strategies [6, 7].

A. J. Adeniran (✉)
Department of Pathology, Yale University School of Medicine, New Haven, CT, USA
e-mail: adebowale.adeniran@yale.edu

G. Cai, A. J. Adeniran (eds.), *Rapid On-site Evaluation (ROSE)*,
https://doi.org/10.1007/978-3-030-21799-0_8

Specimen Adequacy Assessment

Virtually all kidney aspirations are performed percutaneously by radiologists using ultrasonography (US), computed tomography (CT), or magnetic resonance imaging (MRI) for guidance. However, there is increasing use of endoscopic ultrasound-guided fine needle aspiration (EUS-FNA) [8]. Rapid on-site evaluation (ROSE) for assessment of specimen adequacy is very important because it helps in decision-making such as whether additional passes are needed and whether additional tissue such as needle core biopsy is needed. It has been suggested that core biopsy and FNA are complementary and the combination of these techniques is better than either alone [9]. There are no established criteria for adequacy requirement in terms of specimen cellularity. A renal FNA specimen is considered adequate if a specific diagnosis can be made or if there is sufficient cellularity to suggest a limited differential diagnosis [10]. Aspiration of a cystic lesion composed exclusively of macrophages is reported as nondiagnostic rather than negative because a cystic RCC cannot be entirely excluded. The success of a renal FNA is largely dependent on the technique of aspiration, the skill of the aspirator, and the motivation and expertise of the pathologist and cytotechnologist.

Normal Elements in Kidney Cytology

Normal renal parenchymal components are occasionally encountered especially when a small renal mass is targeted and the needle misses the lesion and samples the adjacent normal renal parenchyma. Glomeruli are large, highly cellular globular structures, with sharply demarcated, multilayered clusters of epithelial and endothelial cells. They are much more dense in the center than at the periphery and there are distinctive capillary loops at the edges. Glomeruli may mimic the papillae of papillary RCC.

Proximal convoluted tubules have abundant granular, eosinophilic cytoplasm, and large oval nuclei with small, inconspicuous nucleoli. The cells have ill-defined cell borders, with the granules appearing to be spilling out of the cells. The cells may mimic those of oncocytoma or chromophobe RCC.

The cells of distal convoluted tubules are much smaller than cells from the proximal tubules and they have less cytoplasm. The cytoplasm is clear to slightly granular, and they have a small, round nucleus with an inconspicuous nucleolus. The cell borders are well-defined. The cells may mimic those of a low-grade clear cell or papillary RCC.

Cystic Lesions of the Kidney

Diagnostic Considerations

It has been estimated that up to 85% of asymptomatic renal masses detected by various imaging studies are at least partially cystic [11]. The majority of renal cysts appear radiographically as unilocular cysts with homogeneous watery content and regular, thin, smooth walls. Most of these can be reliably diagnosed as simple benign cysts

[12, 13]. The remainder, however, display atypical imaging features such as multi-locularity; mural nodules; shaggy, irregularly thickened, or calcified cyst wall; or heterogeneous or high-density cyst content [11, 14–16]. For this group, diagnostic possibilities other than simple cysts should be considered. The gross appearance of the aspirated fluid is a poor diagnostic indicator, since fluid from benign cysts and cystic carcinomas may be clear, cloudy, or bloody. Cystic degeneration of tumor tissue, substantial enough to be visible by imaging, is frequently seen in clear cell RCC and papillary RCC [16, 17]. The tumor may be solid with extensive cystic change or it may represent a mural tumor nodule arising from cyst epithelium [14].

1. Cytomorphologic features

   - Macrophages are almost always present, and in most cases, it represents the predominant or the only cell type present.
   - In benign cysts, macrophages display nuclei without atypical features and abundant, uniformly vacuolated, or granular cytoplasm with or without hemosiderin pigment (Figs. 8.1 and 8.2).

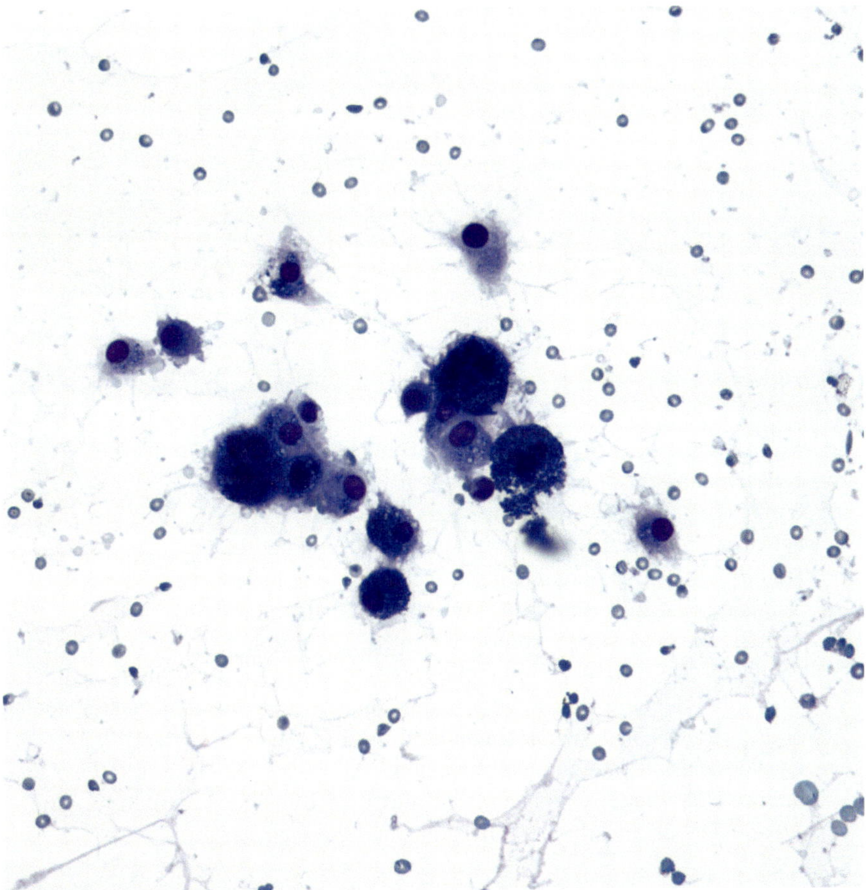

Fig. 8.1 Renal cyst. Macrophages are the predominant cells present, some with hemosiderin pigment (Diff-Quik stain, ×400)

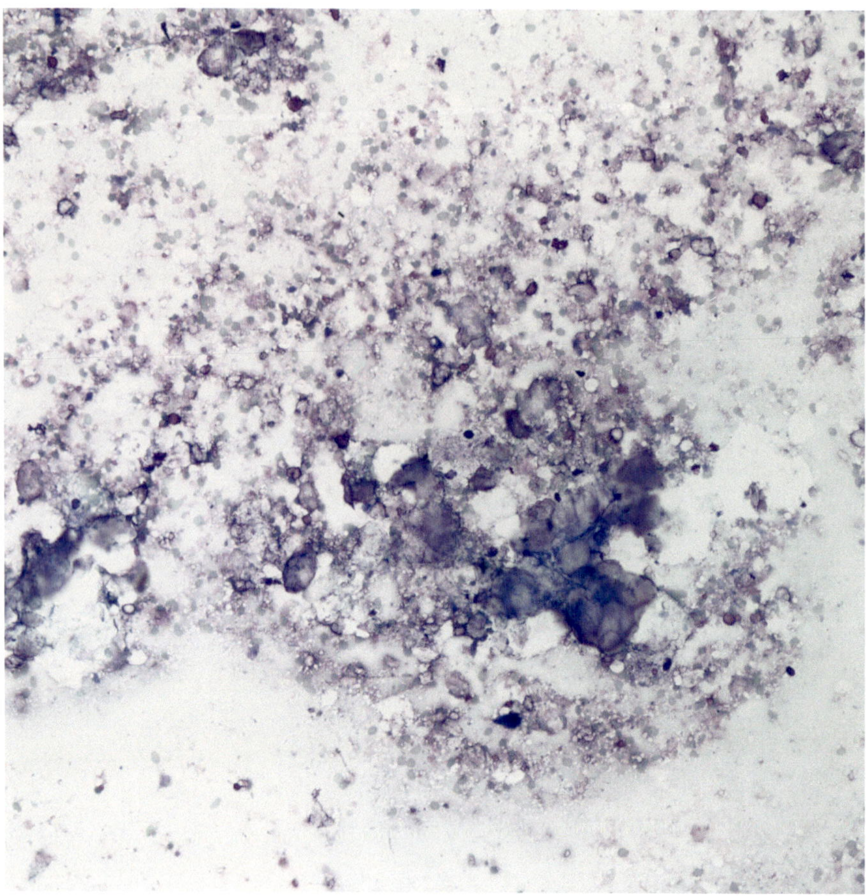

Fig. 8.2 Renal cyst. Predominantly crystals and scattered macrophages (Diff-Quik stain, ×200)

- Macrophages mostly present as single cells but they may be aggregated into cohesive clusters.
- Cyst-lining epithelial cells appear as rare 2-dimensional clusters or isolated epithelial cells with mild nuclear atypia, reticulated or granular cytoplasm, and ill-defined cell borders [11].
- Tubular cells are often seen, consisting mostly of proximal tubular cells, which appear as small, orderly, oriented, 2-dimensional cell clusters with abundant, finely granular, homogeneous cytoplasm and uniform, round nuclei with small nucleoli. Aspirated proximal tubular cells present as naked nuclei or as 2-dimensional tubular fragments.
- Cystic renal cell carcinoma is characterized by abundant clusters and isolated tumor cells with ample, vacuolated, fluffy, or reticulated cytoplasm. Tumor cell clusters are mostly large, irregular, and three-dimensional [11].

2. Tips and pitfalls

- When macrophages are aggregated into cohesive clusters, they may simulate cells of renal cell carcinoma. Immunohistochemistry is very helpful in this scenario as macrophages are positive for CD68, while the cells of renal cell carcinoma will be positive for cytokeratin AE1/AE3.
- The presence of numerous epithelial cells, even with mild atypia, or of few epithelial cells with significant atypia should raise the possibility of a malignant neoplasm or complex cystic lesions.
- Repeated aspiration of any residual solid areas that are visible after evacuation of the cyst usually yields abundant tubular cells, which may be misinterpreted as tumor cells.
- Calcium oxalate crystals are frequently seen in the acquired cystic disease-associated renal cell carcinoma.

Benign or Uncertain Behavior Neoplasms

Oncocytoma

A. Diagnostic considerations

Oncocytoma, a benign tumor of oncocytes, is composed of large epithelial cells with abundant eosinophilic cytoplasm. Grossly, the tumor is usually well-circumscribed and encapsulated with mahogany brown color and a central fibrous scar.

B. Cytomorphologic features

- Cellular specimen with numerous isolated cells with abundant, eosinophilic granular cytoplasm and small, round nuclei with finely granular chromatin and inconspicuous, tiny nucleoli [18].
- Tumor is arranged in rounded nests with well-demarcated cell borders.
- Isolated pleomorphic or bizarre cells consistent with degenerative atypia may be present.

C. Tips and pitfalls

- Hepatocytes from inadvertent sampling of the liver can mimic oncocytes. Although hepatocytes have abundant granular cytoplasm similar to cells of oncocytoma, they show more variation in nuclear and cellular size and they often contain lipofuscin pigment.
- Eosinophilic variant of clear cell RCC and several other different subtypes of RCC can have eosinophilic granular cytoplasm and therefore mimic an oncocytoma. It is essential that additional pass should be collected for cell block preparation for immunohistochemistry to differentiate between oncocytoma and these neoplasms.

- Oncocytic papillary RCC has a similar appearance to oncocytoma, but it also has papillae and abundant macrophages, which are not features of oncocytoma.
- Distinction between chromophobe RCC and oncocytoma can be very difficult on smears alone and additional cell block material is needed for morphology assessment and immunohistochemistry. The neoplastic cells in oncocytoma are arranged in rounded nests, while cells in chromophobe RCC have a trabecular arrangement. Chromophobe RCC is typically positive for CK7 and shows diffuse cytoplasmic staining for Hale's colloidal iron, whereas oncocytoma is negative for CK7 and mostly negative or show focal apical staining for Hale's colloidal iron.
- Hybrid oncocytic tumors comprise of oncocytoma and chromophobe RCC components and the FNA findings depend on the areas sampled. Because of this potential pitfall, it is advisable that these cases should be diagnosed as "oncocytic renal neoplasm." A particular lesion can be favored if possible, but a note should be added that a partial nephrectomy should be considered, if clinically indicated.

Renal Cortical Adenoma

A. Diagnostic considerations

Papillary adenomas are small lesions less than 1.5 cm, which arise in the renal cortex and are often subcapsular. They are usually unencapsulated and histologically, immunohistochemically, and cytologically indistinguishable from type 1 papillary RCC.

B. Cytomorphologic features

- Lesion is composed of densely packed tubules lined by small, regular cuboidal cells with round, uniform, bland nuclei. Pure papillary and tubulopapillary patterns as well as microcyst formation can also be seen [19].

C. Tips and pitfalls

- A diagnosis of papillary adenoma based on FNA should be made with extreme caution, because the presence of capsule or grade heterogeneity may not be visualized.

Metanephric Adenoma

A. Diagnostic considerations

Metanephric adenoma is an uncommon benign neoplasm of the kidney derived from metanephric blastema and composed of well-differentiated epithelial nephroblastic cells [20]. The majority of cases are found during imaging studies for other complaints. There is a close association between metanephric adenoma and polycythemia.

B. Cytomorphologic features

- Cellular smears with cells arranged as short tubules, tight balls, and loose sheets.
- Conspicuous basement membrane-type material surrounds neoplastic cells.
- Tumor cells are small and uniform, with round nuclei, fine chromatin, absent nucleoli, and scant cytoplasm [21].
- Psammoma bodies are common.
- Mitoses are absent or very infrequent.

C. Tips and pitfalls

- Differentiating metanephric adenoma from monophasic Wilm's tumor can be very challenging. Additional passes for cell block material and immunohistochemistry is key. Metanephric adenoma is positive for CD57 and may show nuclear reactivity for WT-1 while negative for CD56, whereas Wilm's tumor is positive for WT-1 and CD56 and may be positive for CD57 in up to 50% of cases.
- Papillary RCC can also be confused with metanephric adenoma. Unlike papillary RCC, metanephric adenoma is negative for epithelial membrane antigen.

Angiomyolipoma

A. Diagnostic considerations

Angiomyolipoma, a benign neoplasm, is regarded as a hamartoma or benign mesenchymoma, and it consists of a mixture of mature adipose tissue, tortuous thick-walled blood vessels, and fascicles of smooth muscle [22, 23]. There is a strong association with tuberous sclerosis, and these patients tend to have multiple small and bilateral angiomyolipomas, and they also demonstrate extrarenal manifestations of tuberous sclerosis complex [10].

B. Cytomorphologic features

- The vascular component is characterized by thick-walled blood vessels lined by endothelial cells.
- The smooth muscle component is composed of clusters of bland small spindle cells, which vary in size and shape, with granular cytoplasm [24].
- The lipomatous component is composed of mature adipose tissue. Areas of fat necrosis, comprising of histiocytes and multinucleated giant cells may be found [23].
- The cells of epithelioid angiomyolipoma are round and range from medium to large cells with prominent nucleoli and abundant cytoplasm, resembling ganglion cells.

C. Tips and pitfalls

- The smooth muscle cells of angiomyolipoma often show atypia and this may be confused with sarcoma or sarcomatoid differentiation in renal cell carcinoma [24].

- Highly cellular smooth muscle cells with predominantly round cell pattern with granular cytoplasm may be confused with RCC with granular cytoplasm.
- Fat-predominant angiomyolipoma can mimic well-differentiated liposarcoma.
- Cells of epithelioid angiomyolipoma, especially in the presence of necrosis and mitoses, can mimic clear cell RCC [25].
- The smooth muscle cells as well as the fat cells are positive for melanoma markers such as HMB-45 and Melan A.

Renal Abscess

A. Diagnostic considerations

Localized bacteria pyelonephritis and renal abscess can have the appearance of a mass on radiologic examination. Both intrarenal and perinephric abscess can be aspirated under US guidance.

B. Cytomorphologic features

- Aspirates yield necrotic material and abundant neutrophils.
- Rare atypical cells may be present.

C. Tips and pitfalls

- If the aspiration yields turbid fluid or frank pus, material should be sent for microbiologic studies.
- The atypical cells can mimic renal cell carcinoma with abundant necrosis. Hence, in the presence of abundant acute inflammation, atypical cells in renal FNA, especially when they are very few, should be interpreted with caution.

Xanthogranulomatous Pyelonephritis

A. Diagnostic considerations

Xanthogranulomatous pyelonephritis is a chronic inflammatory disease of the kidney and is thought to be an atypical host reaction to a bacterial infection, which usually presents as a mass lesion. It is associated with recurrent urinary tract infection and may present as a mass lesion, thereby mimicking carcinoma [26].

B. Cytomorphologic features

- The lesion is composed of histiocytes and multinucleated giant cells [24].
- Histiocytes have foamy, granular, or eosinophilic cytoplasm and small uniform nuclei (Fig. 8.3).
- Necrosis, cholesterol clefts, and lymphocytes are commonly seen.

C. Tips and pitfalls

- Clusters of histiocytes can resemble the cells of clear cell RCC. The histiocytes of xanthogranulomatous pyelonephritis, however, lack nuclear atypia

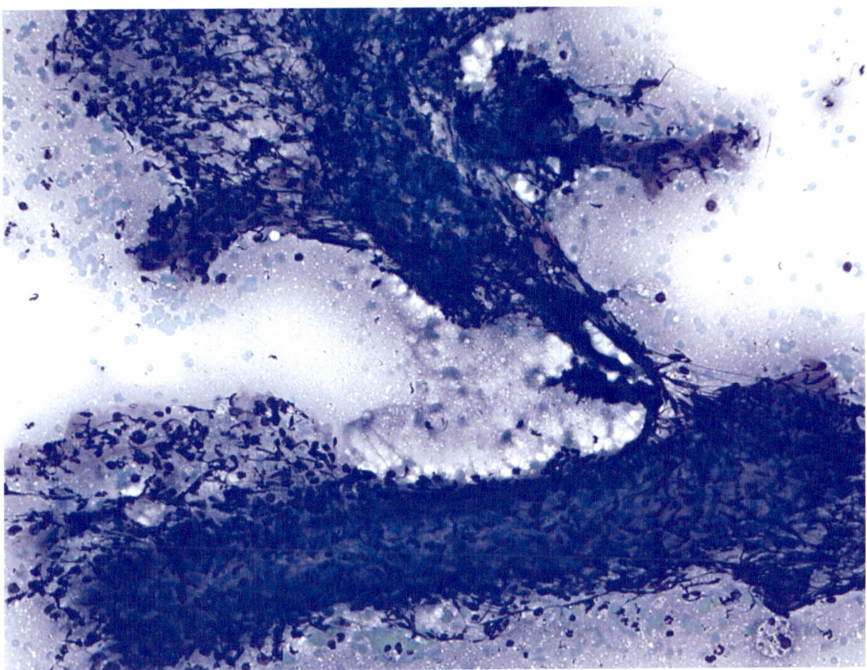

Fig. 8.3 Xanthogranulomatous pyelonephritis. Clusters of histiocytes with small uniform nuclei and foamy cytoplasm. The histiocytes form aggregates resembling clear cell RCC, but they lack nuclear atypia (Diff-Quik stain, ×200)

and have a cytoplasm that has a more microvacuolated appearance than that of typical clear cell RCC.

- Immunohistochemical stains will be helpful in difficult cases, hence the need for additional passes for cell block material. The histiocytes show immunoreactivity for CD68 and negative for cytokeratin AE1/AE3, the precise opposite of the immunoprofile that is seen in clear cell RCC.

Malignant Neoplasms

Clear Cell Renal Cell Carcinoma

A. Diagnostic considerations

Clear cell renal cell carcinoma is the most common variant of RCC, accounting for 75–80% of all RCCs. The tumor cells have a rich network of delicate, thin-walled blood vessels, which accounts for the contrast enhancement pattern on imaging studies and the frequent bloodiness of FNA samples [10]. Grossly, most clear cell RCCs are solitary and randomly distributed in the renal cortex. Multicentricity in the same kidney as well as bilaterality can also be seen and these are often associated with familial and associated conditions such as von Hippel-Lindau disease [27, 28]. The tumor is typically golden yellow in appearance due to the rich lipid content of its cells.

B. Cytomorphologic features

- Aspirates tend to be hypercellular (Fig. 8.4), with bloody and/or necrotic background.
- Cells are interspersed with abundant, thin-walled blood vessels.
- Cells tend to be large with a low to moderate nuclear-cytoplasmic ratio.
- Nuclei tend to be round or slightly irregular, with finely granular, evenly distributed chromatin [29].
- Depending on the degree of differentiation, nucleoli may be absent, sparse, large, or prominent.
- The cytoplasm is abundant, can be clear and foamy, or may be granular and eosinophilic or a mixture of both (Fig. 8.5). Cytoplasm is thin and wispy and

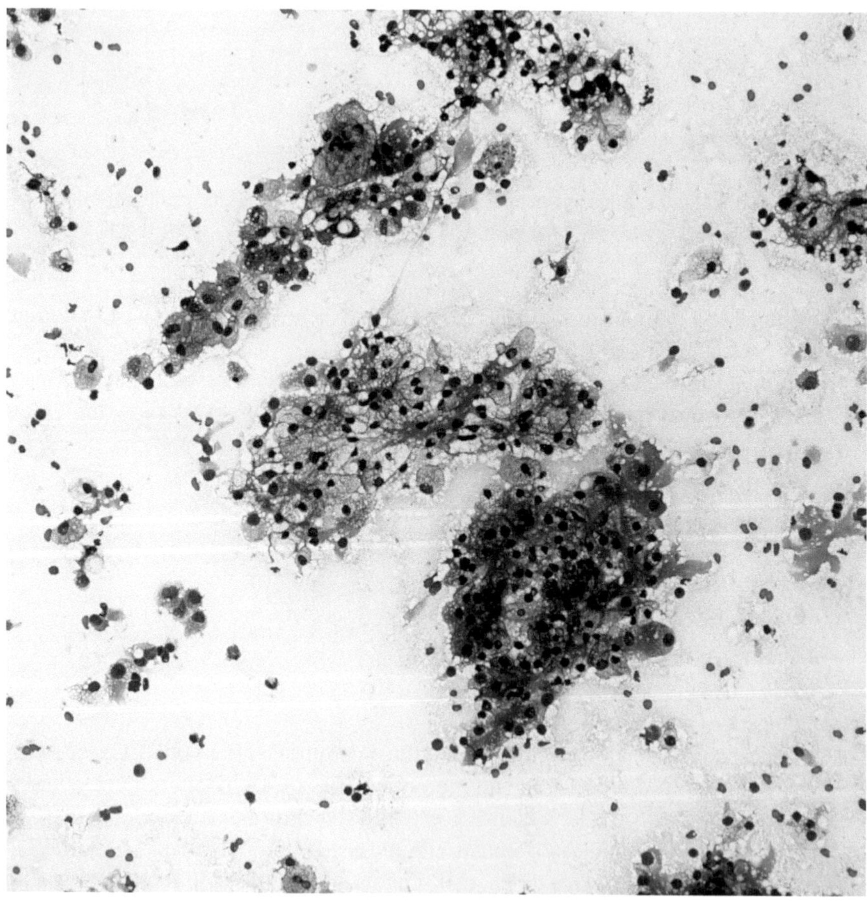

Fig. 8.4 Clear cell RCC. Hypercellular aspirate (Diff-Quik stain, ×200)

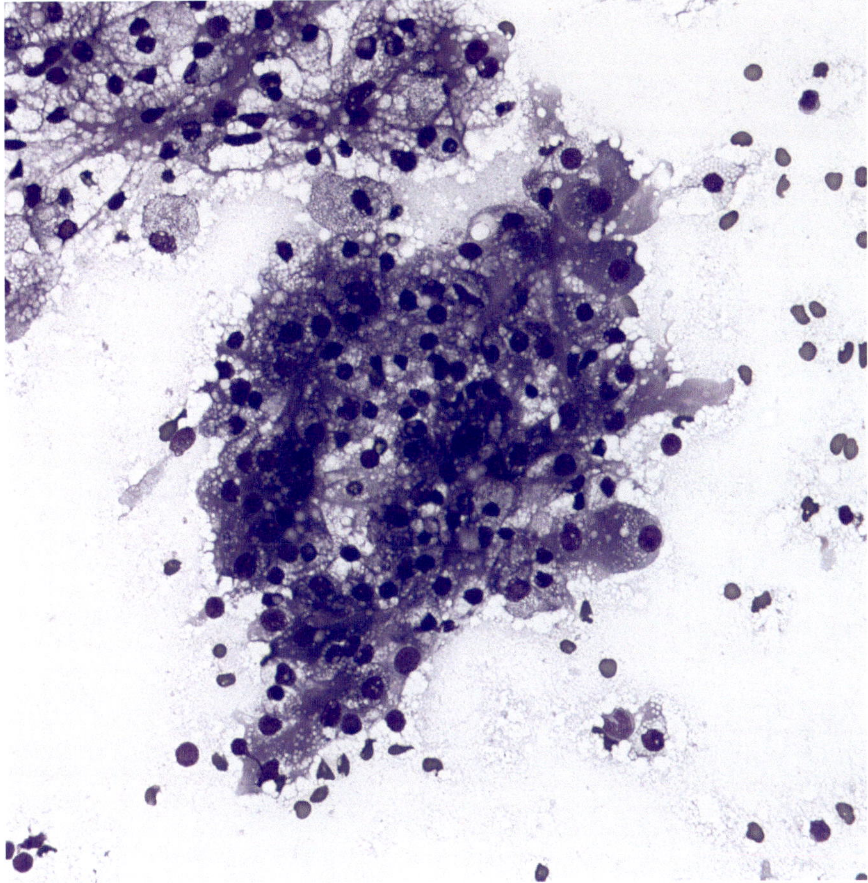

Fig. 8.5 Clear cell RCC. Abundant foamy cytoplasm with peripherally placed small cytoplasmic vacuoles (Diff-Quik stain, ×400)

cell membranes are poorly defined. Small cytoplasmic vacuoles are often peripherally placed [10, 24, 29, 30].

- Necrosis, hemorrhage, cystic degeneration, and calcifications are common.

C. Tips and pitfalls

- Higher-grade tumors have more isolated cells and less vacuolated cytoplasm (Fig. 8.6).
- A small proportion of tumors can have focal or extensive areas of cells with rhabdoid differentiation (Fig. 8.7). This should not be confused with rhabdoid tumor of the kidney.
- Aspirates of benign renal tubular cells can mimic low-grade clear cell RCC. The aspirate is usually flat and shows small groups of cells without vacuolated cytoplasm or branching vessels.

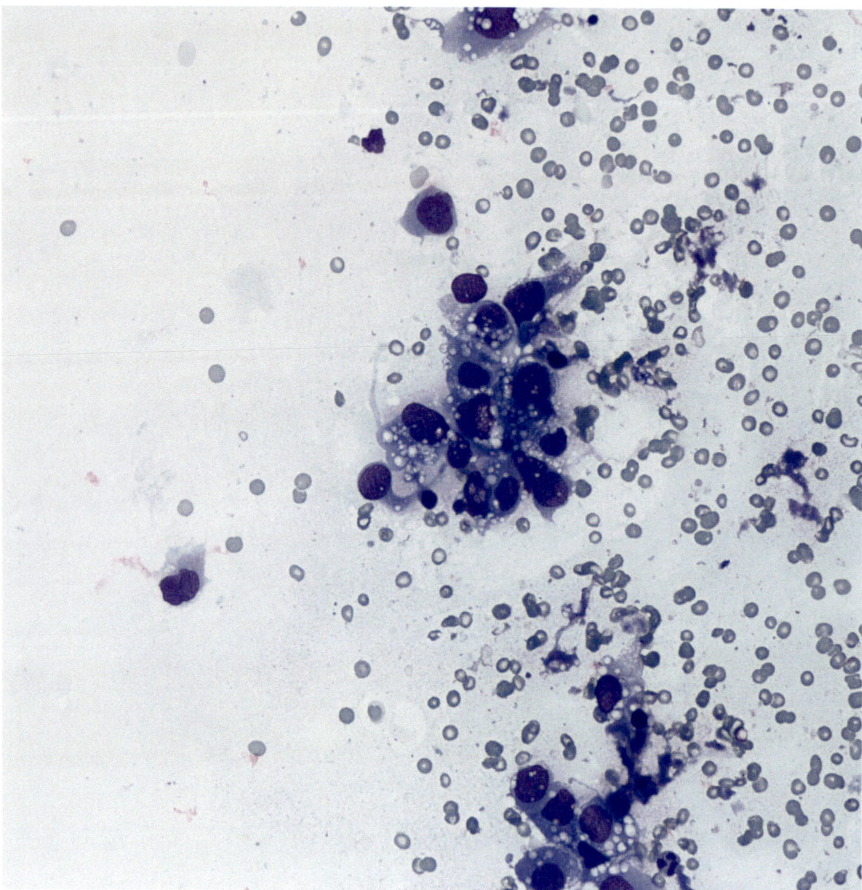

Fig. 8.6 Clear cell RCC. High-grade tumor with more isolated cells and less vacuolated cytoplasm (Diff-Quik stain, ×400)

- Adrenal cortical cells can simulate cells of clear cell RCC. However, the cells of the adrenal cortex are smaller and have a fine bubbly cytoplasm and are frequently stripped of their cytoplasm.
- Predominance of clear cells is also seen in clear cell tubulopapillary RCC and this may be impossible to distinguish from low-grade clear cell RCC based on cytology alone. It is important to collect cell block material for immunohistochemistry. Clear cell RCC typically demonstrates diffuse membranous staining for carbonic anhydrase IX while negative for CK7. In contrast, clear cell tubulopapillary RCC is negative for CK7 and shows cup-like staining for carbonic anhydrase IX.
- Other renal neoplasms with clear cell features such as epithelioid angiomyolipoma and translocation RCC should be considered in the differential diagnosis and immunohistochemical stains should be ordered accordingly.

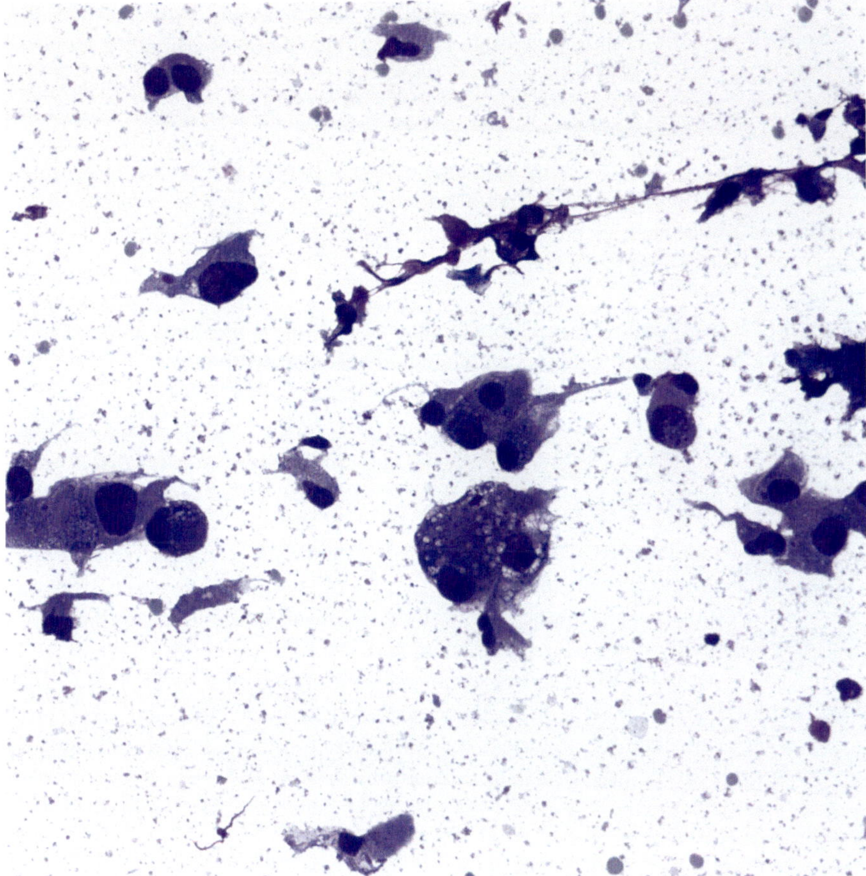

Fig. 8.7 Renal cell carcinoma with rhabdoid features (Diff-Quik stain, ×400)

Epithelioid angiomyolipoma is positive for HMB-45 and negative for carbonic anhydrase IX, while clear cell RCC demonstrates diffuse membranous staining for carbonic anhydrase IX and negative for HMB-45. Translocation RCC is positive for cathepsin K and has a variable but focal positivity for carbonic anhydrase IX, while clear cell RCC is negative for cathepsin K.

Papillary Renal Cell Carcinoma

A. Diagnostic considerations

Papillary RCC accounts for 7–15% of all RCCs [10, 31, 32]. It is associated with renal cortical adenomas and multifocality. Papillary RCC is divided into two morphologic subtypes – types 1 and 2 – which correlate with tumor grade.

Patients with a low-grade/low-stage papillary RCC have an excellent prognosis, while those with a high-grade/high-stage papillary RCC have a poor prognosis [32, 33].

B. Cytomorphologic features

- Aspirates are hypercellular with abundant papillary structures with true fibrovascular cores, spherules, and tubules.
- Type 1 tumors show papillae covered by a single layer of small bland cuboidal cells with uniform round, small nuclei, inconspicuous nucleoli, and scant cytoplasm.
- Type 2 tumors show papillae covered by large eosinophilic cells with enlarged nuclei, prominent nucleoli, and abundant granular cytoplasm.
- Cytoplasm may be clear, eosinophilic, or granular.
- Fibrovascular cores are distended with foamy macrophages.
- Abundant intracytoplasmic hemosiderin and psammoma bodies may be present.

C. Tips and pitfalls

- Type 1 papillary RCC is histologically, immunohistochemically, and cytologically indistinguishable from papillary adenoma. Radiological correlation is essential as the difference between the 2 entities is the size. Papillary adenomas are less than 1.5 cm in diameter.
- Type 1 papillary RCC can be confused with metanephric adenoma. Unlike papillary RCC, metanephric adenoma is negative for epithelial membrane antigen, so obtaining material for cell block for immunohistochemistry is important at the time of on-site evaluation.

Chromophobe Renal Cell Carcinoma

A. Diagnostic considerations

Chromophobe renal cell carcinoma is derived from the intercalated cells of the cortical collecting duct system and it consists of 4% of all RCCs [34]. Patients usually have an excellent prognosis as this entity has a much higher 5-year survival than clear cell RCC [35]. Grossly the cut surface shows a tan brown tumor which may closely mimic an oncocytoma. There are two distinct morphologic variants – the classic and eosinophilic variants.

B. Cytomorphologic features

- Aspirates are cellular with polygonal cells.
- Cells have eccentrically placed nuclei with inconspicuous nucleoli and well-defined cell borders.
- There is marked variation in the size of the nuclei, which have dark chromatin and raisinoid nuclei [36, 37].
- Cells may be binucleated or multinucleated and multiple fused nuclei may also be arranged peripherally (Fig. 8.8).

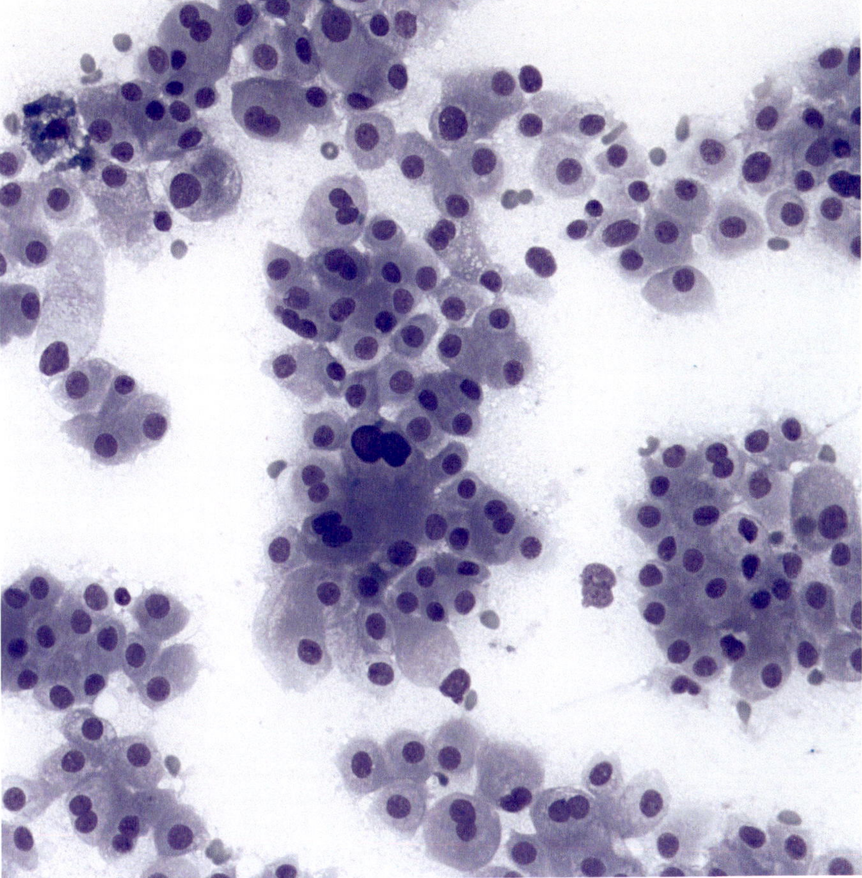

Fig. 8.8 Chromophobe renal cell carcinoma. Cells show frequent binucleation and prominent cell borders (Diff-Quik stain, ×400)

- Cytoplasm is granular and finely reticulated with perinuclear cytoplasmic clearing (Fig. 8.9). In classic variant, the cytoplasm is pale, while it is eosinophilic in the eosinophilic variant [10].
- The cells are reminiscent of koilocytes due to the nuclear features and perinuclear halo.

C. Tips and pitfalls

- Eosinophilic variant of chromophobe RCC can mimic oncocytoma. It has less dense granular cytoplasm than oncocytoma, and it is also characterized by perinuclear cytoplasmic clearing and marked anisonucleosis, features that are not typically seen in oncocytoma. Additional material for cell block preparation is very important as the morphology of tumor cells is better appreciated. In addition, immunohistochemical stains may be helpful in difficult

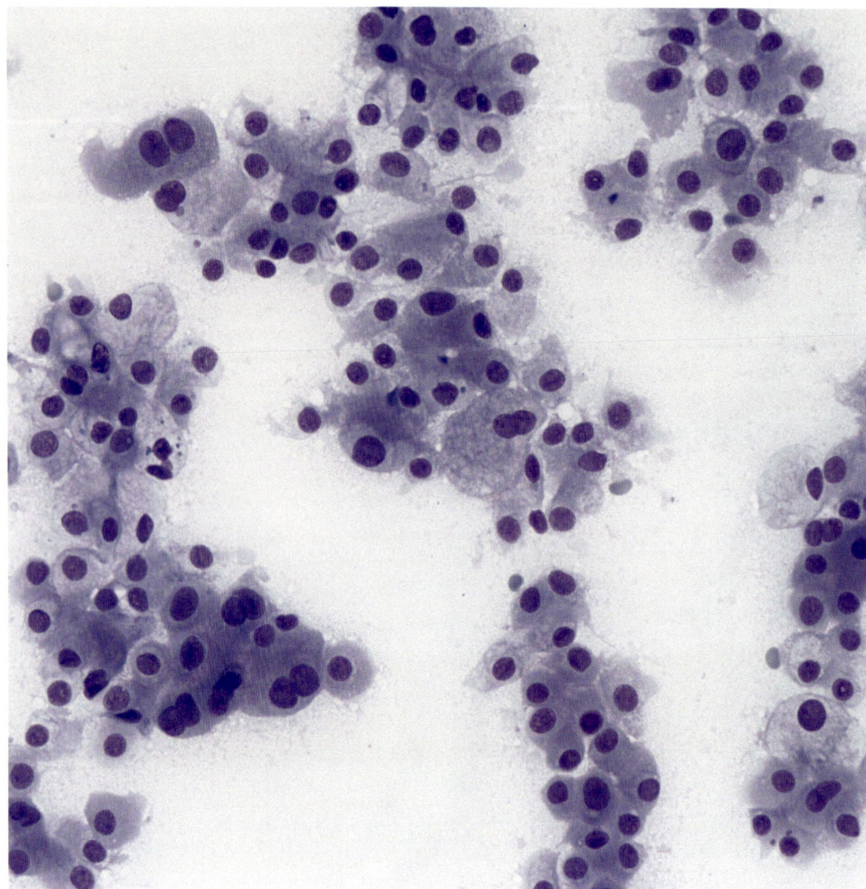

Fig. 8.9 Chromophobe renal cell carcinoma. Granular and finely reticulated cytoplasm with perinuclear cytoplasmic clearing (Diff-Quik stain, ×400)

cases. Chromophobe RCC is positive for CK7, while negative in oncocytoma. Hale's colloidal iron shows a diffuse cytoplasmic staining in chromophobe RCC, while it is usually negative or shows focal apical staining in oncocytoma. In equivocal cases, it is reasonable to interpret the specimen as "oncocytic neoplasm" and defer to partial nephrectomy for definitive classification, if clinically indicated.

- Clear cell RCC can also mimic chromophobe RCC. Clear cell RCC has abundant finely vacuolated cytoplasm with round centrally located nuclei and prominent nucleoli in contrast to the hyperchromatic raisinoid nuclei of chromophobe RCC. Chromophobe RCC is usually positive for CK7 and CD117, two stains that are negative in clear cell RCC.

Sarcomatoid Renal Cell Carcinoma

A. Diagnostic considerations

Sarcomatoid transformation in renal cell carcinomas is considered to be a poor prognostic sign and these tumors are usually highly aggressive [38, 39]. For a tumor to be diagnosed as sarcomatoid RCC, it must consist of a typical RCC component associated with a definite sarcomatoid component. In most cases, sarcomatoid transformation is associated with clear cell RCC, but it has also been documented in papillary, chromophobe, and collecting duct RCCs [40–42]. The greater the proportion of the sarcomatoid component, the worse the prognosis [39]. These tumors are ideal candidates for FNA as many are unresectable at the time of presentation.

B. Cytomorphologic features

- Aspirates are cellular with dimorphic cell population.
- The epithelial component is characterized by individual or small clusters of round cells with moderate to abundant cytoplasm. The nuclei are usually round with prominent nucleoli and nuclear membrane irregularity [43].
- The second population consists of single spindle cells or large clusters of spindle-shaped cells with elongated nuclei, prominent nucleoli, fine chromatin, and little to moderate cytoplasm [43].

C. Tips and pitfalls

- If an epithelial component is not identified, the tumor can be misdiagnosed as a true sarcoma. So, the preparation of cell block material may be of great benefit, especially in equivocal cases. The evaluation of tissue sections from cell blocks makes it easier to assess the sarcomatoid component and also provide a good source of material for immunohistochemical stains. The positivity for keratin and epithelial membrane antigen helps distinguish the tumors from true sarcomas.
- If only the epithelial area is sampled and no sarcomatoid component is represented, the tumor may be indirectly classified as a typical RCC.

Collecting Duct Carcinoma

A. Diagnostic considerations

Collecting duct carcinoma is a rare subtype of renal carcinoma that comprises 1–2% of all RCCs [44]. Unlike most RCCs, it arises in the renal medulla. It occurs in a younger age group than classical RCC and has an aggressive biologic behavior [44, 45].

B. Cytomorphologic features

- Smears have variable cellularity with cells arranged as well-demarcated groups or tightly packed cohesive cells with tubulopapillary growth pattern [44].
- Background is loose and shows loose scattered single cells and fragments of dense connective tissue.
- Nuclei are large, with eccentric or central placement, coarse chromatin, prominent nucleoli, and irregular nuclear contours [44, 46].
- Cytoplasm is scant, eosinophilic granular, or vacuolated.
- Nuclei of tubular cells may protrude into the luminal ends of the cells, giving a hobnail appearance [45].

C. Tips and pitfalls

- In the presence of prominent papillary architecture, it may be difficult to distinguish collecting duct carcinoma from type 2 papillary RCC. These two entities can be distinguished from each other by their location, architecture and immunohistochemical expression. Collecting duct carcinoma is positive for high molecular weight keratin and negative for AMACR, while the converse is true for papillary RCC.
- The cells of collecting duct carcinoma can closely resemble those of urothelial carcinoma. Cells of collecting duct carcinoma are positive for PAX-8 while negative for p63 and GATA-3, which helps distinguish it from urothelial carcinoma.
- Metastatic adenocarcinoma to the kidney can mimic collecting duct carcinoma. With a history of malignancy in other sites, metastasis should be considered and ruled out. Immunohistochemical stains are helpful in this scenario and cell block material should be obtained at the time of on-site assessment. The absence of extrarenal primary neoplasm should prompt consideration of an unusual primary renal tumor.

Mucinous Tubular and Spindle Cell Carcinoma

A. Diagnostic considerations

Mucinous tubular and spindle cell carcinoma (MTSCC) is a low-grade renal cell carcinoma, which is characterized by interconnecting tubular and spindle cells with low-grade nuclei within myxoid/mucinous stroma. Proper classification is important because this tumor behaves in a benign fashion and has excellent prognosis in overwhelming majority of cases [47], although aggressive cases have been reported [48].

B. Cytomorphologic features

- Cellular aspirates showing cohesive tissue fragments, with thick, broad trabecular arrangements as well as branching, pseudo-papillary formations [47] (Fig. 8.10).

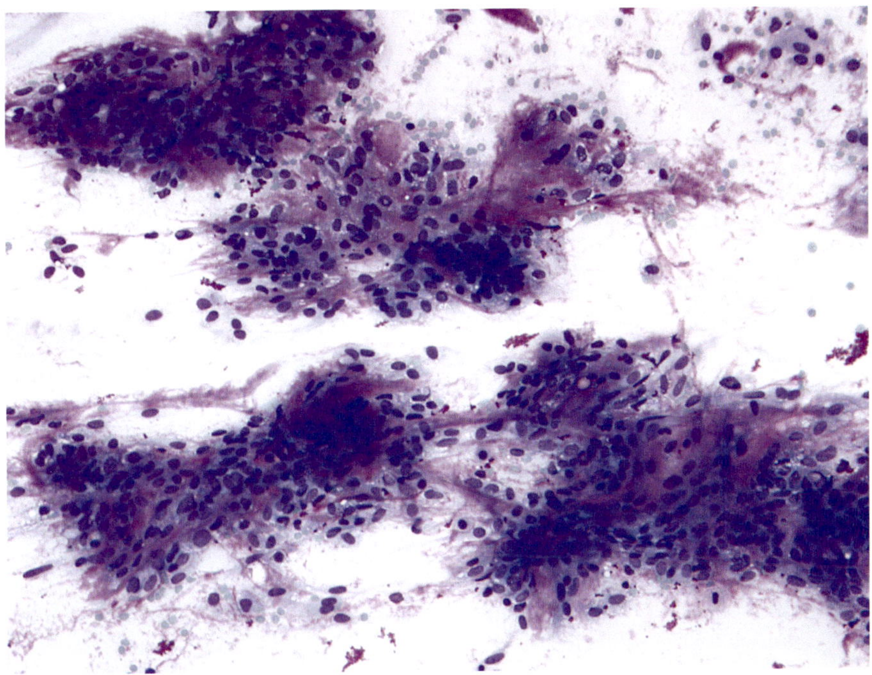

Fig. 8.10 Mucinous tubular and spindle cell carcinoma. Cohesive tissue fragments with branching, pseudo-papillary formations. Cells are uniform, oval to spindled shaped, with abundant myxoid matrix (Diff-Quik stain, ×200)

- Tumor is composed of a mixture of tubular cells and spindle cells.
- Tubular cells are uniform, usually low cuboidal with bland round to oval to slightly elongated nuclei [47, 49].
- Focal moderate nuclear pleomorphism and prominent nucleoli may be present.
- Cytoplasm is delicate with indistinct cell borders. Scattered fine intracytoplasmic vacuoles may be present.
- Metachromatic myxoid/mucinous stroma with linear, basement membrane-like arrangements is also commonly seen but occasional tumors can be mucin-poor [50]. The myxoid stroma stains magenta on Diff-Quik stain, while it stains pale blue on Papanicolaou stain.

C. Tips and pitfalls

- In the absence of myxoid matrix, MTSCC can be confused with papillary RCC because of the pseudo-papillary structures. However, MTSCC lacks true vascular cores and foam cells, two features which are the hallmark features of papillary RCC.
- Branching pseudo-papillary arrangements can also be seen in clear cell RCC but clear cell RCC will be expected to have more cells with vacuolated cytoplasm and perivascular nesting of tumor cells.

- MTSCC can also be confused with sarcomatoid RCC because of the presence of abundance of spindled cells. The spindled cells of MTSCC usually lack significant anisonucleosis and atypia and they also lack necrosis, unlike sarcomatoid carcinoma.

Urothelial Carcinoma

A. Diagnostic considerations

Urothelial carcinoma accounts for 5–10% of all renal tumors. It is similar to its bladder counterparts clinically, histologically, and cytologically. Urothelial carcinoma of the kidney has a significant association with synchronous or metachronous urothelial tumors of other sites. Distinguishing urothelial carcinoma from RCC is important because the management of urothelial carcinoma requires the resection of the ureter along with the kidney.

B. Cytomorphologic features

- The cytologic appearance depends on the grade of the tumor [30, 51, 52].
- Smears from low-grade tumors are usually cellular and are composed of aggregates of cells appearing as sheets, papillae, and single cells. The cells are columnar to polygonal with minimal nuclear atypia. Cells with elongations or cytoplasmic tails may be seen (Fig. 8.11), with occasional intracytoplasmic vacuole at the end of the tail. These are called cercariform cells [53, 54] and are said to be characteristic of low-grade urothelial carcinoma.
- Smears from high-grade tumors are cellular and are composed of large columnar or polygonal cells with dense cytoplasm (Fig. 8.12). The nuclei are large and hyperchromatic, with coarse chromatin, irregular nuclear contours, and high nuclear-to-cytoplasmic ratios. Bizarre multinucleated forms and single cells may be seen (Fig. 8.13).
- Focal squamous differentiation and glandular differentiation with or without production of mucin may be seen.

C. Tips and pitfalls

- High-grade urothelial carcinoma with sarcomatoid transformation may be confused with sarcomatoid RCC. In the absence of recognizable epithelial component, it may be difficult or even impossible to distinguish one from the other and additional material for immunohistochemical stains should be requested at the time of on-site evaluation.
- Urothelial carcinoma with either squamous or glandular differentiation may be confused with metastatic tumors to the kidney. Metastasis should always be ruled out especially when there is a history of extrarenal malignancy.
- It may be difficult to distinguish urothelial carcinoma from papillary RCC especially when there is predominance of papillary architecture. Distinction is made based on the distinctive nuclear features of each entity as well as the

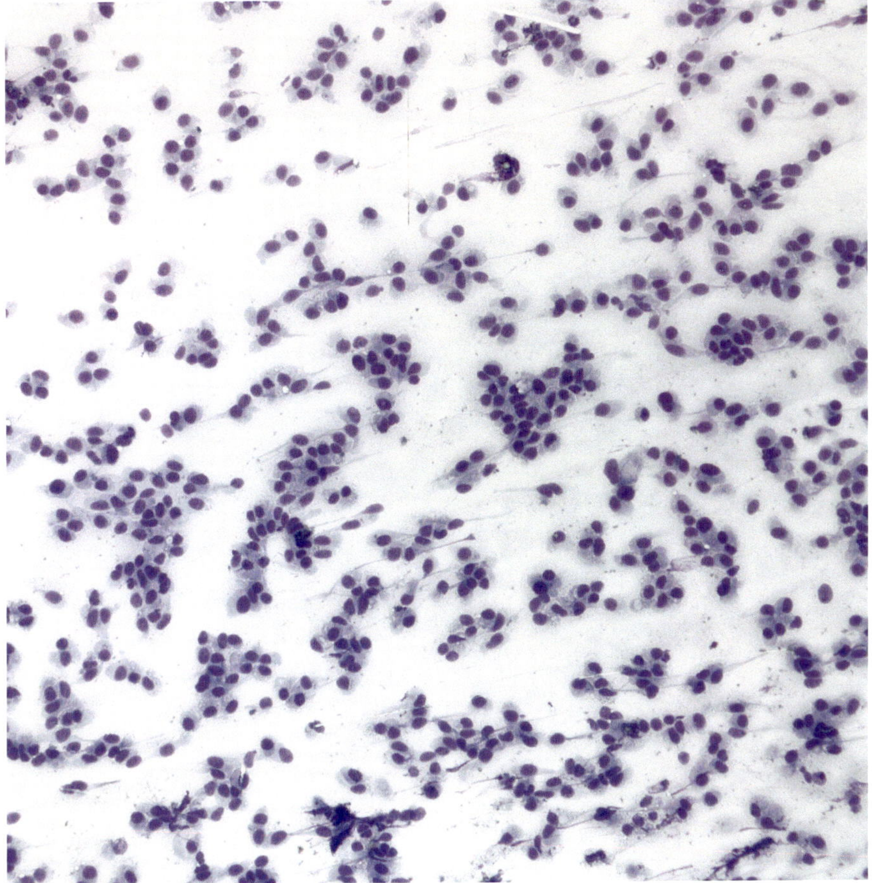

Fig. 8.11 Low-grade urothelial carcinoma. Cellular smear, showing cells with elongated cytoplasm (Diff-Quik stain, ×200)

characteristic features of papillary RCC such as abundant foamy macrophages and psammoma bodies.

- The cells of urothelial carcinoma can closely resemble those of collecting duct carcinoma. This has been discussed earlier.

Metastatic Tumor

A. Diagnostic considerations

Metastases to the kidney account for about 11% of renal tumors [55]. It is extremely uncommon for a kidney metastasis to be the initial manifestation of malignancy. Most tumors that are thought to be metastases in the kidney without a known primary most likely represent unusual primary renal tumors. Metastatic

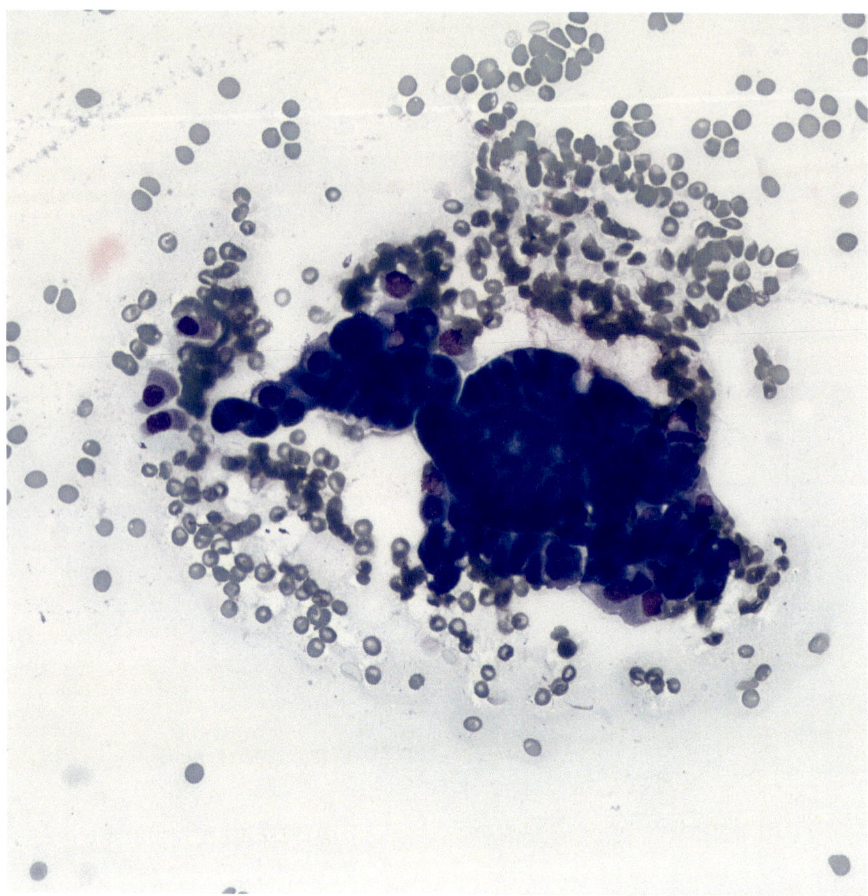

Fig. 8.12 High-grade urothelial carcinoma. Papillary cluster of large columnar cells (Diff-Quik stain, ×400)

tumors are often multifocal and bilateral. The lung is the most common primary site, while other common sites include the stomach, breast, pancreas, and contralateral kidney [55]. Malignant tumors of the adrenal may directly invade the kidney. Lymphomas are almost always metastatic from other sites although they may originate in the kidney.

B. Cytomorphologic features

- Metastatic carcinomas have three-dimensional clusters of tumor cells [56].
- Most metastatic lung tumors show cells with dark nuclei and irregular nuclear outlines, but some may have abundant clear cytoplasm and prominent nucleoli, thereby mimicking high-grade clear cell RCC [10].

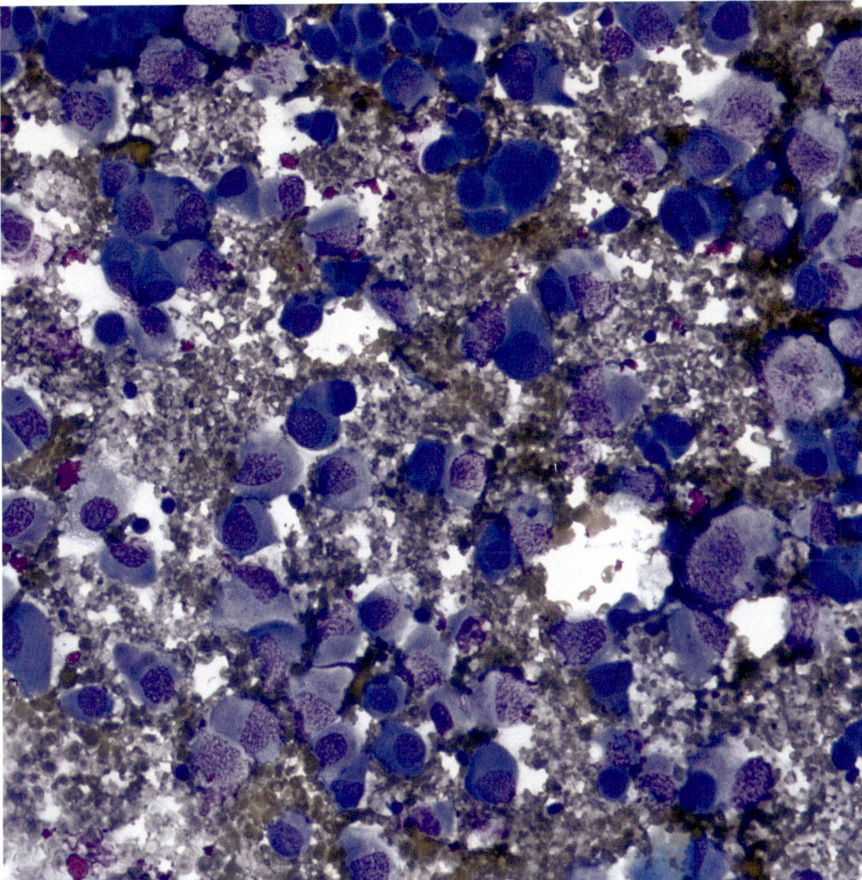

Fig. 8.13 High-grade urothelial carcinoma. Single cells with large, hyperchromatic nuclei, coarse chromatin, and irregular nuclear contours. The nuclear-to-cytoplasmic ratio is high (Diff-Quik stain, ×400)

- For most of the other metastatic tumors, the cells are usually either pleomorphic, large cells or undifferentiated small cells.

C. Tips and pitfalls

- Knowledge of the clinical history as well as judicious use of immunohistochemistry are key to the diagnosis. Although metastatic tumors differ from primary renal cell carcinoma on cytologic smears, the diagnosis is often made by the combination of cytomorphologic features, immunohistochemical stains, radiological appearance, and clinical history.

Adrenal Gland

Introduction

Fine needle aspiration (FNA) is an important procedure in the workup of patients with adrenal gland masses. It is a very effective method for distinguishing between adrenal tumors arising from the cortex and those arising from the medulla. It is also effective in distinguishing benign adrenal nodules from metastatic tumors during staging workup for cancer elsewhere in the body [57, 58]. Its value in the assessment of incidental adrenal nodules in patients without a history of malignancy remains unclear. FNA is generally avoided when a pheochromocytoma is suspected because of episodic hypertension resulting from the procedure.

Specimen Adequacy Assessment

Virtually all aspirations of the adrenal gland are performed by radiologists percutaneously using CT or US imaging guidance; however, endoscopic ultrasound-guided FNA is also becoming increasingly popular [59, 60]. The performance of this procedure requires a skilled operator especially if the lesion is small. To ensure adequate sampling of the suspected lesion, it is recommended that rapid on-site evaluation (ROSE) of direct smears be performed. Depending on the initial impression, additional material may be obtained for cell block. This is needed for subsequent immunohistochemical stains, special stains, or ultrastructural studies. Adrenal FNA has an accuracy of 96–98% and very good negative predictive value, especially for lesions larger than 3 cm [61, 62].

Normal Elements in Adrenal Cytology

Adrenal cortical cells are similar in size to hepatocytes. They are usually arranged in small clusters or cords, and they are polyhedral cells with small, round, vesicular nuclei with evenly distributed chromatin and small but distinct nucleoli (Fig. 8.14). The cytoplasm is faintly vacuolated or granular eosinophilic. Cells from the zona glomerulosa and zona fasciculata show either single prominent or multiple finely dispersed lipid inclusions. The cells from the zona reticularis contain golden-brown lipofuscin pigment. Small spindle-shaped stromal cells are occasionally present.

The cells of normal adrenal medulla are rarely encountered in aspirates of adrenal cortical lesions.

Hepatocytes can be sampled inadvertently during FNA of right adrenal gland. Hepatocytes usually do not have markedly vacuolated cytoplasm or delicate frayed cytoplasmic borders and there is no bubbly lipid-rich background.

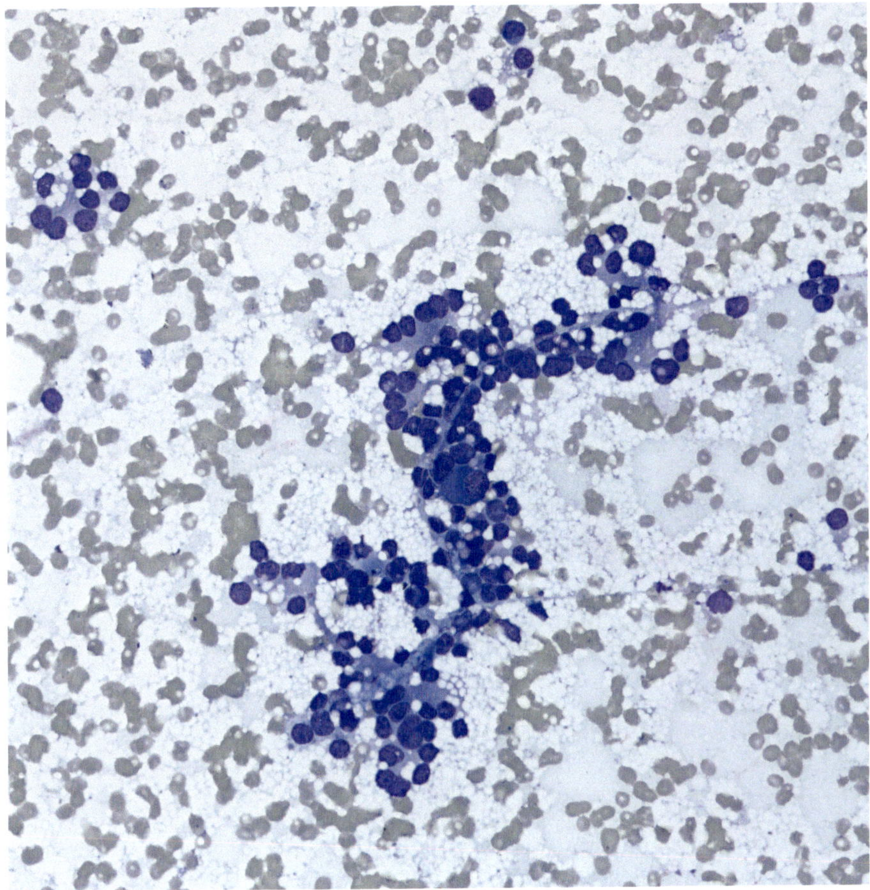

Fig. 8.14 Normal adrenal cortex. Cells with small, round, vesicular nuclei and vacuolated cytoplasm (Diff-Quik stain, ×400)

Benign or Uncertain Behavior Neoplasms

Myelolipoma

A. Diagnostic considerations

Myelolipoma is an uncommon benign neoplasm of the adrenal gland, which consists of mature fat containing normal hematopoietic cells. They are usually incidental findings.

B. Cytomorphologic features

- Smears show mature adipose tissue with immature hematopoietic cells of myeloid and erythroid origin, lymphocytes and megakaryocytes [63] (Fig. 8.15).

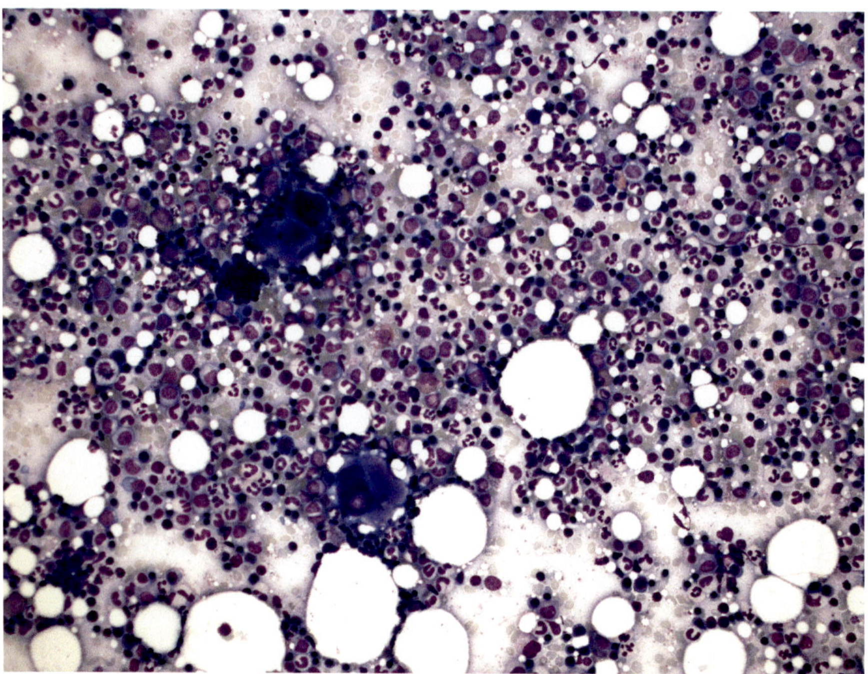

Fig. 8.15 Myelolipoma. Mature adipose tissue with immature hematopoietic cells of myeloid and erythroid origin, lymphocytes and megakaryocytes (Diff-Quik stain, ×200)

C. Tips and pitfalls

- The major differential diagnosis is angiomyolipoma of the kidney. The presence of hematopoietic elements as well as absence of prominent vessels and smooth muscle cells are helpful to make a diagnosis of myelolipoma.
- Retroperitoneal lipoma and liposarcoma should also be considered in the differential diagnosis. These entities also lack hematopoietic components.

Pheochromocytoma

A. Diagnostic considerations

Pheochromocytomas arise from the cells of the adrenal medulla. They are associated with familial neoplastic syndromes such as multiple endocrine neoplasia syndromes 2a and 2b (MEN 2) in 10–20% of cases [10]. Fine needle aspiration of suspected pheochromocytoma should be avoided as this may induce a fatal hypertensive crisis. No single cytologic pattern is diagnostic of this lesion.

B. Cytomorphologic features

- Highly cellular smears with cells arranged in loose clusters and as isolated cells.

- Small polygonal cells are often admixed with large spindled and epithelioid cells.
- Cells show pleomorphic nuclei with irregular nuclear membrane, finely stippled chromatin, prominent nucleoli, and intranuclear cytoplasmic pseudoinclusions [10].
- Cytoplasm is intensely granular and Diff-Quik stain shows red cytoplasmic granules.

C. Tips and pitfalls

- The cytologic features of pheochromocytoma overlap with those of metastatic high-grade malignant neoplasms, and ancillary tests such as immunohistochemistry will be helpful in differentiating this entity from metastatic neoplasms.
- The cytologic picture of pheochromocytoma is rarely conclusive in FNA specimens, and the diagnosis must be supported by clinical, imaging, and biochemical data.

Adrenal Cortical Adenoma

A. Diagnostic considerations

Adrenal cortical adenomas are thought to be very common, occurring in approximately 6% of adults, and their frequency increases with age [64]. They are usually unilateral and solitary masses, which distinguishes them from adrenal cortical hyperplasia which tends to be diffuse and bilateral. The majority of adenomas are nonfunctioning.

B. Cytomorphologic features

- Smears are very cellular and are composed of loose monolayered sheets or discohesive numerous small, round, moderately homogeneous naked nuclei on a pink granular or bubbly background of fragile and ill-defined vacuolated cytoplasm with frayed cellular borders [65].
- Nuclei are evenly spaced and are small and round, with smooth contours, even granular chromatin, and small nucleoli.
- Some of the nuclei may be enlarged but there is no nuclear pleomorphism.

C. Tips and pitfalls

- It is not possible to distinguish adrenal cortical adenoma from a hyperplastic nodule on cytology; hence they are referred to as benign adrenal cortical nodules/adenomas.
- It is often impossible to distinguish adrenal cortical adenoma from well-differentiated adrenal cortical carcinoma. The presence of necrosis and mitoses favor carcinoma. Correlation with radiology is also important as carcinomas tend to be fast growing and infiltrative.

- Clear cell RCC should be considered in the differential diagnosis of adrenal cortical adenoma. Clear cell RCC typically has abnormal nuclear features including the presence of prominent nucleoli and cell pleomorphism.
- Inadvertent sampling of liver tissue may occur during FNA of right adrenal gland. Hepatocytes are generally large polygonal cells with well-defined cell borders. They have prominent nucleoli and granular cytoplasm, which may contain bile pigment as opposed to the microvesicular cytoplasm of adrenal cortical adenoma.
- Superimposition of naked nuclei can mimic nuclear molding seen in small cell carcinoma. The true nuclear molding in small cell carcinoma is associated with necrosis and active mitosis.

Malignant Neoplasms

Adrenal Cortical Carcinoma

A. Diagnostic considerations

Adrenal cortical carcinomas are rare, highly malignant tumor with an annual prevalence estimated at 2–4 cases per million [66, 67]. Most tumors are functional with excess production of glucocorticoid, mineralocorticoid, or sex hormones. Up to 40% of cases have metastases at presentation.

B. Cytomorphologic features

- Cytomorphologic features range from well-differentiated to poorly differentiated tumors.
- Smears of well-differentiated tumors are cellular, and they show uniform tumor cells in loose clusters or single cells, with abundant, eosinophilic granular cytoplasm and large, uniform nuclei with coarse chromatin and prominent nucleoli [68, 69].
- Capillary vessels may be occasionally observed within the cell clusters.
- Smears of poorly differentiated tumors show large anaplastic malignant tumor cells with marked anisocytosis, large pleomorphic nuclei, prominent nucleoli, multinucleation, and abnormal mitoses [68, 69].

C. Tips and pitfalls

- It is often impossible to distinguish adrenal cortical adenoma from well-differentiated adrenal cortical carcinoma (discussed above).
- Clear cell RCC can be confused with adrenal cortical carcinoma. Additional material for immunohistochemistry is necessary. Clear cell RCC typically stains positive for PAX-8 and carbonic anhydrase IX, while adrenal cortical carcinoma is positive for Melan A and inhibin.
- The cells of adrenal cortical carcinoma can closely resemble those of metastatic tumor to the adrenal gland. Metastatic tumors are most likely to be bilateral and multiple. Correlation with history and immunohistochemistry is essential.

Metastatic Tumors

A. Diagnostic considerations

Adrenal gland is the fourth most common site of extranodal metastasis [70]. Metastases are far more common than primary malignant tumors of the adrenal gland [71]. Lung tumors account for the majority of metastases to the adrenal gland. Other common tumors that metastasize to the adrenals include melanoma, lymphoma and RCC [62, 70, 71]. Metastasis to the adrenals correlate with aggressive behavior and widespread dissemination of the primary tumor. Although most metastatic adrenal tumors are multifocal and bilateral, lung tumors and RCC have a tendency to produce a solitary adrenal metastasis. In such cases, FNA plays a key role in distinguishing a primary adrenal lesion from a solitary metastasis.

B. Cytomorphologic features

- Cytologic features depend on the primary tumor (Figs. 8.16, 8.17, 8.18, 8.19, and 8.20).

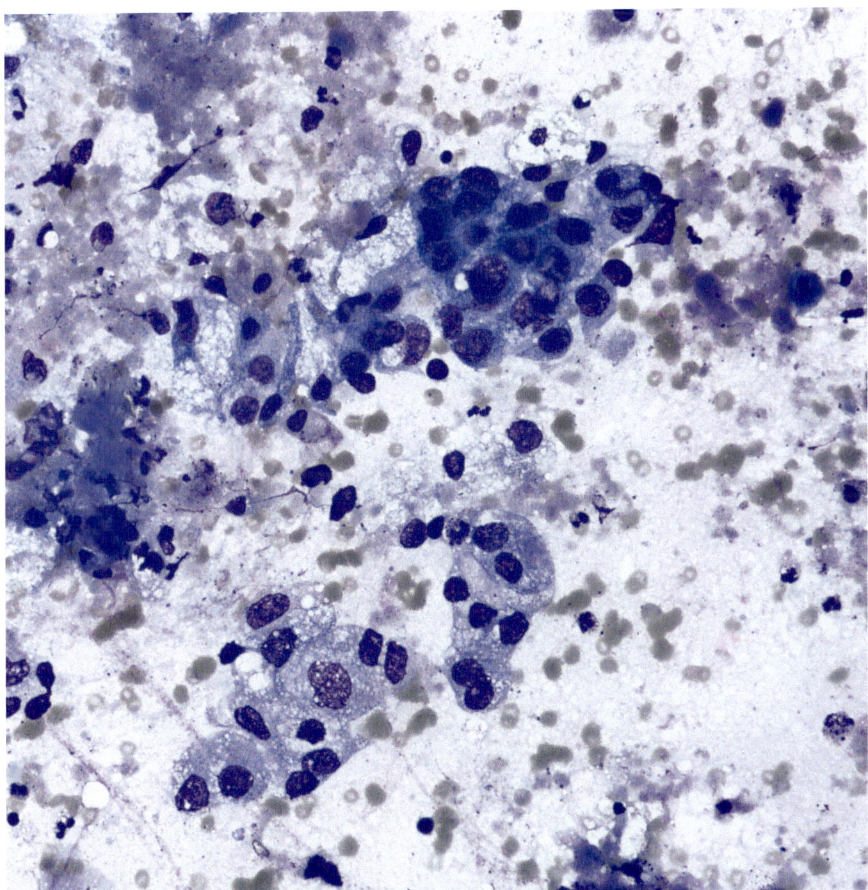

Fig. 8.16 Metastatic adenocarcinoma from the lung (Diff-Quik stain, ×400)

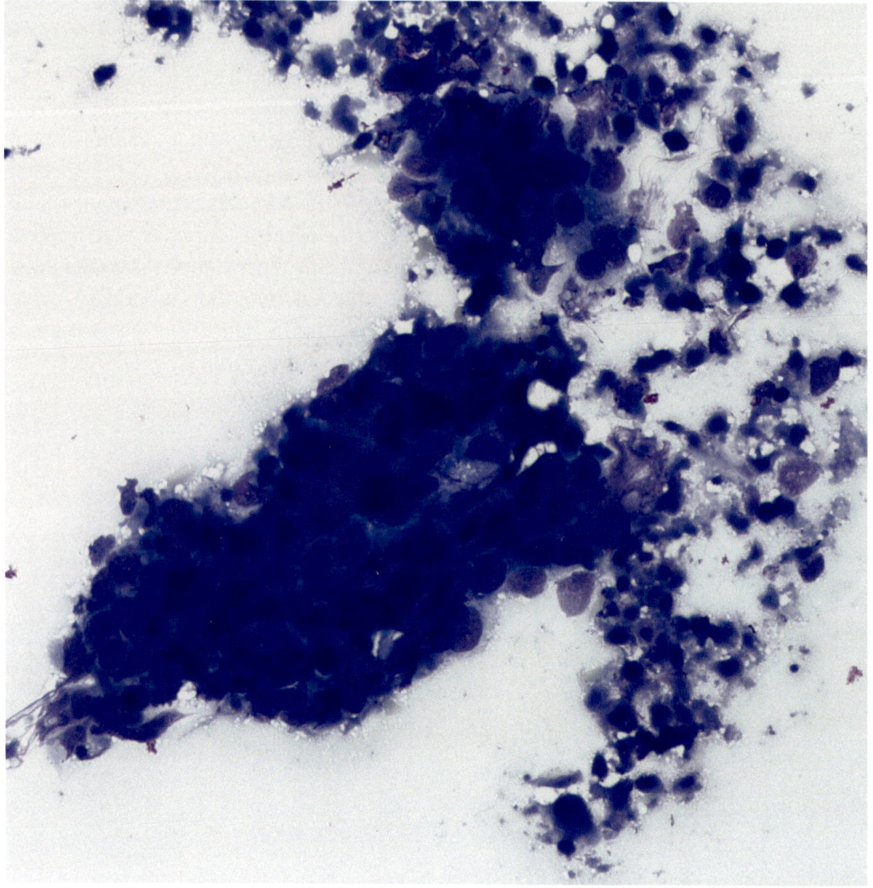

Fig. 8.17 Metastatic squamous cell carcinoma from the lung (Diff-Quik stain, ×400)

- Metastatic adenocarcinoma is the most common.
- Background necrosis or mucin may be seen.

C. Tips and pitfalls

- Cytologic diagnosis of metastasis to the adrenal gland rely on a constellation of clinical history, comparison with previous cytologic or histologic materials, and appropriate additional immunohistochemical stains.

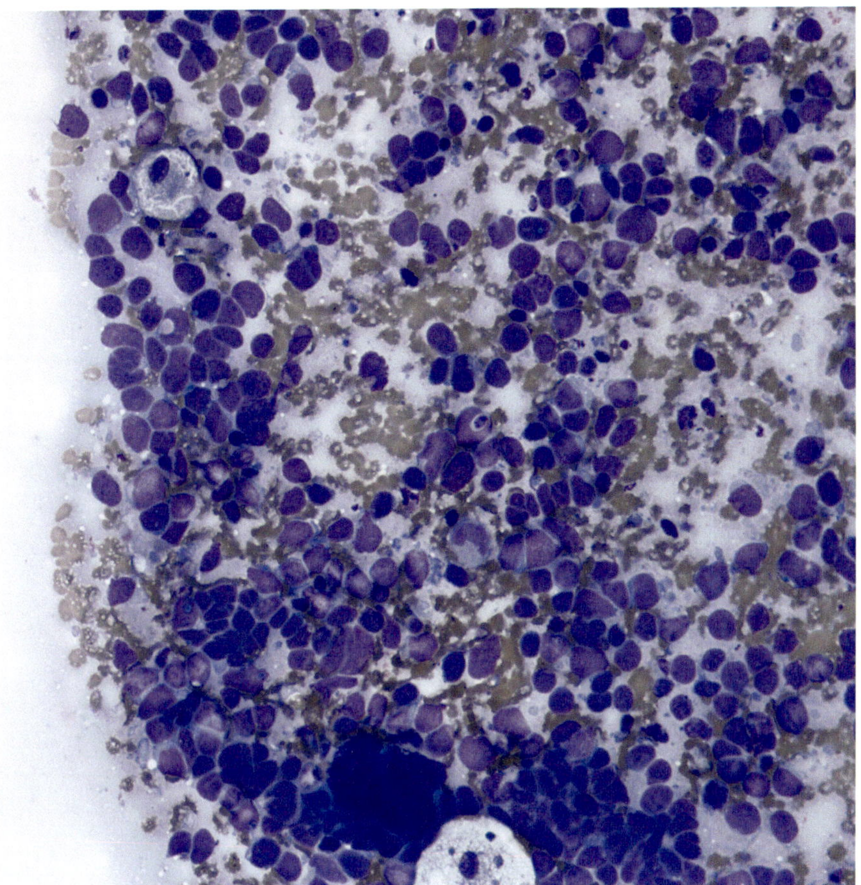

Fig. 8.18 Metastatic small cell carcinoma (Diff-Quik stain, ×400)

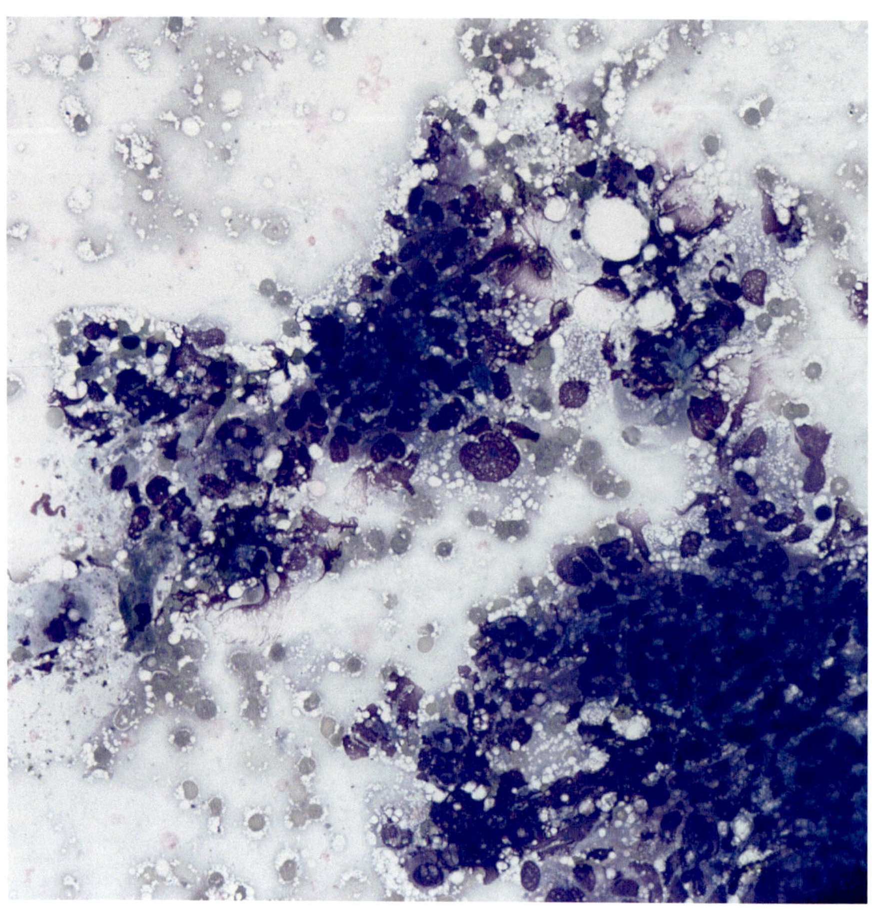

Fig. 8.19 Metastatic clear cell renal cell carcinoma (Diff-Quik stain, ×400)

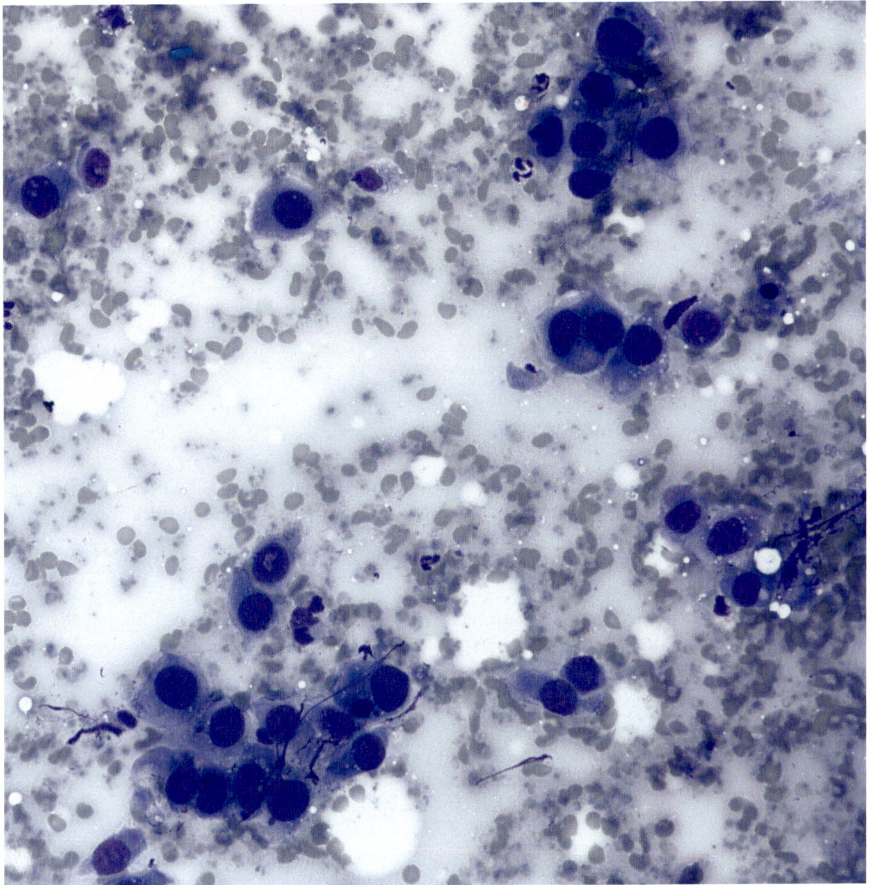

Fig. 8.20 Metastatic high-grade urothelial carcinoma (Diff-Quik stain, ×400)

References

1. Renshaw AA, Granter SR, Cibas ES. Fine-needle aspiration of the adult kidney. Cancer. 1997;81:71–88.
2. Campbell SC, Novick AC, Herts B, et al. Prospective evaluation of fine needle aspiration of small, solid renal masses: accuracy and morbidity. Urology. 1997;50:25–9.
3. Adeniran AJ, Al-Ahmadie H, Iyengar P, Reuter VE, Lin O. Fine needle aspiration of renal cortical lesions in adults. Diagn Cytopathol. 2010;38:710–5.
4. McKiernan J, Yossepowitch O, Kattan MW, Simmons R, Motzer RJ, Reuter VE, Russo P. Partial nephrectomy for renal cortical tumors: pathologic findings and impact on outcome. Urology. 2002;60:1003–9.
5. Tuncali K, vanSonnenberg E, Shankar S, Mortele KJ, Cibas ES, Silverman SG. Evaluation of patients referred for percutaneous ablation of renal tumors: importance of a preprocedural diagnosis. AJR Am J Roentgenol. 2004;183:575–82.
6. Motzer RJ, Bacik J, Schwartz LH, Reuter V, Russo P, Marion S, Mazumdar M. Prognostic factors for survival in previously treated patients with metastatic renal cell carcinoma. J Clin Oncol. 2004;22:454–63.
7. Berg WJ, Schwartz L, Yu R, Mazumdar M, Motzer RJ. Phase II trial of irofulven (6-hydroxymethylacylfulvene) for patients with advanced renal cell carcinoma. Investig New Drugs. 2001;19:317–20.
8. Lopes RI, Moura RN, Artifon E. Endoscopic ultrasound-guided fine-needle aspiration for the diagnosis of kidney lesions: a review. World J Gastrointest Endosc. 2015;7:253–7.
9. Wood BJ, Khan MA, McGovern F, Harisinghani M, Hahn PF, Mueller PR. Imaging guided biopsy of renal masses: indications, accuracy and impact on clinical management. J Urol. 1999;161:1470–4.
10. Renshaw AA, Cibas ES. Kidney and adrenal gland. In: Cibas ES, Ducatman BS, editors. Cytology: diagnostic principles and clinical correlates. Philadelphia: Saunders Elsevier; 2014. p. 423–52.
11. Todd TD, Dhurandhar B, Mody D, Ramzy I, Truong LD. Fine-needle aspiration of cystic lesions of the kidney. Morphologic spectrum and diagnostic problems in 41 cases. Am J Clin Pathol. 1999;111:317–28.
12. Miller MA, Brown JJ. Renal cysts and cystic neoplasms. Magn Reson Imaging Clin N Am. 1997;5:49–66.
13. Bosniak MA. Difficulties in classifying cystic lesions of the kidney. Urol Radiol. 1991;13:91–3.
14. Truong LD, Krishnan B, Cao JT, Barrios R, Suki WN. Renal neoplasm in acquired cystic kidney disease. Am J Kidney Dis. 1995;26:1–12.
15. Clark SP, Kung IT, Tang SK. Fine-needle aspiration of cystic nephroma (multilocular cyst of the kidney). Diagn Cytopathol. 1992;8:349–51.
16. Hartman DS, Davis CJ Jr, Johns T, Goldman SM. Cystic renal cell carcinoma. Urology. 1986;28:145–53.
17. Gibson TE. Interrelationship of renal cysts and tumors: report of three cases. J Urol. 1954;71:241–52.
18. Rodriguez CA, Buskop A, Johnson J, Fromowitz F, Koss LG. Renal oncocytoma: preoperative diagnosis by aspiration biopsy. Acta Cytol. 1980;24:355–9.
19. Grignon DJ, Eble JN. Papillary and metanephric adenomas of the kidney. Semin Diagn Pathol. 1998;15:41–53.
20. Blanco LZ Jr, Schein CO, Patel T, Heagley DE, Cimbaluk DJ, Reddy V, Gattuso P. Fine-needle aspiration of metanephric adenoma of the kidney with clinical, radiographic and histopathologic correlation: a review. Diagn Cytopathol. 2013;41:742–51.
21. Davis CJ Jr, Barton JH, Sesterhenn IA, Mostofi FK. Metanephric adenoma. Clinicopathological study of fifty patients. Am J Surg Pathol. 1995;19:1101–14.
22. Peterson RO. Kidney. In: Urologic pathology. Philadelphia: Lippincott; 1986. p. 1–179.

23. Glenthøj A, Partoft S. Ultrasound-guided percutaneous aspiration of renal angiomyolipoma. Report of two cases diagnosed by cytology. Acta Cytol. 1984;28:265–8.
24. Nguyen GK. Percutaneous fine-needle aspiration biopsy cytology of the kidney and adrenal. Pathol Annu. 1987;22(Pt 1):163–91.
25. Cristallini EG, Paganelli C, Bolis GB. Role of fine-needle aspiration biopsy in the assessment of renal masses. Diagn Cytopathol. 1991;7:32–5.
26. Lizza EF, Elyaderani MK, Belis JA. Atypical presentation of xanthogranulomatous pyelonephritis: diagnosis by ultrasonography and fine needle aspiration biopsy. J Urol. 1984;132: 95–7.
27. Jacobs SC, Berg SI, Lawson RK. Synchronous bilateral renal cell carcinoma: total surgical excision. Cancer. 1980;46:2341–5.
28. Reddy ER. Bilateral renal cell carcinoma--unusual occurrence in three members of one family. Br J Radiol. 1981;54:8–11.
29. Renshaw AA, Lee KR, Madge R, Granter SR. Accuracy of fine needle aspiration in distinguishing subtypes of renal cell carcinoma. Acta Cytol. 1997;41:987–94.
30. Murphy WM, Zambroni BR, Emerson LD, Moinuddin S, Lee LH. Aspiration biopsy of the kidney. Simultaneous collection of cytologic and histologic specimens. Cancer. 1985;56: 200–5.
31. Renshaw AA, Corless CL. Papillary renal cell carcinoma. Histology and immunohistochemistry. Am J Surg Pathol. 1995;19:842–9.
32. Mancilla-Jimenez R, Stanley RJ, Blath RA. Papillary renal cell carcinoma: a clinical, radiologic, and pathologic study of 34 cases. Cancer. 1976;38:2469–80.
33. Lager DJ, Huston BJ, Timmerman TG, Bonsib SM. Papillary renal tumors. Morphologic, cytochemical, and genotypic features. Cancer. 1995;76:669–73.
34. Störkel S, Steart PV, Drenckhahn D, Thoenes W. The human chromophobe cell renal carcinoma: its probable relation to intercalated cells of the collecting duct. Virchows Arch B Cell Pathol Incl Mol Pathol. 1989;56:237–45.
35. Thoenes W, Störkel S, Rumpelt HJ, Moll R, Baum HP, Werner S. Chromophobe cell renal carcinoma and its variants–a report on 32 cases. J Pathol. 1988;155: 277–87.
36. Tejerina E, González-Peramato P, Jiménez-Heffernan JA, Vicandi B, Serrano A, López-Ferrer P, Viguer JM. Cytological features of chromophobe renal cell carcinoma, classic type. A report of nine cases. Cytopathology. 2009;20:44–9.
37. Salamanca J, Alberti N, López-Ríos F, Perez-Barrios A, Martínez-González MA, de Agustín P. Fine needle aspiration of chromophobe renal cell carcinoma. Acta Cytol. 2007;51: 9–15.
38. Bonsib SM, Fischer J, Plattner S, Fallon B. Sarcomatoid renal tumors. Clinicopathologic correlation of three cases. Cancer. 1987;59:527–32.
39. Ro JY, Ayala AG, Sella A, Samuels ML, Swanson DA. Sarcomatoid renal cell carcinoma: clinicopathologic. A study of 42 cases. Cancer. 1987;59:516–26.
40. Akhtar M, Tulbah A, Kardar AH, Ali MA. Sarcomatoid renal cell carcinoma: the chromophobe connection. Am J Surg Pathol. 1997;21:1188–95.
41. Cohen RJ, McNeal JE, Susman M, Sellner LN, Iacopetta BJ, Weinstein SL, Dawkins HJ. Sarcomatoid renal cell carcinoma of papillary origin. A case report and cytogenic evaluation. Arch Pathol Lab Med. 2000;124:1830–2.
42. Baer SC, Ro JY, Ordonez NG, Maiese RL, Loose JH, Grignon DG, Ayala AG. Sarcomatoid collecting duct carcinoma: a clinicopathologic and immunohistochemical study of five cases. Hum Pathol. 1993;24:1017–22.
43. Auger M, Katz RL, Sella A, Ordóñez NG, Lawrence DD, Ro JY. Fine-needle aspiration cytology of sarcomatoid renal cell carcinoma: a morphologic and immunocytochemical study of 15 cases. Diagn Cytopathol. 1993;9:46–51.
44. Caraway NP, Wojcik EM, Katz RL, Ro JY, Ordóñez NG. Cytologic findings of collecting duct carcinoma of the kidney. Diagn Cytopathol. 1995;13:304–9.

45. Kennedy SM, Merino MJ, Linehan WM, Roberts JR, Robertson CN, Neumann RD. Collecting duct carcinoma of the kidney. Hum Pathol. 1990;21:449–56.
46. Ono K, Nishino E, Nakamine H. Renal collecting duct carcinoma. Report of a case with cytologic findings on fine needle aspiration. Acta Cytol. 2000;44:380–4.
47. Owens CL, Argani P, Ali SZ. Mucinous tubular and spindle cell carcinoma of the kidney: cytopathologic findings. Diagn Cytopathol. 2007;35:593–6.
48. Uchida S, Suzuki K, Uno M, Nozaki F, Li CP, Abe E, Yamauchi T, Horiuchi S, Kamo M, Hattori K, Nagashima Y. Mucin-poor and aggressive mucinous tubular and spindle cell carcinoma of the kidney: two case reports. Mol Clin Oncol. 2017;7:777–82.
49. Marks-Jones DA, Zynger DL, Parwani AV, Cai G. Fine needle aspiration biopsy of renal mucinous tubular and spindle cell carcinoma: report of two cases. Diagn Cytopathol. 2010;38: 51–5.
50. Tickoo SK, Chen YB, Zynger DL. Biopsy interpretation of the kidney and adrenal gland. Philadelphia: Wolters Kluwer; 2015.
51. Helm CW, Burwood RJ, Harrison NW, Melcher DH. Aspiration cytology of solid renal tumours. Br J Urol. 1983;55:249–53.
52. Santamaría M, Jauregui I, Urtasun F, Bertol A. Fine needle aspiration biopsy in urothelial carcinoma of the renal pelvis. Acta Cytol. 1995;39:443–8.
53. Powers CN, Elbadawi A. "Cercariform" cells: a clue to the cytodiagnosis of transitional cell origin of metastatic neoplasms? Diagn Cytopathol. 1995;13:15–21.
54. Renshaw AA, Madge R. Cercariform cells for helping distinguish transitional cell carcinoma from non-small cell lung carcinoma in fine needle aspirates. Acta Cytol. 1997;41: 999–1007.
55. Gattuso P, Ramzy I, Truong LD, Lankford KL, Green L, Kluskens L, Spitz DJ, Reddy VB. Utilization of fine-needle aspiration in the diagnosis of metastatic tumors to the kidney. Diagn Cytopathol. 1999;21:35–8.
56. Giashuddin S, Cangiarella J, Elgert P, Levine PH. Metastases to the kidney: eleven cases diagnosed by aspiration biopsy with histological correlation. Diagn Cytopathol. 2005;32: 325–9.
57. de Agustín P, López-Ríos F, Alberti N, Pérez-Barrios A. Fine-needle aspiration biopsy of the adrenal glands: a ten-year experience. Diagn Cytopathol. 1999;21:92–7.
58. Dusenbery D, Dekker A. Fine needle aspiration diagnosis of hepatocellular carcinoma in metastatic sites. Diagn Cytopathol. 1996;14:126–34.
59. Kumar R, Dey P. Fine-needle aspiration cytology of non-neoplastic adrenal pathology. Diagn Cytopathol. 2016;44:472–6.
60. Puri R, Thandassery RB, Choudhary NS, Kotecha H, Misra SR, Bhagat S, Paliwal M, Madan K, Saraf N, Sarin H, Guleria M, Sud R. Endoscopic ultrasound-guided fine-needle aspiration of the adrenal glands: analysis of 21 patients. Clin Endosc. 2015;48:165–70.
61. Silverman SG, Mueller PR, Pinkney LP, Koenker RM, Seltzer SE. Predictive value of image-guided adrenal biopsy: analysis of results of 101 biopsies. Radiology. 1993;187:715–8.
62. Fassina AS, Borsato S, Fedeli U. Fine needle aspiration cytology (FNAC) of adrenal masses. Cytopathology. 2000;11:302–11.
63. Settakorn J, Sirivanichai C, Rangdaeng S, Chaiwun B. Fine-needle aspiration cytology of adrenal myelolipoma: case report and review of the literature. Diagn Cytopathol. 1999;21: 409–12.
64. Jia AH, Du HQ, Fan MH, Li YH, Xu JL, Niu GF, Bai J, Zhang GZ, Ren YB. Clinical and pathological analysis of 116 cases of adult adrenal cortical adenoma and literature review. Onco Targets Ther. 2015;8:1251–7.
65. Wu HH, Cramer HM, Kho J, Elsheikh TM. Fine needle aspiration cytology of benign adrenal cortical nodules. A comparison of cytologic findings with those of primary and metastatic adrenal malignancies. Acta Cytol. 1998;42:1352–8.
66. Belldegrun A, Hussain S, Seltzer SE, Loughlin KR, Gittes RF, Richie JP. Incidentally discovered mass of the adrenal gland. Surg Gynecol Obstet. 1986;163:203–8.

67. Ross NS, Aron DC. Hormonal evaluation of the patient with an incidentally discovered adrenal mass. N Engl J Med. 1990 15;323:1401–5.
68. Sharma S, Singh R, Verma K. Cytomorphology of adrenocortical carcinoma and comparison with renal cell carcinoma. Acta Cytol. 1997;41:385–92.
69. Katz RL, Patel S, Mackay B, Zornoza J. Fine needle aspiration cytology of the adrenal gland. Acta Cytol. 1984;28:269–82.
70. Saboorian MH, Katz RL, Charnsangavej C. Fine needle aspiration cytology of primary and metastatic lesions of the adrenal gland. A series of 188 biopsies with radiologic correlation. Acta Cytol. 1995;39:843–51.
71. Wadih GE, Nance KV, Silverman JF. Fine-needle aspiration cytology of the adrenal gland. Fifty biopsies in 48 patients. Arch Pathol Lab Med. 1992;116:841–6.

Chapter 9
Bone and Soft Tissue

Evita B. Henderson-Jackson and Marilyn M. Bui

Introduction

The disadvantage of small biopsies such as fine needle aspiration (FNA) or core biopsy is their potential for inadequate sampling. The use of rapid on-site evaluation (ROSE) has significant potential to improve adequacy rates. Results of a meta-analysis reported by Schmidt et al. showed on average a 12% improvement in adequacy rate of soft tissue biopsies after implementation of ROSE [1]. With an increasing use of minimally invasive diagnostic techniques, FNA cytology and touch imprint cytology of core biopsies have become an important initial diagnostic tool. There is a high sensitivity (25–100%) and specificity (83–100%) in diagnosing bone and soft tissue lesions by cytology [2–13]. However, the variability in reported sensitivities and specificities with use of cytology may result from study design, type of tissue sampled (bone versus soft tissue), experience of operator obtaining material, experience of cytotechnologist and/or pathologist, presence or absence of ROSE, and the adherent rarity of such lesions. Although the concept of using FNA biopsy for initial diagnosis of primary bone and soft tissue tumors may not be generally accepted by some pathologists, most pathologists are acceptable to use FNA to confirm recurrent/metastatic sarcoma. Despite these challenges, cytology is used to diagnose soft tissue and bone lesions in many different medical institutions [6–8, 14–21]. Additionally, cytology is used to diagnose metastatic carcinoma, lymphoma, and melanoma clinically presenting as a bone or soft tissue lesion. It is important to know that ROSE is critically important to differentiate a sarcoma from a non-sarcoma malignancy, especially when pathologic fracture is associated, because the immediate management for these two entities is completely different. Primary sarcoma with pathologic fracture is contraindicated with intramedullary

E. B. Henderson-Jackson · M. M. Bui (✉)
Department of Anatomic Pathology, H. Lee Moffitt Cancer Center & Research Institute, Tampa, FL, USA
e-mail: Evita.Henderson@moffitt.org; Marilyn.Bui@moffitt.org

G. Cai, A. J. Adeniran (eds.), *Rapid On-site Evaluation (ROSE)*,
https://doi.org/10.1007/978-3-030-21799-0_9

rod for fixation due to the potential of spreading sarcoma via bone marrow. However, metastatic disease and hematopoietic malignancy are considered systemic and indicated with intramedullary rod fixation. This chapter will focus on addressing the benign and malignant tumors of bone and soft tissue, not non-sarcomatous tumors.

We also advocate using cytology as an adjunct during frozen section evaluation to enhance the intraoperative diagnosis of bone and soft tissue tumor [22, 23]. In order for ROSE to be useful in the evaluation of bone and soft tissue tumors, success is dependent upon gathering appropriate clinical and radiological information to complement on-site evaluation. In this chapter, we present a practical approach to the evaluation of immediate on-site cytology of bone and soft tissue lesions to improve adequacy, facilitate proper specimen triage, and enhance accuracy of diagnoses.

Diagnostic Considerations

Specimen Adequacy Assessment

Currently, there are no established adequacy criteria for soft tissue and bone cytology. Study by Palmer et al. arbitrarily defined adequacy in soft tissue cytology fine needle aspiration biopsies as the presence of at least 5 clusters of 10 or more well-visualized cells present on a majority (>50%) of prepared slides [24]. The ultimate reference is whether the clinical, radiologic, and cytologic findings seen explain the presence of the lesion. If there is discordance, the adequacy of the specimen is questionable. The general rule of thumb is that for a homogenous tumor, the adequacy sample size is less than that for a heterogeneous tumor, because the sampling needs to represent various heterogeneous areas of the tumor.

Inadequate or unsatisfactory specimens may result from a variety of causes. The lesion of interest may have been missed and cells from surrounding tissue were aspirated. It is crucial to always correlate with radiological information. Cystic, necrotic, and/or hemorrhagic lesions may be difficult to aspiration because the diagnostic areas prove hard to discern from areas of necrosis, cystic change, and blood. Additionally, lesions that are fibrous with significant collagenous, sclerotic, and/or hyalinized stroma may be difficult to sample because cells are not easily dislodged from stroma [25]. Please also be aware that reactive changes in fatty tissue may mimic liposarcoma and reactive changes in fibroblasts/myofibroblasts within connective tissue may mimic a pleomorphic sarcoma.

Specimen Triage for Ancillary Testing

Some sarcomas have distinct molecular signature such as translocation, gene rearrangement, or mutation. Ancillary testing, especially molecular testing, is warranted for confirmation of a definitive diagnosis. Air-dried touch imprint cytology is an excellent source of specimen for molecular testing [26]. It is important to recognize

Table 9.1 Soft tissue tumors and their common associated chromosomal aberrations

Tumor	Molecular alterations
Alveolar rhabdomyosarcoma	PAX3-FOXO1, PAX7-FOXO1 fusion
Alveolar soft part sarcoma	ASPL-TFE3 fusion
Clear cell sarcoma	EWSR1-ATF1 fusion
Dermatofibrosarcoma protuberans	COL1A1-PDGFR fusion
Desmoplastic small round cell tumor	EWSR1-WT1 fusion
Ewing sarcoma	EWSR1-FLI1, EWSR1-ERG fusion
Extraskeletal myxoid chondrosarcoma	EWSR1-NR4A3 fusion
Fibromatosis	CTNNB1 mutation
Gastrointestinal stromal tumor	GIST, PDGFR mutation, SDH deficient
Liposarcoma (well-differentiated or dedifferentiated)	MDM2 and/or CDK4 amplification
Low-grade fibromyxoid fibrosarcoma	FUS-CREB3L1, FUS-CREB3L2 fusion
Myxoid liposarcoma	FUS-DDIT3 (CHOP), EWSR1-DDIT3 (CHOP) fusion
Myoepithelial tumor	EWSR1, PLAG1 rearrangement
Nodular fasciitis	USP6 rearrangement
Synovial sarcoma	SSX1-SYT, SSX2-XYT fusion
Tenosynovial giant cell tumor	CSF-COL6A3 fusion

these entities during ROSE to triage samples for pertinent molecular testing. Examples of common sarcomas and their corresponding molecular alterations are listed in Table 9.1.

Pattern Recognition Is the Key

The purpose of ROSE is to determine tissue adequacy, delineate the preliminary diagnosis (neoplastic vs. nonneoplastic, benign-low grade vs. malignant-high grade), and recognize the entities that can be worked up by specific ancillary testing, such as translocation studies, so that the tissue can be triaged for appropriate testing. In conjunction with clinical and radiological information, pattern recognition of the cellular and the background morphology is the key to delineate a pertinent list of differential diagnoses.

Evaluation based on cytomorphology patterns can be represented by the following tumor groups: adipocytic, myxoid, spindle cell, epithelioid, round cell, pleomorphic cell, and giant cell-rich neoplasm.

Adipocytic Neoplasms

This is the most commonly encountered group of soft tissue tumor ranging from benign to malignant tumor.

Lipoma

This is the most common soft tissue tumor. Often seen in adults. The tumor rarely grows over the size of 10 cm. It appears homogenous and isodense to fat on imaging.

1. Cytomorphologic features
   - Variably sized tissue fragments.
   - Uniform, univacuolated adipocytes.
   - Small, bland nuclei.
   - Occasional small capillaries.
2. Tips and pitfalls
   - Similar to normal adipose tissue.
   - Should be distinguished from atypical lipomatous tumor or well-differentiated liposarcoma.
   - Tumor often S100 positive, but this stain is not commonly used for diagnosing lipoma because the adipocytic differentiation is apparent on HE stain.

Hibernoma

This is a rare tumor which often occurs in adults and can mimic atypical lipomatous tumor on imaging.

1. Cytomorphologic features
   - Variably sized tissue fragments of adipocytes containing many small capillaries.
   - Numerous adipocytes with multiple small cytoplasmic vacuoles (brown fat).
   - Granular to multivacuolated cytoplasm.
   - Small, bland nuclei.
2. Tips and pitfalls
   - Should be distinguished from atypical lipomatous tumor or well-differentiated liposarcoma, spindle cell/pleomorphic lipoma, lipoma with fat necrosis, and myxoid liposarcoma.
   - Tumor often S100 positive; again the morphology is sufficient to diagnose hibernoma.

Spindle Cell/Pleomorphic Lipoma

It is more often seen in older male patients. Neck and upper trunk are the most common sites.

1. Cytomorphologic features

   - Variably sized tissue fragments of mature adipocytes.
   - Occasional myxoid background with multivacuolated lipoblast-like cells.
   - Spindle cell lipoma demonstrates prominent spindle cells of uniform and bland appearance, ropy collagen fibers, and mast cells.
   - Pleomorphic lipoma demonstrates "floret cells" with dark smudgy chromatin (Fig. 9.1).

2. Tips and Pitfalls

   - Should be distinguished from atypical lipomatous tumor or well-differentiated liposarcoma, myxoid liposarcoma, schwannoma, low-grade myxofibrosarcoma, solitary fibrous tumor, and dermatofibrosarcoma protuberans.
   - Tumor often CD34 positive.

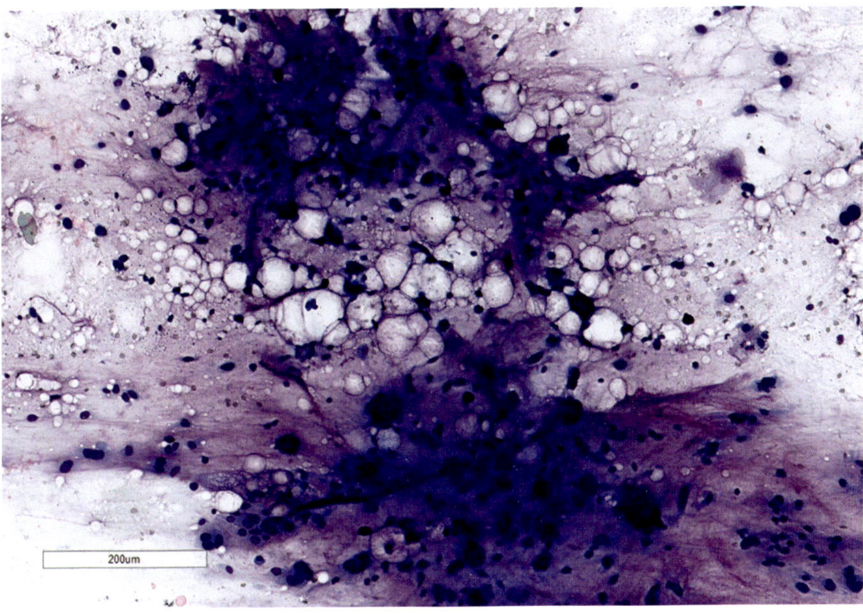

Fig. 9.1 Pleomorphic lipoma (Diff-Quik stain)

Atypical Lipomatous Tumor/Well-Differentiated Liposarcoma

It occurs often in middle-aged adults and accounts for 40–45% of all liposarcomas. It presents with a deep-seated, enlarging mass frequently in thigh, retroperitoneum, paratesticular, and mediastinum areas.

1. Cytomorphologic features (Fig. 9.2)
   - Mature adipocytic cells with variably sized lipid vacuoles.
   - Atypical stromal cell nuclei.
   - Lipoblasts present.
2. Tips and pitfalls
   - Should be distinguished from spindle cell/pleomorphic lipoma, lipoma with fat necrosis, and hibernoma.
   - Tumor often expresses MDM2 or CDK4 by immunostain or has amplification of these genes.

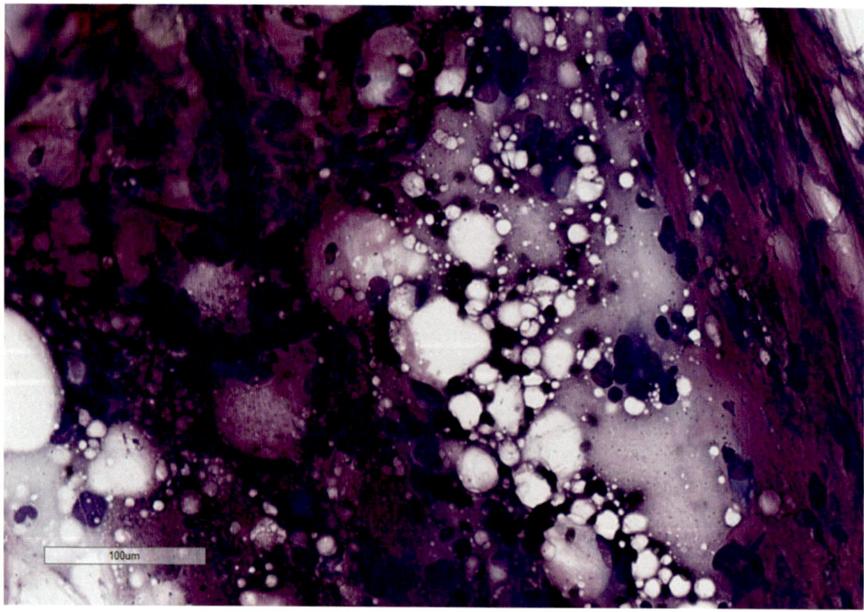

Fig. 9.2 Well-differentiated liposarcoma (Diff-Quik stain)

Myxoid Liposarcoma

It often occurs in the deep soft tissue of lower limbs, especially thigh of young adults.

1. Cytomorphologic features (Figs. 9.3 and 9.4)
   - Tissue fragments containing abundant myxoid matrix material.
   - Delicate, thin-walled capillaries.
   - Primitive round to oval cells.
   - Univacuolate and bivacuolate lipoblasts.
   - Round cell liposarcoma contains increased number of uniform round cells with scant cytoplasm and nucleoli.
2. Tips and pitfalls
   - The differential diagnosis includes spindle cell lipoma with myxoid change, low-grade myxofibrosarcoma, extraskeletal myxoid chondrosarcoma, and myoepithelioma.
   - It almost never occurs in retroperitoneum as a primary tumor. Metastatic disease can involve retroperitoneum.

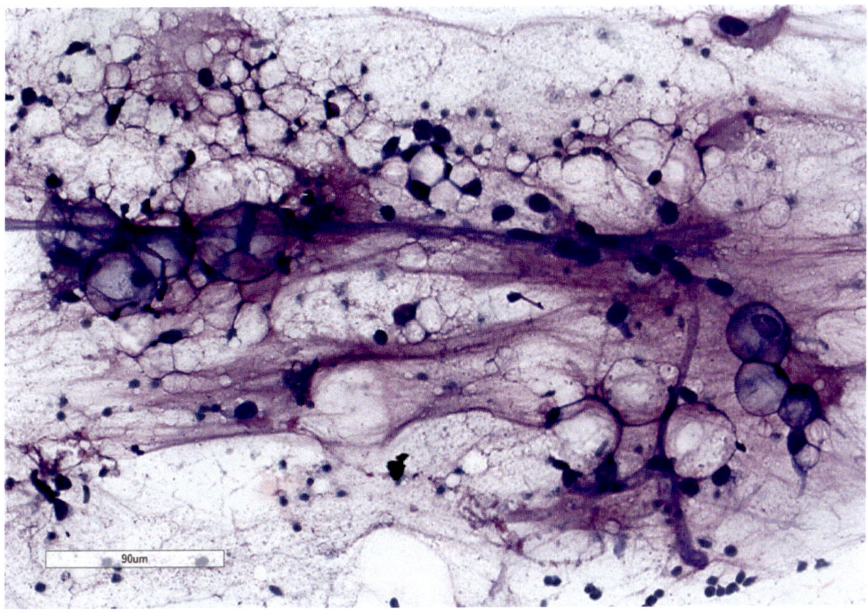

Fig. 9.3 Myxoid liposarcoma (Diff-Quik stain)

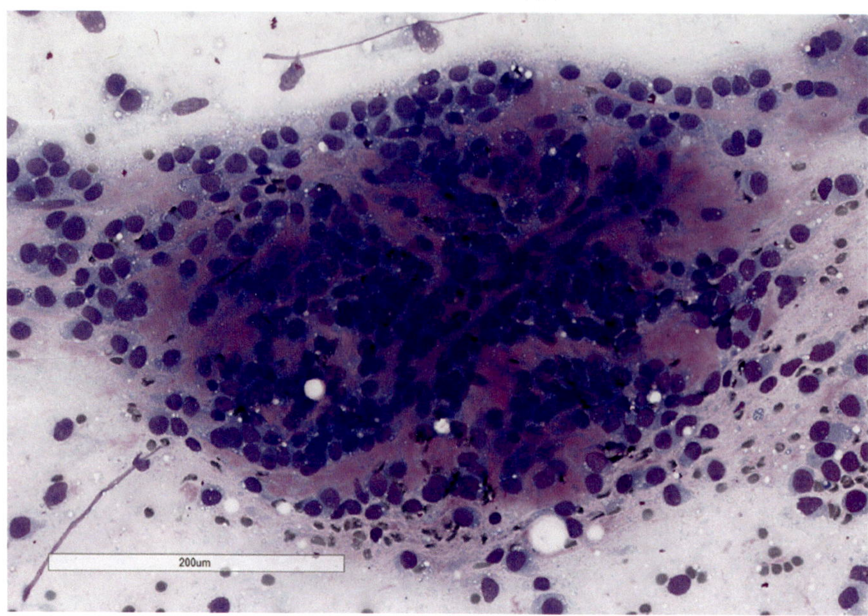

Fig. 9.4 Round cell liposarcoma (Diff-Quik stain)

Dedifferentiated Liposarcoma

It is most commonly seen in the retroperitoneal and intra-abdominal spaces. Imaging shows fatty and nonfatty components in tumor.

1. Cytomorphologic features (Fig. 9.5)
   - Nonlipogenic pleomorphic or spindle cell tissue fragments.
   - Occasional lipoblasts.
2. Tips and pitfalls
   - For small biopsies where the well-differentiated liposarcoma component is missing, think about this entity and perform MDM2 and CDK4 testing to confirm this diagnosis.
   - Dedifferentiated component may exhibit features similar to undifferentiated pleomorphic sarcoma, high-grade myxofibrosarcoma, and pleomorphic liposarcoma.

Pleomorphic Liposarcoma

It is the rarest subtype of liposarcoma and is commonly seen in the late adult life. The tumor is often presented as a fast-growing painless mass.

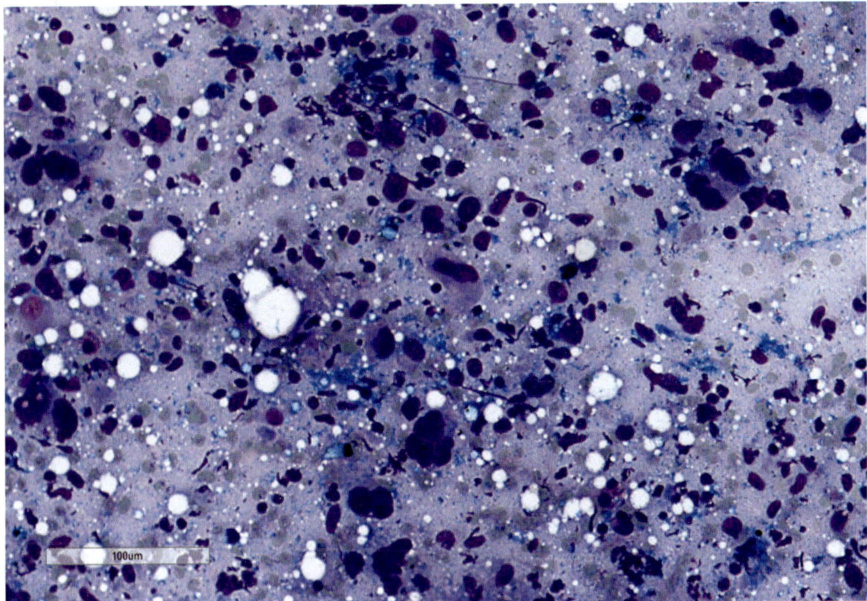

Fig. 9.5 Dedifferentiated liposarcoma (Diff-Quik stain)

1. Cytomorphologic features
   - Cellular smear with clusters and dispersed pleomorphic cells with marked atypia.
   - Variable number of atypical lipoblasts.
   - Mitoses and necrosis.
2. Tips and pitfalls
   - The differential diagnosis includes dedifferentiated liposarcoma, high-grade myxofibrosarcoma, and other pleomorphic sarcomas.

Round Cell Neoplasms

Most of the round cell tumors are high-grade sarcoma. Ewing sarcoma, desmoplastic small round cell tumor (DSRCT), alveolar rhabdomyosarcoma, embryonal rhabdomyosarcoma, undifferentiated round cell sarcoma, mesenchymal chondrosarcoma, round cell liposarcoma, poorly differentiated synovial sarcoma, and osteosarcoma are common encounters. In order to differentiate these tumors during ROSE, attention to tigroid background in Ewing sarcoma, osteoid matrix in osteosarcoma, and prominent fibrous matrix in DSRCT are high-yielded. Synovial sarcoma is typically considered a spindle cell pattern tumor. However, in fluid or touch prep samples, the spindle cells are short and appear round. Except embryonal rhabdomyosarcoma, undifferentiated round cell sarcoma, and osteosarcoma, the other sarcomas have confirmatory molecular signatures; thus triage specimen appropriately for ancillary testing is important. In addition, for this group of tumors, clinical and radiological correlation are very helpful.

Ewing Sarcoma

It is the second most common sarcoma of bone in children and young adults. About 10–20% of cases are extraskeletal. Common presentation is a painful deep soft tissue mass.

1. Cytomorphologic features (Fig. 9.6)
   - Cellular smears with dispersed round cells including naked nuclei.
   - Smaller hyperchromatic degenerating cells.
   - Tigroid background.
   - Nuclear molding.
   - Scant cytoplasm with small intracytoplasmic vacuoles.
2. Tips and pitfalls
   - Differential diagnosis includes synovial sarcoma, desmoplastic blue round cell tumor, rhabdomyosarcoma, undifferentiated round cell sarcoma, mesenchymal chondrosarcoma, and small cell osteosarcoma.
   - Positive markers include CD99, PRKCB II, ERG, FLI1, and NKX2.2.

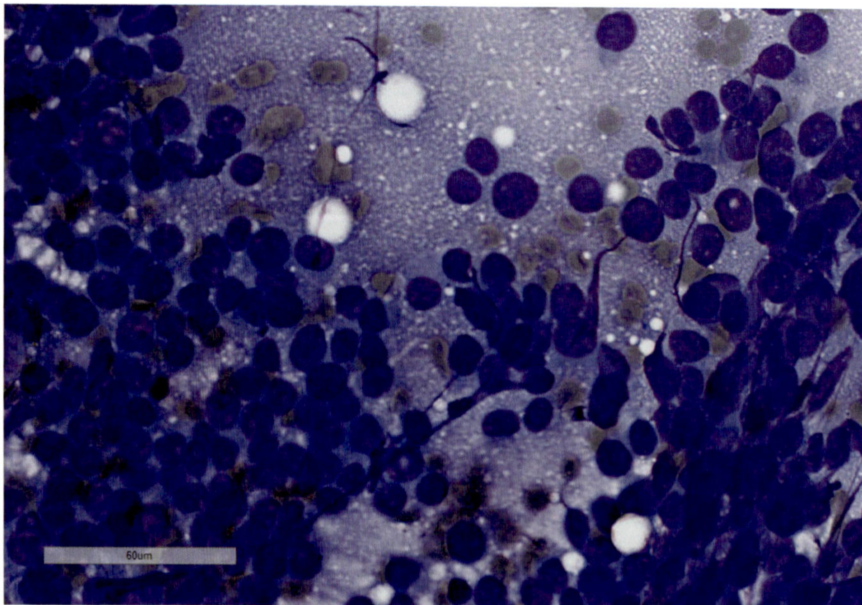

Fig. 9.6 Ewing sarcoma with tigroid background (Diff-Quik stain)

Desmoplastic Small Round Cell Tumor (DSRCT)

It is an aggressive neoplasm with polyphenotypic differentiation. Tumor masses are present on serosal surfaces. Commonly seen in adolescents and young adults, particularly in males.

1. Cytomorphologic features (Fig. 9.7)
    - Sheets or clusters of round cells.
    - Round to ovoid uniform nuclei.
    - Nuclear molding.
    - Collagenous stromal fragments.
2. Tips and pitfalls
    - Differential diagnosis includes synovial sarcoma, Ewing sarcoma, rhabdomyosarcoma, undifferentiated round cell sarcoma, mesenchymal chondrosarcoma, small cell osteosarcoma, neuroblastoma, and round cell liposarcoma.
    - Tumor shows a multi-phenotypic staining pattern, including cytokeratin, EMA, desmin, NSE, and WT1.

Alveolar Rhabdomyosarcoma

Commonly seen in adolescents and young adults. The extremities, head/neck, and trunk are common sites.

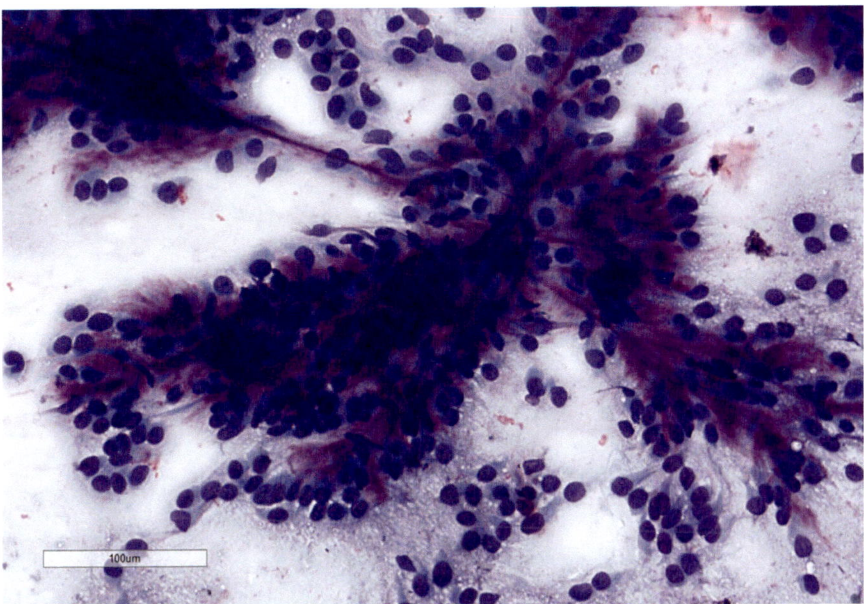

Fig. 9.7 Desmoplastic small round cell tumor (Diff-Quik stain)

1. Cytomorphologic features

   - Discohesive larger round to polygonal cells.
   - Round to irregular nuclei.
   - Multinucleated giant cells "wreath-like".
   - Rhabdomyoblasts, occasional.
   - Mitosis and necrosis.

2. Tips and pitfalls

   - Differential diagnosis includes synovial sarcoma, Ewing sarcoma, desmoplastic blue round cell tumor, undifferentiated round cell sarcoma, mesenchymal chondrosarcoma, small cell osteosarcoma, neuroblastoma, and round cell liposarcoma.
   - Tumor is positive for desmin, myogenin, and Myo D1.

Embryonal Rhabdomyosarcoma

Patients' ages range from infants and children to adults. The head/neck and genitourinary system are common sites.

1. Cytomorphologic features

   - Loosely cohesive and isolated cells.
   - Round- and/or spindle-shaped cells.
   - Cellular pleomorphism.
   - Rare inclusion-line cytoplasmic condensation (myogenic differentiation).

2. Tips and pitfalls

   - Differential diagnosis includes synovial sarcoma, Ewing sarcoma, desmoplastic blue round cell tumor, undifferentiated round cell sarcoma, mesenchymal chondrosarcoma, small cell osteosarcoma, neuroblastoma, and round cell liposarcoma.
   - Tumor is positive for desmin, myogenin, and Myo D1.

Undifferentiated Round Cell Sarcoma

This is a diagnosis of exclusion.

1. Cytomorphologic features

   - Round, ovoid, or spindled cells in clusters or singly.
   - Nuclear pleomorphism.
   - Prominent nucleoli.

- Amphophilic cytoplasm.
- +/− fibrous or myxoid stroma.

2. Tips and pitfalls

- Differential diagnosis includes synovial sarcoma, Ewing sarcoma, desmoplastic blue round cell tumor, rhabdomyosarcoma, mesenchymal chondrosarcoma, small cell osteosarcoma, neuroblastoma, and round cell liposarcoma.
- Tumor is positive for CD99 but lacks the characteristic immunostain pattern of the above tumors.

Mesenchymal Chondrosarcoma

Commonly seen in adolescents and young adults. Craniofacial bones, ribs, ilium, and vertebrae are common sites. One-third cases are extraskeletal.

1. Cytomorphologic features

- Round primitive cells and cartilaginous tissue.
- Cartilaginous matrix.
- Mitoses.

2. Tips and pitfalls

- Differential diagnosis includes synovial sarcoma, Ewing sarcoma, desmoplastic blue round cell tumor, rhabdomyosarcoma, undifferentiated round cell sarcoma, mesenchymal chondrosarcoma, small cell osteosarcoma, neuroblastoma, and round cell liposarcoma.
- Tumor is positive for SOX9 and CD99.

Poorly Differentiated Synovial Sarcoma

Commonly seen in young adults. About 70% occur in deep soft tissue of lower and upper extremities. One-third cases have calcifications on imaging.

1. Cytomorphologic features (Fig. 9.8)

- Cellular smears of uniform round cells.
- Small nucleoli.
- Scant cytoplasm.

2. Tips and pitfalls

- Differential diagnosis includes Ewing sarcoma, synovial sarcoma, desmoplastic blue round cell tumor, rhabdomyosarcoma, undifferentiated round cell

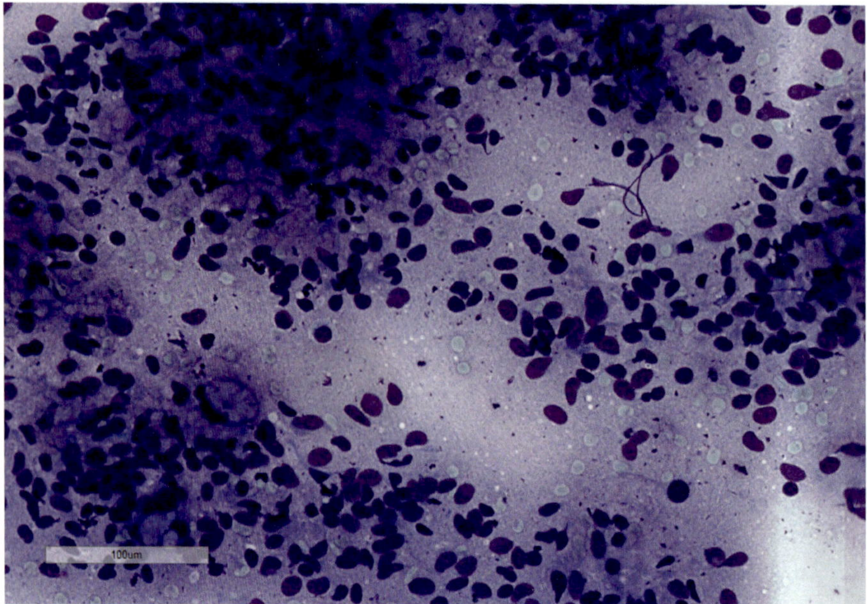

Fig. 9.8 Synovial sarcoma with short spindle cells mimic round cells (Diff-Quik stain)

sarcoma, mesenchymal chondrosarcoma, small cell osteosarcoma, neuroblastoma, and round cell liposarcoma.

- Positive stains include cytokeratin, EMA, TLE-1, bcl-2, and CD99.

Small Cell Osteosarcoma

It affects all ages with most occurring in the second decade of life. Metaphysis of long bones is the most common site.

1. Cytomorphologic features

   - Single cells or clusters of round cells.
   - Cellular pleomorphism.
   - Cytoplasmic vacuolation.
   - metachromatic osteoid-like matrix (rare).

2. Tips and pitfalls

   - Differential diagnosis includes synovial sarcoma, Ewing sarcoma, desmoplastic blue round cell tumor, rhabdomyosarcoma, undifferentiated round cell sarcoma, mesenchymal chondrosarcoma, neuroblastoma, and round cell liposarcoma.
   - Osteoid formation.

Neuroblastoma

Neonates and children are most commonly affected. It arises in adrenal gland or along abdominal sympathetic chain.

1. Cytomorphologic features
   - Dispersed small round primitive cells.
   - "Salt and pepper" chromatin.
   - Fibrillary matrix (neuropil).
   - Homer-Wright rosettes or ganglion-like cells (rare).
2. Tips and pitfalls
   - Differential diagnosis includes synovial sarcoma, Ewing sarcoma, desmoplastic blue round cell tumor, rhabdomyosarcoma, undifferentiated round cell sarcoma, mesenchymal chondrosarcoma, small cell osteosarcoma, and round cell liposarcoma.
   - Tumor is positive for GLUT1 and S100.

High-Grade Myxoid/Round Cell Liposarcoma

The common presentation is young adults with a deep soft tissue mass in lower limbs such as thigh.

1. Cytomorphologic features
   - Singly dispersed and clusters of round cells.
   - Scant or absent lipoblasts, myxoid stroma, and vasculature.
2. Tips and pitfalls
   - Differential diagnosis includes synovial sarcoma, Ewing sarcoma, desmoplastic blue round cell tumor, rhabdomyosarcoma, undifferentiated round cell sarcoma, mesenchymal chondrosarcoma, and neuroblastoma.
   - Triage tissue for molecular testing for confirmation.

Spindle Cell Neoplasms

This is the largest group of tumors ranging from benign to high-grade malignancy. The differential diagnosis includes nodular fasciitis, fibromatosis (desmoid tumor), benign peripheral nerve sheath tumors, malignant peripheral nerve sheath tumor, dermatofibrosarcoma protuberans (DFSP), solitary fibrous tumor (SFT), gastrointestinal stromal tumor (GIST), leiomyoma, leiomyosarcoma, synovial sarcoma, spindle cell/sclerosing rhabdomyosarcoma, fibrosarcoma, dedifferentiated liposarcoma, and undifferentiated spindle cell sarcoma.

Peripheral Nerve Sheath Tumor: Schwannoma/Neurofibroma

Slow-growing and long-standing history of mass involving nerves of skin and subcutaneous tissue. May be painful.

1. Cytomorphologic features (Fig. 9.9)
   - Clusters of spindle cells.
   - Uniform, wavy nuclei.
   - Fibrillary to myxoid/collagenous stroma.
   - Nuclear.
   - Inconspicious nucleoli.
2. Tips and pitfalls
   - Differential diagnosis includes spindle cell lipoma, leiomyoma, fibromatosis, solitary fibrous tumor, low-grade MPNST, low-grade leiomyosarcoma, and low-grade fibromyxoid sarcoma.
   - Tumor is positive for S100 and SOX10. NF-1 is also positive in neurofibroma.

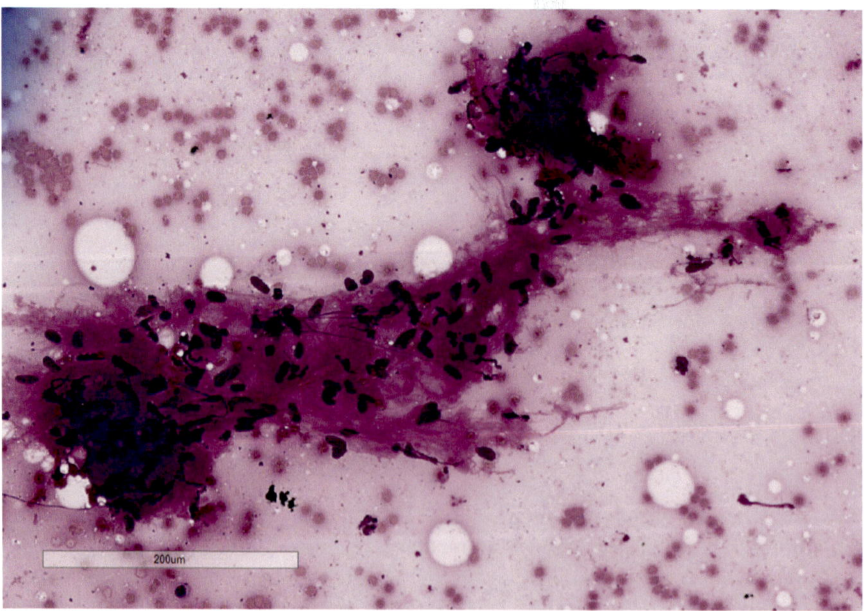

Fig. 9.9 Schwannoma (Diff-Quik stain)

Fibromatosis

Abdominal and extra-abdominal. Associated with Gardner-type familiar adenomatous polyposis. Associated with surgery.

1. Cytomorphologic features (Fig. 9.10)
   - Uniform, bland spindle cells, singly or in slender fascicles.
   - Collagenous stroma.
   - Hypocellular smears.
2. Tips and pitfalls
   - Differential diagnosis includes nodular fasciitis, scar tissue, low-grade fibromyxoid sarcoma, solitary fibrous tumor, gastrointestinal stromal tumor, smooth muscle tumor, and nerve sheath tumor.
   - Beta-catenin is positive.

Nodular Fasciitis

Rapid-growing lesion. History of trauma or surgery. Peripheral calcification of the lesion.

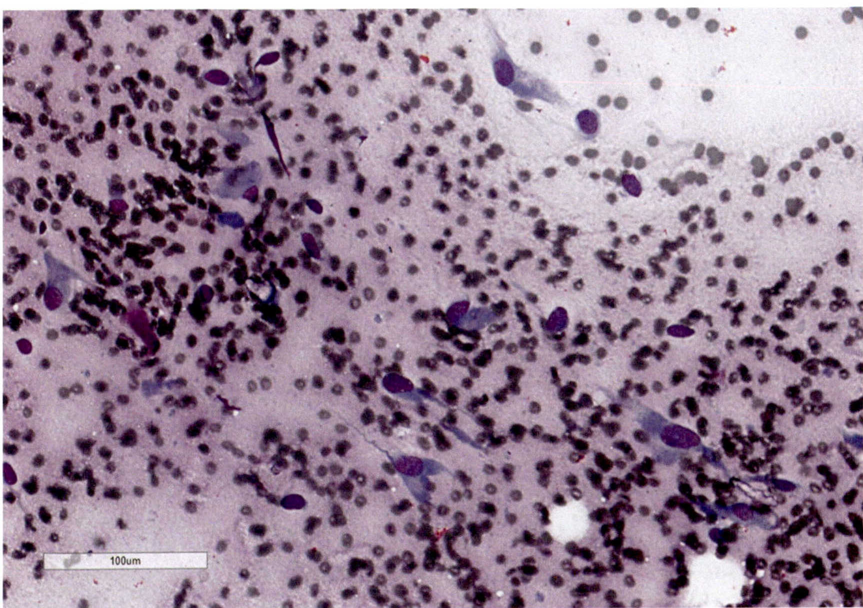

Fig. 9.10 Fibromatosis (Diff-Quik stain)

1. Cytomorphologic features
    - Cellular smears of spindled to stellate cells.
    - Myxoid, inflammatory, or collagenous background.
    - Ganglion-like cells with prominent nuclei.
2. Tips and pitfalls
    - Differential diagnosis includes soft tissue sarcoma, fibromatosis, nerve sheath tumor, fibrous histiocytoma, inflammatory myofibroblastic tumor, myositis ossificans, and myxofibrosarcoma.

Dermatofibrosarcoma Protuberans

Young to middle-aged adults with male predominance. Nodular cutaneous mass of the trunk and proximal extremities.

1. Cytomorphologic features (Fig. 9.11)
    - Dense to loose aggregates of spindle cells (storiform).
    - Myxoid/collagenous stroma.
    - Rare entrapped adipose tissue.
    - Undergo fibrosarcomatous differentiation.

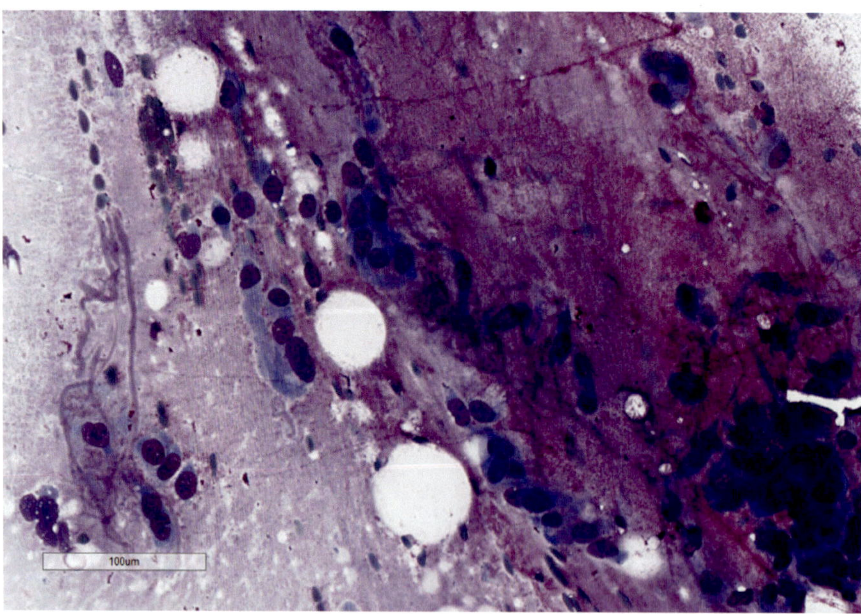

Fig. 9.11 Dermatofibrosarcoma protuberans with fibrosarcomatous transformation and myxoid stroma (Diff-Quik stain)

2. Tips and pitfalls

   - Differential diagnosis includes scar tissue, benign fibrous histiocytoma, nodular fasciitis, neurofibroma, and low-grade fibromyxoid sarcoma.
   - CD34 positive.

Inflammatory Myofibroblastic Tumor

Soft tissue and viscera of children and young adults.

1. Cytomorphologic features

   - Cellular smears of spindle cells with mild atypia.
   - Large polygonal ganglion-like cells.
   - Prominent inflammation.

2. Tips and pitfalls

   - Differential diagnosis includes inflammatory pseudotumor, follicular dendritic cell sarcoma, gastrointestinal stromal tumor, fibromatosis, and leiomyosarcoma.
   - ALK1 positive.

Solitary Fibrous Tumor

Pleural and extrapleural.

1. Cytomorphologic features

   - Variable cellularity.
   - Bland spindle cells with fusiform nuclei and scant cytoplasm.
   - Collagenous stroma.
   - Naked nuclei.

2. Tips and pitfalls

   - Differential diagnosis includes synovial sarcoma, low-grade MPNST, sarcomatoid mesothelioma, spindle cell thymoma, and lipomatous tumor.
   - STAT6 positive.

Gastrointestinal Stromal Tumor (GIST)

Gastric more frequent than intestinal. Reportable if it occurs in the chest or outside the pelvis/retroperitoneum.

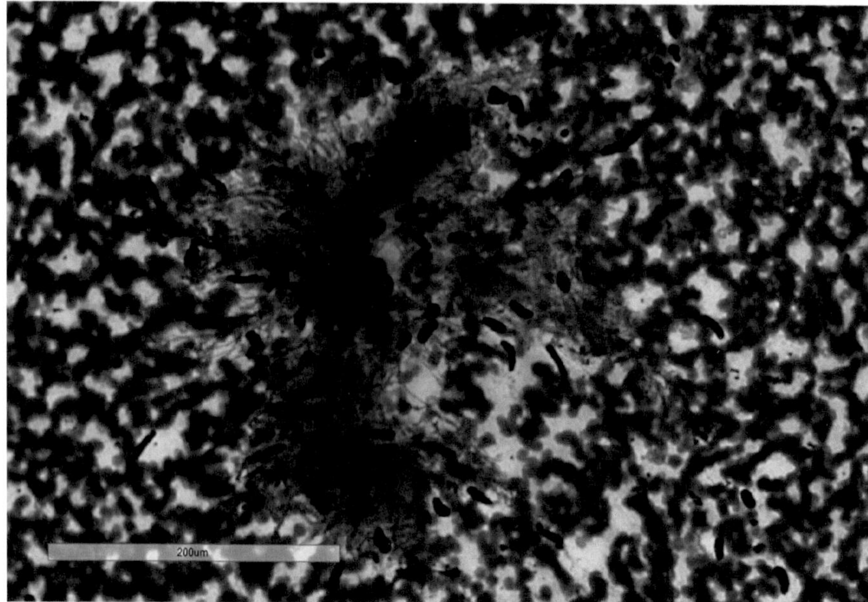

Fig. 9.12 Spindle cell gastrointestinal stromal tumor (Diff-Quik stain)

1. Cytomorphologic features
   - Tight bundles of slender spindle cells (Fig. 9.12).
   - Variable pleomorphism.
   - Epithelioid cells (variant), +/− myxoid stroma (Fig. 9.13).
2. Tips and pitfalls
   - Differential diagnosis includes smooth muscle tumor and nerve sheath tumor.
   - Carcinoma, neuroendocrine tumor, melanoma, or hepatocellular carcinoma should be included in the differential diagnosis of suspect epithelioid variant of gastrointestinal stromal tumor.
   - Often positive for CD117 and DOG1. SDH may be deficient.

Leiomyosarcoma

Middle-aged or older adults. Retroperitoneal or large vessels.

1. Cytomorphologic features
   - Tissue fragments of spindle cells in fascicular arrangement.
   - Elongated, blunt-ended nuclei.
   - Variable nuclear pleomorphism.
   - Mitoses.

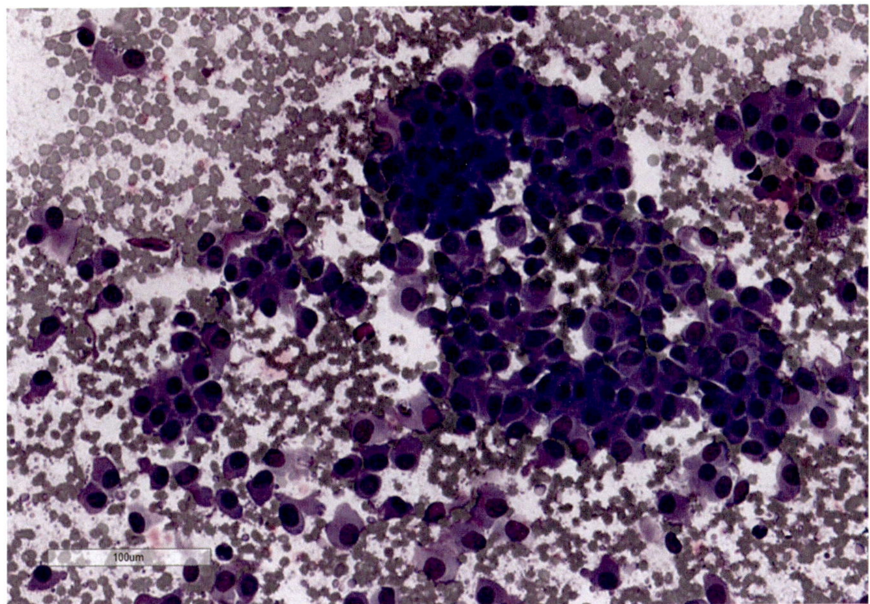

Fig. 9.13 Epithelioid gastrointestinal stromal tumor (Diff-Quik stain)

2. Tips and pitfalls
   - Differential diagnosis includes leiomyoma, nerve sheath tumor, MPNST, GIST, SFT, and fibromatosis.
   - Positive markers include desmin, SMA, SMMS-1, and caldesmin.

Malignant Peripheral Nerve Sheath Tumor (MPNST)

Fifty percent associated with NF1. Patients 20–50s may present with nerve pain.

1. Cytomorphologic features
   - Variable cellularity consisting of fascicles, single cells, and naked nuclei.
   - Spindle cells with wavy nuclei and fibrillary cytoplasm.
   - Polygonal cells (epithelioid variant).
   - Heterologous elements.
2. Tips and pitfalls
   - Differential diagnosis includes schwannoma with ancient change, synovial sarcoma, leiomyosarcoma, melanoma, spindle cell carcinoma, malignant SFT, and DDLPS.
   - H3K27me3 loss.

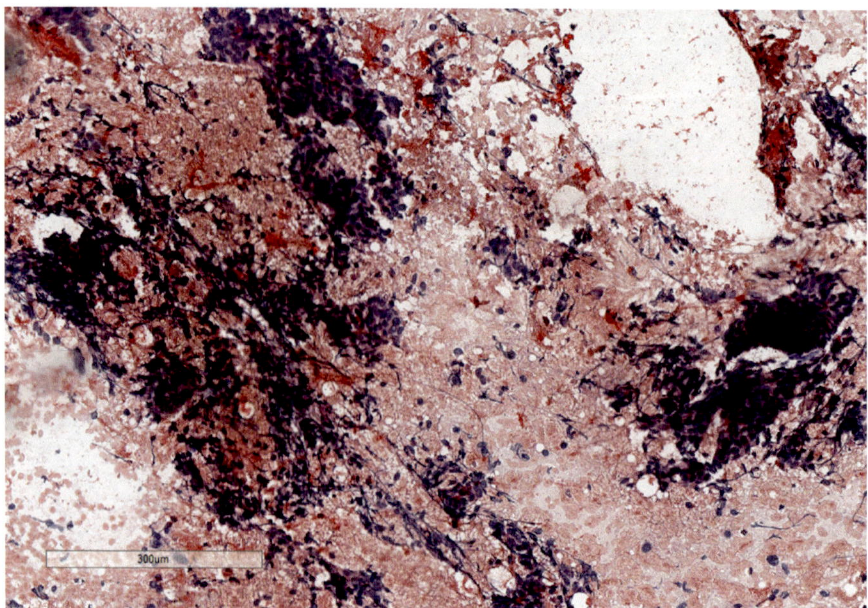

Fig. 9.14 Poorly differentiated monophasic synovial sarcoma (Diff-Quik stain)

Synovial Sarcoma

Deep soft tissue mass of extremities.

1. Cytomorphologic features (Fig. 9.14)
   - Cellular aspirates of clusters and dispersed uniform spindle cells.
   - Bland, ovoid nuclei and scant cytoplasm.
   - +/− mitoses, mast cells.
2. Tips and pitfalls
   - Differential diagnosis includes leiomyosarcoma, MPNST, SFT, and carcinosarcoma.
   - Positive markers include cytokeratin, EMA, TLE-1, bcl-2, and CD99.

Spindle Cell/Sclerosing Rhabdomyosarcoma

Pediatric paratesticular region while adult deep soft tissue of the head and neck.

1. Cytomorphologic features
   - Spindle cells.
   - Cytoplasmic processes with cross-striations.

2. Tips and pitfalls

   - Should be distinguished from smooth muscle tumor.
   - Positive for desmin, myogenin, and Myo D1.

Fibrosarcoma

Middle-aged and older adults. Deep soft tissue of the extremities, trunk, head, and neck.

1. Cytomorphologic features

   - Pleomorphic spindle cells with mitoses.

2. Tips and pitfalls

   - Differential diagnosis includes synovial sarcoma and MPNST.
   - Not reliably diagnosed by aspiration biopsy.

Pleomorphic Neoplasms

Pleomorphic pattern includes differential diagnosis of undifferentiated pleomorphic sarcoma, pleomorphic rhabdomyosarcoma, pleomorphic leiomyosarcoma, dedifferentiated liposarcoma, and myxofibrosarcoma. It is usually sufficient to recognize the malignant nature of these samples to render a preliminary diagnosis of sarcomatoid malignancy during ROSE. Further characterization of the tumor is heavily dependent on ancillary testing. An update on soft tissue tumor by immunohistochemistry is accessible [27].

Undifferentiated Pleomorphic Sarcoma

Diagnosis of exclusion.

1. Cytomorphologic features (Fig. 9.15)

   - Often cellular aspirates with variable clusters and dispersed cells.
   - Marked pleomorphism and anaplasia.
   - Tumor giant cells.
   - Mitoses and necrosis.

2. Tips and pitfalls

   - Differential diagnosis includes sarcomatoid carcinoma, sarcomatoid mesothelioma, melanoma, anaplastic large cell lymphoma, dedifferentiated sarcoma, and pleomorphic sarcoma with specific line of differentiation.

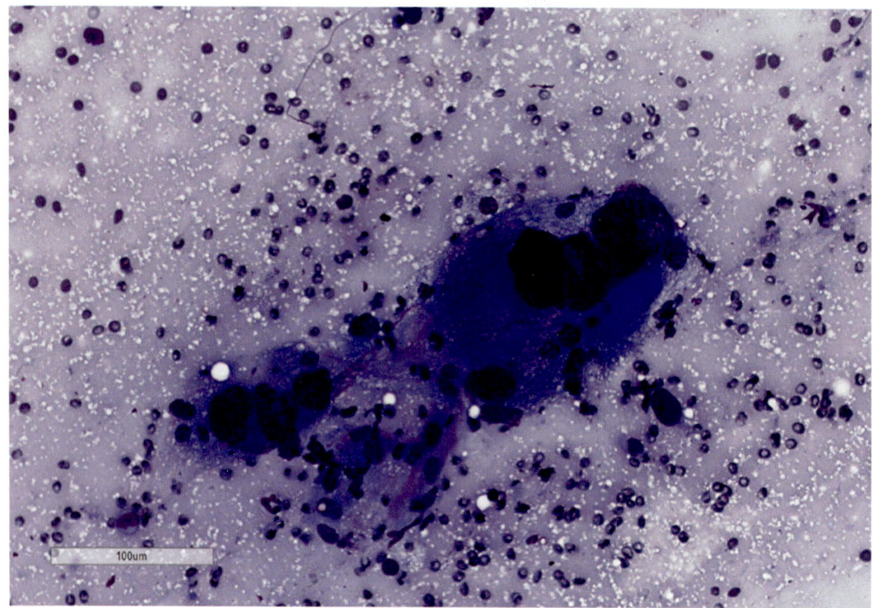

Fig. 9.15 Undifferentiated pleomorphic sarcoma (Diff-Quik stain)

Pleomorphic Rhabdomyosarcoma

Male patients 60–70s. Deep soft tissue mass of lower extremities.

1. Cytomorphologic features
   - Cellular aspirates with numerous dispersed rhabdoid cells.
   - Marked pleomorphism.
   - Bi- and multinucleation.
   - Mitoses and necrosis.
2. Tips and pitfalls
   - Differential diagnosis includes other sarcomas with heterologous rhabdoid differentiation, melanoma, carcinoma, extrarenal rhabdoid tumor, and proximal-type epithelioid sarcoma.

Dedifferentiated Liposarcoma

See the tumors with adipocytic pattern.

Epithelioid Neoplasms

The differential diagnosis of this group includes epithelioid sarcoma, epithelioid hemangioendothelioma (EHE), epithelioid angiosarcoma, clear cell sarcoma of soft tissue, alveolar soft part sarcoma, granular cell tumor, myoepithelial tumor, neoplasm with perivascular epithelioid cell differentiation (PEComa), extrarenal rhabdoid tumor, sclerosing epithelioid fibrosarcoma, and glomus tumor.

Epithelioid Sarcoma, Proximal Type

Superficial location often presenting as nonhealing ulcer. Upper extremities especially hands and fingers.

1. Cytomorphologic features
   - Single round, polygonal, or spindle cells.
   - Eccentric nuclei with dense cytoplasm with small vacuoles.
   - Rhabdoid cells (proximal type).
   - Bi- or multinucleation.
2. Tips and pitfalls
   - Differential diagnosis includes carcinoma, melanoma, myoepithelial carcinoma, EHE, and epithelioid MPNST.
   - Positive cytokeratin, EMA, and CD34.
   - SMARCB1 (INI1) loss.

Epithelioid Hemangioendothelioma (EHE)

Angiocentric soft tissue mass.

1. Cytomorphologic features
   - Round, polygonal to plasmacytoid cells with minimal pleomorphism and binucleation.
   - Nuclear grooves and pseudoinclusions.
   - Intracytoplasmic lumina.
   - Hyaline stroma.
2. Tips and pitfalls
   - Differential diagnosis includes angiosarcoma, carcinoma, melanoma, mesothelioma, epithelioid hemangioma, and epithelioid sarcoma.
   - Positive for cytokeratin, EMA, ERG, FLI1, CD31, and CD34.

Epithelioid Angiosarcoma

Painful and hemorrhagic mass.

1. Cytomorphologic features
   - Large epithelioid cells with moderate to marked pleomorphism and prominent nucleoli.
   - Bloody background, occasional vasoformative structures, and mitoses.
2. Tips and pitfalls
   - Differential diagnosis includes large cell lymphoma, germ cell tumor, epithelioid variant of other sarcomas, carcinoma, melanoma, and mesothelioma.
   - Positive for cytokeratin, EMA, ERG, FLI1, CD31, and CD34.

Clear Cell Sarcoma

Young adults 30–40s. Lower extremities especially the foot and ankle.

1. Cytomorphologic features
   - Round, polygonal or spindle cells with prominent nucleolus.
   - Nuclear pseudoinclusions.
   - Clear/pale cytoplasm.
   - Rare (granular cell variant).
2. Tips and pitfalls
   - Differential diagnosis includes melanoma, clear cell renal cell carcinoma, granular cell tumor, and carcinoma.
   - Positive for S100, HMB45, and MITF.

Alveolar Soft Part Sarcoma

Deep soft tissue of the thigh and buttock of adults. The head and neck especially the tongue and orbit of children.

1. Cytomorphologic features (Fig. 9.16)
   - Large round/polygonal cells with prominent nucleoli.
   - Abundant granular and fragile cytoplasm.
   - Naked nuclei.

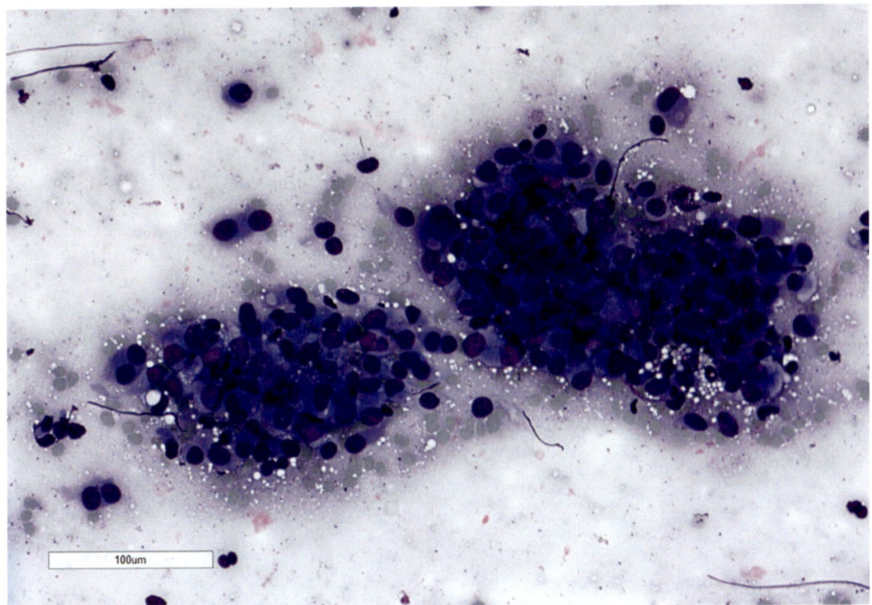

Fig. 9.16 Alveolar soft part sarcoma (Diff-Quik stain)

2. Tips and pitfalls
   - Differential diagnosis includes granular cell tumor, melanoma, paraganglioma, renal cell carcinoma, PEComa, and rhabdomyoma.
   - TFE3 positive.

Granular Cell Tumor

Head and neck including tongue. Adults 40–60s with male predominance.

1. Cytomorphologic features (Fig. 9.17)
   - Cells of uniform appearance with abundant granular cytoplasm.
   - Small nuclei.
   - Bare nuclei in granular background.
2. Tips and pitfalls
   - Differential diagnosis includes renal cell carcinoma, alveolar soft part sarcoma, rhabdomyoma, and Whipple disease.
   - Positive for S100, CD68, MITF, and TFE3.

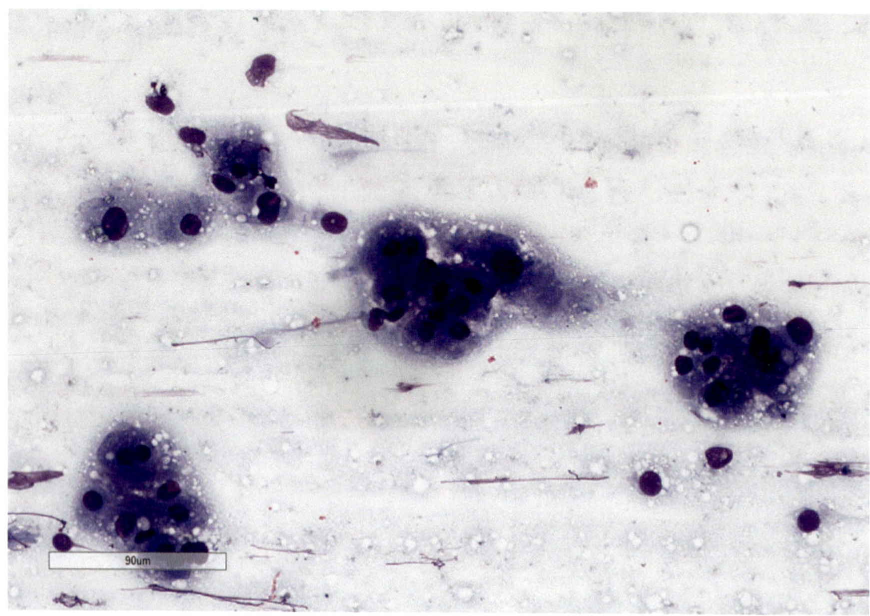

Fig. 9.17 Granular cell tumor (Diff-Quik stain)

Myoepithelial Tumor

Young to middle-aged adults 40s. Subcutaneous tissue more often involved than deep soft tissue.

1. Cytomorphologic features
   - Loose clusters and single cells within fibrillary material.
   - Round, oval, or spindle cells with plasmacytoid appearance.
   - Bland nuclei with fine chromatin (Fig. 9.18).
   - Malignant form exhibits malignant features (Fig. 9.19).
2. Tips and pitfalls
   - Differential diagnosis includes benign mixed tumor, nerve sheath tumor, and smooth muscle tumor.
   - Positive cytokeratin, EMA, S100, calponin, p63, and PLAG1.
   - SMARCB1 (INI1) loss.

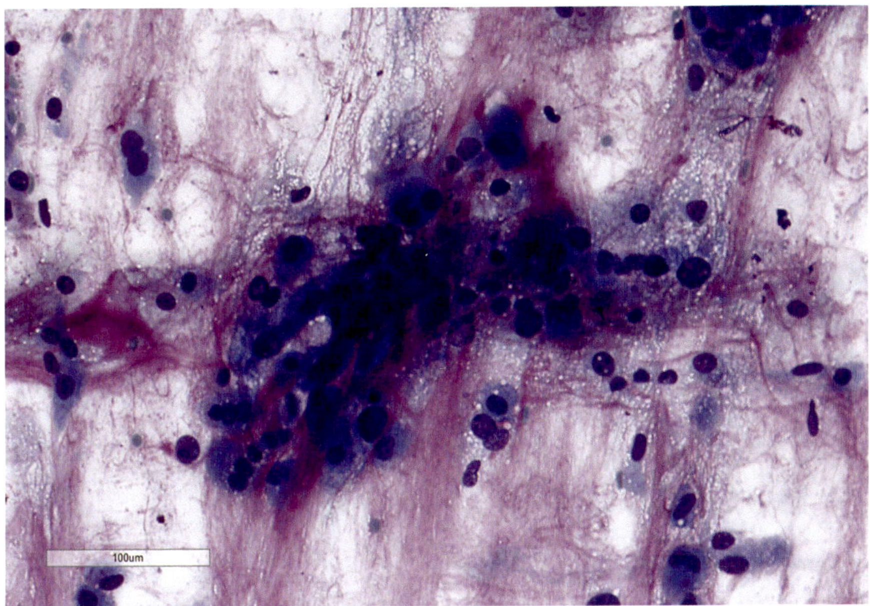

Fig. 9.18 Benign myoepithelial tumor (Diff-Quik stain)

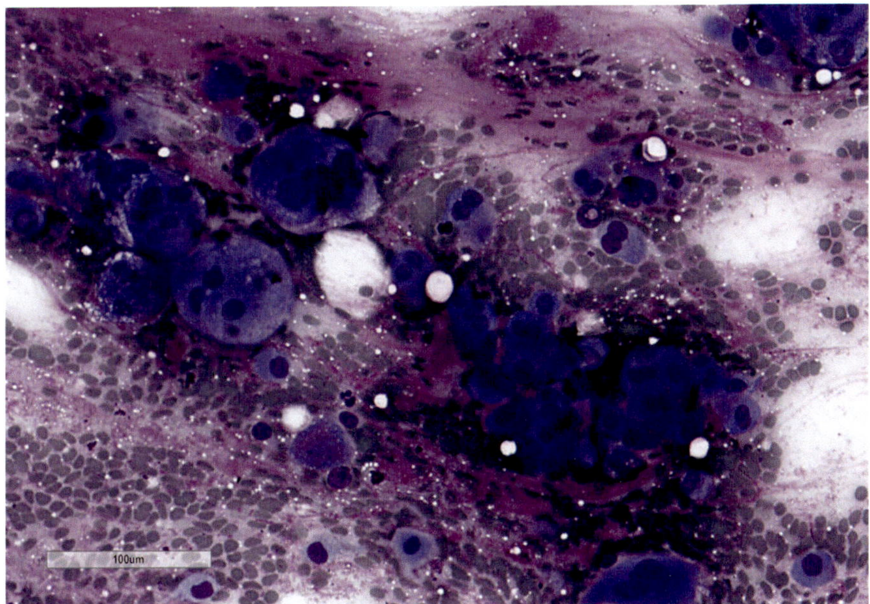

Fig. 9.19 Malignant myoepithelial tumor (Diff-Quik stain)

Giant Cell-Rich Tumors

This group of tumors exhibits strikingly multinucleate giant cells; some can be numerous. Differential diagnosis includes tenosynovial giant cell tumor, localized and diffuse types, giant cell tumor of soft tissue, giant cell tumor of bone, and aneurysmal bone cyst, especially solid variant.

Giant Cell Tumor of Bone

Epiphyseal long bone. Large expansile lesion with sclerotic boarder. Female predominance 20–45s.

1. Cytomorphologic features (Fig. 9.20)
    - Oval/spindle mononuclear cells.
    - Osteoclast-type giant cells.
2. Tips and pitfalls
    - Differential diagnosis includes tenosynovial giant cell tumor and giant cell-rich sarcoma.

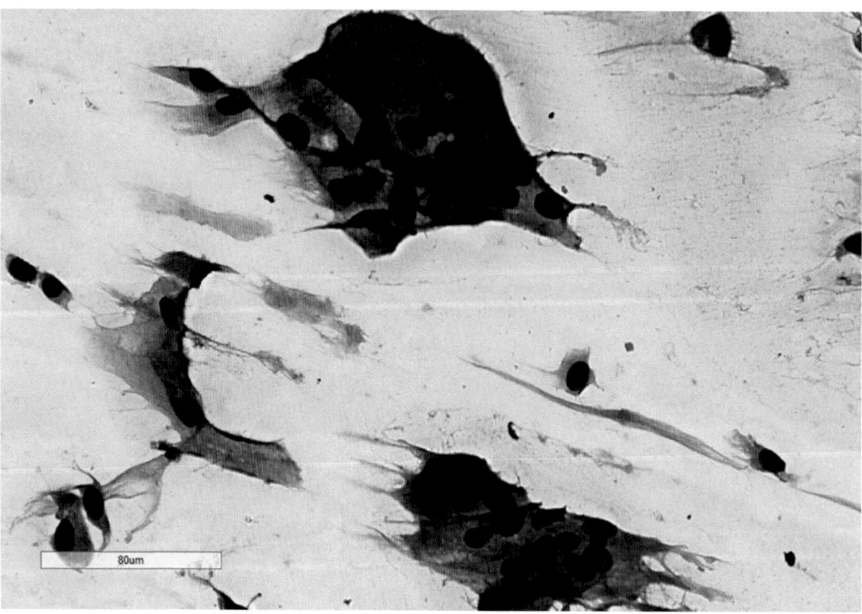

Fig. 9.20 Giant cell tumor of bone (Diff-Quik stain)

Tenosynovial Giant Cell Tumor (TSGCT)

Wide age range with female predominance. Knee is the most common site involved.

1. Cytomorphologic features (Fig. 9.21)
    - Mononuclear cells of varying shapes.
    - Osteoclast-type giant cells.
    - Foamy histiocytes and hemosiderin pigment.
    - Mild anisocytosis/anisokaryosis.
2. Tips and pitfalls
    - Differential diagnosis includes gout, chronic synovitis, melanoma, and giant cell-rich sarcoma.

Myxoid Neoplasms or Other Distinct Matrix-Containing Tumors

This group of tumors exhibits myxoid stroma including differential diagnosis of benign (myxoma) to low-grade (low-grade fibromyxoid sarcoma, low-grade myofibrosarcoma) to high-grade (myxofibrosarcoma, extraskeletal myxoid

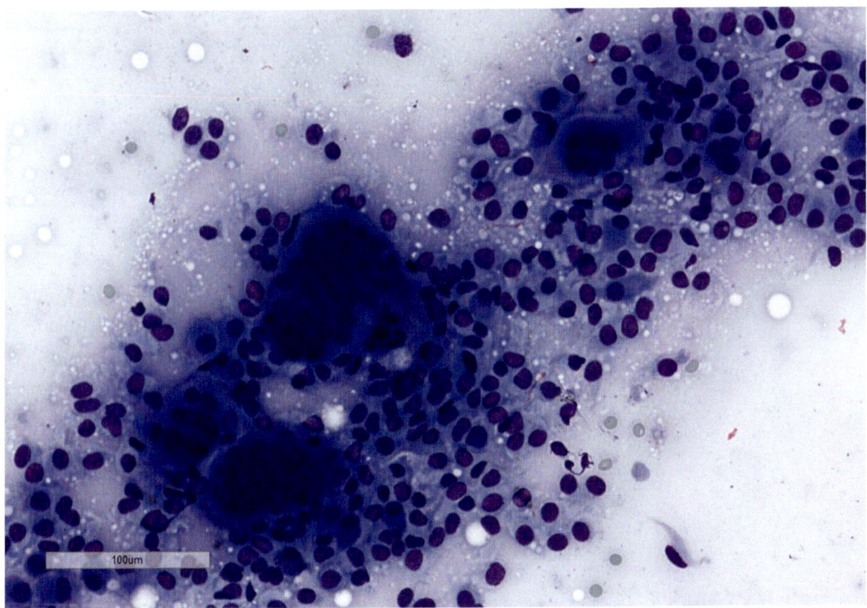

Fig. 9.21 Tenosynovial giant cell tumor (Diff-Quik stain)

chondrosarcoma, dedifferentiated liposarcoma with prominent myxofibrosarcoma-like features, and chordoma) tumor. Myoepithelioma/mixed tumor of soft tissue also has myxoid matrix. Chondroid matrix can also resemble myxoid matrix. Chondrocytes with chondromyxoid matrix are clues for chondroid tumor ranging from enchondroma to chondrosarcoma.

Myxoma

More common in female adult patients 40–70s.

1. Cytomorphologic features (Fig. 9.22)
   - Paucicellular aspirate with scattered bland, uniform cells.
   - Granular matrix material and absent or scant vessels.
   - Atrophic muscle fibers.
2. Tips and pitfalls
   - Differential diagnosis includes ganglion cyst, nodular fasciitis, perineurioma, low-grade myxofibrosarcoma, LGFMS, and myxoid liposarcoma.

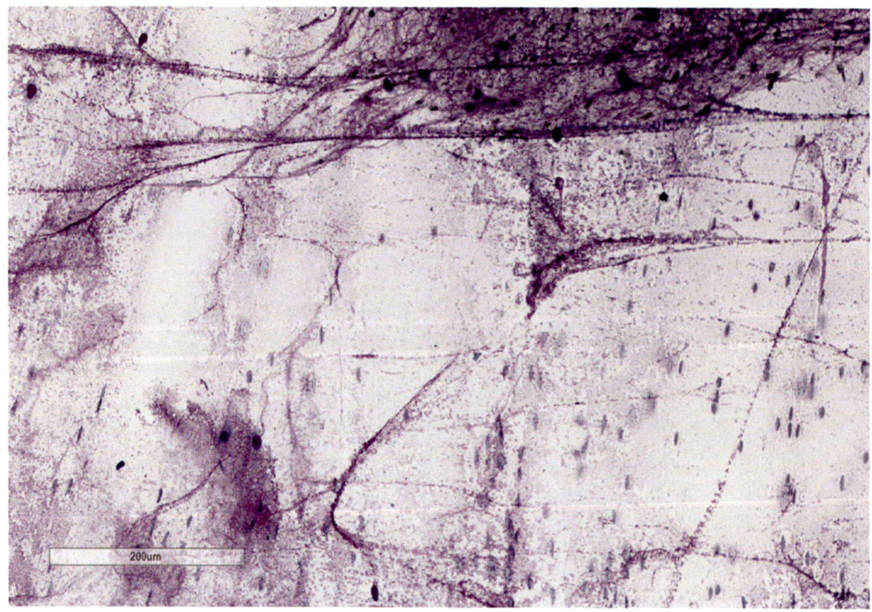

Fig. 9.22 Myxoma (Diff-Quik stain)

Myxoid Liposarcoma

Adult 40–50s. Deep soft tissue mass of extremities, especially thigh. Extremely rare in the retroperitoneum, thinking of metastasis when tumor occurs at this location.

1. Cytomorphologic features
   - Round/oval cells with occasional small cytoplasmic vacuoles.
   - Uni- or bivacuolate lipoblasts.
   - Abundant granular myxoid matrix.
2. Tips and pitfalls
   - Differential diagnosis includes low-grade myxofibrosarcoma, spindle cell lipoma with myxoid changes, and myoepithelial tumor.

Myxofibrosarcoma

Elderly male patients. Extremities. Rare in the retroperitoneum.

1. Cytomorphologic features
   - Variable myxoid stroma with short, curved vessels.
   - Atypical spindle/stellate cells (low grade).
   - Marked nuclear pleomorphism and necrosis (high grade).
   - Pseudolipoblasts.
2. Tips and pitfalls
   - Differential diagnosis includes myxoid liposarcoma, LGFMS, and other high-grade sarcomas.
   - Dedifferentiated liposarcoma, especially in retroperitoneal location.

Low-Grade Fibromyxoid Sarcoma (LGFMS)

Young adults. Proximal extremities or the trunk.

1. Cytomorphologic features
   - Variable myxoid stroma.
   - Spindle cells with fibroblast-like features.
   - Minimal atypia.
   - No significant vascularity.

2. Tips and pitfalls
    - Differential diagnosis includes cellular myxoma, perineurioma, low-grade myxofibrosarcoma, low-grade MPNST, SFT, and fibromatosis.
    - MUC4 positive.

Extraskeletal Myxoid Chondrosarcoma (EMC)

Deep-seated large soft tissue mass of the thigh in adults in 50s.

1. Cytomorphologic features (Fig. 9.23)
    - Monotonous population of epithelioid to spindle cells within magenta fibrillary stroma.
    - Cords or lacelike arrangement.
    - Round, oval nuclei with fine stippled chromatin and nuclear grooves.
    - Scant to moderate cytoplasm with well-defined borders.
2. Tips and pitfalls
    - Myoepithelial tumor and ossifying fibromyxoid tumor are among the main differential diagnoses.

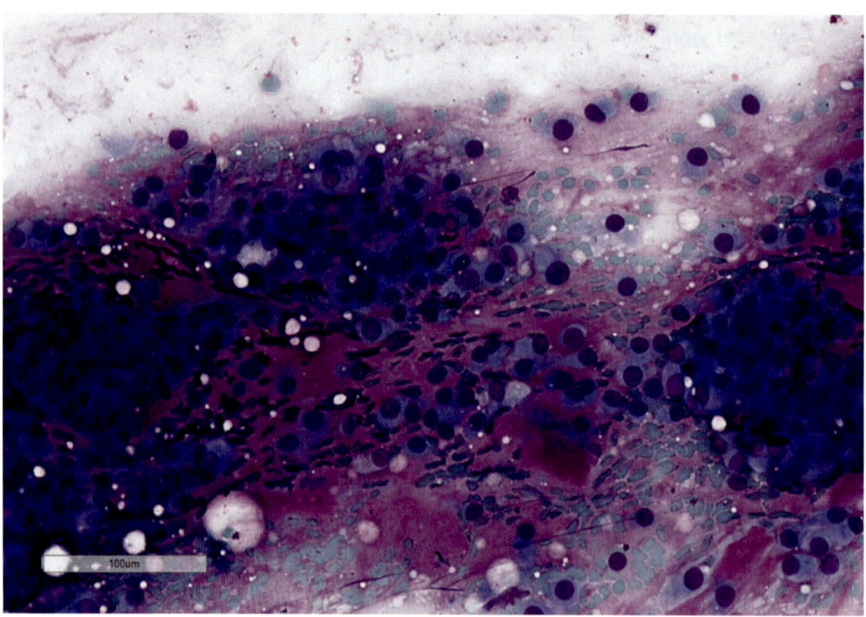

Fig. 9.23 Extraskeletal myxoid chondrosarcoma (Diff-Quik stain)

Myxoinflammatory Fibroblastic Sarcoma

Distal extremities, especially fingers, middle-aged patients.

1. Cytomorphologic features

    - Mix of spindle and mononuclear cells with large atypical Reed-Sternberg-like cells.
    - Myxoid matrix and background inflammation.
    - Pseudolipoblasts.

2. Tips and pitfalls

    - Differential diagnosis includes nodular fasciitis, reactive lesion, myxofibrosarcoma, liposarcoma, inflammatory myofibroblastic tumor, and Hodgkin lymphoma.

Dedifferentiated Liposarcoma with Myxofibrosarcoma Features

See the tumor with adipocytic pattern.

Osteosarcoma

Adolescent or young adult. Long bones of the extremities. Most common radiation-induced sarcoma in older patients. Tumor involves the bone and soft tissue.

1. Cytomorphologic features (Fig. 9.24)

    - Cellular aspirate of dyscohesive, single cells.
    - Plasmacytoid appearance with basophilic to vacuolated cytoplasm.
    - Round-oval nuclei.
    - +/− multinucleated giant cells; +/− immature osteoid.
    - Pleomorphism and/or mitoses.

2. Tips and pitfalls

    - Differential diagnosis includes primary undifferentiated sarcoma of bone, chondrosarcoma, melanoma, anaplastic large cell lymphoma, metastatic carcinoma, fracture callus, myositis ossificans, and osteoblastoma.
    - SATB2 positive.

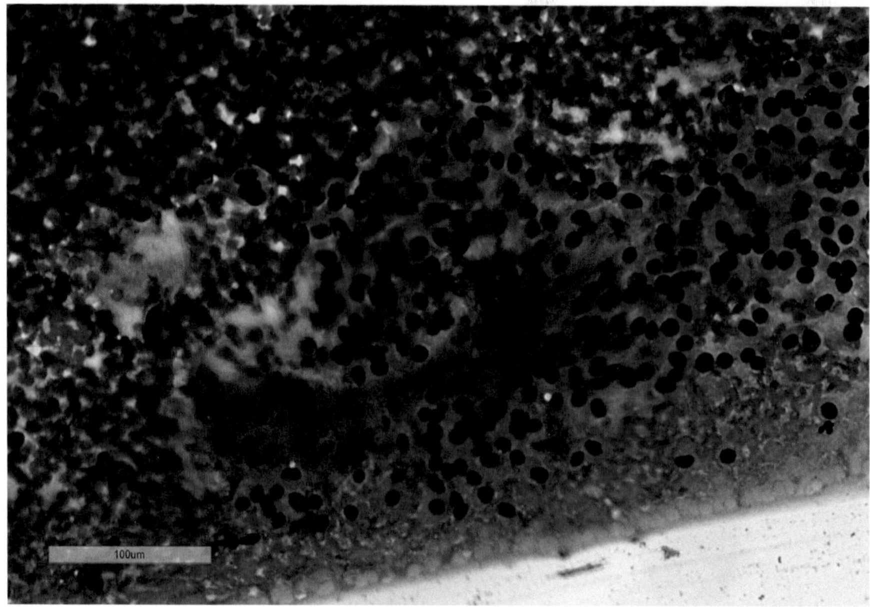

Fig. 9.24 Osteosarcoma (Diff-Quik stain)

Enchondroma

Wide age range. Hand bone or long bone. No cortical breakthrough or soft tissue involvement.

1. Cytomorphologic features
   - Low cellularity.
   - Chondromyxoid matrix.
   - Lacunar spaces with small chondrocytes and bland, dark nuclei.
2. Tips and pitfalls
   - Differential diagnosis includes low-grade chondrosarcoma and chondromyxoid fibroma.

Chondrosarcoma

Older patients. Pelvis, femur, humerus, and rib. Cortical breakthrough and soft tissue involvement.

1. Cytomorphologic features (Fig. 9.25)
   - Hyaline or myxoid cartilaginous tissue fragments.
   - Lacunar spaces with bland cells (low grade).

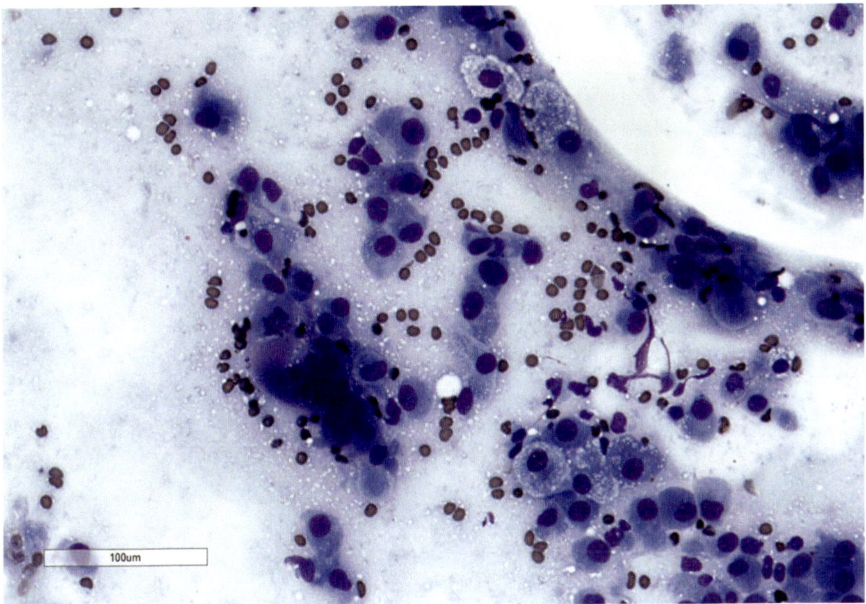

Fig. 9.25 Chondrosarcoma (Diff-Quik stain)

- Increased cellularity, anaplasia, binucleation, +/– mitoses (high grade).
- Spindle/pleomorphic cells (dedifferentiation).
- Small round blue cells (mesenchymal chondrosarcoma).

2. Tips and pitfalls

- Differential diagnosis includes chondroblastic osteosarcoma and enchondroma.

Chordoma

Base of the skull, vertebral bodies, and sacrococcygeal bone. Patients of 50–70s.

1. Cytomorphologic features

- Fibrillary/granular myxoid matrix.
- Cords or clusters of round/cuboidal cells (Fig. 9.26).
- Physaliphorous cells (Fig. 9.27).

2. Tips and pitfalls

- Differential diagnosis includes myxoid chondrosarcoma, myxopapillary ependymoma, and metastatic mucinous adenocarcinoma.
- Positive for cytokeratin, EMA, S-100, and brachyury.
- SMARCB1 (INI1) loss.

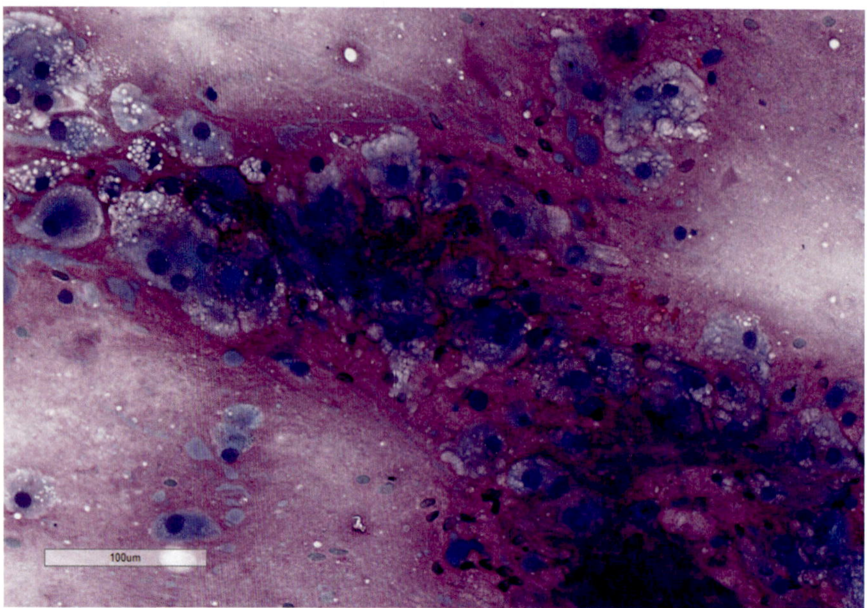

Fig. 9.26 Chordoma (Diff-Quik stain)

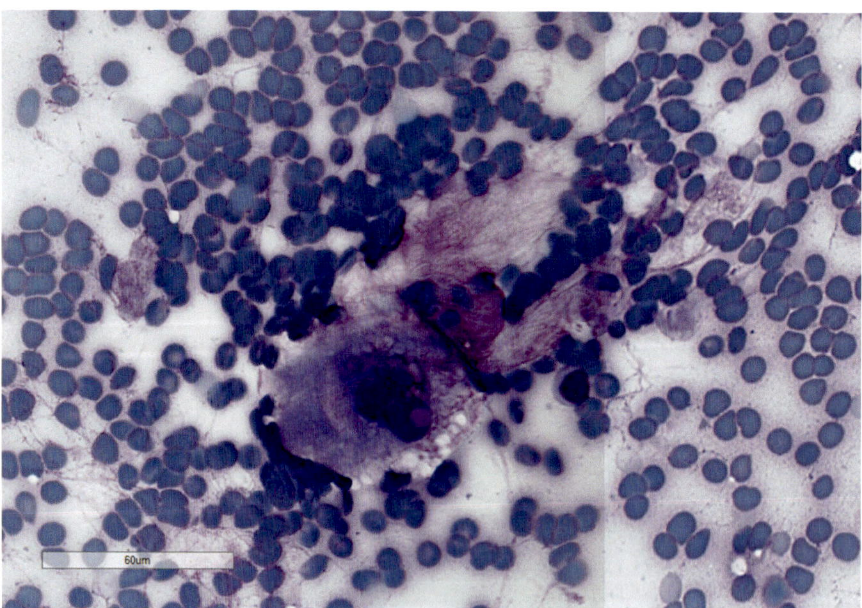

Fig. 9.27 Chordoma with physaliphorous cell (Diff-Quik stain)

References

1. Schmidt RL, Witt BL, Lopez-Calderon LE, Layfield LJ. The influence of rapid onsite evaluation on the adequacy rate of fine-needle aspiration cytology: a systematic review and meta-analysis. Am J Clin Pathol. 2013;139(3):300–8.
2. Khalbuss WE, Teot LA, Monaco SE. Diagnostic accuracy and limitations of fine-needle aspiration cytology of bone and soft tissue lesions: a review of 1114 cases with cytological-histological correlation. Cancer Cytopathol. 2010;118(1):24–32.
3. Jorda M, Rey L, Hanly A, Ganjei-Azar P. Fine-needle aspiration cytology of bone: accuracy and pitfalls of cytodiagnosis. Cancer. 2000;90(1):47–54.
4. Akerman M, Rydholm A, Persson BM. Aspiration cytology of soft-tissue tumors. The 10-year experience at an orthopedic oncology center. Acta Orthop Scand. 1985;56(5):407–12.
5. Kitagawa Y, Ito H, Sawaizumi T, Matsubara M, Yokoyama M, Naito Z. Fine needle aspiration cytology for soft tissue tumours of the hand. J Hand Surg Br. 2003;28(6):582–5.
6. Dey P, Mallik MK, Gupta SK, Vasishta RK. Role of fine needle aspiration cytology in the diagnosis of soft tissue tumours and tumour-like lesions. Cytopathology. 2004;15(1):32–7.
7. Wakely PE Jr, Kneisl JS. Soft tissue aspiration cytopathology. Cancer. 2000;90(5):292–8.
8. Layfield LJ, Anders KH, Glasgow BJ, Mirra JM. Fine-needle aspiration of primary soft-tissue lesions. Arch Pathol Lab Med. 1986;110(5):420–4.
9. Nagira K, Yamamoto T, Akisue T, Marui T, Hitora T, Nakatani T, et al. Reliability of fine-needle aspiration biopsy in the initial diagnosis of soft-tissue lesions. Diagn Cytopathol. 2002;27(6):354–61.
10. Rekhi B, Gorad BD, Kakade AC, Chinoy R. Scope of FNAC in the diagnosis of soft tissue tumors–a study from a tertiary cancer referral center in India. Cytojournal. 2007;4:20.
11. Amin MS, Luqman M, Jamal S, Mamoon N, Anwar M. Fine needle aspiration biopsy of soft tissue tumours. J Coll Physicians Surg Pak. 2003;13(11):625–8.
12. Bommer KK, Ramzy I, Mody D. Fine-needle aspiration biopsy in the diagnosis and management of bone lesions: a study of 450 cases. Cancer. 1997;81(3):148–56.
13. Hirachand S, Lakhey M, Singha AK, Devkota S, Akhter J. Fine needle aspiration (FNA) of soft tissue tumours (STT). Kathmandu Univ Med J (KUMJ). 2007;5(3):374–7.
14. Kilpatrick SE, Cappellari JO, Bos GD, Gold SH, Ward WG. Is fine-needle aspiration biopsy a practical alternative to open biopsy for the primary diagnosis of sarcoma? Experience with 140 patients. Am J Clin Pathol. 2001;115(1):59–68.
15. Layfield LJ. Cytologic diagnosis of osseous lesions: a review with emphasis on the diagnosis of primary neoplasms of bone. Diagn Cytopathol. 2009;37(4):299–310.
16. Maitra A, Ashfaq R, Saboorian MH, Lindberg G, Gokaslan ST. The role of fine-needle aspiration biopsy in the primary diagnosis of mesenchymal lesions: a community hospital-based experience. Cancer. 2000;90(3):178–85.
17. Kilpatrick SE, Geisinger KR. Soft tissue sarcomas: the usefulness and limitations of fine-needle aspiration biopsy. Am J Clin Pathol. 1998;110(1):50–68.
18. Fleshman R, Mayerson J, Wakely PE Jr. Fine-needle aspiration biopsy of high-grade sarcoma: a report of 107 cases. Cancer. 2007;111(6):491–8.
19. Handa U, Bal A, Mohan H, Bhardwaj S. Fine needle aspiration cytology in the diagnosis of bone lesions. Cytopathology. 2005;16(2):59–64.
20. Sapi Z, Antal I, Papai Z, Szendroi M, Mayer A, Jakab K, et al. Diagnosis of soft tissue tumors by fine-needle aspiration with combined cytopathology and ancillary techniques. Diagn Cytopathol. 2002;26(4):232–42.
21. Domanski HA, Akerman M, Carlen B, Engellau J, Gustafson P, Jonsson K, et al. Core-needle biopsy performed by the cytopathologist: a technique to complement fine-needle aspiration of soft tissue and bone lesions. Cancer. 2005;105(4):229–39.

22. Bui MM, Smith P, Agresta SV, Cheong D, Letson GD. Practical issues of intraoperative frozen section diagnosis of bone and soft tissue lesions. Cancer Control. 2008;15(1):7–12.
23. Khalbuss WE, Parwani AV. Cytopathology of soft tissue and bone lesions. In: Essentials in cytopathology. New York: Springer; 2011.
24. Palmer HE, Mukunyadzi P, Culbreth W, Thomas JR. Subgrouping and grading of soft-tissue sarcomas by fine-needle aspiration cytology: a histopathologic correlation study. Diagn Cytopathol. 2001;24(5):307–16.
25. Domanski HA. Fine-needle aspiration cytology of soft tissue lesions: diagnostic challenges. Diagn Cytopathol. 2007;35(12):768–73.
26. Dogan S, Becker JC, Rekhtman N, Tang LH, Nafa K, Ladanyi M, et al. Use of touch imprint cytology as a simple method to enrich tumor cells for molecular analysis. Cancer Cytopathol. 2013;121(7):354–60.
27. Wei S, Henderson-Jackson E, Qian X, Bui MM. Soft tissue tumor immunohistochemistry update: illustrative examples of diagnostic pearls to avoid pitfalls. Arch Pathol Lab Med. 2017;141(8):1072–91.

Part IV
Bronchoscopy-Guided Biopsies

Chapter 10
Lung

Guoping Cai

Introduction

The causes for localized lung lesions are diverse and range from nonneoplastic to neoplastic and from benign to malignant. Image-guided biopsy such as fine needle aspiration (FNA) and tissue biopsy is the choice of diagnostic approach, which helps identify the underlying etiologies for the lesions of interest and therefore provides a guidance for clinical management [1–3]. Depending on the location of lung lesions, different biopsy routes may be used. Centrically located lung lesions are often approached through bronchoscopy, while transthoracic biopsy is typically used for a peripheral lung lesion. With advances in bronchoscopy techniques such as electromagnetic navigation bronchoscopy, peripheral lung lesions may also be sampled by a transbronchial approach [1, 4–7]. In addition, bronchial brushing can be applied to the lesions involving bronchial mucosa although the sensitivity seems lower [1]. Imaging-guided biopsy, either FNA or tissue biopsy, has been shown to have a high sensitivity and specificity in diagnosing malignant neoplasms of the lung [1].

Direct smears prepared from FNA or bronchial brushing and imprints prepared from tissue biopsy can be used for rapid on-site evaluation (ROSE), which has been shown to improve overall diagnostic performances of biopsy procedures [8–12]. The findings from ROSE evaluation provide real-time feedbacks to the physician who performs the biopsy so that the physician can adjust targeting site and determine pass number to ensure adequate specimens are obtained. As a result, ROSE can help decrease the nondiagnostic rate and therefore reduce repeat biopsies. ROSE also provide a preliminary diagnosis, which may be used as the basis to determine whether additional sites should be biopsied. In the era of personalized medicine, it is extremely important to secure sufficient material for ancillary studies including molecular testing if ROSE impression is non-small cell carcinoma [12–15].

G. Cai (✉)
Department of Pathology, Yale University School of Medicine, New Haven, CT, USA
e-mail: guoping.cai@yale.edu

G. Cai, A. J. Adeniran (eds.), *Rapid On-site Evaluation (ROSE)*,
https://doi.org/10.1007/978-3-030-21799-0_10

Diagnostic Considerations

Specimen Adequacy Assessment

There are no well-established criteria for adequacy assessment of lung lesions [12, 16]. In general, the presence of malignant cells on biopsy specimen is considered adequate. However, there is no numeric requirement for cell numbers in the absence of malignant cells. The ultimate reference for adequacy assessment may rely on the fact whether the findings from the biopsy can explain, at a relative confident level, the clinical presentations of the lesion, which may be the result of an inflammatory/infectious process, a benign tumor or malignant neoplasm. In other words, a nondiagnostic specimen is the one which provides no useful diagnostic information about the lesion [16, 17].

In patients with clinical suspicion for lung cancer or other lung lesions with associated mediastinal lymphadenopathy, mediastinal lymph nodes are often subjected to biopsy for establishing a primary diagnosis or serving as staging workup [8, 9, 18–20]. Not uncommonly the biopsy of the lymph nodes ends up with a negative result, which may reflect a true negative lymph node or represent a sampling error. There is an increasing need for establishing specimen adequacy assessment criteria, especially in cases with a negative result. Indeed, there are reports recommending requirement for a minimal number of lymphocytes [12, 21, 22]. Alsharif et al. have suggested that an adequate specimen should contain greater than 40 lymphocytes at X40 magnification or abundant pigment-laden macrophages if malignancy or granulomas are not identified [21]. The lymphocyte adequacy proposed by Nayak et al. is more than 5 low-power fields (X100 magnification) containing at least 100 lymphocytes per field or any smear with germinal center fragment [22].

Normal Elements and Contaminants in Lung Cytology

Normal elements of the lung biopsy specimen include bronchial epithelial cells, pneumocytes, and alveolar macrophages. Depending on the route a biopsy is approached, different normal elements may be present as contaminants. For example, bronchial epithelial cells are often seen as contaminants in transbronchial biopsy of lymph nodes, while transthoracic biopsy of a lung lesion can have mesothelial cells present.

1. Bronchial epithelial cells (Fig. 10.1)
    - Columnar epithelial cells with cilia and/or terminal bars, arranged singly or as groups with a pickle fence appearance.
    - Bronchial cells are bipolar and have vacuolated cytoplasm and round to oval nuclei with smooth nuclear membrane, evenly distributed chromatin, and small nucleolus.

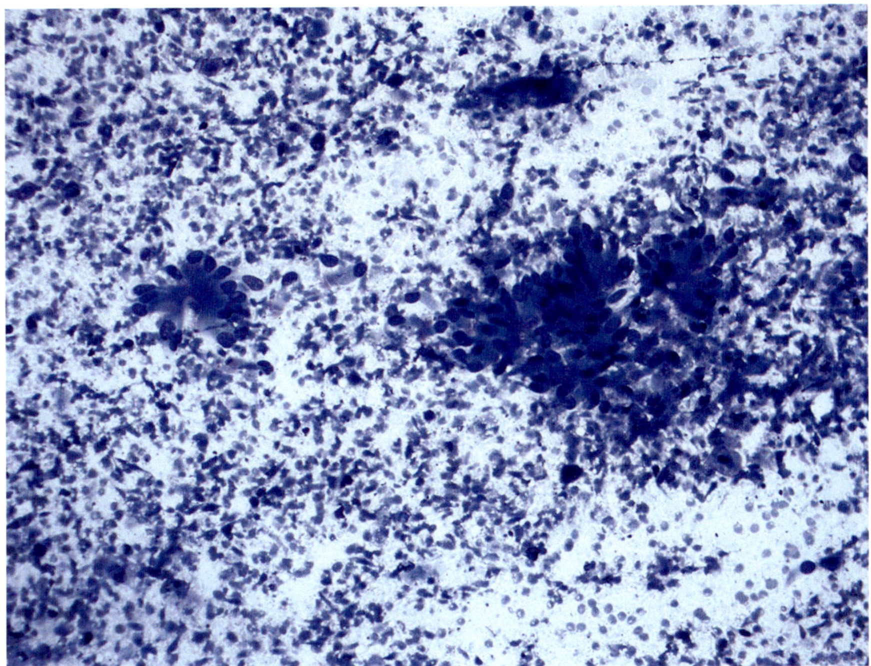

Fig. 10.1 Benign bronchial epithelial cells. Groups of uniform columnar cells with attached cilia (Diff-Quik stain, ×200)

- When arranged in groups, bronchial cells can be intermixed with mucin-containing goblet cells.
- Reserve cells, which are located in basal layer of bronchial epithelium, may be seen. Reserve cells are small and have high nuclear-to-cytoplasmic ratios, arranged in small cohesive clusters (Fig. 10.2).
- Bronchial cells can undergo changes of squamous metaplasia showing dense cytoplasm and focal keratinization.

2. Pneumocytes (Fig. 10.3)

   - Relatively uniform cells arranged in small groups or flat sheets.
   - Vacuolated cytoplasm and round nuclei with smooth nuclear membrane, evenly distributed chromatin, and inconspicuous nucleolus.
   - Reactive pneumocytes can show prominent nucleolus.

3. Alveolar macrophages (Fig. 10.4)

   - Dispersed single cells with or without anthracotic pigment.
   - Large cells with abundant vacuolated cytoplasm and folded oval nuclei with pale chromatin and small nucleolus.
   - Reactive macrophages can show increased nuclear-to-cytoplasmic ratios and conspicuous nucleolus, even sometimes arranged in groups or clusters, mimicking adenocarcinoma.

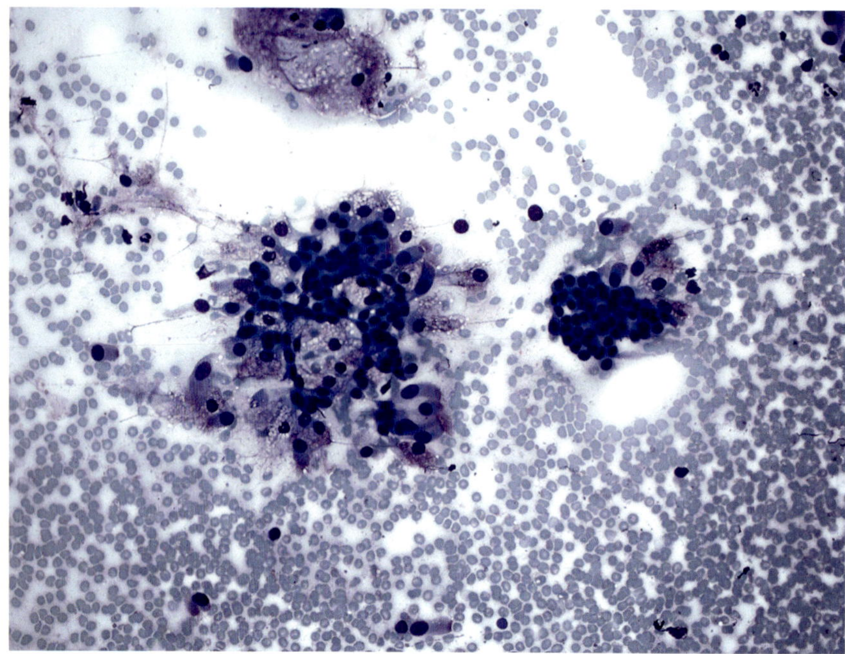

Fig. 10.2 Benign bronchial epithelial cells and reserve/basal cells. Groups of uniform columnar cells with adjacent reserve/basal cells. Reserve cells are small and have scant cytoplasm, arranged in cohesive flat sheets (Diff-Quik stain, ×200)

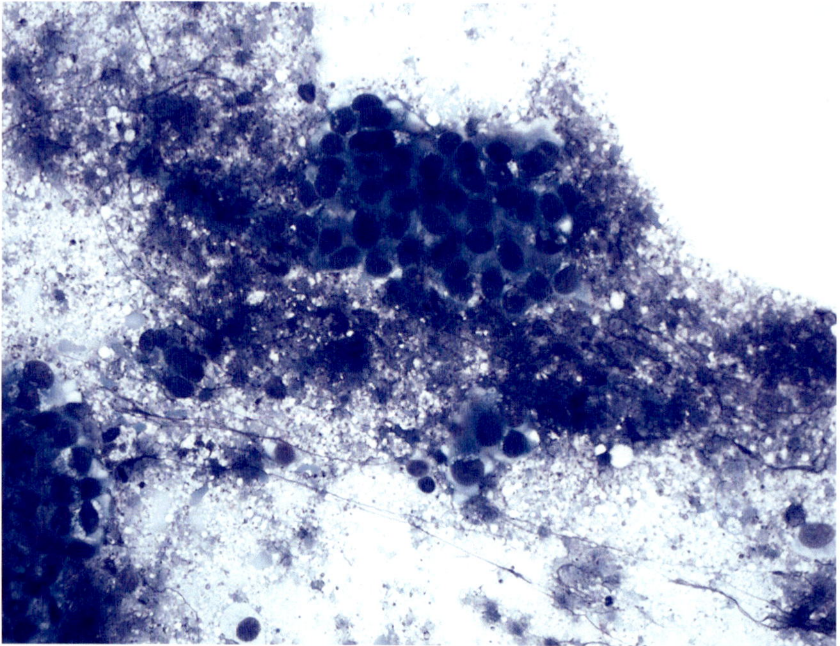

Fig. 10.3 Reactive pneumocytes. Relatively uniform cuboidal cells arranged in flat sheets (Diff-Quik stain, ×400)

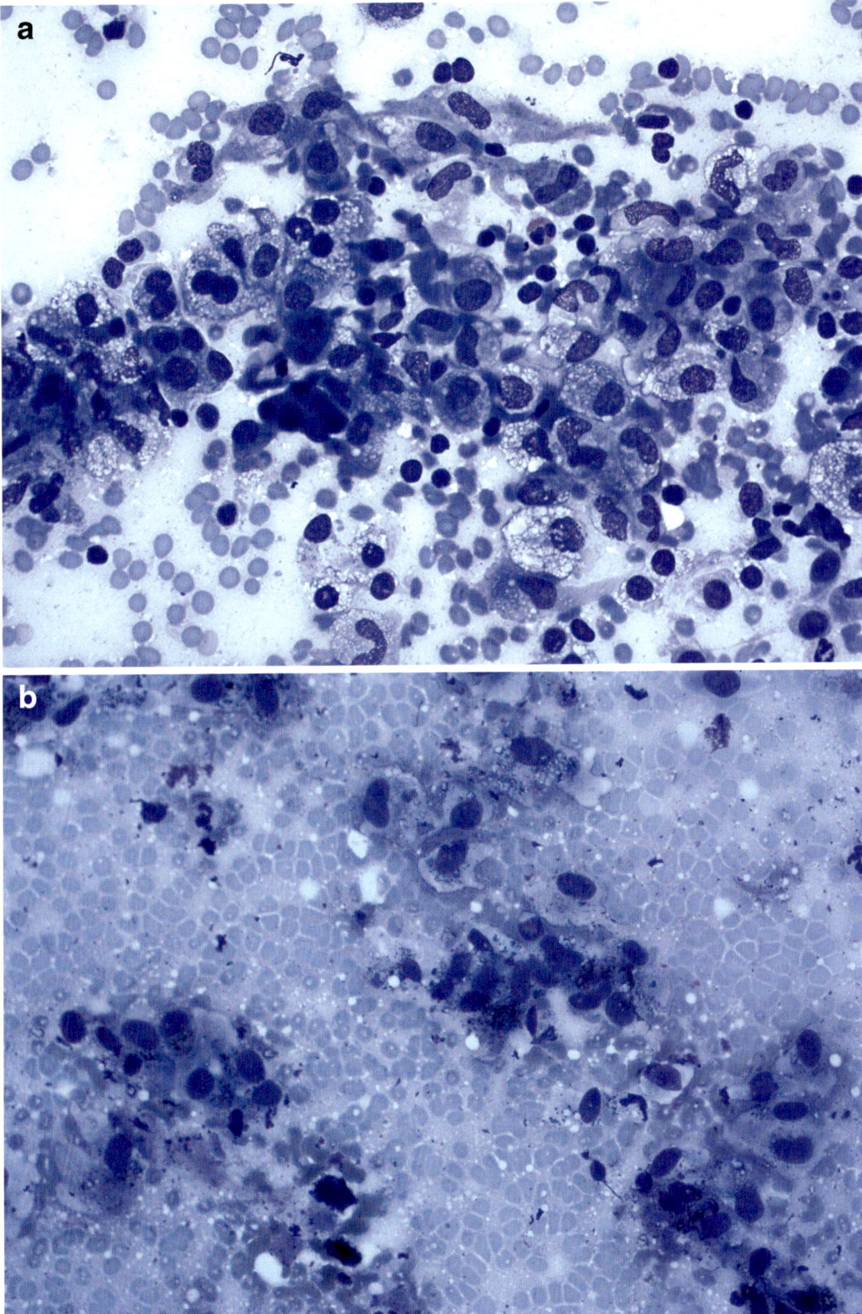

Fig. 10.4 Macrophages. Single and dyscohesive groups of cells with vacuolated cytoplasm and indented nuclei (**a** Diff-Quik stain, ×400). Macrophages contain cytoplasmic anthracotic pigments (**b** Diff-Quik stain, ×400)

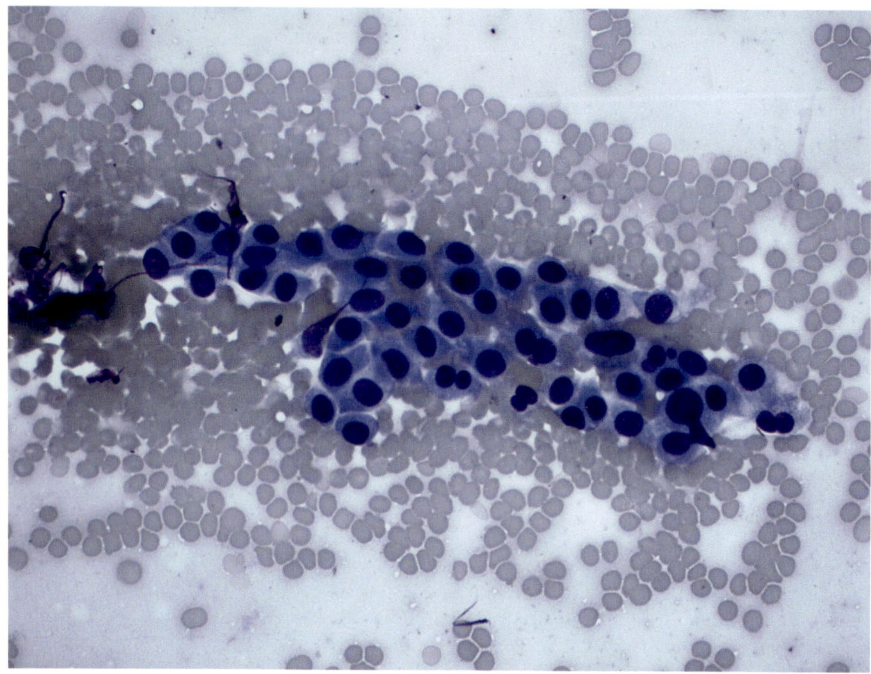

Fig. 10.5 Mesothelial cells. Relative uniform epithelial cells with round to oval nuclei arranged in flat sheet. Spaces between cells are noticeable (Diff-Quik stain, ×400)

4. Mesothelial cells (Fig. 10.5)
   - Uniform cells arranged in flat sheets with sizable spaces between the cells (as known as windows).
   - Cells are polygonal in shape and have dense cytoplasm and round to oval nuclei with inconspicuous nucleolus.

Specimens and Specimen Triage

- Cytological specimens of respiratory system include FNA smears, imprints of biopsy tissue, bronchial brushing smears, bronchial washing, and bronchoalveolar lavage.
- FNA and tissue biopsy are the preferred sampling methods although bronchial brushing can be used for bronchial mucosal lesions.
- Bronchial washing or lavage specimens are primarily used to identify infectious causes and are often not available for on-site evaluation.
- Appropriate specimen triage is essential for a diagnosis [12], especially in respiratory systems where infections account for a significant numbers of lung lesions.

- In cases suspicious for infections, it is important to save part of specimens, in a sterile fashion, for microbiology culture study.
- In cases suspicious for lymphoproliferative disorders, part of specimens should be saved in RPMI for flow cytometry study.
- In cases suspicious for tumors other than lymphoproliferative disorders, specimens should be saved as much as possible for ancillary study, particularly in cases suspicious for non-small cell carcinomas.

Nonneoplastic Lung Diseases

There are a number of possible nonneoplastic causes underlying a lung lesion, including inflammatory and infectious. These diseases often diffusely involve the lung and are seldom subjected to a biopsy unless they are presented as localized lesions. The common findings from these entities include variable inflammatory cells and absence of malignant features with or without necrosis [16]. Since a tumor can be associated with significant inflammation, multiple passes may be required to rule out malignancy.

Infection

1. Fungal infection

   Fungal infections in the lung are caused by fungal organisms, and *Pneumocystis*, *Aspergillus*, *Histoplasma*, *Cryptococcus*, and *Blastomyces* are among the common pathogens.

   A. Cytomorphologic features

   - Acute inflammation, granulomatous inflammation, or mixed inflammation.
   - Fungal organisms can sometimes be seen on Diff-Quik stain.
   - Hypha form organisms include *Aspergillus* (Fig. 10.6), *Mucor*, etc.
   - Yeast form organisms include *Histoplasma*, *Cryptococcus*, *Blastomyces*, and coccidioides (Fig. 10.7).
   - *Candida* shows dimorphic features with pseudohyphae and yeasts.
   - *Pneumocystis* shows foamy alveolar casts with trophozoites (negative cyst outline with a tiny punctate dot in the center) (Fig. 10.8).
   - Organisms are best viewed on special stains (Gomori methenamine silver, GMS, or periodic acid–Schiff, PAS, stains).
   - Reactive changes can be seen in epithelial cells (reactive bronchial cells, pneumocytes, or squamous metaplasia).
   - Necrosis may be present.

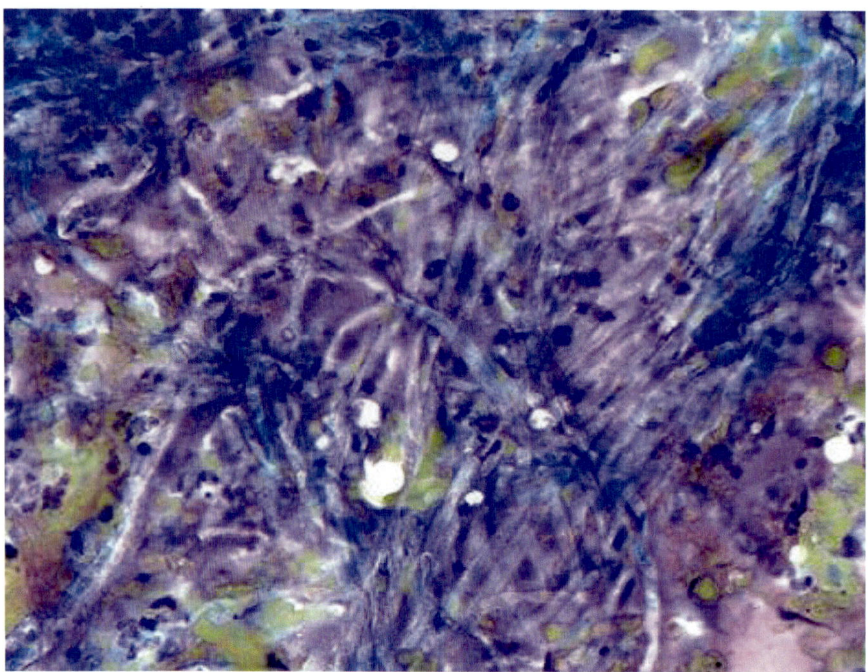

Fig. 10.6 *Aspergillus*. Branching hyphae with even width as negative images in an inflammatory background (Diff-Quik stain, ×400)

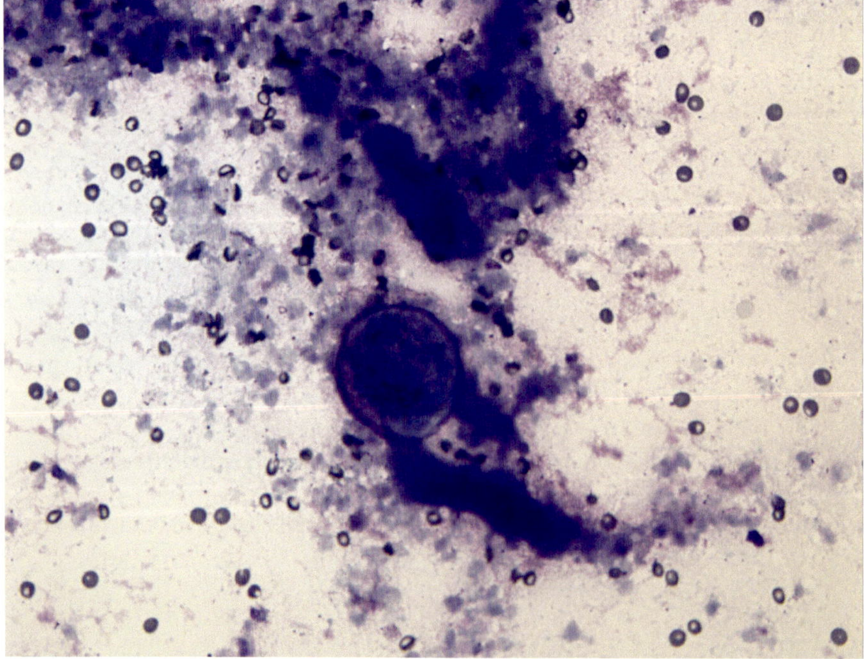

Fig. 10.7 Coccidiosis. A large spherule structure in a necrotic background (Diff-Quik stain, ×200)

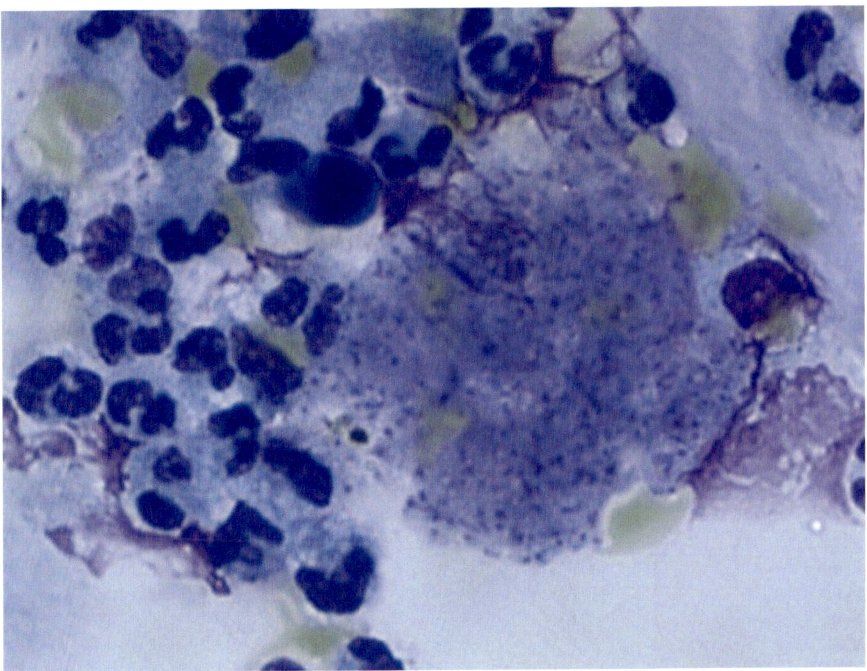

Fig. 10.8 *Pneumocystis jiroveci*. A foamy alveolar cast with trophozoites, each as a tiny negative cystic space with a punctate dot in the center in an inflammatory background (Diff-Quik stain, ×400)

B. Tips and pitfalls

- Cytomorphologic features are not specific for any specific type of infection.
- Triage specimens for microbiology culture studies and save specimens for special stains.
- Multiple passes are needed to rule out malignancy.

2. Mycobacterial infection

Mycobacterial infection in the lung often present with one or multiple lung nodules or mass-like lesions.

A. Cytomorphologic features

- Granulomatous inflammation with abundant necrosis (Fig. 10.9).
- Acute inflammation and multinucleated giant cells can be seen.
- In atypical mycobacterial infection (often in immunocompromised patients), organisms are abundant and may be seen as negative images on Diff-Quik stain.
- Organisms are best viewed on acid-fast stain.
- Reactive bronchial cells or pneumocytes may be present.

B. Tips and pitfalls

- Findings are not specific unless organisms are identified.
- There is a very low yield to identify mycobacterial organisms even with special stain unless it is atypical mycobacterial infection.
- Positive culture result is often needed to confirm diagnosis.

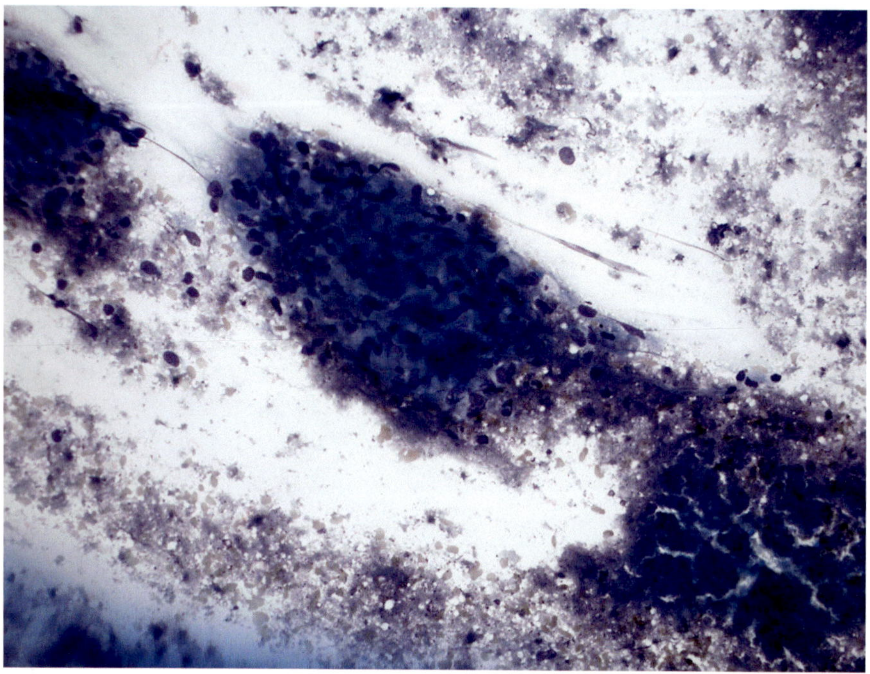

Fig. 10.9 Necrotizing granulomatous inflammation. Clusters of epithelioid histiocytes and a few intermixed lymphocytes in a necrotic background (Diff-Quik stain, ×200)

3. *Actinomyces/Nocardia* infection

   Actinomyces and *Nocardia* are two filamentous bacteria, the infection of which may cause a mass-like lung lesion.

   A. Cytomorphologic features

      - Acute or mixed inflammation.
      - Filamentous bacteria can be seen on Diff-Quik stain.
      - Sulfur granules often present in actinomycosis infection.
      - *Actinomyces* are Gram-positive bacteria, while *Nocardia* are best viewed by Fite stain.
      - Reactive bronchial cells or pneumocytes may be present.

   B. Tips and pitfalls

      - Findings are not specific unless organisms are identified.
      - Positive culture result may be needed to confirm diagnosis.

Inflammation

1. Organizing pneumonia

   Organizing pneumonia is a form of pneumonia which is often the result of resolution or remodeling following bacterial or other infections. Histologically, organizing pneumonia can present as a localized lesion with fibroblast proliferation and mixed inflammation.

A. Cytomorphologic features (Fig. 10.10)

- Variable mixed inflammatory cells.
- Fragments of fibrotic lung tissue and clusters of fibroblast may be seen.
- Reactive bronchial cells and pneumocytes.

B. Tips and pitfalls

- Cytomorphologic features are not specific.
- Ruling out infectious organisms is important.

2. Granulomatous inflammation

Granulomatous inflammation may be associated with a specific type infectious pneumonia such as fungal or mycobacterial infection, in which necrosis is often present. Non-necrotizing granulomatous infection is most commonly seen in patients with sarcoidosis.

A. Cytomorphologic features

- Granulomatous inflammation is characterized by clusters of epithelioid histiocytes and intermixed lymphocytes in the clusters as well as in the background (Fig. 10.11).
- Multinucleated giant cells may be present.

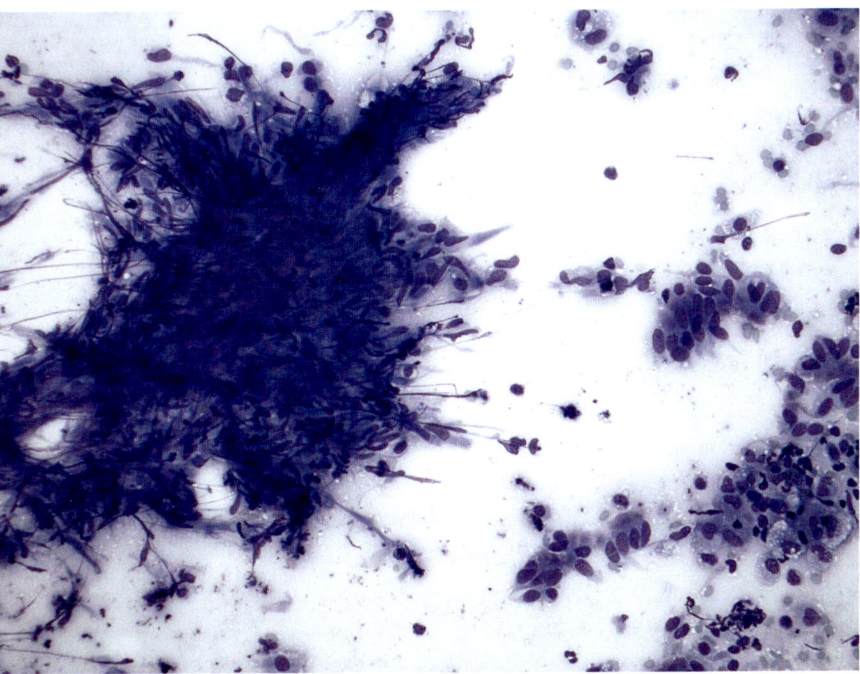

Fig. 10.10 Organizing pneumonia. Clusters of fibrous/myofibroblastic tissue with lymphocytes, macrophages, and reactive bronchial cells (Diff-Quik stain, ×200)

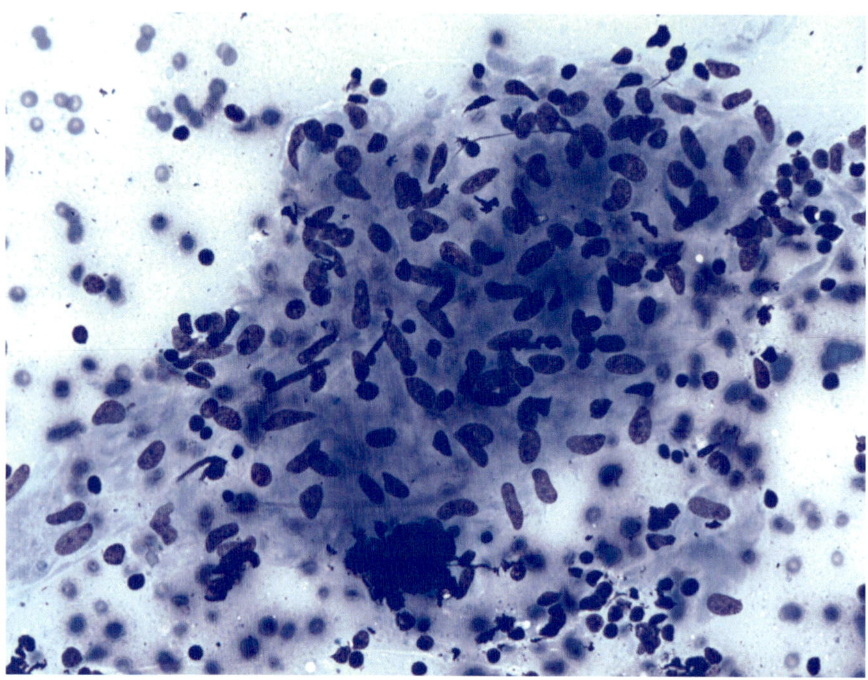

Fig. 10.11 Non-necrotizing granulomatous inflammation. A tight cluster of epithelioid histiocytes and intermixed lymphocytes (Diff-Quik stain, ×400)

- Necrosis may be present.
- Granulomas seen in sarcoidosis are tight clusters of epithelioid histiocytes without background necrosis.
- Reactive bronchial cells and pneumocytes may be present.

B. Tips and pitfalls

- In cases with necrosis, an infectious etiology should be considered. Specimen triage for microbiopsy culture studies is recommended.
- Sarcoidosis is a clinical diagnosis which require additional clinical information and pertinent tests. Thus, even the cytomorphologic features suggest sarcoidosis, it will best be classified as non-necrotizing granulomatous information.

Benign Tumors or Tumors with Uncertain Behavior

Although infrequently, these tumors can be encountered during on-site evaluation. Recognition of these lesions is important for differential diagnosis of a lung mass and is also crucial for assessing whether adequate specimens are obtained.

Hamartoma

Pulmonary hamartomas are benign tumors composed of at least two mesenchymal elements such as cartilage, fat, and smooth muscle combined with entrapped respiratory epithelium.

1. Cytomorphologic features (Fig. 10.12)

   - Abundant benign-appearing epithelial cells intermixed with matrix material.
   - Epithelial cells: clusters or sheets of uniform ciliated columnar cells, similar to ciliated bronchial cells.
   - Matrix: myxoid, fibromyxoid, fibrocartilaginous, or cartilaginous material or in their combination; mature cartilage tissue may be seen.
   - Mature adipose tissue may be present.

2. Tips and pitfalls

   - Should not be confused with normal bronchial contaminants, especially when the biopsy is performed via a transbronchial route. Pay attention to the quantity of both epithelial and matrix elements.

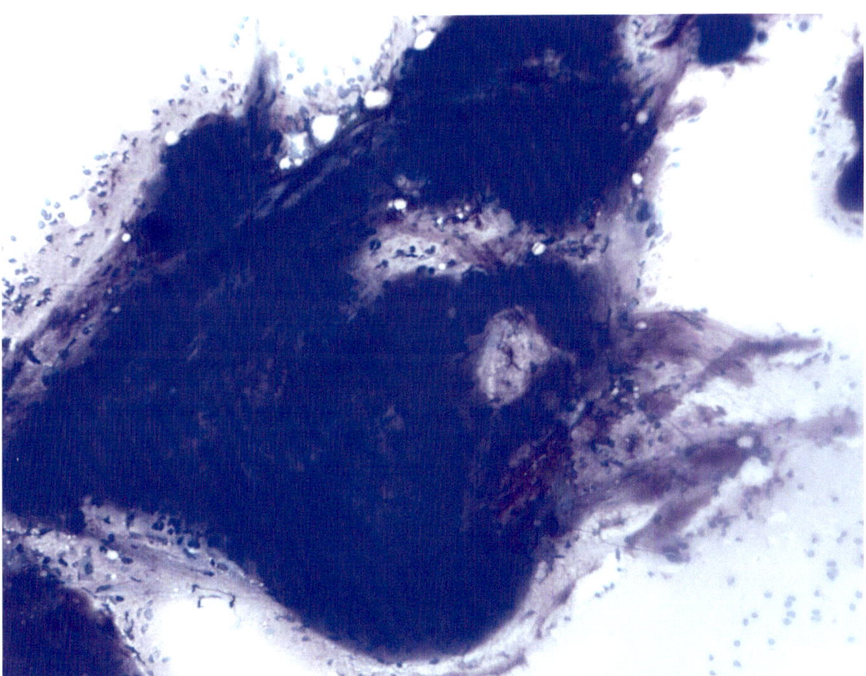

Fig. 10.12 Pulmonary hamartoma. Abundant metachromatic myxoid material with intermixed bland spindle cells and a few bronchial epithelial cells (Diff-Quik stain, ×200)

- Be aware of the potential false-positive interpretation as adenocarcinoma [23]. Note the cilia and uniformity of epithelial cells in hamartoma.
- Salivary gland tumors, particularly pleomorphic adenoma, should be included in the differential diagnosis.

Inflammatory Myofibroblastic Tumor

Inflammatory myofibroblastic tumor is a distinct mesenchymal lesion with an indolent clinical course, characterized by myofibroblastic proliferation intermixed with abundant inflammatory cells including lymphocytes and plasma cells. It occurs in adults as well as in pediatric population.

1. Cytomorphologic features [24] (Fig. 10.13)
   - Abundant mixed inflammatory cells composed of lymphocytes, plasma cells, eosinophils, and histiocytes.
   - Scattered intermediate- to large-sized atypical cells.
   - Atypical cells have delicate cytoplasm and round to oval nuclei with conspicuous nucleolus and rare intranuclear pseudoinclusions.
   - No necrosis.

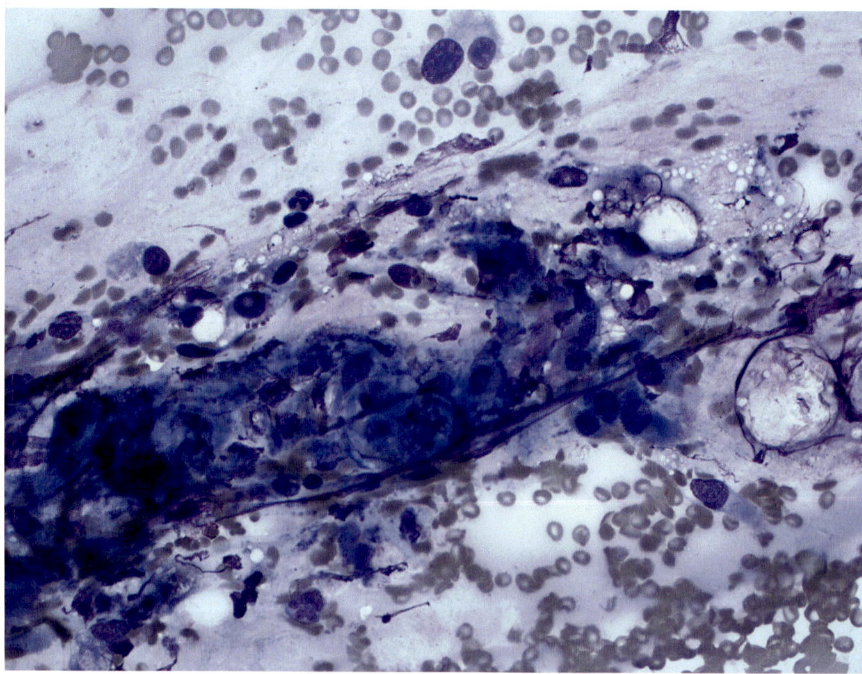

Fig. 10.13 Inflammatory myofibroblastic tumor. A few atypical intermixed with scattered lymphocytes, histiocytes, and reactive bronchial cells. Atypical cells have delicate cytoplasm and oval nuclei with conspicuous nucleolus (Diff-Quik stain, ×400)

2. Tips and pitfalls
   - Searching for atypical cells in the mixed inflammatory background is the key to avoid a false-negative diagnosis.
   - There may be some overlapping cytomorphologic features with organizing pneumonitis.
   - The differential diagnosis should include Langerhans cell histiocytosis and Hodgkin lymphoma.

Solitary Fibrous Tumor

Solitary fibrous tumors are more commonly seen in the pleura rather than in the lung. Even a pleural solitary fibrous tumor can have a significant inward growth into the lung, which may mimic a lung tumor. Solitary fibrous tumor typically shows uniform fibroblastic spindle cells with prominent branching vasculatures. However, variable morphologic features can be seen.

1. Cytomorphologic features [25]
   - Abundant uniform spindle cells, arranged in single cells, loosely cohesive groups, and clusters.
   - Spindle cells have delicate cytoplasm and oval or elongated nuclei with inconspicuous nucleolus.
   - Fibromyxoid matrix may be present.
   - Pleomorphism, mitoses, and necrosis can be seen in malignant form of the tumor.
2. Tips and pitfalls
   - The differential diagnosis should include other spindle cell tumors such as spindle cell carcinoid tumor, monomorphic synovial sarcoma, leiomyoma/leiomyosarcoma, schwannoma, sarcomatoid mesothelioma, and sarcomatoid carcinoma.
   - Diagnostic clues include its pleura-based location and bland uniform spindle cell population. Final diagnosis and distinction from other spindle cell tumors may rest on immunophenotypic analysis.

Sclerosing Pneumocytoma

Sclerosing pneumocytoma is a benign tumor which has a dual population of tumor cells, the epithelial cells lining the alveolar surface and the epithelioid cells within the expanded alveolar septa.

1. Cytomorphologic features [25, 26]
   - Dual populations of epithelial cells and epithelioid cells.

- Epithelial cells are polygonal or cuboid in shape and have vacuolated cytoplasm, round nuclei, conspicuous nucleolus, and occasional intranuclear pseudoinclusions.
- Epithelioid cells have indistinct cell borders and oval nuclei.

2. Tips and pitfalls

- Difficult to diagnose on cytology alone. The diagnosis requires confirmation of dual cell populations by immunocytochemistry.
- The differential diagnosis includes adenocarcinoma, alveolar adenoma, and reactive pneumocytes in the setting of pneumonitis.

Primary Malignant Neoplasms

Lung cancer is the leading cause of cancer-related death worldwide. The most common types of lung cancer include adenocarcinoma, squamous cell carcinoma, and small cell carcinoma, which in combination account for 85–90% of all primary lung malignant neoplasms. Traditionally, non-small cell carcinoma is an acceptable diagnostic term for the tumors other than small cell carcinoma in small biopsy or cytology specimens. With a paradigm shift in treatment of lung cancers, especially lung adenocarcinomas, it is crucial to further classify non-small cell carcinoma. The cases with a diagnosis of adenocarcinoma will be subjected to molecular testing, the results of which help triage patients for appropriate clinical management. Therefore, it is important during on-site evaluation to secure sufficient specimens to ancillary studies including molecular testing.

Adenocarcinoma

Adenocarcinoma is the most common subtype of primary lung cancers. Currently, adenocarcinomas are classified as adenocarcinoma in situ, minimally invasive adenocarcinoma, and invasive adenocarcinoma, which can only be rendered on resection specimens [27–29]. Furthermore, diagnosis of invasive carcinomas has been recommended to include the description of a predominant growth pattern such as lepidic, acinar, papillary, micropapillary, solid, etc. [27, 28]. Again, it is difficult, if not impossible, to pinpoint these growth patterns on cytological material [29]. A well-differentiated adenocarcinoma more likely has a lepidic or acinar growth pattern, while a cytological diagnosis of poorly differentiated adenocarcinoma is probably a tumor with a solid growth pattern on histology.

1. Well- to moderately differentiated adenocarcinoma

   A. Cytomorphologic features (Fig. 10.14)

      - Cellular smear with tumor cells arranged in acinar configurations, sheets and clusters, some as single cells.

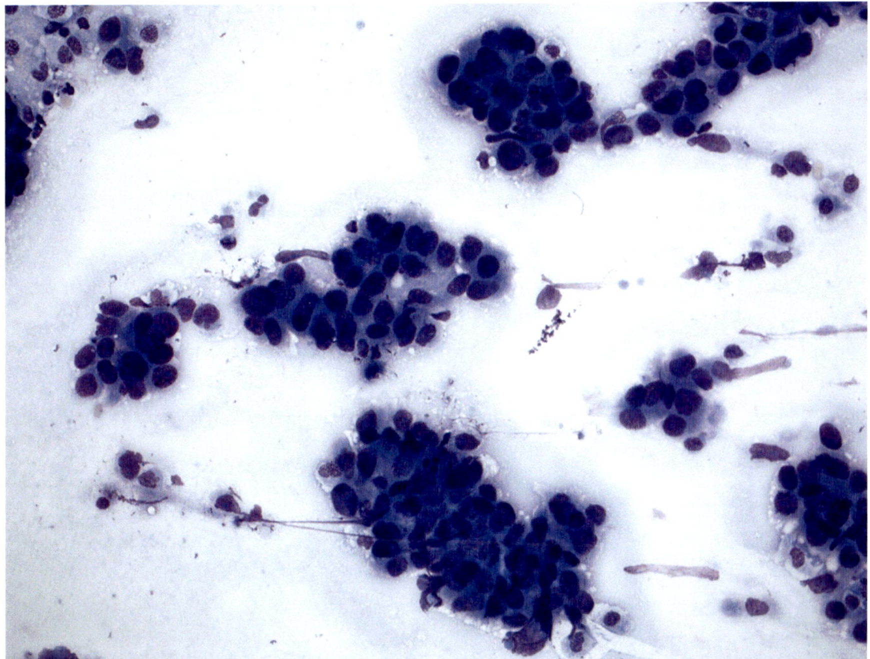

Fig. 10.14 Well-differentiated adenocarcinoma. Groups and clusters of tumor cells with variable-sized nuclei and vacuolated cytoplasm, some arranged in acinar patterns (Diff-Quik stain, ×200)

- Tumor cells are varying in size.
- Tumor cells have vacuolated or granular cytoplasm and round to oval nuclei with conspicuous nucleolus.
- Focal necrosis may be present.

B. Tips and pitfalls

- Should be differentiated from reactive pneumocytes, atypical adenomatous hyperplasia, and alveolar adenoma.
- Pay attention to cytological atypia and clinical presentation including the size of the lesion.
- Some metastatic adenocarcinomas such as breast carcinoma and pancreatic adenocarcinoma may have bland cytomorphology.

2. Poorly differentiated adenocarcinoma

A. Cytomorphologic features (Fig. 10.15)

- Cellular smear with tumor cells arranged in dyscohesive groups and clusters, abundant single cells.
- Marked pleomorphism with prominent nucleolus.
- Focal cytoplasmic vacuolization may be seen.
- Necrosis present.

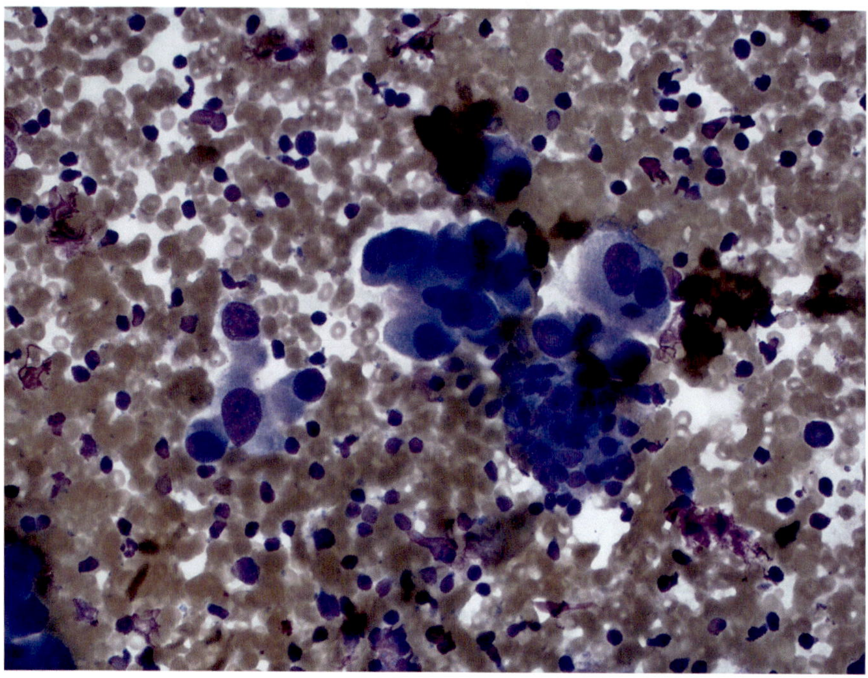

Fig. 10.15 Poorly differentiated adenocarcinoma. Dyscohesive clusters of tumor cells with nuclear pleomorphism, vacuolated cytoplasm, and conspicuous nucleolus. Vague acinar arrangement is present (Diff-Quik stain, ×400)

B. Tips and pitfalls

- May be difficult to distinguish from other lung cancers such as poorly differentiated squamous cell carcinoma and large cell carcinoma. It is appropriate to use the term of non-small cell carcinoma during the on-site evaluation.
- Similar cytomorphologic features can also be seen in some metastatic adenocarcinoma.

3. Adenocarcinoma, morphologic variants

Although uncommon, morphologic variants of adenocarcinomas can be encountered, including invasive mucinous adenocarcinoma, colloid adenocarcinoma, fetal adenocarcinoma, and enteric adenocarcinoma.

A. Cytomorphologic features

- Mucinous adenocarcinoma and colloid adenocarcinoma show sheets and clusters of mucinous epithelial cells with variable amount of mucin in the background (Fig. 10.16).
- Fetal adenocarcinoma has sheets and clusters of epithelial cells with prominent glycogen-rich cytoplasmic vacuoles.
- Enteric adenocarcinoma demonstrates columnar epithelial cells arranged in an acinar or cribriform pattern. Scant or abundant necrosis can be seen.

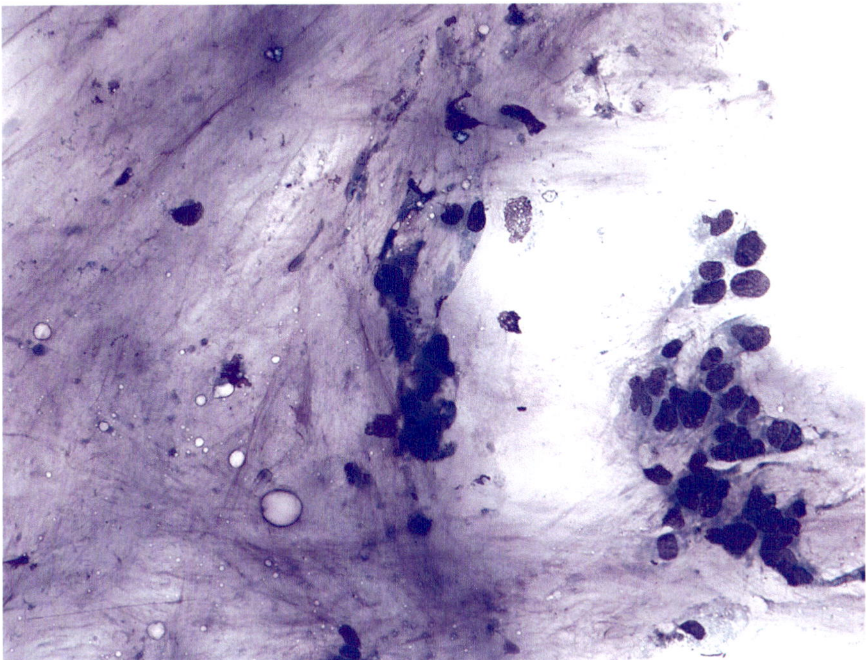

Fig. 10.16 Mucinous adenocarcinoma. Loosely cohesive clusters of tumor cells with variable-sized nuclei and vacuolated cytoplasm in a background of abundant mucin material (Diff-Quik stain, ×200)

B. Tips and pitfalls

- Mucinous and colloid adenocarcinomas should be differentiated from reactive process with abundant mucus accumulation.
- The main differential diagnosis for fetal adenocarcinoma includes endometriosis, PEComatous tumors, and metastatic renal cell carcinoma.
- Enteric adenocarcinoma shares similar cytomorphologic and immunophenotypic features with colorectal adenocarcinoma. It is important to check patient's history to exclude a metastasis.

Squamous Cell Carcinoma

Squamous cell carcinoma is the second most common primary lung cancer. Dependent on keratinization and atypia, squamous cell carcinomas can be classified as well-, moderately, and poorly differentiated tumors. A well- or moderately differentiated squamous cell carcinoma can be recognized by morphological analysis, while a diagnosis of poorly differentiated squamous cell carcinoma needs confirmation by immunohistochemical studies.

1. Well- to moderately differentiated squamous cell carcinoma

   A. Cytomorphologic features (Figs. 10.17 and 10.18)

      - Cellular smears with cohesive clusters of tumor cells.
      - Tumor cells are polygonal and have increased nuclear-to-cytoplasmic ratios, dense cytoplasm, hyperchromatic nuclei, and inconspicuous nucleolus.
      - Keratinizing squamous cells with pleomorphic nucleic are often present.
      - Necrosis is often present.

   B. Tips and pitfalls

      - Should be differentiated from squamous metaplasia, dysplasia, or squamous cell carcinoma in situ, especially when evaluating brushing or washing specimens.
      - Pay attention to clusters of non-keratinizing squamous cells with high nuclear-to-cytoplasmic ratios and hyperchromasia.
      - Rule out the possibility of metastatic squamous cell carcinoma.

2. Poorly differentiated squamous cell carcinoma

   A. Cytomorphologic features (Fig. 10.19)

      - Cellular smears with tumor cells arranged singly, in small groups, or in clusters.

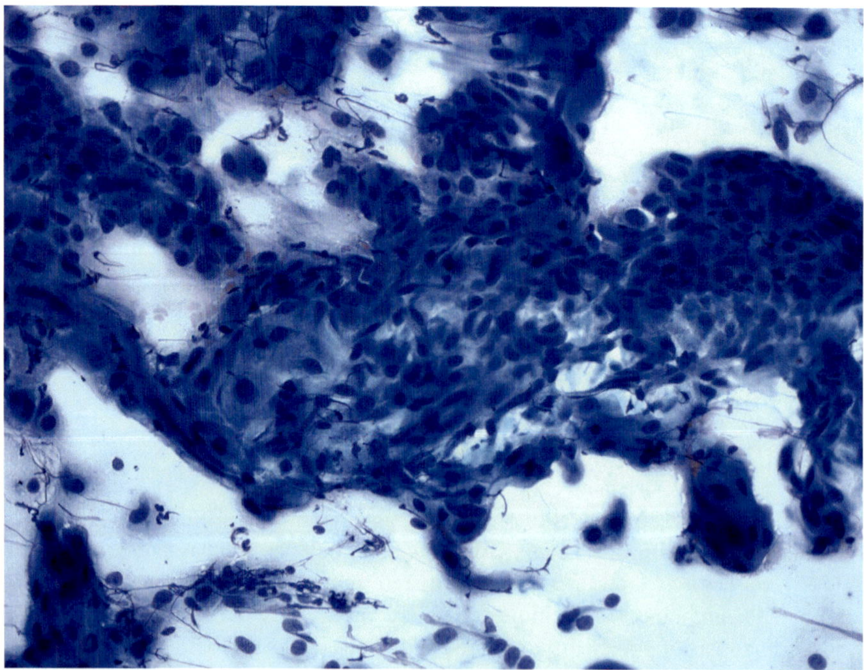

Fig. 10.17 Well-differentiated squamous cell carcinoma. Large cohesive clusters of tumor cells with round to oval nuclei and dense cytoplasm (Diff-Quik stain, ×200)

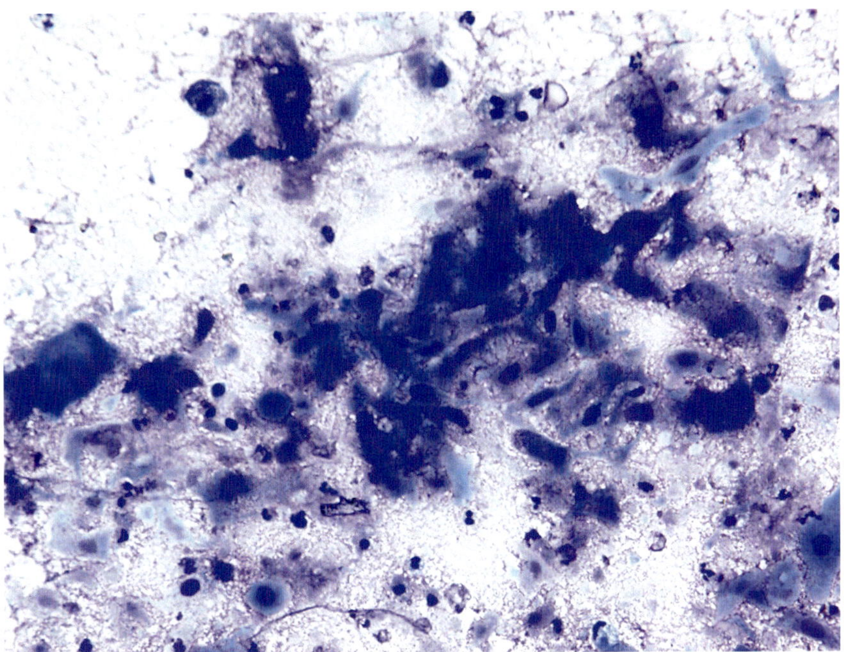

Fig. 10.18 Keratinizing well-differentiated squamous cell carcinoma. Single and dyscohesive groups of pleomorphic tumor cells with dense cytoplasm in a necrotic and inflammatory background (Diff-Quik stain, ×400)

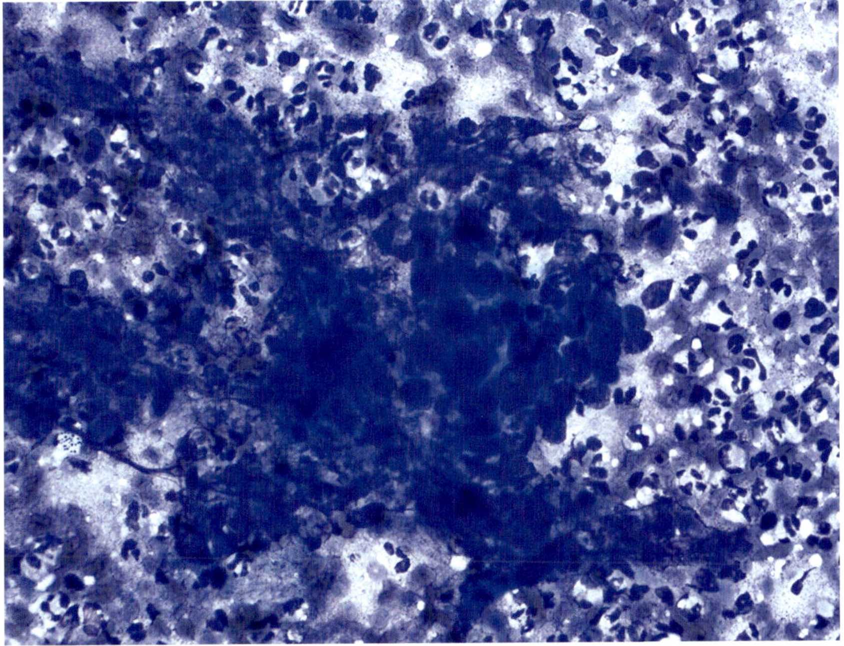

Fig. 10.19 Poorly differentiated squamous cell carcinoma. Clusters of tumor cells with dense cytoplasm and variable-sized nuclei in a necrotic and inflammatory background (Diff-Quik stain, ×400)

- Tumor cells have high nuclear-to-cytoplasmic ratios, dense cytoplasm, and pleomorphic hyperchromatic nuclei with conspicuous nucleolus.
- Focal keratinizing squamous cells may be seen.
- Abundant necrosis present.

B. Tips and pitfalls

- Difficult to distinguish from other poorly differentiated non-small cell lung carcinomas morphologically [30].
- Rule out the possibility of metastatic squamous cell carcinoma or urothelial carcinoma.

3. Basaloid squamous cell carcinoma

Basaloid squamous cell carcinoma is a poorly differentiated carcinoma that has a lobular growth pattern with peripheral palisading. Although the tumor cells lack atypical squamous morphology, they stain positive for squamous markers.

A. Cytomorphologic features (Fig. 10.20)

- Sheets and clusters of tumor cells with relatively uniform morphology.
- Tumor cells are intermediate in size and have scant cytoplasm, round nuclei, and inconspicuous nucleolus. Prominent nucleolus can be seen in a subset of cases.
- Necrosis and apoptosis are often seen.

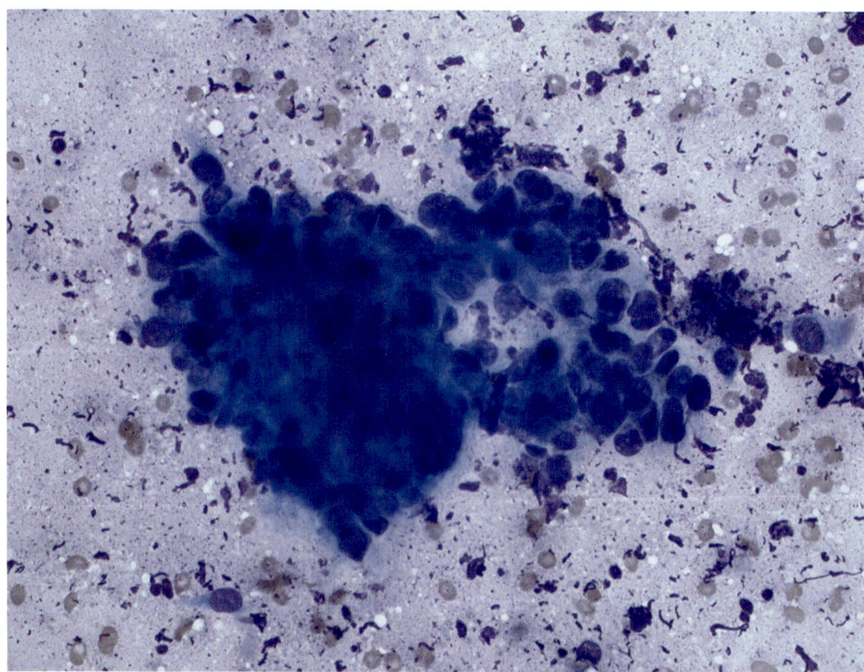

Fig. 10.20 Basaloid squamous cell carcinoma. Clusters of tumor cells with large relatively uniform nuclei and scant cytoplasm (Diff-Quik stain, ×400)

B. Tips and pitfalls

- May share some cytomorphologic features with small cell carcinoma such as high nuclear-to-cytoplasmic ratios, but tumor cells are more cohesive and lack nuclear streaming artifacts.
- Also, should be differentiated from large cell neuroendocrine carcinoma, adenoid cystic carcinoma, and poorly differentiated squamous cell carcinoma.

Small Cell Carcinoma

Small cell carcinoma accounts for 10–15% of primary malignant lung neoplasms. It is characterized by proliferation of small tumor cells with scant cytoplasm, speckled chromatin, and absence of nucleolus. Tumor cells stain positive for neuroendocrine markers.

1. Cytomorphologic features (Fig. 10.21)

- Cellular specimen with single or loosely cohesive clusters of relatively uniform tumor cells.
- Tumor cells are small to intermediate in size and have scant cytoplasm.
- Round, oval, or spindle nuclei with speckled chromatin and absence of nucleolus or inconspicuous nucleolus.
- Nuclear pleomorphism may be seen in some cases.
- Nuclear molding and nuclear streaming artifacts.
- Abundant necrosis and apoptosis.

2. Tips and pitfalls

- Differential diagnosis includes other neuroendocrine tumors such as large cell neuroendocrine carcinoma and carcinoid tumors.
- Small cell carcinoma has overlapping cytomorphologic features with basaloid squamous cell carcinoma and metastatic Merkel cell carcinoma.
- In cases with dominant dispersed single cell pattern, non-Hodgkin lymphoma should be included in the differential diagnosis. The latter has lymphoglandular bodies in the background. This distinction may still be challenging, especially in lymph node sampling.

Large Cell Neuroendocrine Carcinoma

Large cell neuroendocrine carcinoma is considered to be a high-grade neuroendocrine carcinoma, which has morphic features of rosettes and peripheral palisading as well as expresses neuroendocrine markers.

1. Cytomorphologic features [16] (Fig. 10.22)

- Cellular specimen with sheets or clusters of relatively uniform tumor cells, some arranged in acinar/rosette pattern.

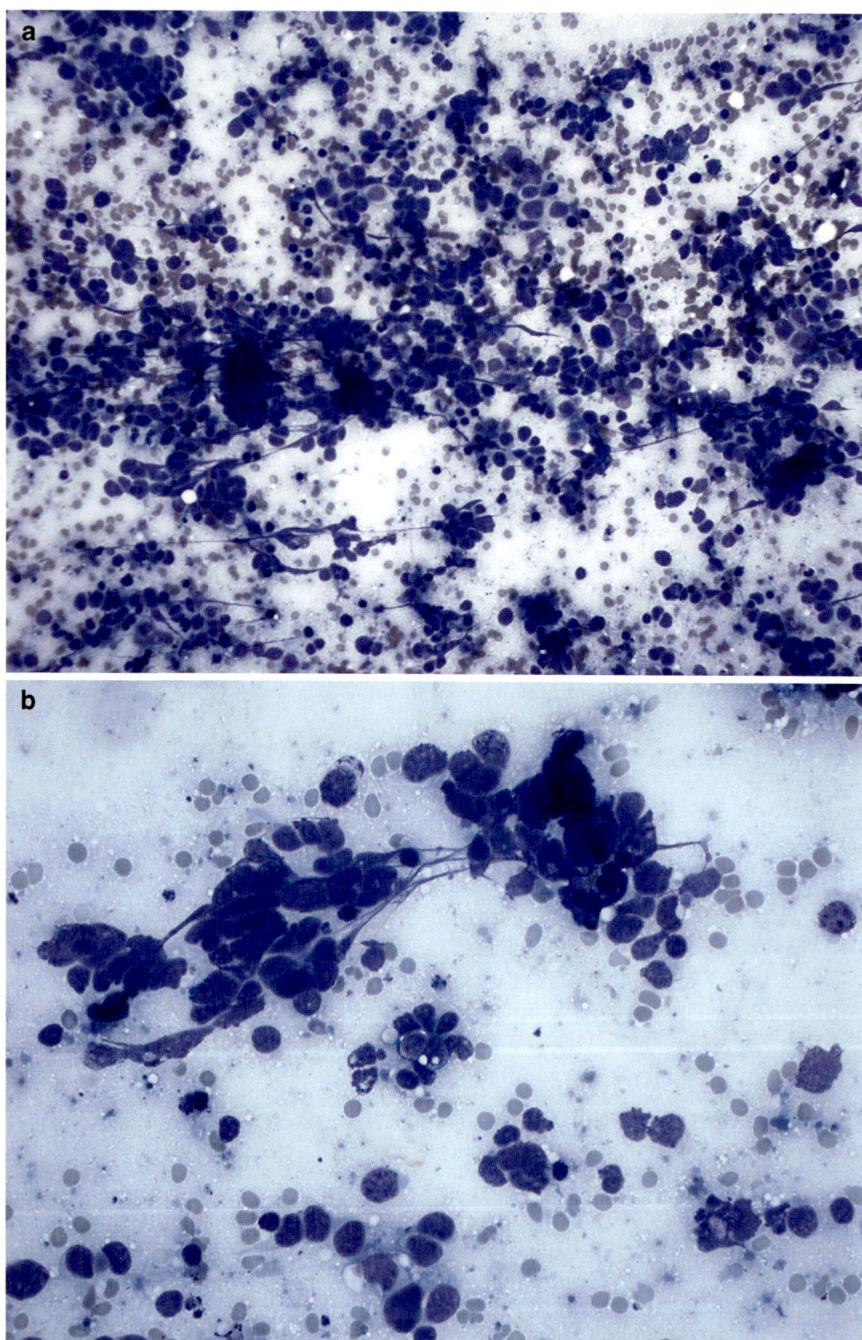

Fig. 10.21 Small cell carcinoma. Single and loosely cohesive clusters of tumor cells (**a** Diff-Quik stain, ×200) with scant cytoplasm, nuclear molding, and nuclear streaming (**b** Diff-Quik stain, ×400)

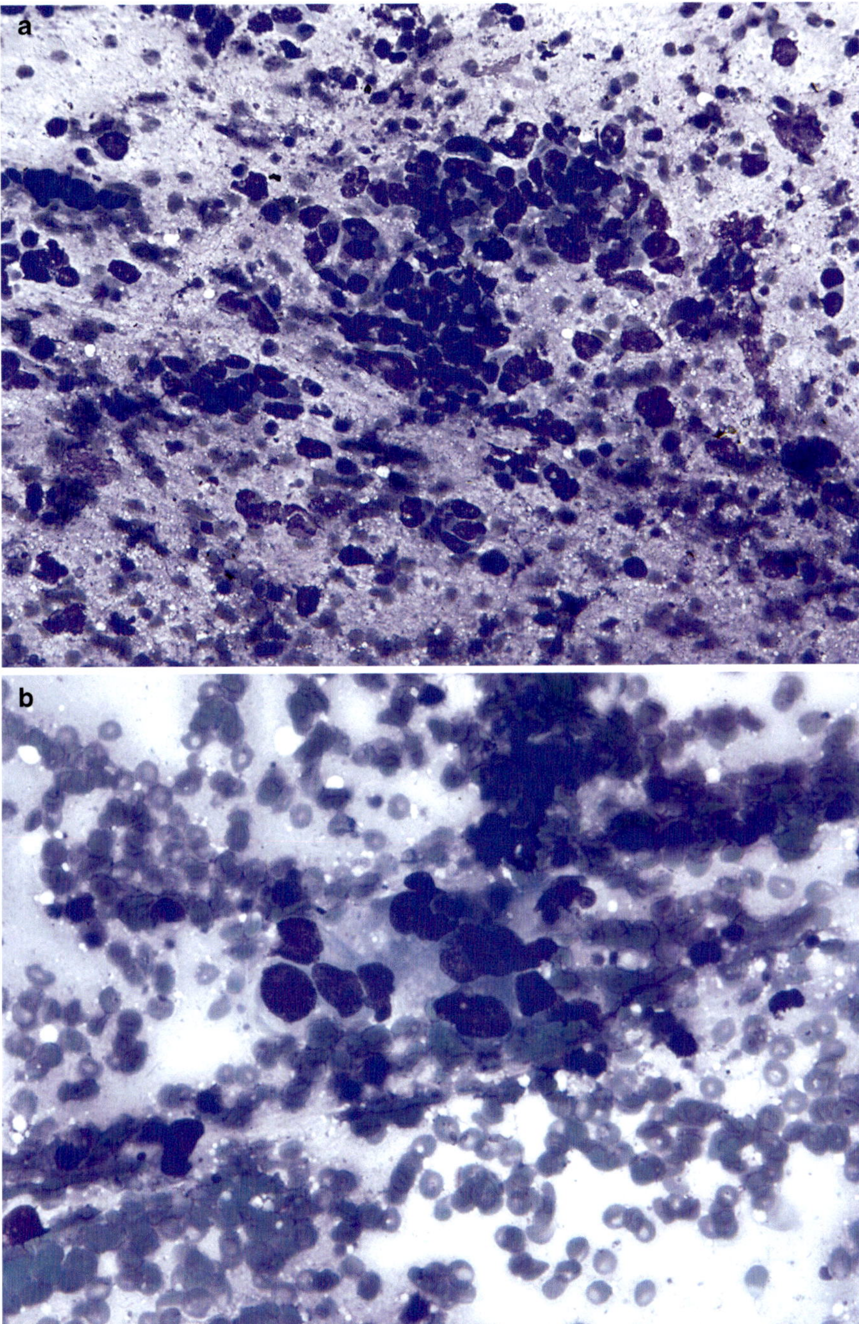

Fig. 10.22 Large cell neuroendocrine carcinoma. Loosely cohesive clusters of tumor cells with relatively uniform nuclei (**a** Diff-Quik stain, ×200) and moderate amount of cytoplasm and conspicuous nucleolus (**b** Diff-Quik stain, ×400)

- Tumor cells are intermediate in size and have scant to moderate amount of delicate cytoplasm, round nuclei, and prominent nucleolus.
- Focal necrosis may be present.

2. Tips and pitfalls

- Large cell neuroendocrine carcinoma cytomorphologically overlaps with other lung cancers, especially small cell carcinoma, adenocarcinoma, and basaloid squamous cell carcinoma [31].
- The feature of uniform tumor cells with prominent nucleolus is the clue.
- It would be reasonable to be classified as non-small cell carcinoma during the on-site evaluation if there are no features suggesting small cell carcinoma.
- In cases with prominent nucleolus, small cell carcinoma should be included in the differential diagnosis.

Typical Carcinoid Tumor/Atypical Carcinoid Tumor

Typical and atypical carcinoid tumors are the two subtypes of well-differentiated neuroendocrine neoplasms, which differ in their mitotic counts and absence or presence of necrosis. The tumors can be found in the trachea, bronchus, and central or peripheral lung. When occurred in the peripheral lung, the tumors are more likely to be atypical. It is however difficult to differentiate typical from atypical carcinoid tumors based on limited cytological material.

1. Cytomorphologic features [16] (Fig. 10.23)

- Single, dyscohesive or loosely cohesive groups of relative uniform tumor cells.
- Fragments of tumor cells with embedded capillary vasculatures may be present.
- In most cases, tumor cells have moderate amount of cytoplasm and round to oval, eccentrically placed nuclei with speckled chromatin and inconspicuous nucleolus.
- Spindle cell or oncocytic morphology can be seen in a minority of cases.
- Necrosis and mitosis are uncommon.

2. Tips and pitfalls

- Check patient's history and rule out metastatic neuroendocrine tumors, particularly of gastrointestinal tract origin.
- Carcinoid tumors have overlapping morphology with salivary gland-type tumors, paraganglioma, and metastatic lobular breast carcinoma.
- Spindle cell carcinoid tumors should be differentiated from solitary fibrous tumor due to their spindle cell morphology and peripheral location.

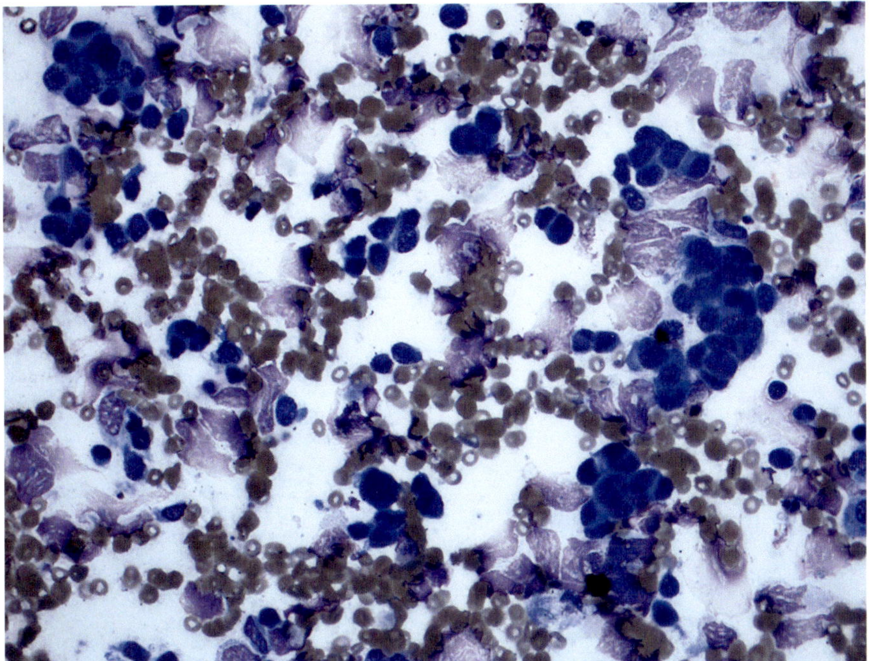

Fig. 10.23 Well-differentiated neuroendocrine tumor. Single and dyscohesive groups of tumor cells with slightly enlarged uniform nuclei (Diff-Quik stain, ×400)

Sarcomatoid Carcinoma

Sarcomatoid carcinomas include pleomorphic carcinoma, carcinosarcoma, and pulmonary blastoma.

1. Cytomorphologic features

   - Pleomorphic carcinoma is a poorly differentiated carcinoma with a component of squamous cell carcinoma, adenocarcinoma, or small cell carcinoma as well as a component of spindle cells or giant cells (Fig. 10.24).
   - Carcinosarcoma is a biphasic tumor consisting of a squamous or adenocarcinoma component intermixed with a sarcoma-containing heterologous element.
   - Pulmonary blastoma is also a biphasic tumor having components of fetal adenocarcinoma and primitive mesenchymal stroma.

2. Tips and pitfalls

   - Presence of dual morphologic elements is the clue; however, it is difficult, if not impossible, to diagnose these entities during the on-site evaluation.
   - Should be differentiated from sarcoma and other poorly differentiated carcinoma.

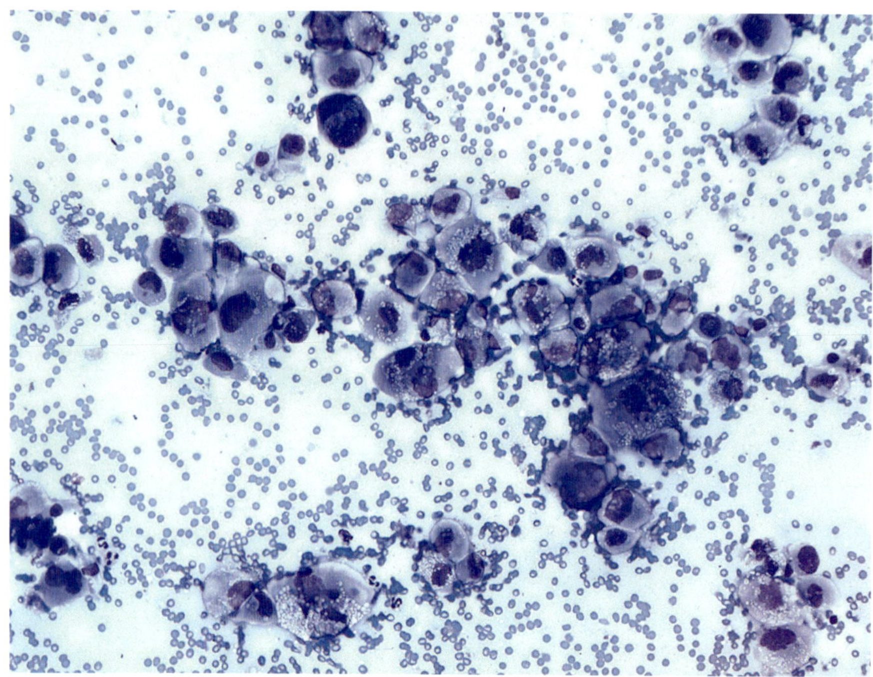

Fig. 10.24 Pleomorphic carcinoma. Single and dyscohesive groups of pleomorphic tumor cells with binucleated and multinucleated tumor giant cells (Diff-Quik stain, ×200)

Salivary Gland-Type Tumors

Salivary gland-type tumors of the lung are uncommon, accounting for less than 1% of all lung tumors. These tumors arise predominantly in the central airway.

1. Cytomorphologic features

   - Salivary gland-type tumors include mucoepidermoid carcinoma, adenoid cystic carcinoma, epithelial–myoepithelial tumor, myoepithelial tumor, and pleomorphic adenoma.
   - Morphologically similar to the tumors seen in the salivary glands (Figs. 10.25 and 10.26).
   - There are often cellular elements as well as matrix/metachromatic material.

2. Tips and pitfalls

   - Should be differentiated from other non-small cell carcinomas
   - May have overlapping morphology with carcinoid tumors

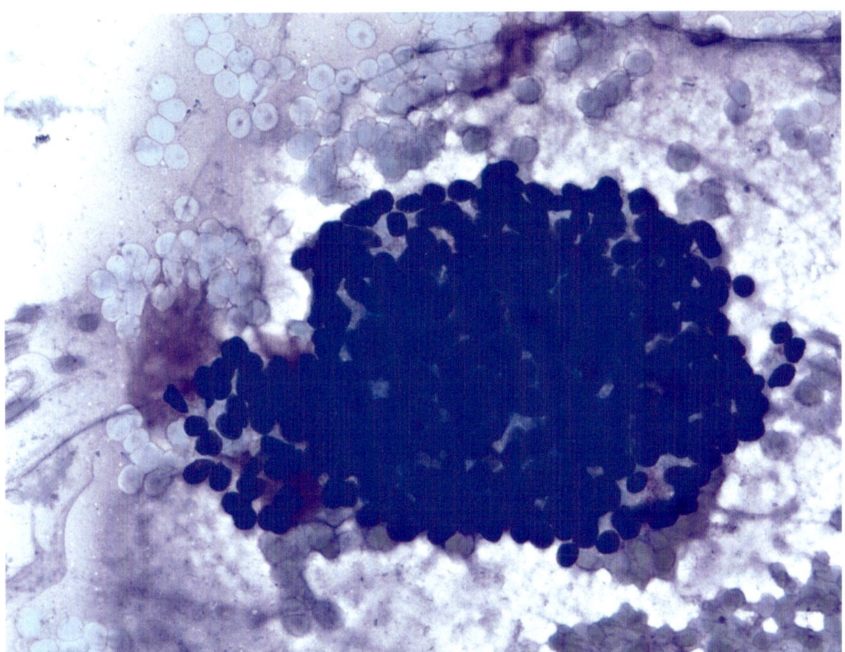

Fig. 10.25 Adenoid cystic carcinoma. A cohesive cluster of relatively small uniform tumor cells with scant cytoplasm. Scant metachromatic material is seen at the edge of the tumor cluster (Diff-Quik stain, ×200)

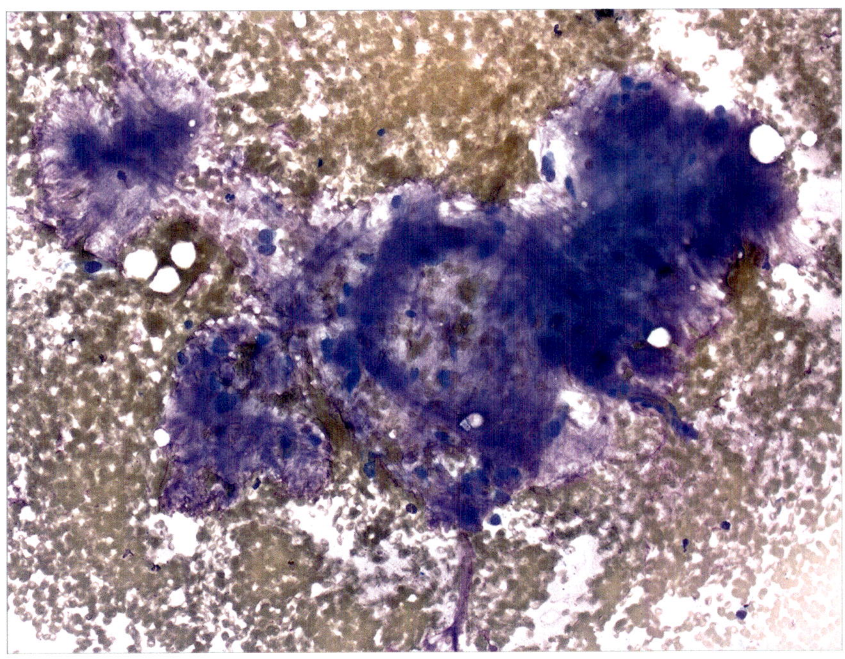

Fig. 10.26 Pleomorphic adenoma. Abundant metachromatic material intermixed with scattered bland epithelioid cells (Diff-Quik stain, ×200)

Other Uncommon Carcinomas

Included are adenosquamous carcinoma, large cell carcinoma, lymphoepithelioma-like carcinoma, and NUT carcinoma. Diagnosis of these entities may need extensive sampling, immunohistochemical analysis, and exclusion of other non-small cell carcinomas.

1. Cytomorphologic features

   - Adenosquamous cells show dual cell population of adenocarcinoma and squamous cells recognized by morphology and confirmed by immunostaining.
   - Large cell carcinoma shows single or loosely groups of large pleomorphic tumor cells. The tumor cells have no morphologic and immunophenotypic features of adenocarcinoma, squamous cell carcinoma, or small cell carcinoma.
   - Lymphoepithelioma-like carcinoma shares the same features of nasopharyngeal carcinoma (Fig. 10.27).

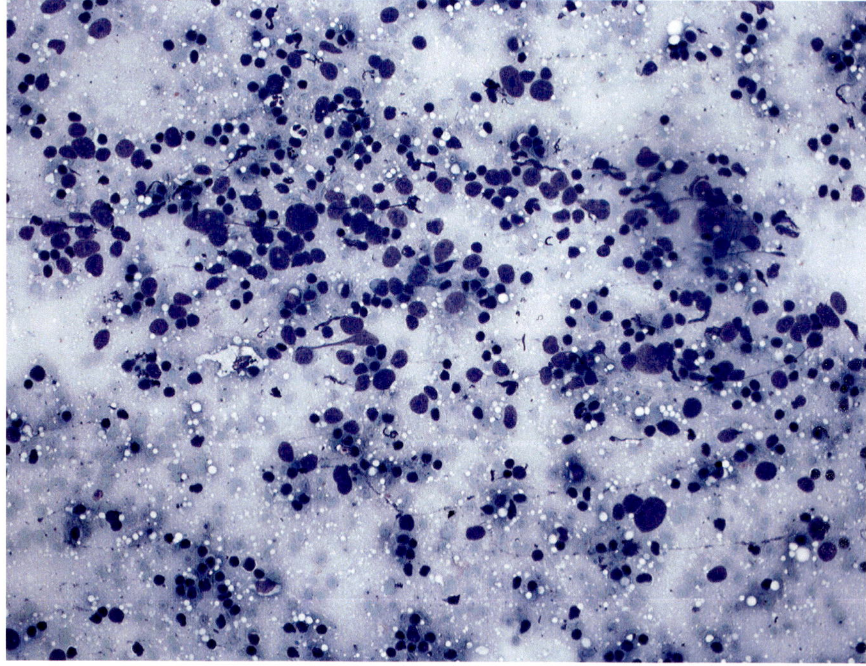

Fig. 10.27 Lymphoepithelioma-like carcinoma. Single and dyscohesive groups of tumor cells intermixed with lymphocytes. The tumor cells are large and pleomorphic and have delicate cytoplasm and prominent nucleolus (Diff-Quik stain, ×200)

- NUT carcinoma is a poorly differentiated aggressive carcinoma showing monomorphic tumor cells with irregular nuclear contours and prominent nucleolus.

2. Tips and pitfalls

- Cytomorphologic features may not be specific and immunostains are often required to support the diagnosis.
- During on-site evaluation, these can classified as poorly differentiated non-small cell carcinoma.

Sarcomas

Sarcomas primary to the lung are rare with synovial sarcoma being the most common type. In fact, after bone and soft tissue, lung is the most common site for synovial sarcoma.

1. Cytomorphologic features [25]

- Sarcomas of the lung share the same morphologic features arisen in the bone and soft tissue.
- Synovial sarcoma can have a biphasic (epithelial and spindle cell components) or a monophasic morphologic (spindle cells only).

2. Tips and pitfalls

- Since primary lung sarcoma is a rare occurrence, it is essential to rule out a metastatic sarcoma.

Metastatic Tumors

The lung is one of the most common sites for metastatic tumors, which are mostly carcinomas followed by sarcomas, melanoma, and germ cell tumors. In addition, lymphoproliferative disorders seen in the lung could be a primary or secondary involvement. Most metastatic tumors present as multiple lung lesions while a solitary lung metastasis can occur. Some tumors such as breast carcinoma, renal cell carcinoma, and melanoma can present as an endobronchial lesion when metastatic to the lung. Many patients with metastatic diseases have a known history of the corresponding malignancy although metastasis can occur as an initial presentation. In cases with only cytological specimens available, a metastasis should always be included in the differential diagnosis since cytology specimens lack the architectural features helpful for determination of primary versus metastatic.

Metastatic Carcinoma

Metastatic carcinomas are originated from extrapulmonary sites such as gastrointestinal tract, gynecological tract, breast, kidney, urothelium, head and neck, and prostate.

1. Cytomorphologic features
   - Metastatic carcinomas show identical cytomorphologic features as their primaries (Figs. 10.28 and 10.29).
2. Tips and pitfalls
   - Knowledge of patient's prior history of malignancy is important.
   - Review of imaging findings should always be encouraged; however, it should be kept in mind that multiple lung lesions could represent synchronous primary tumors or intrapulmonary metastasis of a lung tumor.
   - Immunophenotypic analysis may be needed to rule out a metastasis.

Metastatic Sarcoma

Primary sarcomas of the lung are rare. It is imperative to rule out a metastasis before diagnosis of a lung sarcoma is rendered.

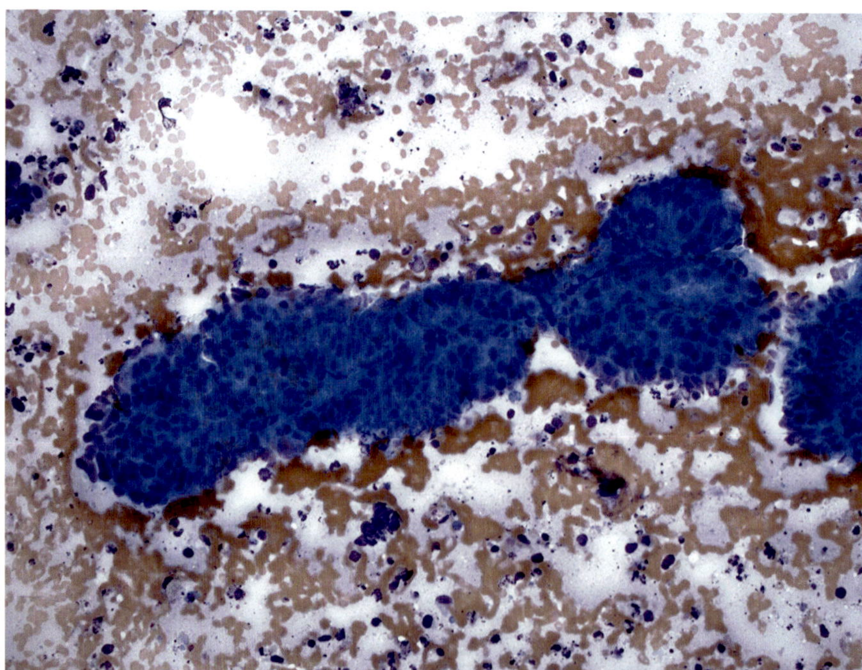

Fig. 10.28 Metastatic colorectal carcinoma. Cohesive clusters of columnar cells with an acinar pattern in a necrotic and inflammatory background (Diff-Quik stain, ×200)

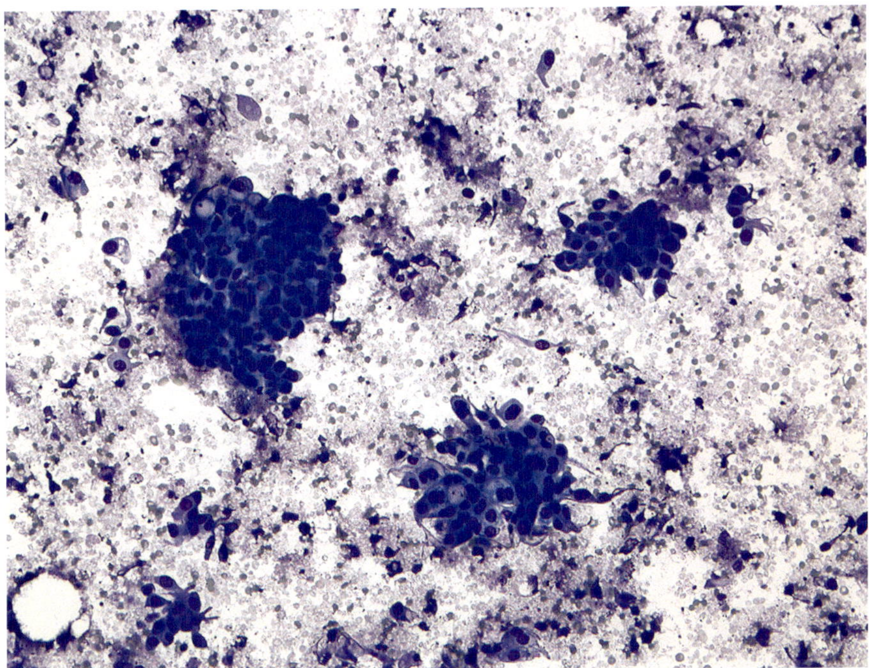

Fig. 10.29 Metastatic urothelial carcinoma. Single and clusters of tumor cells with dense cytoplasm and focal vague papillary architecture (Diff-Quik stain, ×200)

1. Cytomorphologic features
    - Metastatic sarcomas show the same cytomorphologic features as their primaries.
2. Tips and pitfalls
    - Patient's prior history of malignancy and imaging findings are crucial for ruling out a metastasis.

Metastatic Melanoma

The patients with metastatic melanoma to the lung may or may not have a documented history of melanoma. Primary tumors such as mucosa-associated melanoma and skin melanoma with regression could be occult. Melanoma can rarely arise in the lung as an ectopic tumor.

1. Cytomorphologic features (Fig. 10.30)
    - Dispersed single cells with eccentrically located nuclei and prominent nucleolus.
    - Binucleation, intranuclear pseudoinclusions, and melanin pigments can be seen.
    - Spindle cell melanoma is a morphologic variant.

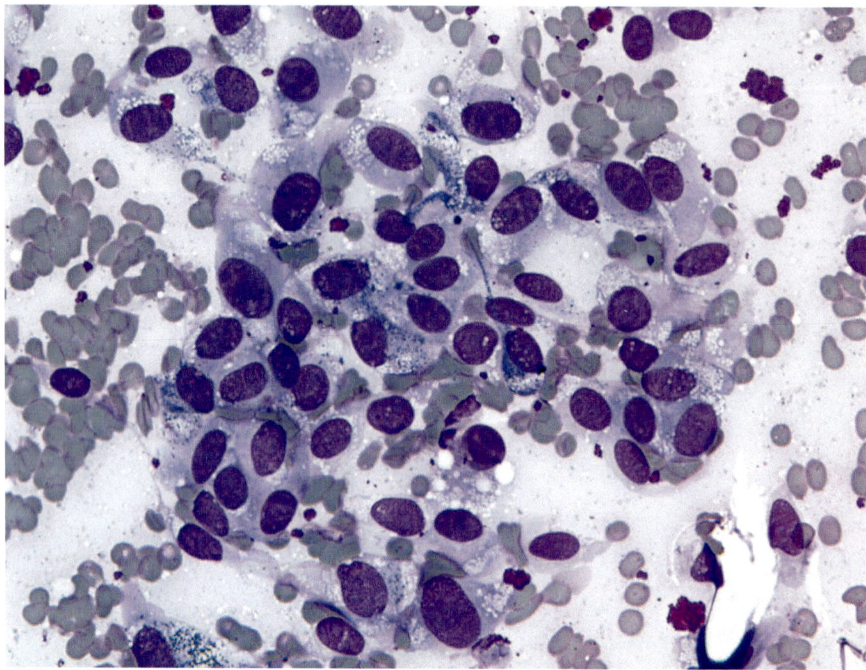

Fig. 10.30 Metastatic melanoma. Single and dyscohesive groups of tumor cells with oval nuclei and conspicuous nucleolus. Some tumor cells contain cytoplasmic melanin pigments (Diff-Quik stain, ×400)

2. Tips and pitfalls
   - Classical cytomorphologic features are the clues for an accurate diagnosis; presence of melanin pigments, although uncommon, is helpful.
   - Differential diagnosis may include carcinoid tumor, metastatic lobular breast carcinoma, and plasma cell neoplasm.

Lymphoproliferative Disorders

Lymphoproliferative disorders can involve the lung as a primary or secondary tumor. The most common primary lymphoproliferative disorder is the extranodal marginal zone lymphoma of mucosa-associated lymphoid tissue (MALT lymphoma) followed by diffuse large B-cell lymphoma [32, 33]. The tumors of histiocytic origin include Langerhans cell histiocytosis.

1. Cytomorphologic features
   - Abundant dispersed single cells.
   - The cells of MALT lymphoma are small and monotonous and have eccentrically located nuclei and inconspicuous nucleolus (Fig. 10.31).

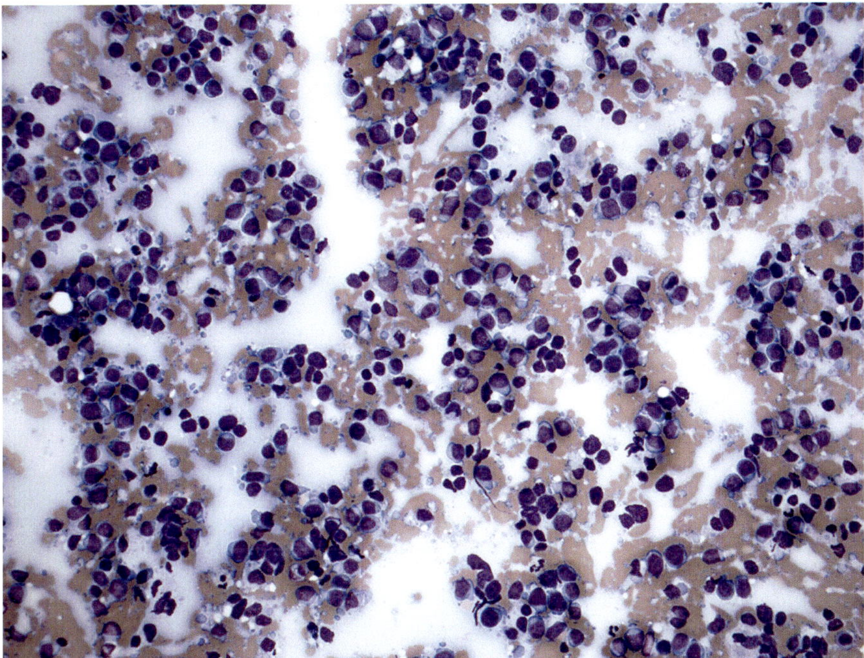

Fig. 10.31 Mucosa-associated lymphoid tissue (MALT) lymphoma. Dispersed single relative uniform lymphoid cells with eccentrically located nuclei. Abundant lymphoglandular bodies are seen in the background (Diff-Quik stain, ×200)

- The cells of diffuse large B-cell lymphoma are large and pleomorphic and have scant cytoplasm and enlarged pleomorphic nuclei with irregular nuclear membranes and conspicuous nucleolus.
- The cells of Langerhans cell histiocytosis are large and have abundant cytoplasm and delicate nuclei with prominent nuclear membrane folding.

2. Tips and pitfalls

- It is important to recognize these lesions during the on-site evaluation.
- Triaging specimens for flow cytometry and cell block is essential for an accurate diagnosis and differentiate from a reactive process or other tumors.

References

1. Rivera MP, Mehta AC, Wahidi MM. Establishing the diagnosis of lung cancer: diagnosis and management of lung cancer, 3rd ed: American College of Chest Physicians evidence-based clinical practice guidelines. Chest. 2013;143(5 Suppl):e142S–65S.
2. Eapen GA, Shah AM, Lei X, Jimenez CA, Morice RC, Yarmus L, Filner J, Ray C, Michaud G, Greenhill SR, Sarkiss M, Casal R, Rice D, Ost DE, American College of Chest Physicians Quality Improvement Registry, Education, and Evaluation (AQuIRE) Participants. Complications, consequences, and practice patterns of endobronchial ultrasound-guided transbronchial needle aspiration: results of the AQuIRE registry. Chest. 2013;143(4):1044–53.

3. VanderLaan PA, Wang HH, Majid A, Folch E. Endobronchial ultrasound-guided transbronchial needle aspiration (EBUS-TBNA): an overview and update for the cytopathologist. Cancer Cytopathol. 2014;122(8):561–76.
4. Loo FL, Halligan AM, Port JL, Hoda RS. The emerging technique of electromagnetic navigation bronchoscopy-guided fine-needle aspiration of peripheral lung lesions: promising results in 50 lesions. Cancer Cytopathol. 2014;122(3):191–9.
5. Ost DE, Ernst A, Lei X, Kovitz KL, Benzaquen S, Diaz-Mendoza J, Greenhill S, Toth J, Feller-Kopman D, Puchalski J, Baram D, Karunakara R, Jimenez CA, Filner JJ, Morice RC, Eapen GA, Michaud GC, Estrada-Y-Martin RM, Rafeq S, Grosu HB, Ray C, Gilbert CR, Yarmus LB, Simoff M, AQuIRE Bronchoscopy Registry. Diagnostic yield and complications of bronchoscopy for peripheral lung lesions. Results of the AQuIRE registry. Am J Respir Crit Care Med. 2016;193(1):68–77.
6. Shepherd RW. Bronchoscopic pursuit of the peripheral pulmonary lesion: navigational bronchoscopy, radial endobronchial ultrasound, and ultrathin bronchoscopy. Curr Opin Pulm Med. 2016;22(3):257–64.
7. Mondoni M, Sotgiu G, Bonifazi M, Dore S, Parazzini EM, Carlucci P, Gasparini S, Centanni S. Transbronchial needle aspiration in peripheral pulmonary lesions: a systematic review and meta-analysis. Eur Respir J. 2016;48(1):196–204.
8. Nakajima T, Yasufuku K, Saegusa F, Fujiwara T, Sakairi Y, Hiroshima K, Nakatani Y, Yoshino I. Rapid on-site cytologic evaluation during endobronchial ultrasound-guided transbronchial needle aspiration for nodal staging in patients with lung cancer. Ann Thorac Surg. 2013;95(5):1695–9.
9. da Cunha Santos G, Boerner SL, Geddie WR. Maximizing the yield of lymph node cytology: lessons learned from rapid onsite evaluation of image- and endoscopic-guided biopsies of hilar and mediastinal lymph nodes. Cancer Cytopathol. 2011;119(6):361–6.
10. Oki M, Saka H, Kitagawa C, Kogure Y, Murata N, Adachi T, Ando M. Rapid on-site cytologic evaluation during endobronchial ultrasound-guided transbronchial needle aspiration for diagnosing lung cancer: a randomized study. Respiration. 2013;85(6):486–92.
11. Kubik MJ, Bovbel A, Goli H, Saremian J, Siddiqi A, Masood S. Diagnostic value and accuracy of imprint cytology evaluation during image-guided core needle biopsies: review of our experience at a large academic center. Diagn Cytopathol. 2015;43(10):773–9.
12. Jain D, Allen TC, Aisner DL, Beasley MB, Cagle PT, Capelozzi VL, Hariri LP, Lantuejoul S, Miller R, Mino-Kenudson M, Monaco SE, Moreira A, Raparia K, Rekhtman N, Roden AC, Roy-Chowdhuri S, da Cunha Santos G, Thunnissen E, Troncone G, Vivero M. Rapid on-site evaluation of endobronchial ultrasound-guided transbronchial needle aspirations for the diagnosis of lung cancer: a perspective from Members of the Pulmonary Pathology Society. Arch Pathol Lab Med. 2018;142(2):253–62.
13. Yarmus L, Akulian J, Gilbert C, Feller-Kopman D, Lee HJ, Zarogoulidis P, Lechtzin N, Ali SZ, Sathiyamoorthy V. Optimizing endobronchial ultrasound for molecular analysis. How many passes are needed? Ann Am Thorac Soc. 2013;10(6):636–43.
14. Trisolini R, Cancellieri A, Tinelli C, de Biase D, Valentini I, Casadei G, Paioli D, Ferrari F, Gordini G, Patelli M, Tallini G. Randomized trial of endobronchial ultrasound-guided transbronchial needle aspiration with and without rapid on-site evaluation for lung cancer genotyping. Chest. 2015;148(6):1430–7.
15. Stoy SP, Segal JP, Mueller J, Furtado LV, Vokes EE, Patel JD, Murgu S. Feasibility of endobronchial ultrasound-guided transbronchial needle aspiration cytology specimens for next generation sequencing in non-small-cell lung cancer. Clin Lung Cancer. 2018;19(3):230–8.
16. Layfield LJ, Baloch Z, Elsheikh T, Litzky L, Rekhtman N, Travis WD, Zakowski M, Zarka M, Geisinger K. Standardized terminology and nomenclature for respiratory cytology: the Papanicolaou Society of Cytopathology guidelines. Diagn Cytopathol. 2016;44(5):399–409.
17. Suen KC, Abdul-Karim FW, Kaminsky DB, et al. Guidelines of the Papanicolaou Society of Cytopathology for the examination of cytologic specimens obtained from the respiratory

tract. Papanicolaou Society of Cytopathology Task Force on Standards of Practice. Diagn Cytopathol. 1999;21(1):61–9.
18. Wallace MB, Pascual JM, Raimondo M, Woodward TA, McComb BL, Crook JE, Johnson MM, Al-Haddad MA, Gross SA, Pungpapong S, Hardee JN, Odell JA. Minimally invasive endoscopic staging of suspected lung cancer. JAMA. 2008;299(5):540–6.
19. Vilmann P, Clementsen PF, Colella S, Siemsen M, De Leyn P, Dumonceau JM, Herth FJ, Larghi A, Vazquez-Sequeiros E, Hassan C, Crombag L, Korevaar DA, Konge L, Annema JT. Combined endobronchial and esophageal endosonography for the diagnosis and staging of lung cancer: European Society of Gastrointestinal Endoscopy (ESGE) guideline, in cooperation with the European Respiratory Society (ERS) and the European Society of Thoracic Surgeons (ESTS). Endoscopy. 2015;47(6):545–59.
20. Navani N, Nankivell M, Lawrence DR, Lock S, Makker H, Baldwin DR, Stephens RJ, Parmar MK, Spiro SG, Morris S, Janes SM, Lung-BOOST Trial Investigators. Lung cancer diagnosis and staging with endobronchial ultrasound-guided transbronchial needle aspiration compared with conventional approaches: an open-label, pragmatic, randomised controlled trial. Lancet Respir Med. 2015;3(4):282–9.
21. Alsharif M, Andrade RS, Groth SS, Stelow EB, Pambuccian SE. Endobronchial ultrasound-guided transbronchial fine-needle aspiration: the University of Minnesota experience, with emphasis on usefulness, adequacy assessment, and diagnostic difficulties. Am J Clin Pathol. 2008;130(3):434–43.
22. Nayak A, Sugrue C, Koenig S, Wasserman PG, Hoda S, Morgenstern NJ. Endobronchial ultrasound-guided transbronchial needle aspirate (EBUS-TBNA): a proposal for on-site adequacy criteria. Diagn Cytopathol. 2012;40(2):128–37.
23. Hughes JH, Young NA, Wilbur DC, Renshaw AA, Mody DR, Cytopathology Resource Committee, College of American Pathologists. Fine-needle aspiration of pulmonary hamartoma: a common source of false-positive diagnoses in the College of American Pathologists Interlaboratory Comparison Program in Nongynecologic Cytology. Arch Pathol Lab Med. 2005;129(1):19–22.
24. Hosler GA, Steinberg DM, Sheth S, Hamper UM, Erozan YS, Ali SZ. Inflammatory pseudotumor: a diagnostic dilemma in cytopathology. Diagn Cytopathol. 2004;31(4):267–70.
25. Hummel P, Cangiarella JF, Cohen JM, Yang G, Waisman J, Chhieng DC. Transthoracic fine-needle aspiration biopsy of pulmonary spindle cell and mesenchymal lesions: a study of 61 cases. Cancer. 2001;93(3):187–98.
26. Zeng J, Zhou F, Wei XJ, Kovacs S, Simsir A, Shi Y. Sclerosing hemangioma: a diagnostic dilemma in fine needle aspiration cytology. Cytojournal. 2016;13:9.
27. Kadota K, Villena-Vargas J, Yoshizawa A, Motoi N, Sima CS, Riely GJ, Rusch VW, Adusumilli PS, Travis WD. Prognostic significance of adenocarcinoma in situ, minimally invasive adenocarcinoma, and nonmucinous lepidic predominant invasive adenocarcinoma of the lung in patients with stage I disease. Am J Surg Pathol. 2014;38(4):448–60.
28. Travis WD, Brambilla E, Nicholson AG, Yatabe Y, Austin JHM, Beasley MB, Chirieac LR, Dacic S, Duhig E, Flieder DB, Geisinger K, Hirsch FR, Ishikawa Y, Kerr KM, Noguchi M, Pelosi G, Powell CA, Tsao MS, Wistuba I, WHO Panel. The 2015 World Health Organization classification of lung tumors: impact of genetic, clinical and radiologic advances since the 2004 classification. J Thorac Oncol. 2015;10(9):1243–60.
29. Travis WD, Brambilla E, Noguchi M, Nicholson AG, Geisinger K, Yatabe Y, Ishikawa Y, Wistuba I, Flieder DB, Franklin W, Gazdar A, Hasleton PS, Henderson DW, Kerr KM, Petersen I, Roggli V, Thunnissen E, Tsao M. Diagnosis of lung cancer in small biopsies and cytology: implications of the 2011 International Association for the Study of Lung Cancer/American Thoracic Society/European Respiratory Society classification. Arch Pathol Lab Med. 2013;137(5):668–84.
30. Yildiz-Aktas IZ, Sturgis CD, Barkan GA, Souers RJ, Fraig MM, Laucirica R, Khalbuss WE, Moriarty AT. Primary pulmonary non-small cell carcinomas: the College of American Pathologists Interlaboratory Comparison Program confirms a significant trend toward subcat-

egorization based upon fine-needle aspiration cytomorphology alone. Arch Pathol Lab Med. 2014;138(1):65–70.

31. Crapanzano JP, Loukeris K, Borczuk AC, Saqi A. Cytological, histological, and immunohistochemical findings of pulmonary carcinomas with basaloid features. Diagn Cytopathol. 2011;39(2):92–100.
32. Wong PW, Stefanec T, Brown K, White DA. Role of fine-needle aspirates of focal lung lesions in patients with hematologic malignancies. Chest. 2002;121(2):527–32.
33. Ko HM, Geddie WR, Boerner SL, Rogalla P, da Cunha Santos G. Cytomorphological and clinicopathological spectrum of pulmonary marginal zone lymphoma: the utility of immunophenotyping, PCR and FISH studies. Cytopathology. 2014;25(4):250–8.

Chapter 11
Mediastinum

Rita Abi-Raad and Guoping Cai

Introduction

The mediastinum is a site of various pathologic disorders, including lesions spreading from organs located in and outside the mediastinum. Just as the advent of new radiologic techniques has facilitated procurement of surgical material for treatment planning, fine needle aspiration (FNA) has been shown to be an excellent tool for diagnosis of mediastinal lesions, sparing more invasive surgeries [1–3]. Diagnostic accuracy ranges from 80% to 100% [4–7] with increased specificity and sensitivity when rapid on-site evaluation (ROSE) is available [3, 6, 8–10]. Immediate assessment of cytology specimens by a cytopathologist at the time of the procedure has been shown to reduce the frequency of nondiagnostic specimens regardless of tumor size [11, 12], while improving agreement with final interpretation [13].

FNA biopsy is used primarily to diagnose malignancies, metastasis representing 60% of the neoplasms, and primary mediastinal tumors representing the next largest category [6]. Reactive lymphadenopathy and infectious and granulomatous diseases are the most benign conditions that can manifest with mediastinal lymphadenopathy. Mediastinal neoplasms, as well as nonneoplastic conditions, can be sampled by FNA under the guidance of endoscopy ultrasound (EUS), endobronchial ultrasound (EBUS), or computed tomography (CT) depending on the location and accessibility of the lesion. It is important to discuss the clinical aspect and imaging characteristics with clinicians at the time of biopsy, so that adequacy can be assessed, and with on-site preliminary findings, biopsy material be triaged for appropriate ancillary testing. FNA has been considered to be a substitute to core biopsy [4] in some studies, others however have suggested that carcinomatous lesions can be diagnosed by FNA, while core or excisional biopsy is recommended for lymphoma, thymoma, neural masses, and benign masses [14].

R. Abi-Raad (✉) · G. Cai
Department of Pathology, Yale University School of Medicine, New Haven, CT, USA
e-mail: rita.abiraad@yale.edu; guoping.cai@yale.edu

G. Cai, A. J. Adeniran (eds.), *Rapid On-site Evaluation (ROSE)*,
https://doi.org/10.1007/978-3-030-21799-0_11

Diagnostic Considerations

Specimen Adequacy Assessment

The majority of mediastinal lesions are of epithelial and lymphoid origin [4]. There are no well-established criteria for specimen adequacy. The reference would be whether the findings of FNA biopsy can explain the lesion based on patient's history, imaging study findings, and clinical suspicion. The presence of cellular debris and macrophages alone may be considered adequate if imaging studies suggest a cystic lesion [15].

Sampling error is the major issue in the diagnosis of mediastinal lesions. Necrotic and fibrotic lesions yield much less cellular material and often lead to inadequate sampling [6]. Proximity to major vessels and deep-seated small lesions are the major technical obstacles for adequate sampling. Biopsy of a highly vascular lesion may result in blood dilution of specimen, which leads to a nondiagnostic or indeterminate diagnosis.

Contaminants

- Contamination from the surrounding non-lesional tissue may sometimes impose a diagnostic challenge and result in a misdiagnosis.
- The types of contaminants are related to the method of FNA biopsy techniques utilized.
- Transthoracic FNA: contamination with mesothelial cells, skeletal muscle, and fibroconnective tissue.
- Transbronchial FNA: contamination with bronchial epithelial cells.
- Transesophageal or transgastric FNA: contamination with esophageal squamous epithelium or gastric mucosa.

Approach for Solid Lesions

- Approximately 80% of mediastinal tumors are solid lesions [2].
- The mediastinum is divided into several hypothetical compartments, with specific tumor types occurring in specific compartments. Thymic neoplasms and metastatic tumor in the lymph nodes are the common lesions seen in the anterior compartment, while the tumors seen in the posterior compartment are most likely of neurogenic origin.
- The subtypes of mediastinal lesions also differ in different age groups. Metastatic tumors are most likely seen in elderly patients. In younger patients, certain types of lymphomas including Hodgkin lymphoma, anaplastic large cell lymphoma, and lymphoblastic lymphoma are common findings.
- Adequate sampling as well as appropriate specimen triage are important to render a definite diagnosis. In cases suspicious for lymphoproliferative disorders, part of the specimen should be saved in RPMI preservative for flow cytometry study.

- It may be difficult to make distinction between a thymic tumor, particularly a lymphocyte-rich thymic tumor, and a lymphoproliferative disorder. It is reasonable to save some of the specimen for flow cytometry in indeterminate cases.

Approach for Cystic Lesions

- Cystic lesions comprise approximately 15–20% of primary mediastinal masses in adults [2].
- Most of these are either foregut duplication cysts or pericardial cysts, less commonly cystic neoplasms of the mediastinum. Other rare mediastinal cysts include lymphangiomas, thymic cysts, thoracic duct cysts, and lateral thoracic meningoceles [16–19].
- Correlate with radiologic findings. Cyst contents only in a complex cystic lesion/cystic lesion with a solid component is considered inadequate sampling.
- Keep in mind that a cystic lesion could be a malignant tumor. Malignant tumors can undergo cystic degeneration and thus present as partially cystic tumors.
- Contaminants present on the aspirates may cause erroneous interpretation of cystic lesions.

Lesions of Anterior/Superior Mediastinal Compartments – Tumors of Thymic Epithelium

Thymoma

Thymomas exhibit a wide variety of morphological appearances and show an admixture, in a variable proportion, of neoplastic thymic epithelium and nonneoplastic lymphoid infiltrate [20]. Currently, thymomas are classified as (1) Type A, thymoma composed of bland spindle to oval cells with few to no lymphocytes; (2) Type AB, thymoma with a mixture of lymphocyte-rich and lymphocyte-poor spindle cell components; (3) Type B1, predominantly composed of immature T cells with scattered polygonal epithelial cells; (4) Type B2, thymoma with prominent polygonal epithelial cells with a roughly even admixture of numerous lymphocytes; and (5) Type B3, thymoma composed of sheets of polygonal epithelial cells with mild to moderate atypia and scant lymphocytes.

A. Cytomorphologic features [21, 22]

   - Aspirates are usually moderately to markedly cellular.
   - The key diagnostic feature is the presence of a dual population: a mixture of round/oval or spindle epithelial cells and lymphocytes in variable proportion (Fig. 11.1).
   - The epithelial cells show inconsistency in size, shape, and number with variable amount of cytoplasm and nuclear pleomorphism.

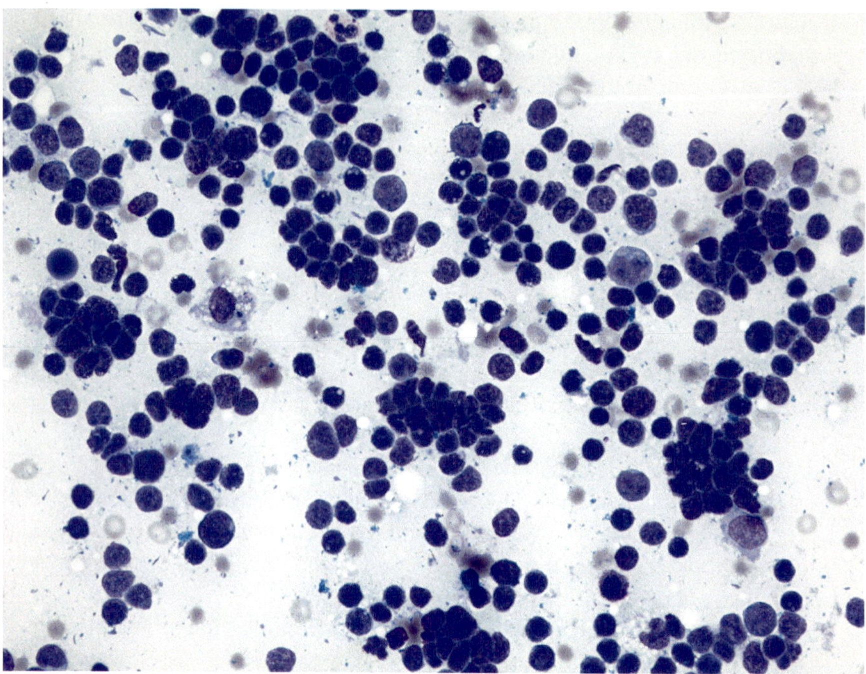

Fig. 11.1 Type B2 thymoma. Dual population of single and clusters of epithelial cells, closely intermingled with lymphocytes (Diff-Quik stain, ×400)

- The lymphoid population is comprised predominantly of small, mature lymphocytes admixed with occasional larger lymphocytes.
- The lymphocytes intermingle with the neoplastic epithelial cells with clusters of epithelial cells frequently present.
- Lymphocyte-rich thymoma (Type B1) shows abundant monomorphic population of small, mature lymphocytes with inconspicuous nucleoli and scattered epithelial cells.
- Predominant epithelial subtypes show many cohesive clusters, single epithelial cells, and stripped nuclei with lesser number of lymphocytes.
- Large, round to polygonal cells with abundant cytoplasm, large vesicular nuclei, prominent nucleoli, and occasional mitotic figures are seen in Type B3 thymomas.
- Foci displaying squamoid features can also be present.

B. Tips and pitfalls [23]

- An accurate cytologic diagnosis of thymoma can be made if the characteristic dual population of epithelial and lymphoid elements is recognized.
- Nonneoplastic thymic epithelial cells may be noted in FNA smears in cases of thymic hyperplasia, and these cases are difficult to diagnose on

cytology alone. Thymic hyperplasia usually occurs in children, whereas thymoma often occurs in adults.

- Spindle cell thymoma can present difficulty on FNA as they can be misidentified as other spindle cell lesions, such as nerve sheath tumors, carcinoid, and low-grade sarcoma, or misinterpreted, as the sclerosis seen in a large cell lymphoma. The presence of a dual population of epithelial cells and lymphocytes favors thymoma.
- The differential diagnosis includes predominantly lymphoma, especially in lymphocyte-rich thymoma, and seminoma. Patients with thymoma tend to be older. A dual epithelial and lymphoid population with cohesive clusters of cells, presence of tissue fragments, and lack of lymphoglandular bodies favor thymoma. In lymphoma, smears should not include epithelial cells, and the lymphoid cells appear monomorphic and cytologically atypical. Seminoma cells have more round nuclei with greatly thickened nuclear membranes, prominent nucleoli, and clear cytoplasm [24]. A characteristic feature is the presence of a tigroid background comprised of interwoven, lacy material and absence of tissue fragments [25]. True intercellular cohesion will be essentially nonexistent in lymphoma and minimal in seminoma.
- The differential diagnosis of aspirates showing a predominance of epithelial cells includes metastatic carcinoma. Carcinoma may contain many tightly packed cohesive cell clusters and neoplastic tissue fragments, but the neoplastic cells generally are far more atypical and pleomorphic. Clinical history of primary malignancy is very helpful in this situation. Additional material should be submitted for cell block analysis.

Thymic Carcinoma

Malignant thymic epithelial neoplasms have diverse morphologic variants, but they do clearly exhibit malignant cytologic features [20, 26].

A. Cytomorphologic features

- Cellular aspirates with variable cell morphologies.
- Significant nuclear enlargement, nuclear pleomorphism, mitotic activities, and background necrosis are the most common findings.

B. Tips and pitfalls

- The differential diagnosis of aspirates showing a predominance of atypical epithelial cells includes metastatic tumors.
- Primary thymic carcinoma must be differentiated from metastatic poorly differentiated carcinoma and germ cell tumors such as embryonal carcinoma.
- Clinical history of primary malignancy is very helpful in this situation. Additional material should be submitted for cell block analysis.

Thymic Carcinoid Tumor

Very rarely encountered in FNA of the mediastinum [20].

A. Cytomorphologic features

- Cellular smear composed of cell clusters and numerous single tumor cells.
- Cells have round to oval nuclei, finely granular chromatin, and a scant granular cytoplasm.

B. Tips and pitfalls

- Thymoma is the most frequent misdiagnosis for carcinoid tumor of the thymus. Carcinoid tumor may be distinguished from thymoma by formation of rosettes, cytoplasmic granularity, salt and pepper chromatin pattern, and absence of tissue fragments. Also the presence of lymphocytes favors thymoma [22]. Additional material for cell block is needed for immunocytochemistry analysis.
- Small cell carcinoma is within the differential for thymic carcinoid tumor. The presence of necrosis, pleomorphism, and prominent nuclear molding and crush artifact favor small cell carcinoma [27].
- Lymphoma also demonstrates a pattern of dispersed single cells. A separate aliquot for flow cytometry analysis is recommended.

Thymic Cyst

A. Cytomorphologic features

- Background contains inflammatory cells, erythrocytes, debris, calcium deposits, and cholesterol crystals.
- Epithelial cells can be present. These are cuboidal, columnar, ciliated columnar, or squamous cells.

B. Tips and pitfalls

- Differential diagnosis includes cystic disorders such as cystic thymoma, cystic germ cell tumor, lymphangioma, and cystic lymphoma of the thymus gland.
- FNA smear showing cyst contents only from a complex cystic lesion is considered inadequate.

Lesions of Anterior/Superior Mediastinal Compartments – Others

Lymphomas of the Mediastinum

Most common primary lymphomas of the mediastinum are Hodgkin lymphoma, diffuse large B-cell lymphoma, and lymphoblastic lymphoma [20, 24, 28].

1. Hodgkin lymphoma

   A. Cytomorphologic features

      - Scattered extremely large mononucleated or binucleated (Reed-Sternberg cells)
      - Background mixed inflammatory infiltrate including lymphocytes, eosinophils, and histiocytes

   B. Tips and pitfalls

      - Nodular sclerosis subtype, the most common type of Hodgkin disease in the mediastinum, may have a low cellularity due to dense fibrosis.
      - It is difficult to further classify Hodgkin lymphoma on cytological specimens.
      - Classical Reed-Sternberg cells may be absent, which can make the diagnosis by FNA difficult.

2. Non-Hodgkin lymphomas
   Diffuse large B-cell lymphoma and lymphoblastic lymphoma are among the non-Hodgkin lymphomas commonly seen in the mediastinum.

   A. Cytomorphologic features

      - Smears are usually cellular and composed of dispersed single cells.
      - Monotonous-appearing cells, twice the size of small, mature-appearing lymphocytes, with scant cytoplasm, convoluted nuclei, fine powdery chromatin, and inconspicuous nucleoli are seen in lymphoblastic lymphomas.
      - The smears of diffuse large B-cell lymphoma show a pleomorphic population of atypical lymphoid cells [29] (Fig. 11.2).
      - Background lymphoglandular bodies

   B. Tips and pitfalls

      - The differential diagnosis for lymphoblastic lymphoma includes follicular hyperplasia of lymph nodes, thymic hyperplasia, and thymoma. Lymphoblastic lymphoma is the most common malignant lymphoma of childhood, while thymoma rarely occurs in children.
      - Diffuse large B-cell lymphoma can also be confused with poorly differentiated carcinomas. Metastatic poorly differentiated carcinoma may also show large number of pleomorphic cells. However, the malignant cells often show cohesive clusters.
      - Another differential diagnosis with lymphoma is small cell carcinoma which usually shows single cells with round to oval nuclei having minimal cytoplasm. Crushing artifacts, nuclear molding, and single rows of cells indicate the possibility of small cell carcinoma. Cytologically, the lack of lymphoglandular bodies and the presence of cohesive aggregates of epithelial cells and tissue fragments are not features of lymphomas.

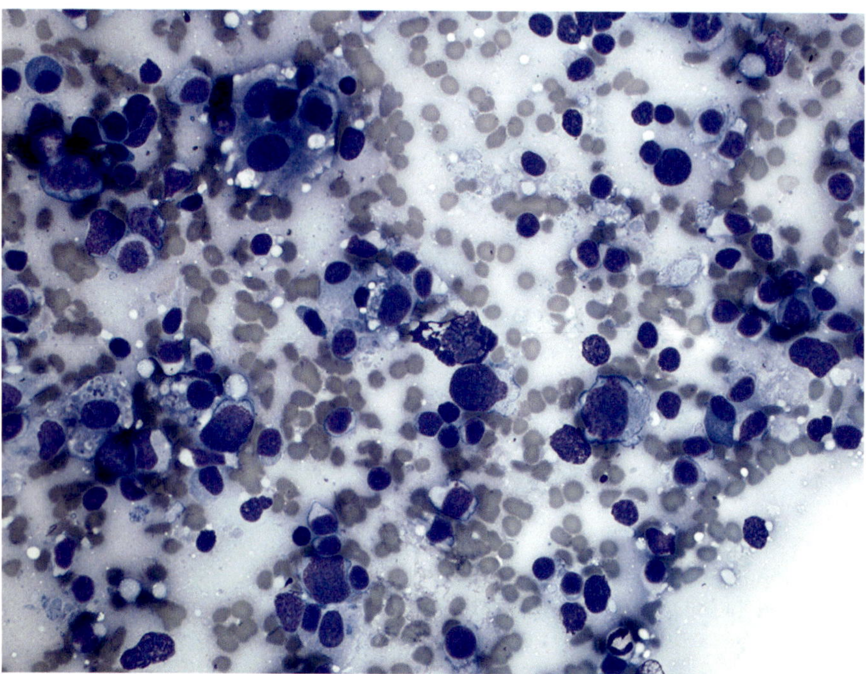

Fig. 11.2 Diffuse large B-cell lymphoma of the mediastinum. Polymorphous population of lymphocytes with scattered large atypical cells (Diff-Quik stain, ×400)

Nonneoplastic Lymphadenopathy

- FNA has a role in diagnosing nonmalignant, inflammatory, or infectious causes, such as sarcoidosis; however, many of these cases are given descriptive diagnosis due to lack of specific findings [6].
- Sarcoidosis is probably the lesion in which FNA has a better diagnostic yield. One study has found that sarcoidosis can be identified by FNA with a sensitivity and specificity of 89 and 96%, respectively [30].
- Typical features of sarcoidosis include granulomas consisting of epithelioid histiocytes with carrot-shaped nuclei and abundant cytoplasm with absence of necrosis [13] (Fig. 11.3).

Germ Cell Tumors (GCTs)

Extragonadal germ cell tumors are relatively uncommon, accounting for 20% of all mediastinal tumors. Anterior mediastinum is the most common extragonadal site of GCTs in adults and second most common extragonadal site in children

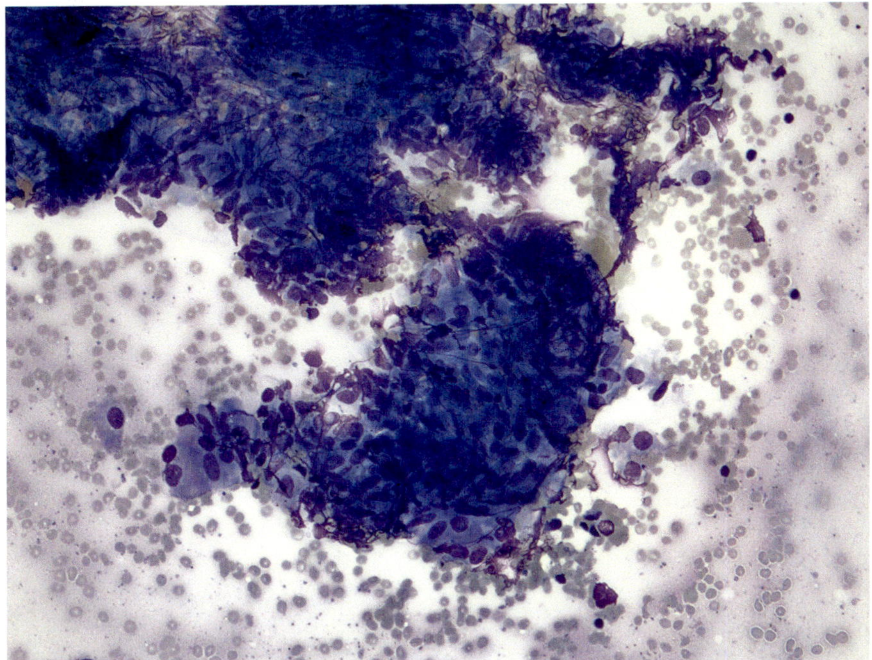

Fig. 11.3 Sarcoidosis. Polymorphous lymphocytes and epithelioid histiocytes forming non-necrotizing granulomas (Diff-Quik stain, ×200)

[25, 31]. It is not possible to distinguish between primary and secondary mediastinal GCTs based on morphologic features alone. The most common primary germ cell tumor of the mediastinum is mature cystic teratoma. Seminoma is the second most common example of pure germ cell tumors of the mediastinum. Non-seminomatous germinal cell tumors include embryonal carcinoma, yolk sac tumor, and choriocarcinoma.

A. Cytomorphologic features

- Mature cystic teratoma shows discrete benign squamous cells on a clean background.
- Typical seminomas/germinomas consist of uniform, large, round neoplastic cells with large vesicular nuclei and prominent nucleoli admixed with small lymphocytes in a tigroid background on Diff-Quik stain (Fig. 11.4). The tigroid background is characteristic of seminoma, although not specific, but may not be present in every case. It is reported that the tigroid background is noted only in highly cellular specimens and is absent in specimens with low cellularity [25, 32].
- Embryonal carcinoma yields cellular smears of cohesive groups of pleomorphic hyperchromatic epithelioid cells with prominent nucleoli. The cytoplasm is usually scant with indistinct cell borders, resulting in a syn-

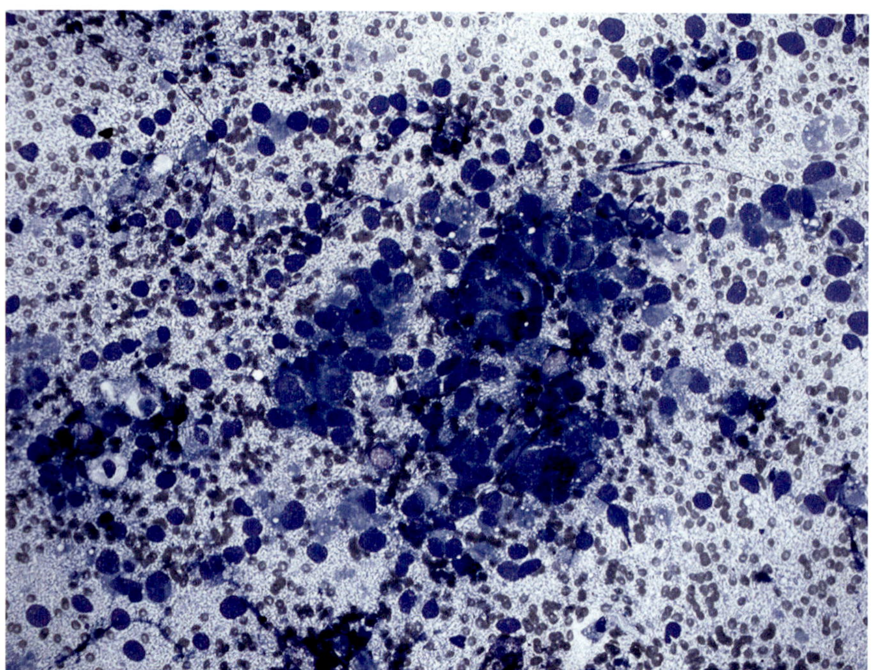

Fig. 11.4 Germ cell tumor/germinoma. Clusters of large atypical cells admixed with small lymphocytes in a tigroid background (Diff-Quik stain, ×200)

cytial growth pattern. In addition, the neoplastic cells can also demonstrate a papillary and/or glandular arrangement. Necrosis is frequently noted [33, 34].

- Yolk sac tumors yield cohesive clusters of pleomorphic epithelioid cells with large nuclei, vacuolated cytoplasm, and extracellular hyaline matrix (spheres or hyaline globules) [35]. Schiller-Duval bodies are only occasionally noted in cytologic preparations. The finding of metachromatic basement membrane-like extracellular material is helpful in recognizing the presence of a yolk sac tumor component in aspirates [36, 37]. Necrosis can be quite prominent.
- The finding of multinucleated tumor giant cells (syncytiotrophoblasts) suggests choriocarcinoma. Aspirates of choriocarcinoma reveal single and cohesive groups of pleomorphic cells with bizarre nuclei and prominent nucleoli, often in a hemorrhagic background.

B. Tips and pitfalls

- When FNA yields undifferentiated malignant cells, particularly in young adult males, then the diagnosis of germ cell tumor needs to be considered. Material for cell block and immunocytochemical stains should be obtained.

- Mixed germ cell tumors are relatively frequent in the mediastinum and consist of two or more of histologic subtypes of germ cell tumors. Recognition of all the components of mixed germ cell tumors based on FNA material may not be possible because of sampling limitation.
- The differential diagnosis in seminoma includes large cell lymphoma. The presence of loosely cohesive tumor cell groups, rounded nuclei, prominent nucleoli, and a tigroid background favor seminoma. Nuclear atypia such as cleaved nuclei, nuclear projections, and abundant lymphoglandular bodies are helpful features in lymphomas.
- When the lymphoid component of seminoma is prominent, the differential diagnosis should include thymoma. The presence of a mixture of epithelioid and spindled cells points to a thymoma.
- In non-seminomatous germ cell tumors, markedly atypical epithelioid cells arranged in papillary or glandular structures in a hemorrhagic and/or necrotic background can be confused with a thymic carcinoma or metastatic carcinoma to the mediastinum. It may be difficult to differentiate these entities based on morphologic features alone unless diagnostic cytologic features such as Schiller-Duval bodies are present. Mediastinal germ cell tumors typically occur during young adulthood or early middle age, whereas thymic carcinomas seldom occur in patients younger than 30 years, and metastatic carcinomas tend to occur in elderly patients [23].

Thyroid/Parathyroid Tissue or Tumors

Thyroid and parathyroid tissue may be found in the superior/anterior mediastinum as a primary ectopic lesion, a lesion extending from cervical neck area into the mediastinal space, or a metastatic neoplasm [38, 39]. Goiters tissue, thyroid cysts, parathyroid cyst, and parathyroid neoplasms are among the most frequently diagnosed disorders on FNA samples.

A. Cytomorphologic features

- Intrathoracic goiter shows clusters and sheets of bland thyroid follicular cells in a honeycombed tissue pattern or colloid-containing follicles.
- Mediastinal parathyroid adenoma (Fig. 11.5) shows cellular smears, loosely cohesive clusters, disorganized sheets, papillary fragments, and microfollicles. The cells are small, round to ovoid, associated with mild to moderate anisokaryosis tissue and focal nuclear overlapping. The cytoplasm is pale and finely vacuolated, the nuclei are hyperchromatic, and occasional nucleoli are noted.

B. Tips and pitfalls

- The differential includes metastatic thyroid or parathyroid malignancy. Clinical history and radiologic tissue correlation are helpful.

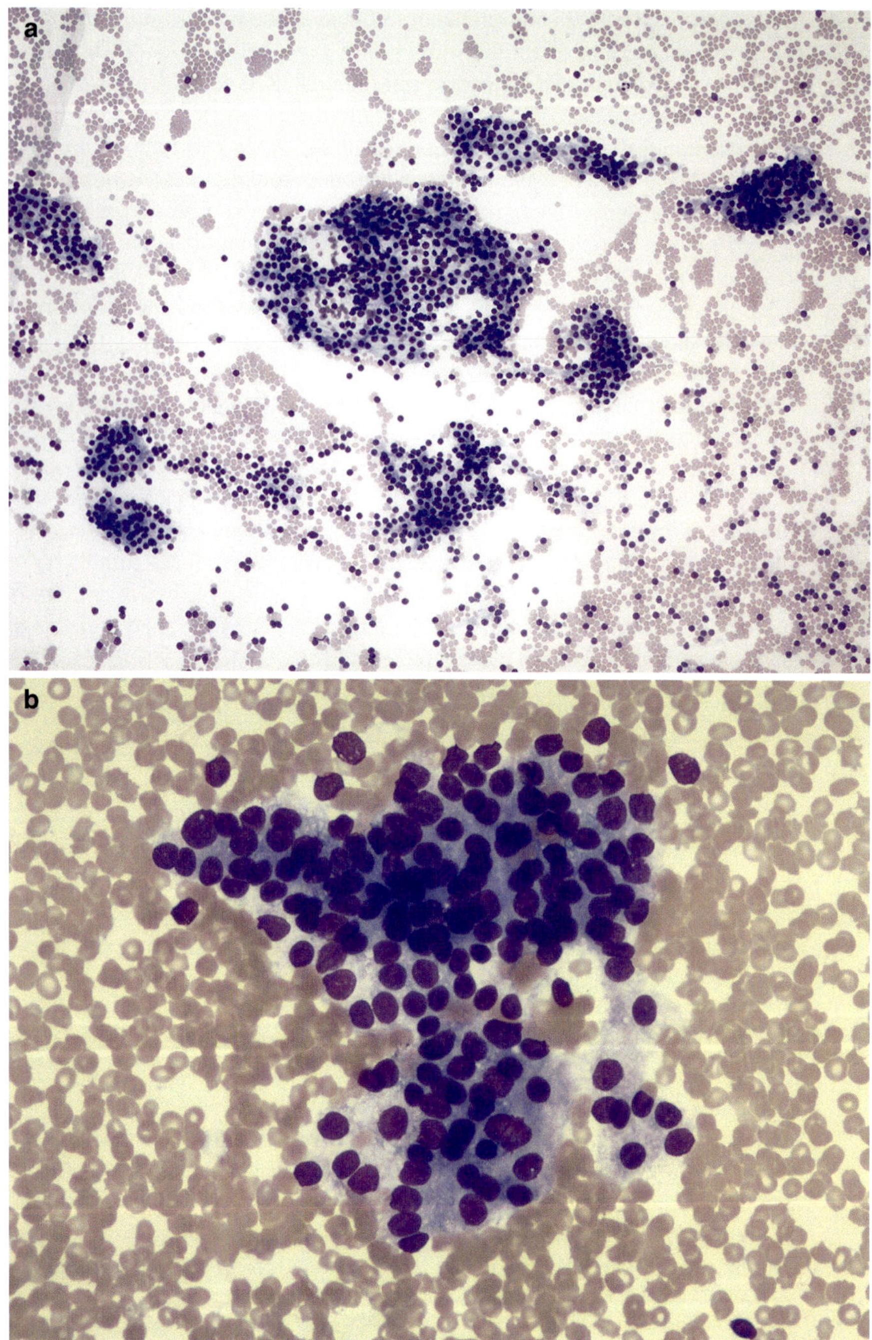

Fig. 11.5 Parathyroid adenoma of the mediastinum. Loosely cohesive clusters of small, round to ovoid cells (**a** Diff-Quik stain, ×100) with pale, finely vacuolated cytoplasm and bland nuclei (**b** Diff-Quik stain, ×400)

- Additional material for immunocytochemical study is needed to confirm the thyroid or parathyroid origin of the cells.
- Thyroglobulin or PTH concentration tissue measurement in the aspirated material may be also helpful in cases of suspected thyroid or parathyroid lesion.

Lesions of Middle Mediastinal Compartment

Pericardial Mesothelial Cyst

A. Cytomorphologic features

- Low cellularity
- Mesothelial cells arranged in regular flattened sheets
- Monomorphic nuclei with fine chromatin and smooth borders and low N:C ratio
- Scattered histiocytes

B. Tips and pitfalls

- Should be differentiated from other cystic lesions in a low-cellularity specimen

Paraganglioma [40–42]

A. Cytomorphologic features

- Cells are round to oval, plasmacytoid and spindled, scattered, in clusters, and in acinar and perivascular pattern.
- Cytoplasm is moderate to abundant with fine pink granules and vacuoles.
- Nuclei are single to multiple and round to oval, with vesicular chromatin and prominent nucleoli.

B. Tips and pitfalls

- Can be confused with malignant epithelial tumor, soft tissue tumors, and thyroid and parathyroid neoplasms.
- Plasmacytoid appearance and intracytoplasmic reddish-pink granules in paraganglionic tumors may lead to a misdiagnosis of medullary carcinoma thyroid. However, significant discohesion, anisonucleosis, and amyloid seen in medullary carcinoma help.
- A misdiagnosis of neurogenic tumor is possible when there is predominance of ovoid- or spindle-shaped nuclei in some paragangliomas. The uniform and

benign-looking chromatin pattern of the nucleus in paraganglioma helps in distinguishing it from metastatic carcinoma.

- Additional material for cell block and immunocytochemistry is recommended.

Lesions of Posterior Mediastinal Compartment

Neurogenic Tumor [24, 43–46]

The common neurogenic tumors in the mediastinum are neurofibromas, schwannomas, ganglioneuromas, and malignant peripheral nerve sheath tumors.

A. Cytomorphologic features

- Both neurofibroma and schwannoma present as spindle cell lesions with low to moderate cellularity, predominantly cohesive clusters and single spindle cells with ill-defined fibrillar cytoplasm and stripped wavy nuclei with moderate nuclear pleomorphism and bland chromatin (Fig. 11.6). The smear background may contain a fibrillar eosinophilic material, as well as collagen.

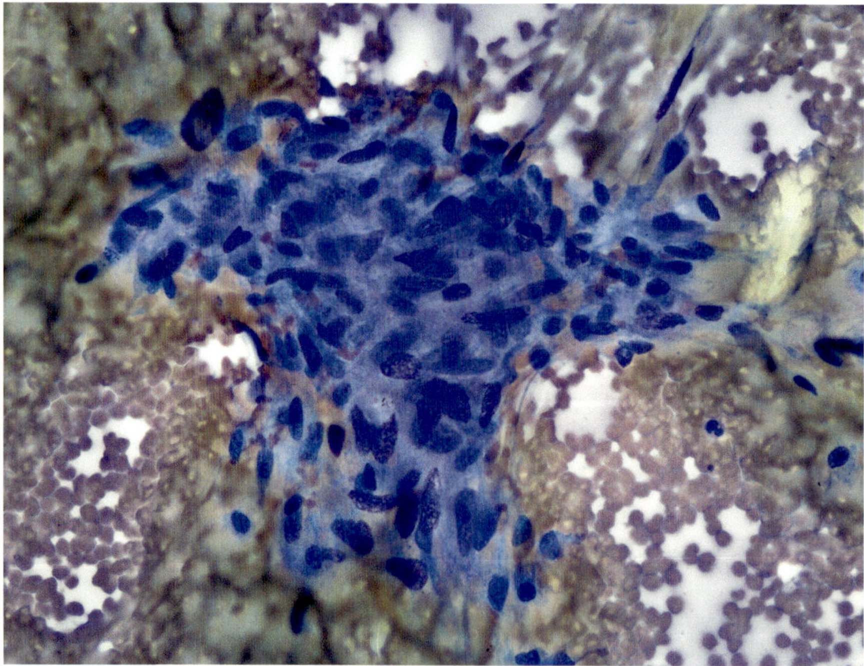

Fig. 11.6 Schwannoma. Cohesive cluster of spindle cells with ill-defined fibrillar cytoplasm (Diff-Quik stain, ×400)

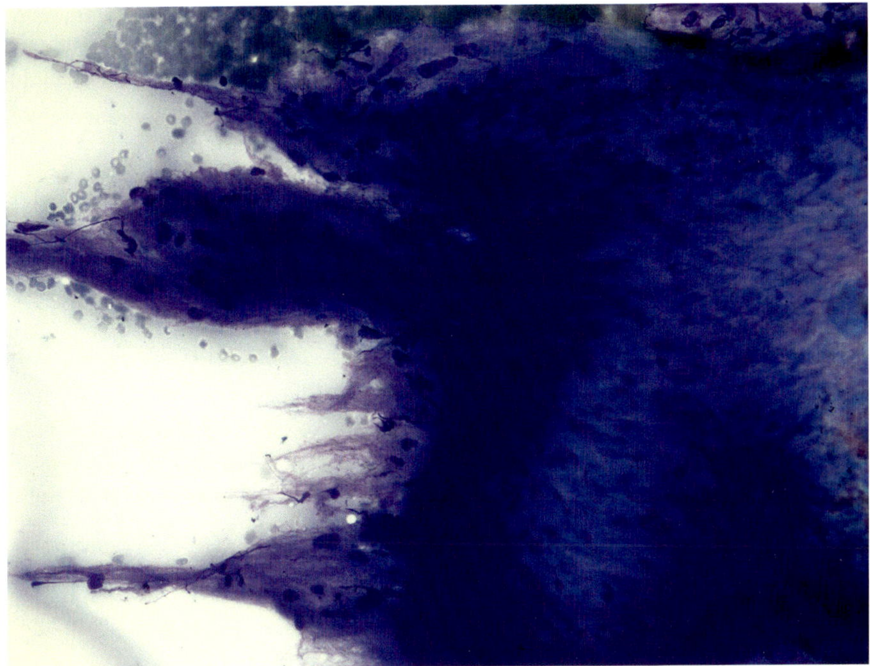

Fig. 11.7 Ganglioneuroma. Spindle cells with scattered epithelioid cells suggestive of ganglioneuroma (Diff-Quik stain, ×200)

- Cellular pleomorphism, bizarre cells, and mitotic activities indicate the possibility of malignant tumor.
- Smears from ganglioneuroma yield sparse spindle cells and scattered ganglion cells (Fig. 11.7).
- Neuroblastoma is composed of numerous small malignant cells characterized by a single round hyperchromatic nucleus and a high N:C ratio, with pseudorosettes embedded in an eosinophilic filamentous material.
- Ganglioneuroblastoma, in addition to the features of neuroblastoma, shows cells which show ganglionic differentiation (larger with more vesicular chromatin, prominent nucleoli, and distinct polygonal cytoplasm).

B. Tips and pitfalls

- Cellular schwannoma shows high cellularity with dense cell bundles and fascicles, storiform areas, moderate mitotic activity, and moderate nuclear atypia. The differential diagnosis includes a malignant tumor [47].
- The differential diagnosis of a peripheral nerve sheath tumor includes primary and metastatic soft tissue sarcomas, spindle cell variant of thymoma, and spindle cell variant of carcinoid tumor.

- Nerve sheath tumors should be differentiated from metastatic sarcomas. A prior history of resected soft tissue sarcoma is helpful.
- In all cases, additional material for cell block immunocytochemistry should be obtained.

Foregut Cyst [1, 2, 44]

Foregut cyst including esophageal reduplication and bronchogenic cysts.

A. Cytomorphologic features

- Degenerated cellular debris and scattered macrophages (Fig. 11.8).
- The presence of numerous squamous cells supports the diagnosis of an esophageal reduplication cyst.
- The presence of numerous goblet cells with an absence of squamous cells supports the diagnosis of bronchogenic cyst.

B. Tips and pitfalls

- The differential diagnosis includes tumors with cystic change such as teratoma, thymoma, germinoma, and squamous cell carcinoma.
- Radiologic correlation with cytologic features is necessary.

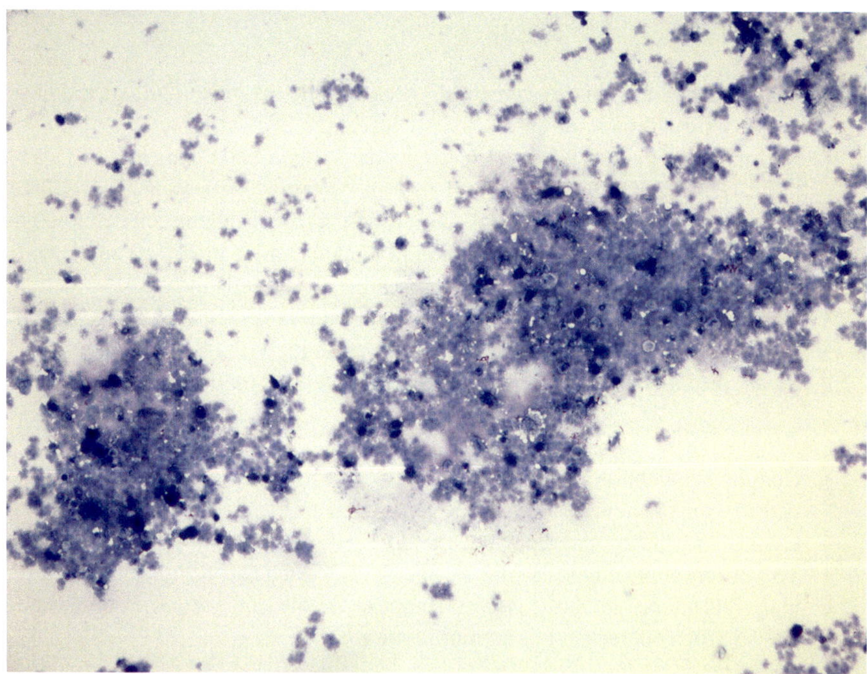

Fig. 11.8 Duplication cyst. Degenerated cellular debris and macrophages (Diff-Quik stain, ×200)

References

1. Hucl T, Wee E, Anurhada S, Gupta R, Ramchandani M, Rakesh K, Shrestha R, Reddy D, Lakhtakia S. Feasibility and efficiency of a new 22G core needle: a prospective comparison study. Endoscopy. 2013;45:792–8.
2. Panelli F, Erickson R, Prasad V. Evaluation of mediastinal masses by endoscopic ultrasound and endoscopic ultrasound-guided fine needle aspiration. Am J Gastroenterol. 2001;96(2): 401–8.
3. Emery S, Savides T, Behling C. Utility of immediate evaluation of endoscopic ultrasound-guided transesophageal fine needle aspiration of mediastinal lymph nodes. Acta Cytol. 2004;48(5):630–4.
4. Goel D, Prayaga A, Sundaram C, Raghunadharao D, Rajappa S, Rammurti S, Rao T, Kumar R. Utility of fine needle aspiration cytology in mediastinal lesions. A clinicopathologic study of 161 cases from a single institution. Acta Cytol. 2008;52(4):404–11.
5. Kramer H, Sanders J, Post W, Groen H, Suurmeijer A. Analysis of cytological specimens from mediastinal lesions obtained by endoscopic ultrasound-guided fine-needle aspiration. Cancer Cytopathol. 2006;108:206–11.
6. Powers C, Silverman J, Geisinger K, Frable W. Fine-needle aspiration biopsy of the mediastinum. A multi-institutional analysis. Am J Clin Pathol. 1996;105(2):168–73.
7. Assaad M, Pantanowitz L, Otis C. Diagnostic accuracy of image-guided percutaneous fine needle aspiration biopsy of the mediastinum. Diag Cytopathol. 2007;35(11):705–9.
8. Silverman J, Finley J, O'brien K, Dabbs D, Park H, Larkin E, Norris H. Diagnostic accuracy and role of immediate interpretation of fine needle aspiration biopsy specimens from various sites. Acta Cytol. 1989;33(6):791–6.
9. DiMaio CJ, Kolb JM, Benias PC, Shah H, Shah S, Haluszka O, Sharzehi K, Lam E, Gordon S, Hyder S, Kaimakliotis P, Allaparthi S, Gress F, Sethi A, Shah A, Nieto J, Kaul V, Kothari S, Kothari T, Ho S, Izzy M, Sharma N, Watson R, Muthusamy V, Pleskow D, Berzin T, Sawhney M, Sawhney M, Aljahdi E, Ryou M, Wong C, Gupta P, Yang D, Gonzalez S, Adler D. Initial experience with a novel EUS-guided core biopsy needle (SharkCore): results of a large North American multicenter study. Endosc Int Open. 2016;4:E974–9.
10. Catalano M, Rosenblatt M, Chak A, Sivak M, Scheiman J, Gress F. Endoscopic ultrasound-guided fine needle aspiration in the diagnosis of mediastinal masses of unknown origin. Am J Gastroenterol. 2002;97(10):2559–65.
11. Jhala N, Jhala D, Eltoum I, Vickers S, Wilcox C, Chhieng D, Eloubeidi M. Endoscopic ultrasound-guided fine-needle aspiration biopsy: a powerful tool to obtain samples from small lesions. Cancer. 2004;102:239–46.
12. Klapman JB, Logrono R, Dye CE, Waxman I. Clinical impact of on-site cytopathology interpretation on endoscopic ultrasound-guided fine needle aspiration. Am J Gastroenterol. 2003;98:1289–94.
13. Eloubeidi M, Tamhane A, Jhala N, Chhieng D, Jhala D, Crowe R, Eltoum I. Agreement between rapid onsite and final cytologic interpretations of EUS-guided FNA specimens: implications for the endosonographer and patient management. Am J Gastroenterol. 2006;101: 2841–7.
14. Morrissey B, Adams H, Gibbs A, Crane M. Percutaneous needle biopsy of the mediastinum: review of 94 procedures. Thorax. 1993;48:632–7.
15. Jhala N, Jhala D, Chhieng D, Eloubeidi M, Eltoum I. Endoscopic ultrasound-guided fine-needle aspiration: a cytopathologist's perspective. Am J Clin Pathol. 2003;120:351–67.
16. Kawashima A, Fishman E, Kuhlman J, Nixon M. CT of posterior mediastinal masses. Radiographics. 1991;11(6):1045–67.
17. LeBlanc J, Guttentage A, Shepard J, McLoud T. Imaging of mediastinal foregut cysts. Can Assoc Radiol J. 1994;45:381–6.
18. Murayama S, Murakami J, Watanabe H, Sakai S, Hinaga S, Soeda H, Nakata H, Masuda K. Signal intensity characteristics of mediastinal cystic masses on T1-weighted MRI. J Comput Assist Tomogr. 1995;19:188–91.

19. Wick M. Mediastinal cysts and intrathoracic thyroid tumors. Semin Diagn Pathol. 1990;7(4):285–94.
20. Marx A, Chan J, Coindre JM, Detterbeck F, Girard N, Harris N, Jaffe E, Kurrer M, Merom E, Moreira A, Mukai K, Orazi A, Ströbel P. The 2015 World Health Organization classification of tumors of the thymus. Continuity and changes. J Thorac Oncol. 2015;10:1383–95.
21. Dahlgren S, Sandstedt B, Sundstrom C. Fine needle aspiration cytology of thymic tumors. Acta Cytol. 1983;27:1–6.
22. Chhieng D, Rose D, Ludwig M, Zakowski M. Cytology of thymomas: emphasis on morphology and correlation with histologic subtypes. Cancer. 2000;90(1):24–32.
23. Zakowski M, Huang J, Bramlage M. The role of fine needle aspiration cytology in the diagnosis and management of thymic neoplasia. J Thorac Oncol. 2010;5(10):S281–5.
24. Geisinger K. Differential diagnostic considerations and potential pitfalls in fine-needle aspiration biopsies of the mediastinum. Diagn Cytopathol. 1995;13:436–42.
25. Chhieng D, Lin O, Moran C, Eltoum I, Jhala N, Jhala D, Simsir A. Fine-needle aspiration biopsy of nonteratomatous germ cell tumors of the mediastinum. Am J Clin Pathol. 2002 Sep;118(3):418–24.
26. Finley JL, Silverman JF, Strausbauch PH, Dobbs DJ, West RL, Weaver MD, et al. Malignant thymic neoplasm: diagnosis by fine-needle aspiration biopsy with histological, immunocytochemical, and ultrastructural confirmation. Diagn Cytopathol. 1986;2:118–25.
27. Gal A, Kornstein M, Cohen C, Duarte I, Miller J, Mansour K. Neuroendocrine tumors of the thymus: a clinicopathological and prognostic study. Ann Thorac Surg. 2001;72(4):1179–82.
28. Hoda R, Picklesimer L, Green K, Self S. Fine-needle aspiration of a primary mediastinal large B-cell lymphoma: a case report with cytologic, histologic, and flow cytometric considerations. Diag Cytopathol. 2005;32(6):370–3.
29. Silverman J, Raab S, Park H. Fine-needle aspiration cytology of primary large cell lymphoma of the mediastinum: cytomorphologic findings with potential pitfalls in diagnosis. Diagn Cytopathol. 1993;9:209–14.
30. Wildi SM, Judson MA, Fraig M, Fickling WE, Schmulewitz N, Varadarajulu S, Roberts SS, Prasad P, Hawes RH, Wallace MB, Hoffman BJ. Is endosonography guided fine needle aspiration (EUS-FNA) for sarcoidosis as good as we think? Thorax. 2004;59(9):794–9.
31. Dehner L. Germ cell tumors of the mediastinum. Semin Diagn Pathol. 1990;7:266–84.
32. Caraway N, Fanning C, Amato R, Sneige N. Fine-needle aspiration cytology of seminoma: a review of 16 cases. Diagn Cytopathol. 1995;12:327–33.
33. Stanley M, Powers C, Pitman M, Korourian S, Bardales R, Khurana K. Cytology of germ cell tumors: extragonadal, extracranial masses and intraoperative problems. Cancer. 1997;81:220–7.
34. Kapila K, Hadju S, Whitmore W, Golbey R, Beattie E. Cytologic diagnosis of metastatic germ-cell tumors. Acta Cytol. 1983;27:245–51.
35. Collins K, Geisinger K, Wakely P, Olympio G, Silverman J. Extragonadal germ cell tumors: a fine-needle aspiration biopsy study. Diagn Cytopathol. 1995;12(3):223–9.
36. Akhtar M, Ali M, Sackey K, Jackson D, Bakry M. Fine-needle aspiration biopsy diagnosis of endodermal sinus tumor: histologic and ultrastructural correlations. Diagn Cytopathol. 1990;6:184–92.
37. Mizrak B, Ekinci C. Cytologic diagnosis of yolk sac tumor: a report of seven cases. Acta Cytol. 1995;39:936–40.
38. Noussios G, Anagnostis P, Natsis K. Ectopic parathyroid glands and their anatomical, clinical and surgical implications. Exp Clin Endocrinol Diabetes. 2012;120(10):604–10.
39. Santangelo G, Pellino G, De Falco N, Colella G, D'Amato S, Maglione M, De Luca R, Canonico S, De Falco M. Prevalence, diagnosis and management of ectopic thyroid glands. Int J Surg. 2016;28(1):S1–6.
40. Varma K, Jain S, Mandal S. Cytomorphologic spectrum in paraganglioma. Acta Cytol. 2008;52(5):549–56.

41. Kapila K, Tewari MC, Verma K. Paraganglioma: diagnostic dilemma on fine needle aspirate. Indian J Cancer. 1993;30:152–7.
42. Handa U, Kundu R, Mohan H. Cytomorphologic spectrum in aspirates of extra-adrenal paraganglioma. J Cytol. 2014;31(2):79–82.
43. Hoffman O, Gillespie D, Aughenbaugh G, Brown L. Primary mediastinal neoplasms (other than thymoma). Mayo Clinic Proc. 1993;68:880–91.
44. Slagel D, Powers C, Melaragno M, Geisinger K, Frable W, Silverman J. Spindle-cell lesions of the mediastinum: diagnosis by fine-needle aspiration biopsy. Diagn Cytopathol. 1997;17:167–76.
45. Domanski H. Fine-needle aspiration of ganglioneuroma. Diagn Cytopathol. 2005;32(6):363–6.
46. Silverman J, Dabbs D, Ganick D, Holbrook C, Geisinger K. Fine needle aspiration cytology of neuroblastoma, including peripheral neuroectodermal tumor, with immunocytochemical and ultrastructural confirmation. Acta Cytol. 1988;32(3):367–76.
47. Woodruff J, Goodwin T, Erlandson R. Cellular schwannoma. A variety sometimes mistaken for a malignant tumor. Am J Surg Pathol. 1981;5:733–44.

Part V
Endoscopy-Guided Biopsies

Chapter 12
Pancreas

Guoping Cai

Introduction

Pancreatic lesions comprise a variety of entities ranging from nonneoplastic diseases to malignant neoplasms. Over the last two decades, there has been an increase in the reported incidence of pancreatic tumors, especially cystic neoplasms, due to improvement of imaging techniques [1]. Pancreatic lesions are often evaluated with fine needle aspiration (FNA) biopsy under the guidance of imaging techniques such as computed tomography (CT) and endoscopy. Endoscopic ultrasound-guided fine needle aspiration (EUS-FNA) biopsy is a preferred method [2, 3]. A number of studies have repeatedly shown that EUS-FNA has moderate sensitivity and high specificity in diagnosing pancreatic malignancies [4–9]. There is a very low complication rate, slightly higher in cystic than solid lesions [10, 11].

Several factors may affect the diagnostic yield of EUS-FNA, such as the nature of the lesion, endoscopist's skill, and availability of rapid on-site evaluation (ROSE). The purposes of ROSE are to determine sampling adequacy, to perform specimen triage, and to render a preliminary diagnosis. ROSE has been shown to improve adequacy of biopsy material, decrease the number of needle passes, and increase diagnostic accuracy [12–16]. In addition, ROSE may also help reduce the need for a repeated procedure [17].

Specimen Adequacy Assessment

Assessment of specimen adequacy is important because it has an impact on the decisions whether additional passes should be performed, whether additional diagnostic approaches such as thin core needle biopsy should be taken, and whether

G. Cai (✉)
Department of Pathology, Yale University School of Medicine, New Haven, CT, USA
e-mail: guoping.cai@yale.edu

G. Cai, A. J. Adeniran (eds.), *Rapid On-site Evaluation (ROSE)*,
https://doi.org/10.1007/978-3-030-21799-0_12

additional sites should be sampled. However there are no established criteria regarding the cellularity of specimen. The ultimate reference is dependent upon whether the findings seen in the specimen can explain the presence of the lesion of interest [18]. A nondiagnostic specimen is one that provides no diagnostic or useful information about the lesion sampled. This determination certainly requires incorporation of clinical and imaging findings. The specimen with normal elements only is more likely considered as inadequate in a patient with a discrete mass lesion and associated pancreatic ductal obstruction. However, it may be considered adequate if the patient has an ill-define lesion with the differential diagnosis including chronic pancreatitis. Cyst contents only may be considered an adequate sample if the lesion of interest is a simple cyst.

Normal Elements in Pancreatic Cytology

The normal elements of the pancreas including ductal epithelial cells and acinar cells can be seen in the sampling of a nonneoplastic or neoplastic pancreatic lesion. The presence of these normal elements may sometimes be helpful for identification of abnormal cells because these normal cells can be used as reference to defining abnormalities.

1. Pancreatic acinar cells (Fig. 12.1)
   - Arranged in acinar pattern or sometimes seen as large tissue fragments.
   - Uniform cells with abundant granular cytoplasm.
   - Round nuclei equal to slightly larger than the size of red blood cells.
2. Pancreatic ductal cells (Fig. 12.2)
   - Arranged in cohesive honeycomb sheets.
   - Uniform cuboidal epithelial cells with moderate amount of vacuolated cytoplasm.
   - Round nuclei with minimal variation in size.

Gastrointestinal Contaminants

Benign gastrointestinal epithelial cells are often present as contaminants when the lesion of pancreas is sampled by EUS-FNA. Selection of a trans-gastric and transduodenal approach is determined upon the location of lesion. Pancreatic or uncinate lesion is often biopsied via transduodenal route, while a trans-gastric approach is the choice for the lesion located in the tail or body of the pancreas. Recognition of gastrointestinal contaminants may help avoid diagnostic pitfalls, especially in the lesion with relatively bland cytomorphology. It should

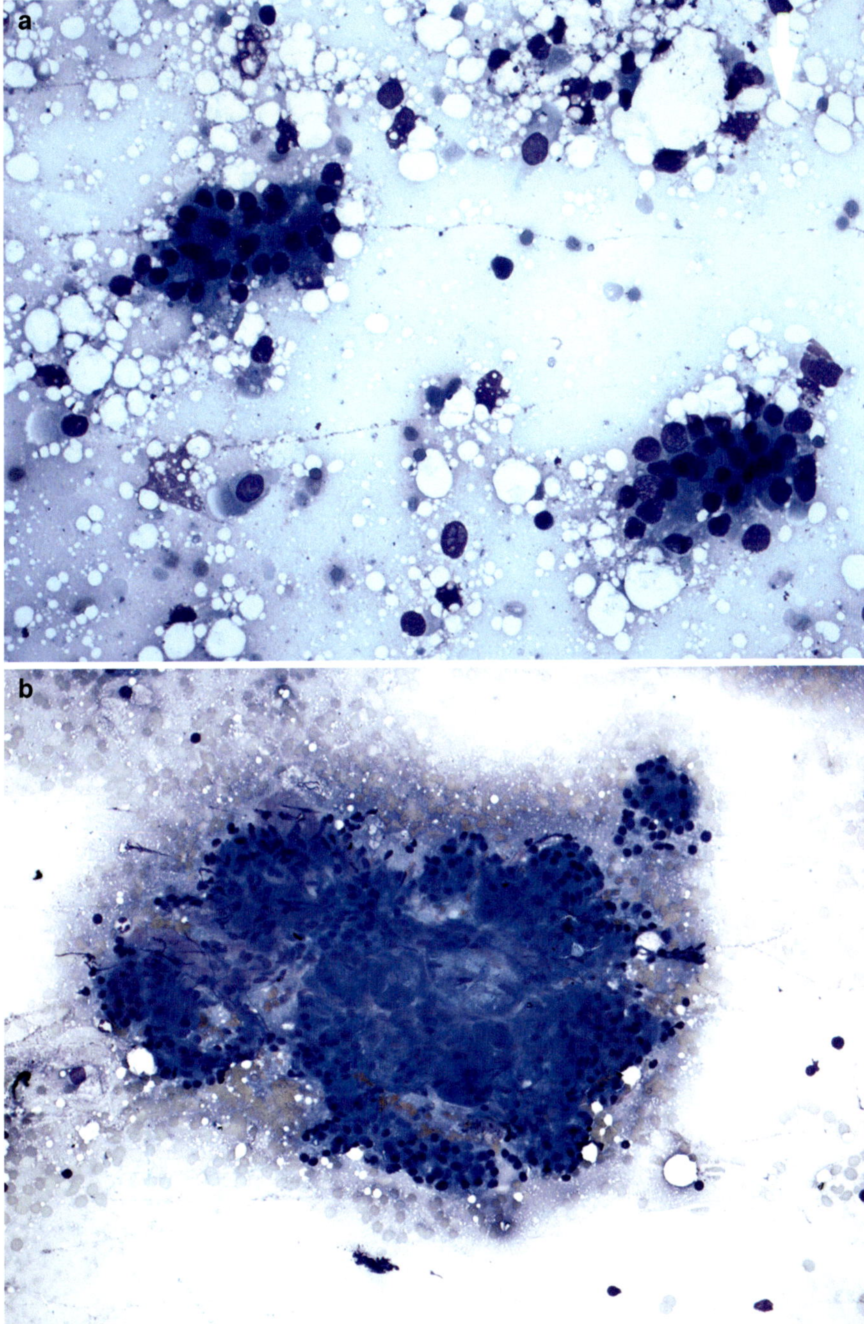

Fig. 12.1 Benign pancreatic acinar cells. Uniform cells with granular cytoplasm arranged in an acinar pattern (**a** Diff-Quik stain, ×400) and as a small tissue fragment (**b** Diff-Quik stain, X200)

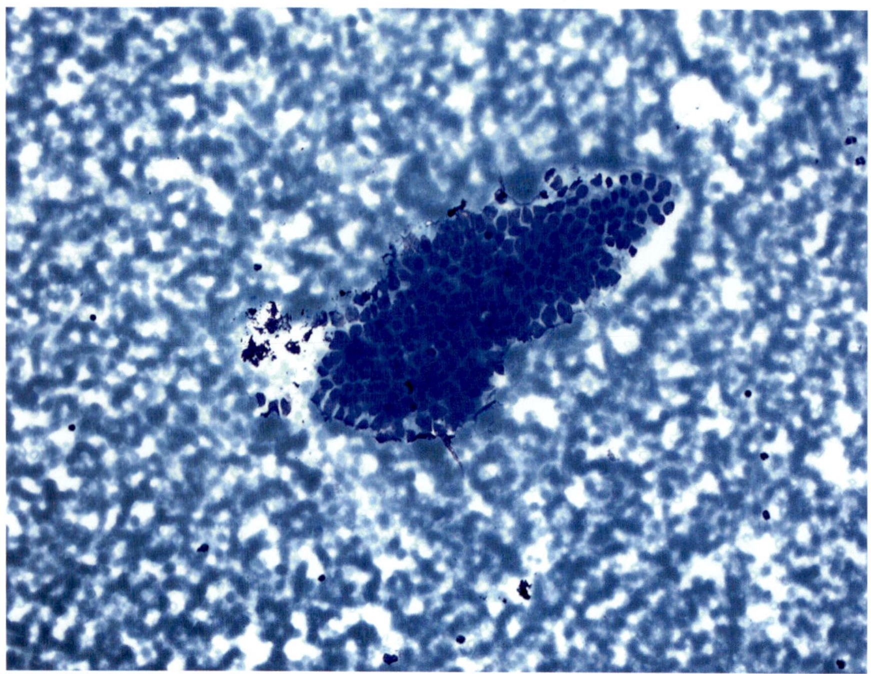

Fig. 12.2 Benign ductal cells. Uniform cells with vacuolated cytoplasm arranged in a honeycomb pattern (Diff-Quik stain, ×200)

also be kept in mind that benign mesothelial cells may be present as contaminants in the specimens sampled by EUS-FNA or transabdominal CT-guided biopsy.

1. Duodenal epithelium (Fig. 12.3)
   - Arranged in large flat sheets or cohesive clusters with papillary configuration.
   - Uniform columnar cells with vacuolated cytoplasm.
   - Scattered goblet cells with abundant cytoplasm and eccentrically located nuclei identified within flat sheets or clusters of epithelial cells, displaying a starry sky appearance.
2. Gastric epithelium (Fig. 12.4)
   - Large monolayered sheets, small clusters, groups, or dyscohesive cells can sometimes present.
   - Small uniform cells with vacuolated cytoplasm.
   - May see sheets of uniform cells with large cytoplasmic vacuoles, representative of foveolar epithelial cells.
   - Round to oval, bland nuclei.

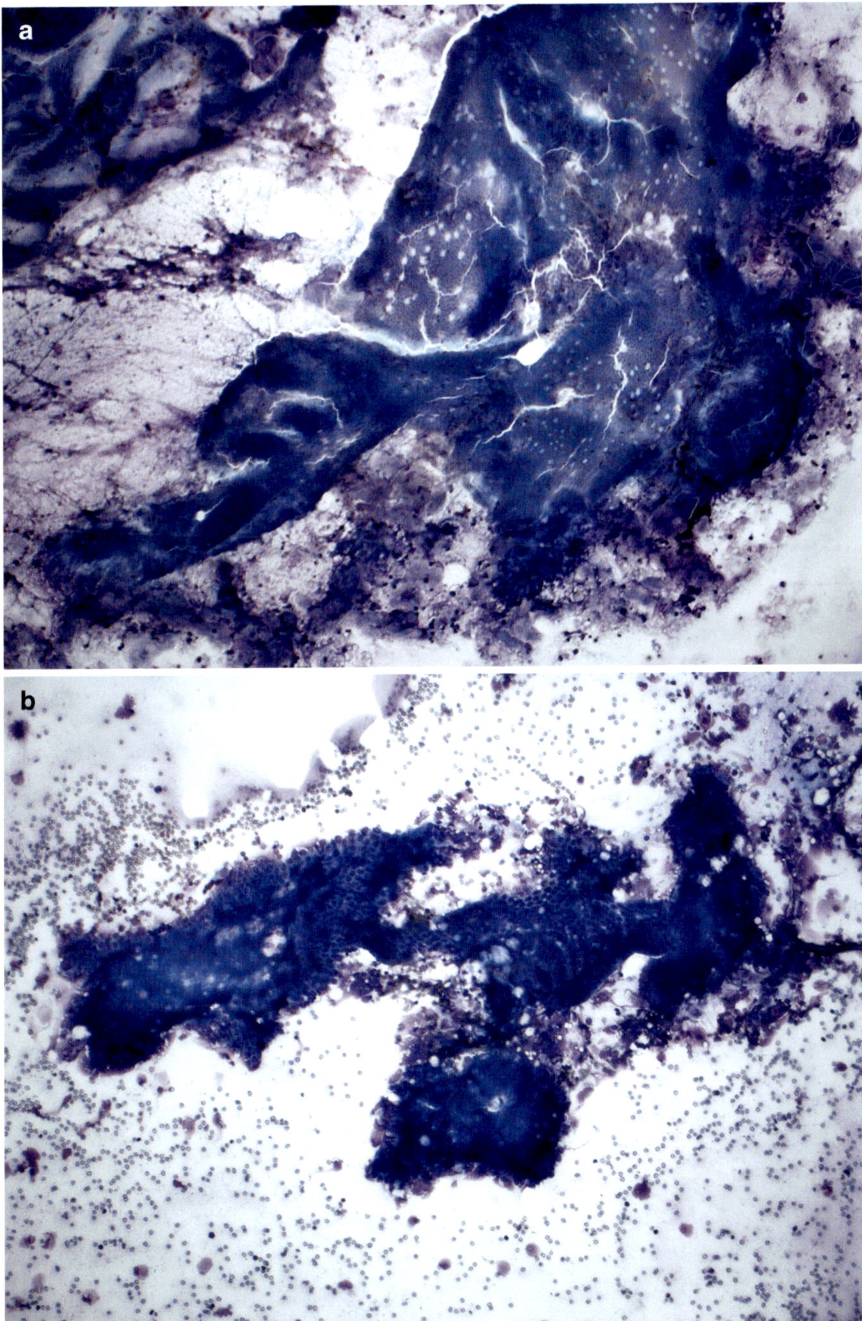

Fig. 12.3 Duodenal epithelial contaminant. Uniform columnar cells are arranged in large cohesive clusters with papillary configuration (**a** Diff-Quik stain, ×100) or flat sheets (**b** Diff-Quik stain, ×100). Goblet cells are scattered within the epithelium, giving a starry sky appearance

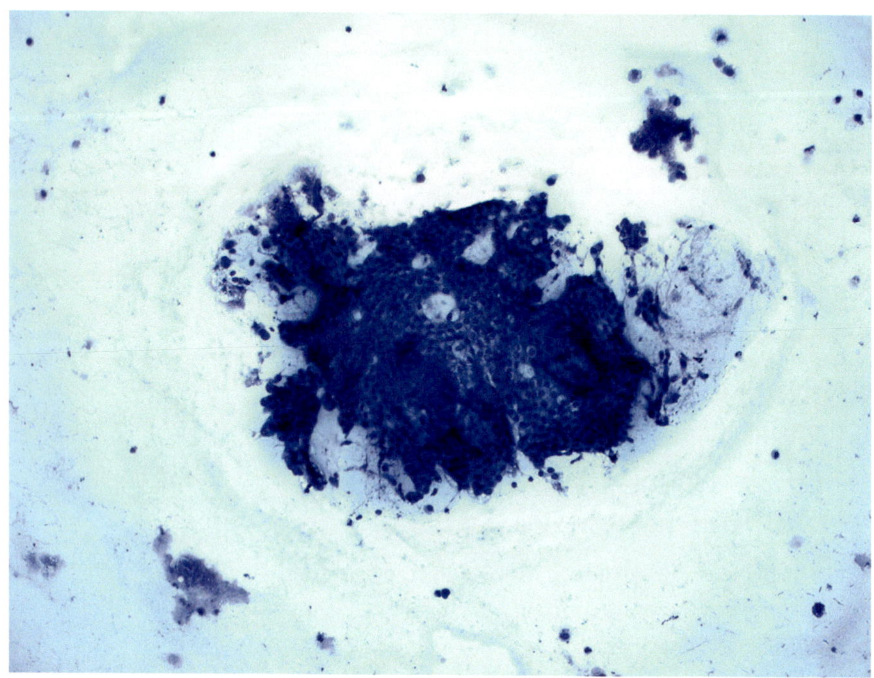

Fig. 12.4 Gastric epithelial contaminant. Relatively uniform cuboidal to columnar cells arranged in cohesive sheets with a few "punch-out" holes (Diff-Quik stain, ×100)

Solid Pancreatic Lesions

Solid pancreatic masses are more likely subjected to imaging-guided biopsy. The majority of solid pancreatic masses are malignant tumors with ductal adenocarcinoma being the most common malignancy. However, benign mimics of malignancy does exit. Endoscopic ultrasound-guided fine needle aspiration biopsy (EUS-FNA) helps rule in or rule out a neoplastic process and, if neoplastic, further classify the tumor [6–8]. ROSE has been shown to improve the performance of EUS-FNA in diagnosing pancreatic malignancies [12–15].

Diagnostic Considerations

- It is important to categorize solid pancreatic lesions into ductal adenocarcinoma, lymphoid lesions, and other neoplasms. A definite diagnosis and further classification may be desirable but not be required.
- Diagnosis of ductal adenocarcinoma is primarily based on cytomorphologic evaluation, and ancillary tests have a limited role in substantiating the diagnosis.

Thus, well-prepared smears with Diff-Quik and Papanicolaou stains are critical for rendering a definite diagnosis. Therefore, repeating smear preparations from multiple passes may be required.
- Precise diagnosis of lymphoproliferative disorders may require flow cytometry studies [18, 19]. Therefore, in case there is a suspicion for a lymphoid lesion during on-site evaluation, additional samples should be saved in RPMI solution to be sent to flow cytometry lab. Primary pancreatic lymphoproliferative disorders are rare, and most patients have known history of the diseases.
- Other tumors such as acinar cell carcinoma, neuroendocrine tumor, solid pseudopapillary tumor, as well as secondary tumors involving the pancreas often need ancillary immunocytochemistry study results for their diagnosis and classification. When these entities are considered to be included in the differential diagnosis, biopsy specimens should be saved as much as possible for preparation of a cell block.

Features of Commonly Seen Entities

1. Chronic pancreatitis

   The patients with chronic pancreatitis often have typical clinical presentations and imaging findings and are seldom subjected to biopsy. However, some patients may present with a localized mass-like lesion, thus raising the possibility of malignancy. The primary goal of biopsy is to rule out malignancy although the findings from biopsy may provide a hint or clues for diagnosis of specific-type pancreatitis such as autoimmune pancreatitis [20, 21]. Cytologically, chronic pancreatitis may show some features overlapping with pancreatic adenocarcinoma and should be considered as a diagnostic pitfall [22, 23].

   A. Cytomorphologic features (Fig. 12.5)

      - Mixed populations of ductal epithelial cells and acinar cells.
      - Ductal epithelial cells with evenly spaced distribution or arranged in honeycomb pattern.
      - Ductal epithelial cells showing reactive changes such as increased nuclear size, high nuclear-to-cytoplasmic ratio, and conspicuous nucleolus.
      - Acinar cells mostly arranged in acinar pattern.
      - Acinar cells showing reactive changes such as increased nuclear size and conspicuous nucleolus.
      - Mixed inflammatory cells including lymphocytes and plasma cells.
      - Scant fibrous tissue fragments with embedded crushed inflammatory cells.
      - Necrosis and calcification may be present.

   B. Tips and pitfalls

      - Pay attention to patient's history and imaging findings, presence of mixed ductal cells and acinar cells, as well as background inflammatory cells.

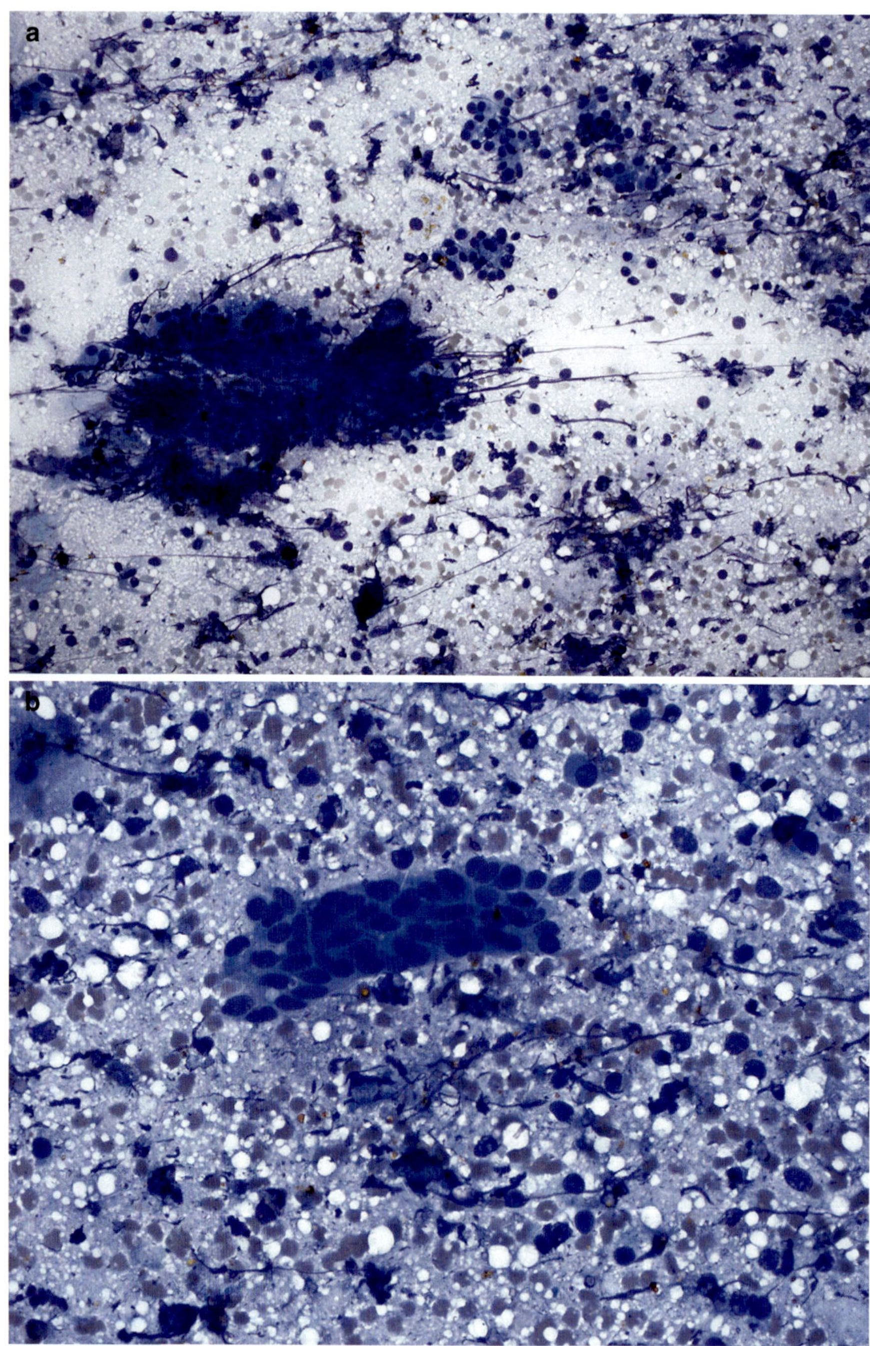

Fig. 12.5 Chronic pancreatitis. Benign-appearing acinar cells (**a** Diff-Quick stain, ×200) and ductal cells (**b** Diff-Quik stain, ×400) intermixed with lymphocytes and plasma cells

Table 12.1 Clinical and cytomorphologic features of chronic pancreatitis and well-differentiated ductal adenocarcinoma

	Chronic pancreatitis	Ductal adenocarcinoma
Patient population	A wide range of age	Elderly
Symptoms	Asymptomatic or pain	Pain, jaundice, and weight loss
Cell population	Mixed ductal and acinar cells	Predominant ductal cells
Cell organization	Flat orderly sheet (honeycomb)	Flat disorganized sheet (drunken honeycomb)
Cell size	Uniformly enlarged	Variation in size
Nucleus	Round to oval with smooth contours	Round to oval with irregular contours
Single cell	Absent	Few to many
Inflammatory cell	Often abundant	May present
Necrosis	Absent	Absent

- Well-differentiated ductal adenocarcinoma is the main differential diagnosis, which has predominant ductal cells, and the ductal cells are variable in size and arranged in a disorganized fashion (Table 12.1).
- In cases with scant inflammatory cells and acinar cell predominance, differential diagnosis may include acinar cell neoplasm and neuroendocrine neoplasm.

2. Ductal adenocarcinoma, well differentiated

   Ductal adenocarcinoma is the most common malignancy, accounting for more than 85% of all pancreatic carcinomas [24]. Ductal adenocarcinoma is often seen in middle-aged or elderly patients with a slightly higher prevalence in males. Pain, jaundice, and weight loss are the classical triad for carcinoma of pancreatic head. The carcinoma arising in the body or tail may have only subtle clinical symptoms. Ductal adenocarcinoma could be well, moderately, or poorly differentiated, among which well-differentiated carcinoma imposes the biggest diagnostic challenge [4, 5, 9, 23–25].

   A. Cytomorphologic features (Fig. 12.6)

      - Moderate to high cellularity with predominant population of ductal-type epithelial cells.
      - Cohesive groups of ductal epithelial cells arranged in flat sheet with a disorganized "drunken honeycomb" pattern.
      - Tumor cells have cytoplasmic vacuoles, nuclear enlargement, and anisonucleosis.
      - Rare single cells may be present.
      - Mucinous material present or absent.
      - Necrosis absent.

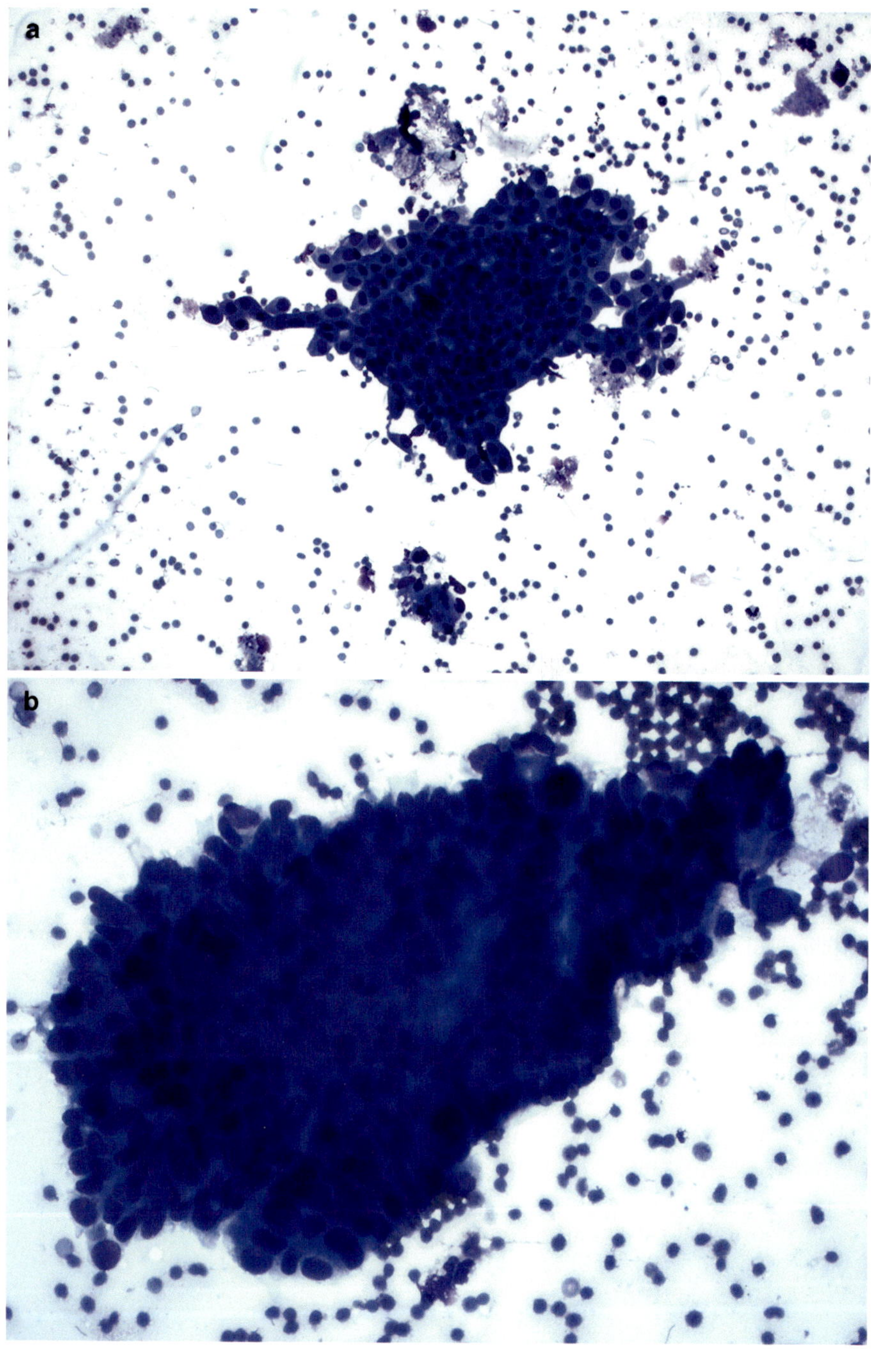

Fig. 12.6 Well-differentiated ductal adenocarcinoma. Ductal epithelial cells arranged in cohesive slightly disorganized flat sheets (**a** Diff-Quik stain, ×200) with focal nuclear overlapping and variation in size (**b** Diff-Quik stain, ×400). A few dyscohesive cells are seen at the edge

B. Tips and pitfalls

- The main differential diagnosis is chronic pancreatitis. The ductal cells in pancreatitis can show reactive changes including nuclear enlargement, nuclear overlapping, and prominent nucleolus but are often uniformly enlarged (Table 12.1).
- In cases with equivocal features, a preliminary diagnosis should be deferred after ample specimen has been collected. Abnormal nuclear features such as nuclear membrane irregularity and chromatin clearing, best appreciated on Papanicolaou stain, may aid final diagnosis.
- In cases with significant amount of mucin material, the differential diagnosis may also include mucinous cystic neoplasm and intraductal papillary mucinous neoplasm.

3. Ductal adenocarcinoma, moderately to poorly differentiated

As compared to well-differentiated ductal adenocarcinoma, moderately to poorly differentiated carcinoma displays significant cytological atypia that helps render diagnosis of malignancy.

A. Cytomorphologic features (Fig. 12.7)

- Moderate to high cellularity.
- Loosely cohesive groups and three-dimensional clusters as well as many single cells.
- Tumor cells have cytoplasmic vacuoles, enlarged nuclei, nuclear overlapping, and marked nuclear anisonucleosis.
- Mucinous material present or absent.
- Necrosis present.

B. Tips and pitfalls

- Although diagnosis of malignancy is not an issue in poorly differentiated carcinoma, careful search for features of ductal differentiation is important for elucidation of tumor origin.
- Metastatic carcinoma or sarcoma should be kept in the differential diagnosis when encountering a poorly differentiated tumor, especially in patients with a known history of other malignancies.
- Presence of uncommon cytomorphologic features such as abundant extracellular mucin and extensive necrosis should also prompt consideration of a metastatic disease.

4. Poorly differentiated ductal carcinoma, morphologic variants

Poorly differentiated pancreatic carcinoma, although rare, can display a variety of morphologic features. Among the most noticeable morphologic variants are anaplastic carcinoma, adenosquamous carcinoma, and small cell carcinoma [26–28].

A. Cytomorphologic features

- Anaplastic carcinoma is characterized as high-cellularity specimen with abundant large, pleomorphic single cells. Multinucleated tumor cells as well as osteoclast-like giant cells may be present. Necrosis is often seen (Fig. 12.8).

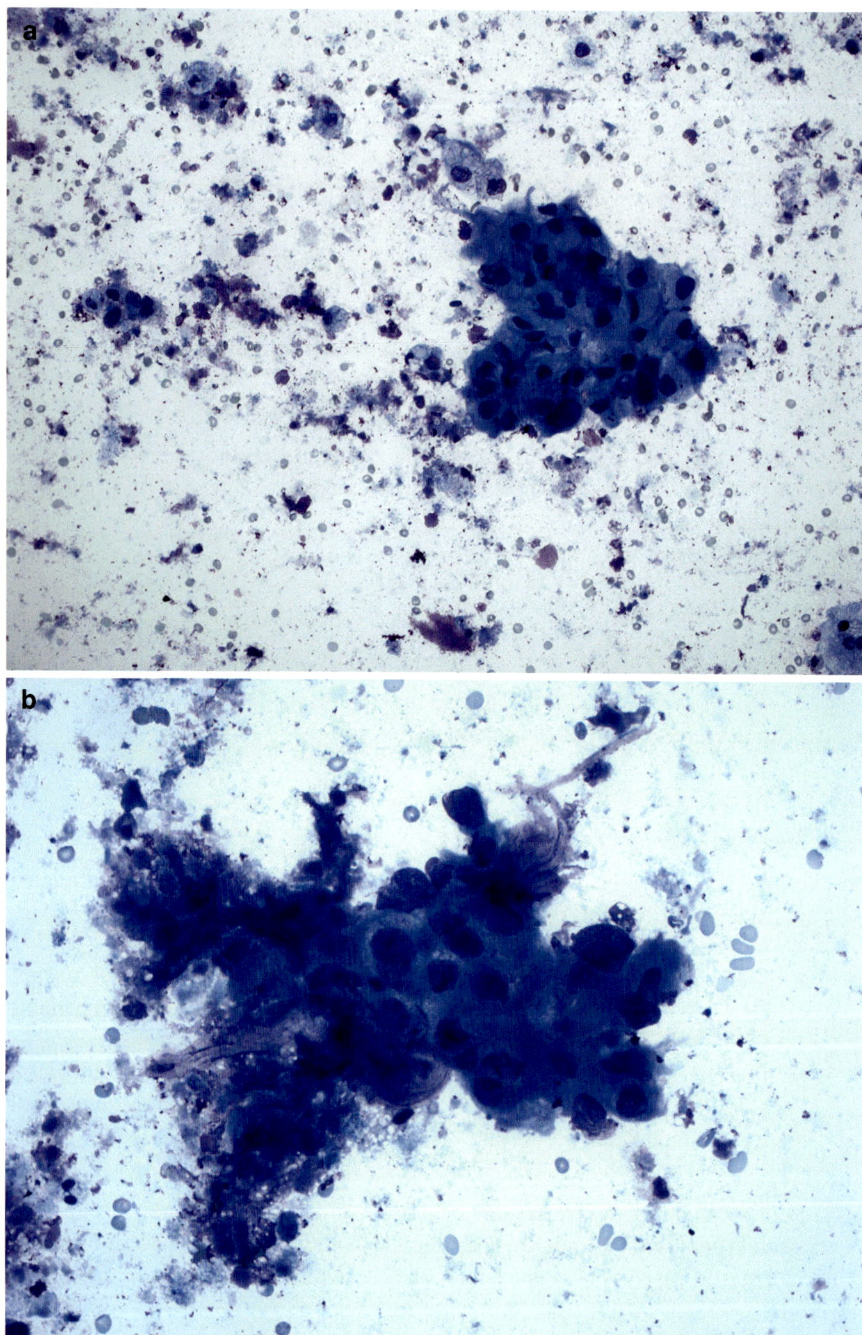

Fig. 12.7 Moderately differentiated ductal adenocarcinoma. Single and clusters of epithelial cells with vacuolated cytoplasm (**a** Diff-Quik stain, ×200) and pleomorphic nuclei (**b** Diff-Quik stain, ×400). Necrosis is present

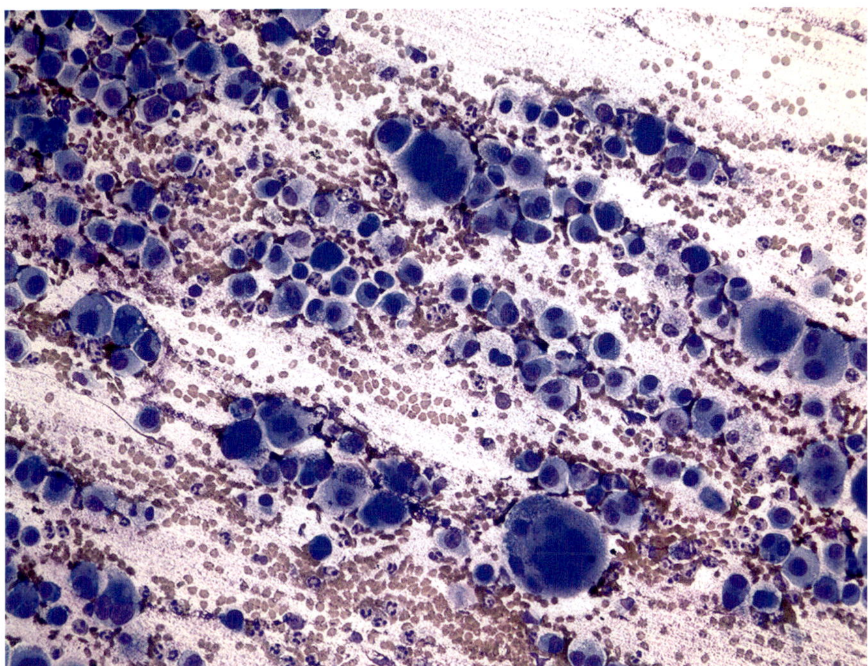

Fig. 12.8 Anaplastic carcinoma. Single and dyscohesive groups of cells with large pleomorphic nuclei, prominent nucleolus, and frequent multinucleated tumor giant cells (Diff-Quik stain, ×200)

- Adenosquamous carcinoma shows a duo populations of tumor cells. Some tumor cells have moderate amount of vacuolated cytoplasm arranged in clusters and acinar or single cell patterns (adenocarcinoma component), while other tumor cells have dense cytoplasm arranged in sheets, clusters, or single cell patterns with focal keratinization (squamous carcinoma component).
- Small cell carcinoma of the pancreas shares the same cytomorphologic features with the tumor arising in the lung. The classic features include abundant single and dyscohesive clusters of small- to intermediate-size tumor cells with high nuclear-to-cytoplasmic ratios, nuclear molding, and smearing rushing artifacts. Apoptosis, mitosis, and necrosis are present (Fig. 12.9).

B. Tips and pitfalls

- Diagnosis of these morphologic variants is straightforward and does not impose diagnostic challenge. Due to their rarity, exclusion of a metastatic disease should always be considered.
- Anaplastic carcinoma should be differentiated from metastatic sarcoma, while a lung primary should be ruled out before rendering a diagnosis of pancreatic small cell carcinoma.

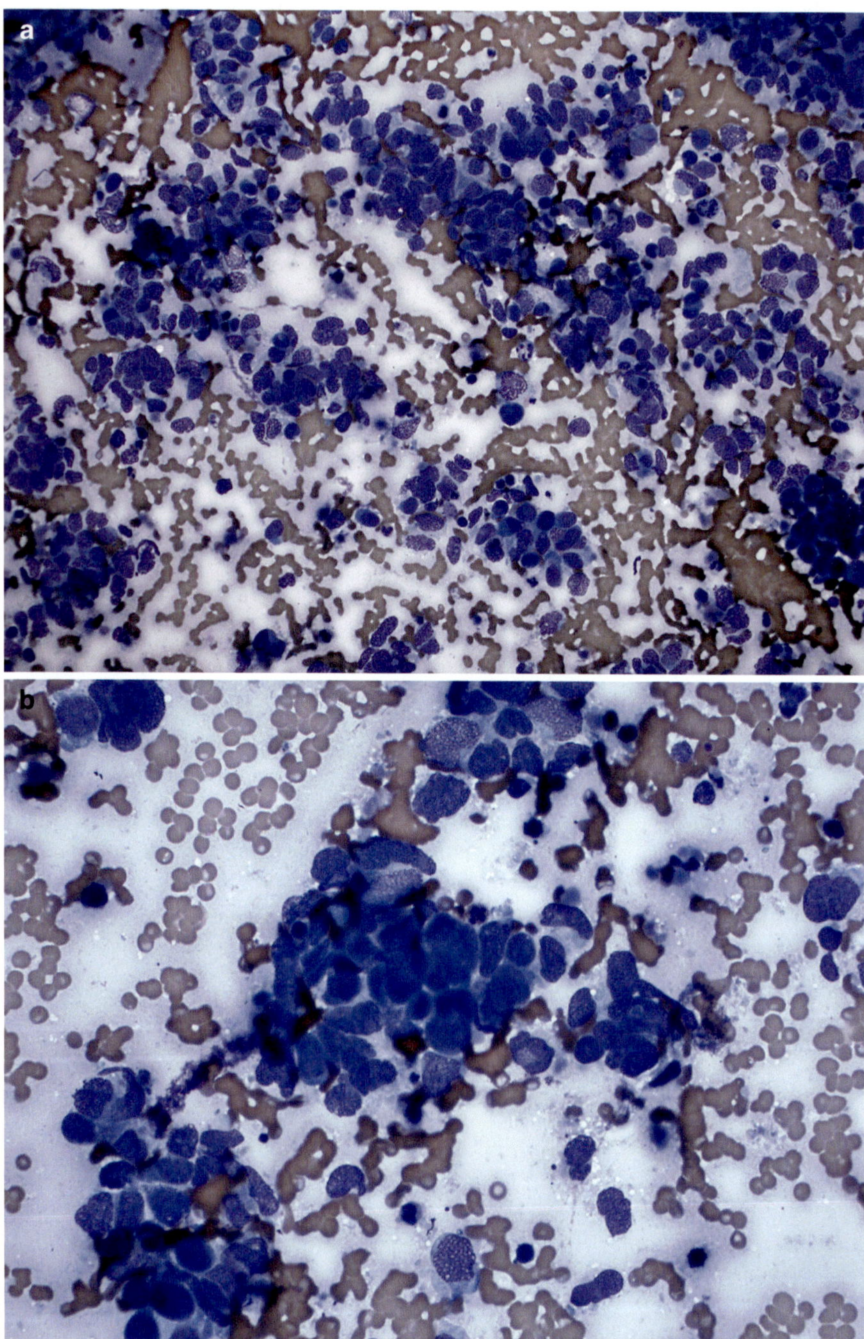

Fig. 12.9 Small cell carcinoma. Single and loosely cohesive clusters of cells (**a** Diff-Quik stain, ×200) with high nuclear-to-cytoplasmic ratios, nuclear molding, and inconspicuous nucleolus (**b** Diff-Quik stain, ×400). Scattered apoptotic bodies are seen

- In adenosquamous carcinoma, demonstration of a due population of tumor cells may be challenging during on-site evaluation. Papanicolaou stain and immunocytochemical studies may be helpful for identifying squamous carcinoma component.
- Small cell carcinomas, primary or metastatic, share the same cytomorphologic features. Knowledge of a prior history, clinical presentation, and imaging findings is crucial for determination of primary site.

5. Acinar cell carcinoma

   Acinar cell carcinoma is an uncommon tumor, accounting for only 1–2% of pancreatic neoplasms [29, 30]. It is seen more often in elderly male patients. The patients are often asymptomatic or present with nonspecific symptoms. Lipase hypersecretion symptoms related to release of pancreatic exocrine enzymes is seen in a small number of patients.

   A. Cytomorphologic features [31, 32] (Fig. 12.10)

      - High cellularity.
      - Arranged in acinar, cord, or trabecular patterns.
      - Single cells present, sometimes as naked nuclei.
      - Relatively uniform cells with enlarged round nuclei and prominent nucleolus.
      - Modest amount of granular cytoplasm.

   B. Tips and pitfalls

      - Acinar cell carcinoma should be differentiated from the lesions with non-neoplastic acinar cells. Acinar cells are characterized by granular cytoplasm and round nuclei arranged in an acinar pattern. The acinar cells of acinar cell carcinoma have enlarged nuclei (twice size of red blood cells) and prominent nucleoli and may be arranged in cords or trabeculae in addition to acinar pattern.
      - Neuroendocrine neoplasm should be included in the differential diagnosis because it can have a rosette growth pattern, mimicking acinar appearance [9]. However, the neuroendocrine tumor cells often have plasmacytoid features and inconspicuous nucleolus. Prominent capillary vasculatures may be seen (Table 12.2).
      - Solid pseudopapillary tumor may share some of cytomorphologic features with acinar cell carcinoma, but it almost exclusively occurs in young woman. The tumor cells have oval nuclei with nuclear grooves. Papillary architectures are frequently seen (Table 12.2).

6. Neuroendocrine neoplasm

   This is an uncommon tumor, accounting for 2–3% of pancreatic neoplasm. It is often seen in middle-aged and elderly patients without gender preference. The patients could be symptomatic or asymptomatic dependent on the functional status of tumors. In functional tumors, the symptoms are related to secretion of insulin, glucagon, or gastrin. Neuroendocrine tumors are preferentially located in the body and tail of the pancreas.

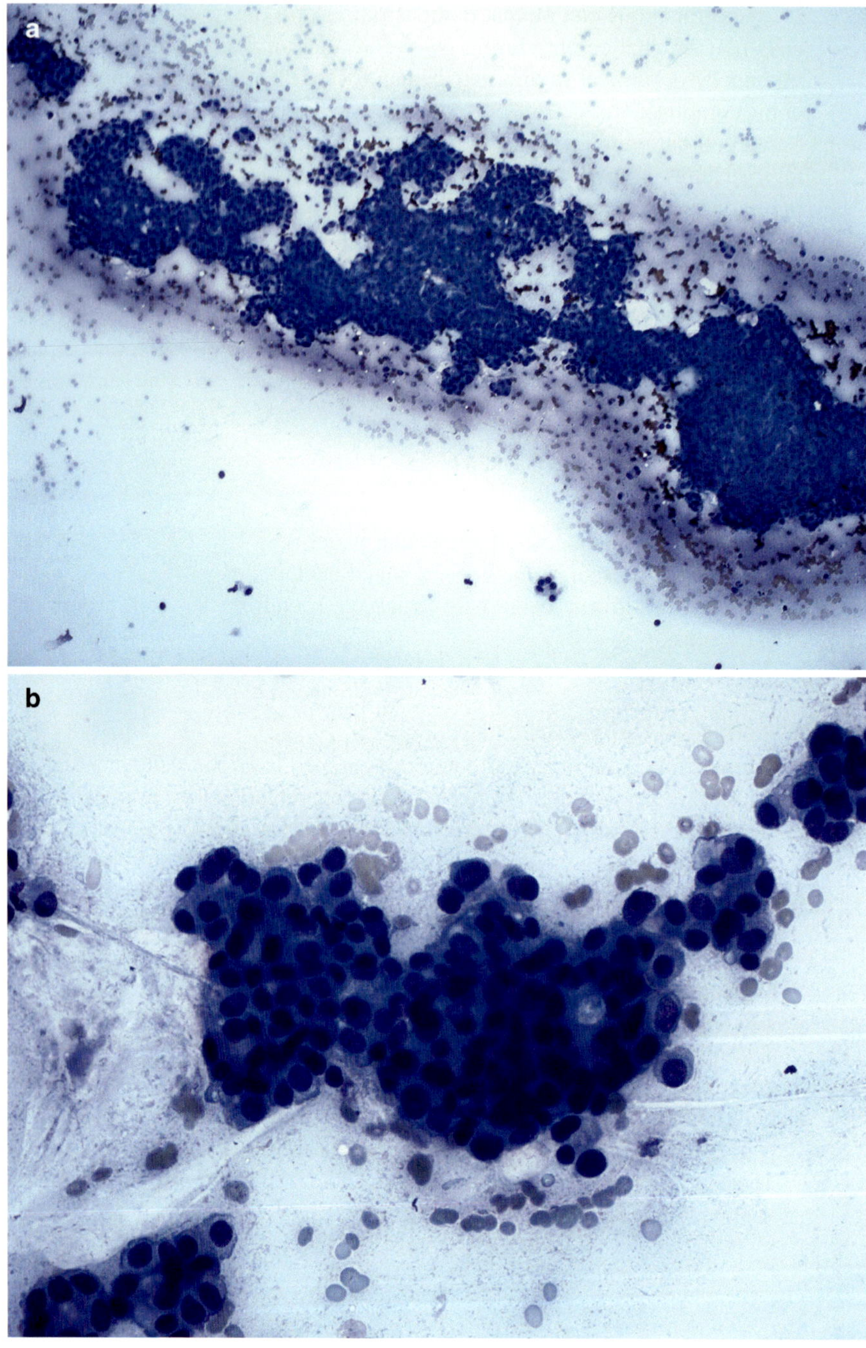

Fig. 12.10 Acinar cell carcinoma. Relatively uniform cells arranged in acinar, trabeculae, and sheets (**a** Diff-Quik stain, ×100) and with granular cytoplasm and enlarged nuclei (**b** Diff-Quik stain, ×400)

Table 12.2 Clinical and cytomorphologic features of solid non-ductal pancreatic tumors

	Acinar cell carcinoma	Neuroendocrine neoplasm	Solid pseudopapillary tumor
Patient population	Elderly, male > female	Middle age or elderly, male = female	Almost exclusively young female
Symptoms	Asymptomatic or nonspecific	Maybe symptomatic related to functional status of tumor	Asymptomatic or nonspecific
Cellularity	High	Moderate to high	High
Cell organization	Acinar, cord, and trabecular	Single cells, loose groups, papillary groups	Single cells, loose groups, papillary groups
Cell size	Enlarged, uniform	Uniform	Uniform
Nucleus	Round, prominent nucleolus	Round, inconspicuous nucleolus	Oval, nuclear grooves, inconspicuous nucleolus
Cytoplasm	Granular	Plasmacytoid	Delicate, indistinct cell border
Single cells	Present	Abundant	Abundant
Necrosis	May present	Absent	May present

A. Cytomorphologic features [33–35] (Fig. 12.11)

- Modest to high cellularity.
- Dyscohesive or loosely cohesive groups of tumor cells.
- Abundant single cells.
- Relatively uniform cells with eccentrically placed round or oval nuclei (plasmacytoid) and inconspicuous nucleolus.
- Scant to modest amount of cytoplasm, sometimes could be granular or vacuolated.
- Bloody background.

B. Tips and pitfalls

- Relatively uniform plasmacytoid cells arranged singly or in dyscohesive groups are the diagnostic clues for neuroendocrine neoplasm. Saving specimen for immunocytochemical studies is highly recommended.
- Poorly differentiated neuroendocrine carcinomas include small cell carcinoma and large cell neuroendocrine carcinoma, which may impose a diagnostic challenge [28, 36].
- The differential diagnosis may include acinar cell carcinoma and solid pseudopapillary tumor (Table 12.2). The cells of solid pseudopapillary tumor have delicate cytoplasm and oval nuclei with nuclear grooves, while the cells of acinar cell carcinoma have granular cytoplasm and prominent nucleolus, primarily arranged in an acinar pattern.
- In cases with a predominant single cell pattern, plasma cell neoplasm involving the pancreas should also be included in the differential diagnosis [37]. The cells of plasma cell neoplasm often have cytoplasmic clearing near the nucleus (perinuclear hof).

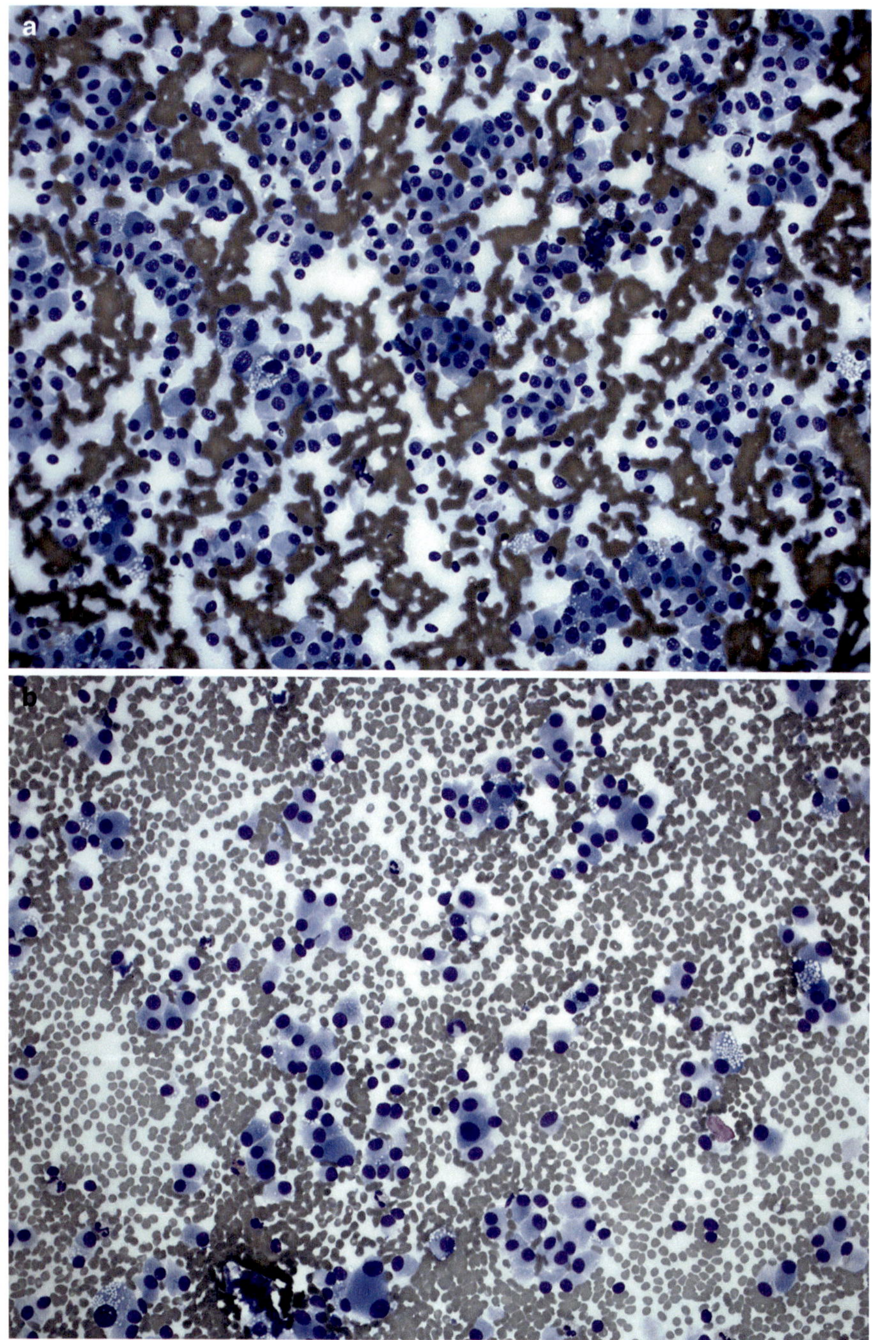

Fig. 12.11 Well-differentiated neuroendocrine neoplasm. Single and loosely cohesive clusters of relatively uniform cells (**a** Diff-Quik stain, ×200) with abundant cytoplasm and eccentrically located nuclei (**b** Diff-Quik stain, ×400). Focal fine cytoplasmic vacuoles are present

- Neuroendocrine neoplasm has prominent capillary vasculatures with clinging cells, which mimics the cytomorphologic features of accessory spleen [38, 39].

7. Solid pseudopapillary tumor

   Solid pseudopapillary tumor is a rare neoplasm of the pancreas [40]. It almost exclusively occurs in young female patients although it does occur in man or elderly woman. The patients are often asymptomatic or present with nonspecific symptoms. The tumor could present as a partially cystic lesion.

   A. Cytomorphologic features [41, 42] (Fig. 12.12)

   - High cellularity.
   - Prominent vasculatures or capillary networks with loosely attached cells.
   - Abundant single cells or dyscohesive cell groups.
   - Relatively uniform cells with delicate cytoplasm, oval nuclei, nuclear grooves, and inconspicuous nucleolus.
   - Focal necrosis may be present.

   B. Tips and pitfalls

   - Solid pseudopapillary tumor should be on the top of differential diagnosis list in a young female patient presenting with a solid pancreatic mass. Classic cytomorphologic features include prominent vasculatures with loosely attached cells as well as abundant single cells in the background.
   - The differential diagnosis may include acinar cell carcinoma and neuroendocrine neoplasm (Table 12.2).

Cystic Pancreatic Lesions

There are a number of cystic lesions in the pancreas, which may be a nonneoplastic or a neoplastic process. The vast majority of these lesions are pseudocysts. Fine needle aspiration biopsy is performed when there is an uncertainty about the nature of cystic lesions based on clinical presentations and imaging findings such as a suspected pseudocyst with thickened wall and differential diagnosis including mucinous versus non-mucinous cyst [3, 43–45]. Fine needle aspiration biopsy is also used to monitor progression of a mucinous cyst [44, 45]. In general, on-site evaluation has a limited value unless the lesion of interest has a significantly thickened cystic wall or has a solid component.

Diagnostic Considerations

- A multimodal approach has been recommended for evaluation of cystic lesions, which includes clinical/imaging findings, cytomorphologic features, and cyst fluid analysis [18, 46, 47].

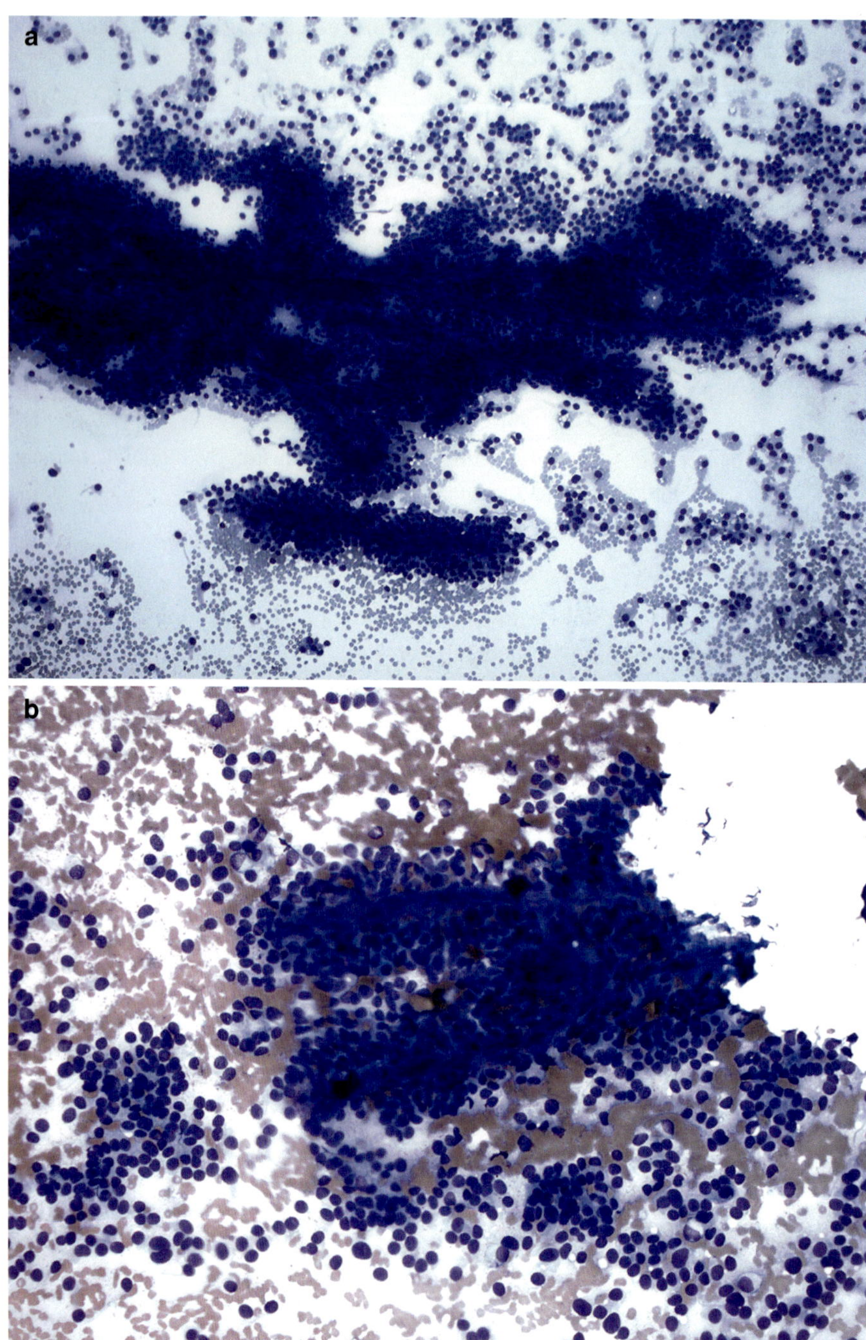

Fig. 12.12 Solid pseudopapillary tumor. Uniform cells seen scattered in the background and clinging around the capillary vasculatures (**a** Diff-Quik stain, ×100) and with oval nuclei and delicate cytoplasm (**b** Diff-Quik stain, ×200)

- During on-site evaluation, it is important to know if the patient has a history of pancreatitis, where the lesion is located (such as the relationship with main pancreatic duct), how the lesion looks like on imaging studies, and what are the clinical impression.
- Pay close attention to appearance of aspirated fluid, including its color and viscosity.
- A portion or supernatant of aspirated fluid should be saved freshly and submitted for cyst fluid chemical analysis.
- Neuroendocrine neoplasm and solid pseudopapillary tumor can present as a cystic pancreatic lesion. If the cytomorphology suggests these tumors, the specimen should be saved as much as possible for preparation of a cell block.
- In patients with suspicion for a mucinous lesion, attention should be paid to presence of cytologic atypia which may suggest malignant transformation.

Features of Commonly Seen Entities

1. Pseudocyst

   Pseudocyst is the most commonly encountered cystic lesion, accounting for 75–90% of all pancreatic cystic lesions evaluated. Most patients have documented history of acute pancreatitis.

   A. Cytomorphologic features

   - Scattered inflammatory cells, predominantly histiocytes, some containing hemosiderin pigments.
   - Cellular debris, bile pigments.
   - No cyst lining cells.
   - Normal elements of pancreatic tissue such as acinar cells and ductal cells may be present.

   B. Tips and pitfalls

   - Diagnosis of pseudocyst is straightforward in patients with typical clinical presentation. Assessment of cytomorphology with amylase analysis may be helpful in borderline cases.
   - Pseudocyst may sometimes be confused with other cystic neoplasms due to misinterpretation of sampled normal acinar cells, ductal cells, or gastrointestinal contaminants.

2. Serous cystadenoma

   Serous cystadenoma is a benign neoplasm and is seen commonly in elderly women [48–50]. Histopathologically, serous cystadenoma can have a microcystic or a macrocystic growth pattern. Tumor with a microcystic growth has a characteristic sunburst appearance on ultrasound examination.

   A. Cytomorphologic features [51–53] (Fig. 12.13)

   - Low cellularity.
   - Tumor cells arranged in honeycomb sheet or acinar pattern.

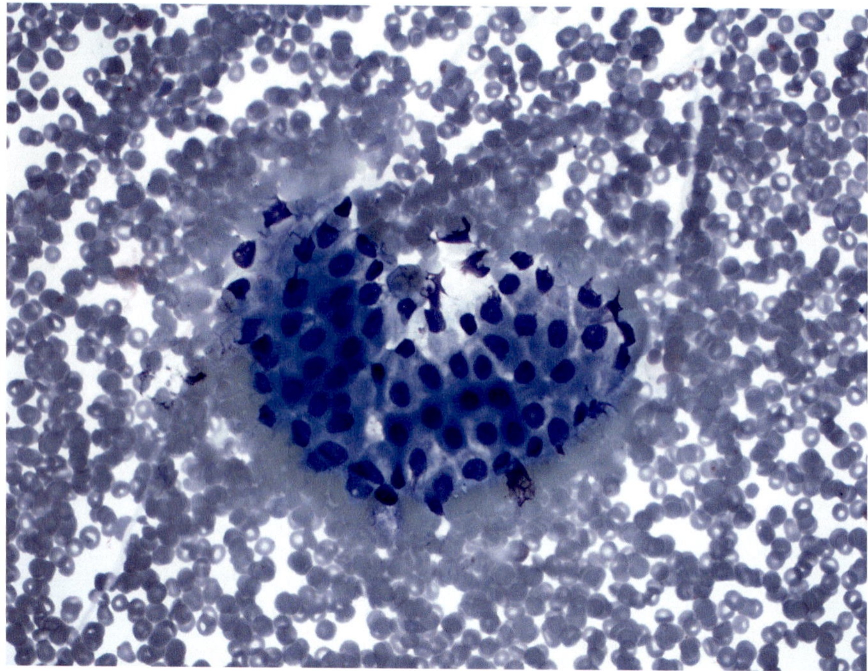

Fig. 12.13 Serous cystadenoma. Paucicellular specimen with benign-appearing non-mucinous epithelial cell arranged in flat sheet (Diff-Quik stain, ×400)

- Uniform cuboidal cells with distinct cell borders.
- Moderate or abundant vacuolated cytoplasm and round nuclei.
- Clean background.

B. Tips and pitfalls

- Diagnosis of serous cystadenoma can be challenging due to low cellularity and bland appearance of tumor cells, particularly during on-site evaluation. It is however important to separate this entity from a mucinous lesion. Cyst fluid analysis for CEA level may be helpful for the differential diagnosis.
- It is crucial to recognize which epithelial cells are representative of the lesion. Be aware that normal acinar cells, ductal cells, or gastrointestinal, particularly gastric, contaminants can be confused with the cells of interest [51].

3. Mucinous cystic neoplasm

Mucinous cystic neoplasm is a relatively common tumor, accounting for about 6% of all primary pancreatic neoplasms. It almost exclusively occurred in middle-aged women. The tumor has potential of progression including malignant transformation [49, 50, 54].

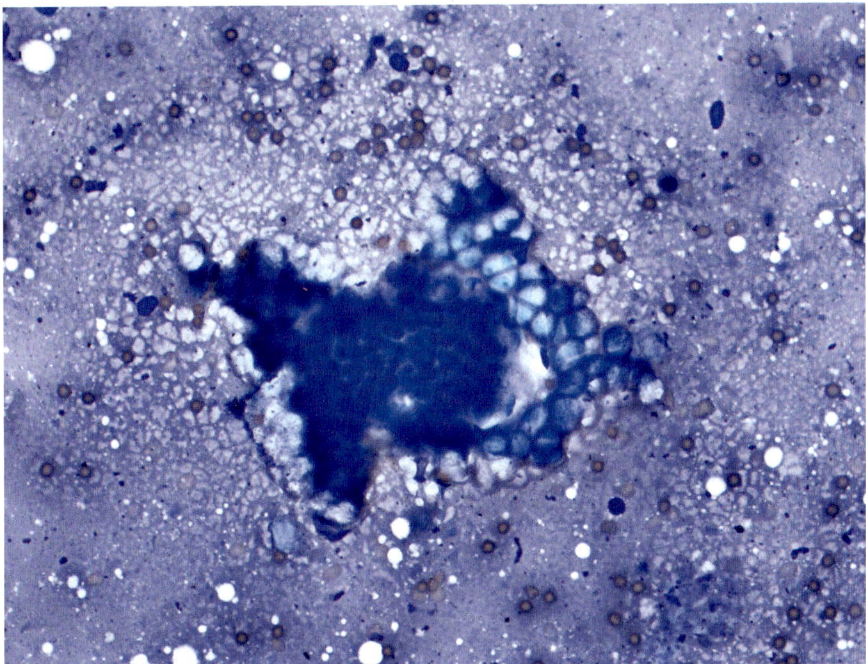

Fig. 12.14 Mucinous cystic neoplasm. Paucicellular specimen with benign-appearing mucinous epithelial cells arranged in flat sheet (Diff-Quik stain, ×200)

A. Cytomorphologic features [55–57] (Fig. 12.14)

- Scant to moderate cellularity.
- Arranged in honeycomb sheet, occasionally in papillary clusters or single cells.
- Low columnar cells with cytoplasmic vacuoles.
- Mild cytologic atypia including nuclear enlargement and nuclear overlapping.
- Ovarian-type stromal fragments often absent.
- Malignant transformation should be considered when many single cells or dyscohesive cell clusters and severe cytologic atypia such as pleomorphism, anisonucleosis, single cells, and necrosis are identified.
- Mucinous material, often thick, present.

B. Tips and pitfalls

- Aspirates from a middle-age woman showing clusters of mucinous epithelial cells with mucin in the background is suggestive of a mucinous cystic neoplasm.
- Recognition of possible gastrointestinal contaminants helps avoid diagnostic pitfalls.

- Mucinous cystic neoplasm shares some cytomorphologic features with intraductal papillary mucinous neoplasm [55]. Presence of large papillary clusters, non-mucinous epithelial cells, and male gender favors intraductal papillary mucinous neoplasm.
- Accurate grading of atypia may be challenging, which bears a low interobserver agreement on interpretation [56].
- Mucinous ductal adenocarcinoma should be included in the differential diagnosis when malignant transformation from a mucinous cystic neoplasm is considered.

4. Intraductal papillary mucinous neoplasm

   Intraductal papillary mucinous neoplasm is commonly seen in elderly patients, more frequently seen in males than females. It can arise in main pancreatic duct or/and its side branches [49, 50, 58]. The main duct tumor predominantly occurs in the head and presents as intraductal tumor growth within dilated pancreatic duct. During endoscopy, mucin oozing out from the ampulla of Vater can be seen. Based on biological behavior, tumor can be classified as benign, borderline, or malignant neoplasm.

   A. Cytomorphologic features [55–57, 59, 60] (Fig. 12.15)

   - Moderate to high cellularity.
   - Arranged in sheets, clusters, or papillary groups.
   - Relatively bland cuboidal or columnar epithelial cells with or without intracytoplasmic mucin and round to oval nuclei.
   - Background mucin present.
   - Significant cytologic atypia including pleomorphism, single cells, and necrosis are seen in malignant neoplasm.

   B. Tips and pitfalls

   - Main duct intraductal papillary mucinous neoplasm has characteristic sonographic and endoscopic findings, which in combination of cytomorphologic features help render a diagnosis.
   - Intraductal papillary mucinous neoplasm has different types of epithelium such as intestinal type and pancreaticobiliary type, which may add to diagnostic challenge and potential confusion with gastrointestinal contaminants in a low-cellularity specimen [61].
   - It is difficult to distinguish side branch intraductal papillary mucinous neoplasm from mucinous cystic neoplasm based on cytomorphology alone.

Tumors Secondarily Involving the Pancreas

Although uncommon, pancreatic lesion could represent a tumor secondarily involving the pancreas [62–68]. The secondary tumors may include metastatic carcinoma, metastatic sarcoma, metastatic melanoma, or lymphoproliferative disorders. FNA could result in a highly specific diagnosis [69].

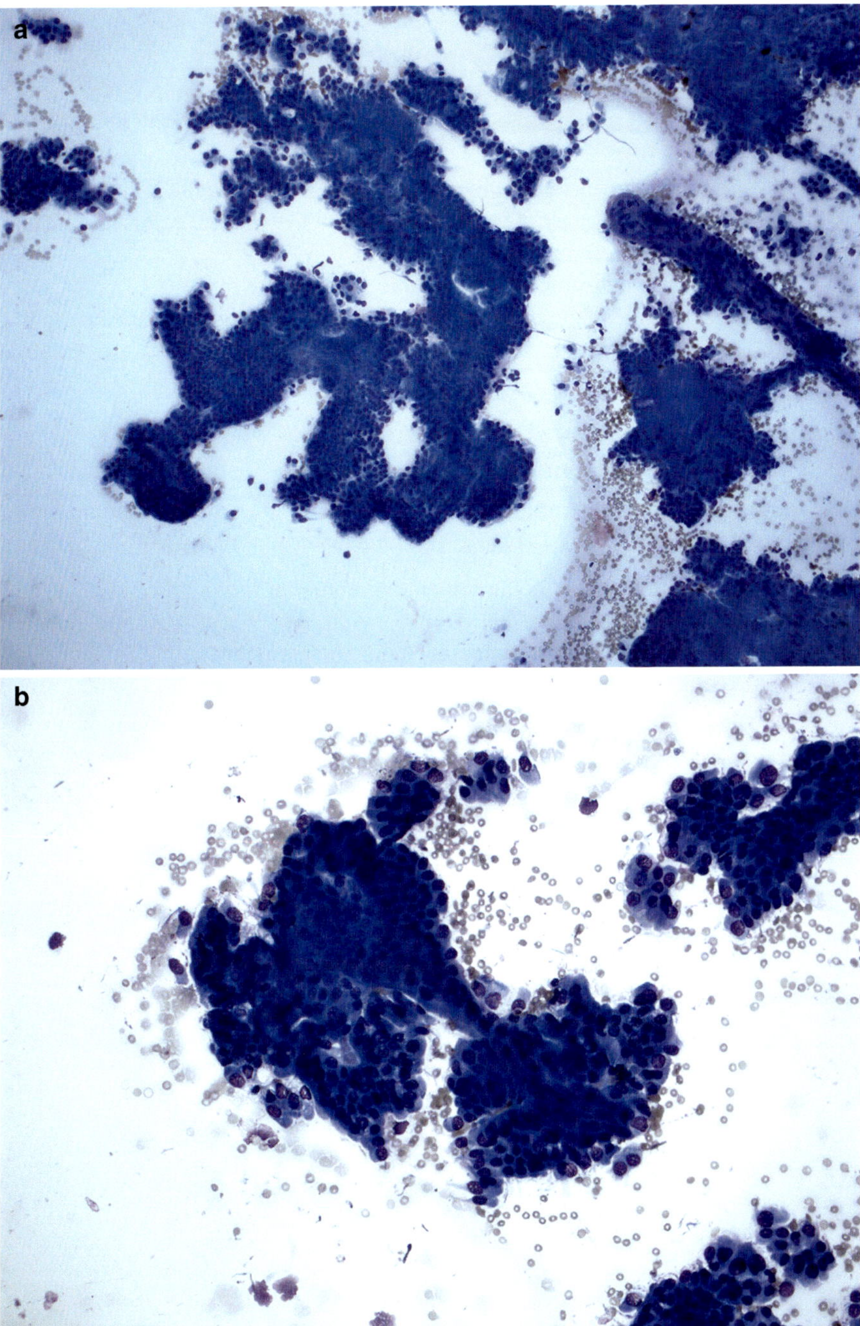

Fig. 12.15 Intraductal papillary mucinous neoplasm. Relatively uniform columnar epithelial cells with papillary architectures (**a** Diff-Quik stain, ×100) and arranged in cohesive clusters or small groups (**b** Diff-Quik stain, ×200)

Diagnostic Considerations

- Most patients have a documented history of malignant neoplasm(s).
- Patients have broad demographic features, depending on the type of malignant tumors.
- The most common metastatic tumors are renal cell carcinoma. Other primary sites include the lung, breast, skin, and urothelium. Gastric and colon cancers can metastasize to or directly involve the pancreas.
- Lymphoproliferative disorders or metastatic sarcoma are rare.
- Patients present with single or multiple lesions without a preferential location.

Lesions with Features of Adenocarcinoma

Metastatic adenocarcinoma should be differentiated from ductal adenocarcinoma of the pancreas and be considered in patients with a history of malignancy.

- Lung and colon adenocarcinoma are among common tumors metastatic to the pancreas [62, 63, 65, 68].
- Lung adenocarcinoma shows significant cytologic atypia including anisonucleosis, single cells, and necrosis (Fig. 12.16).

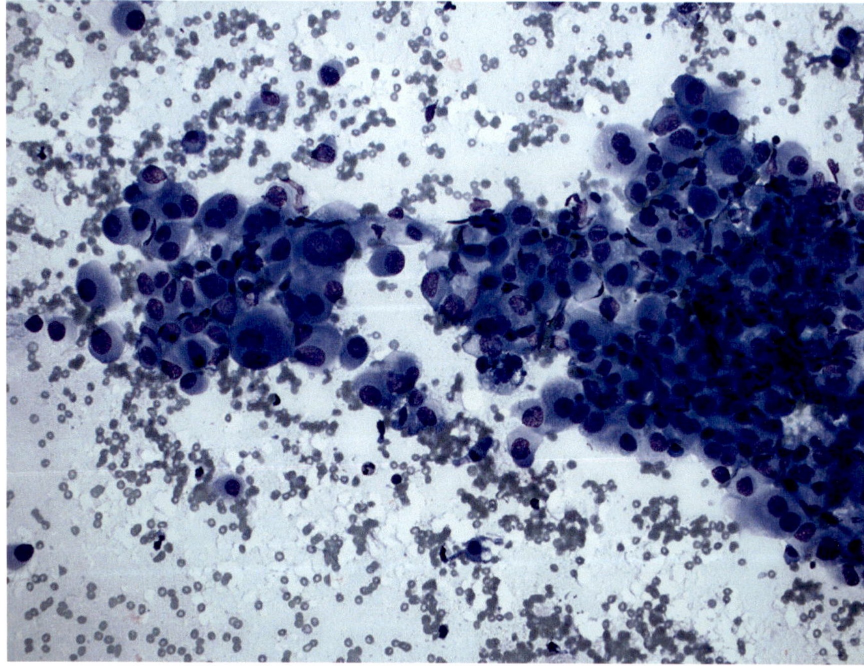

Fig. 12.16 Metastatic lung adenocarcinoma. Loosely cohesive clusters of cells with vacuolated cytoplasm and pleomorphic nuclei (Diff-Quik stain, ×200)

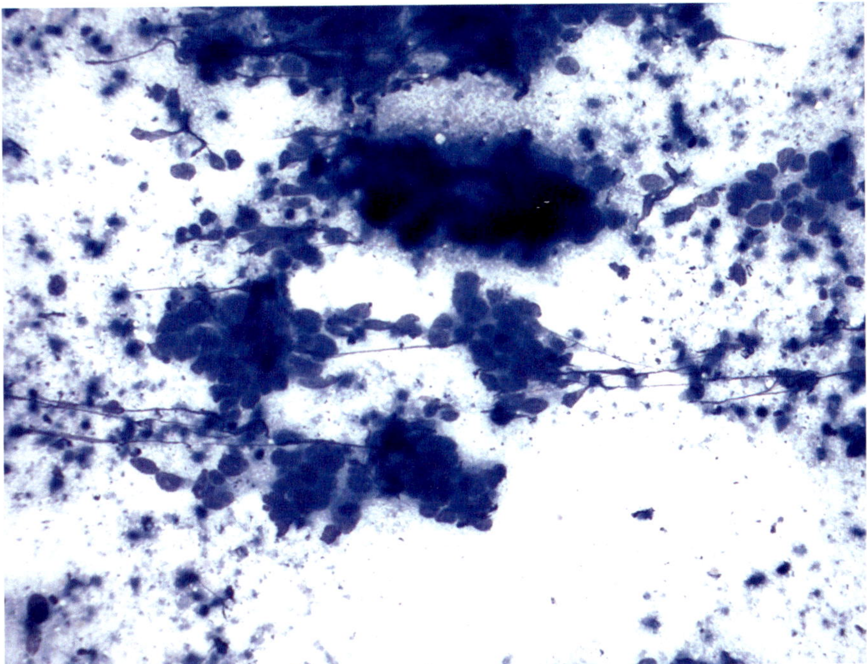

Fig. 12.17 Metastatic colon adenocarcinoma. Clusters of columnar cells with vacuolated cytoplasm and conspicuous nucleolus arranged in an acinar pattern in a necrotic background (Diff-Quik stain, ×200)

- Colon adenocarcinoma has columnar cells arranged in acinar pattern in a background of necrosis (Fig. 12.17).
- Although cytomorphologic features may suggest a possibility, final diagnosis may rest on the results of immunocytochemical studies.

Lesions with Large Pleomorphic Cells

Anaplastic carcinoma of the pancreas is rare. When smears show abundant large pleomorphic cells, metastatic poorly differentiated carcinoma or metastatic sarcoma should be included in the differential diagnosis [68, 70]. Metastatic melanoma could also be a possibility [62, 63].

- Patients with suspected metastatic carcinoma or sarcoma often have a documented history of malignancy.
- If carcinoma, tumor cells show some degree of cohesiveness and are at least focally grouped or clustered.
- Sarcoma tumor cells are dyscohesive and matrix material may be present (Fig. 12.18).
- Melanoma cells are present as single cells and often have prominent nucleolus. Melanin pigment can sometime be seen within tumor cells or histiocytes.

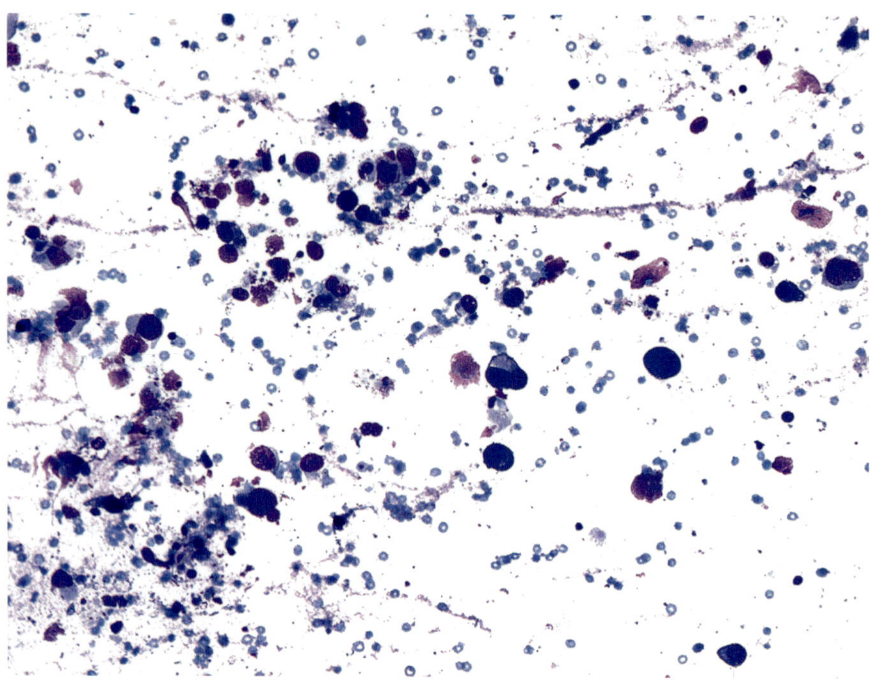

Fig. 12.18 Metastatic high-grade sarcoma. Dispersed single cells with high nuclear-to-cytoplasmic ratios and pleomorphic nuclei (Diff-Quik stain, ×400)

Lesions with Clear Cell Features

Metastatic renal cell carcinoma is the most common tumors metastatic to the pancreas, which may have overlapping cytomorphologic features with ductal adenocarcinoma because of clear cytoplasm [71–73]. Neuroendocrine neoplasm may sometimes show cytoplasmic vacuoles [74, 75].

- Smears of renal cell carcinoma show clusters of tumor cells with abundant clear cytoplasm and prominent nucleolus, which may be associated with capillary vasculatures. Fine lipid droplets may be seen in the cytoplasm as well as background (Fig. 12.19).
- The neuroendocrine tumor cells are single or dyscohesive clusters and have eccentrically located nuclei with inconspicuous nucleolus.

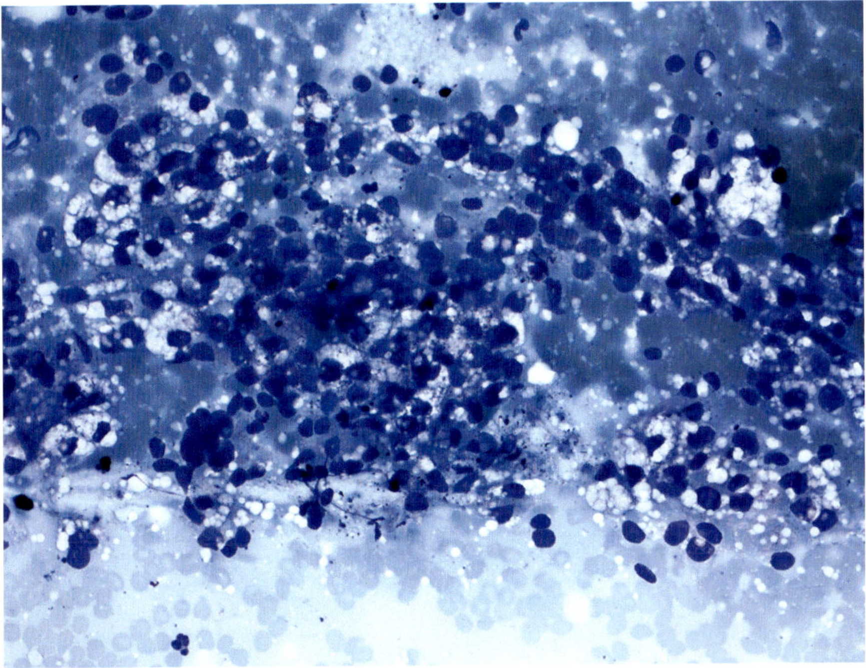

Fig. 12.19 Metastatic clear cell renal cell carcinoma. Loose cohesive clusters of epithelial cells with abundant vacuolated cytoplasm and variation in nuclear size. Lipid droplets present in cytoplasm as well as in the background (Diff-Quik stain, ×400)

Lesions with Plasmacytoid Cells

The differential diagnosis includes neuroendocrine neoplasm as well as plasma cell neoplasm and metastatic melanoma [37, 62, 63, 68].

- Neuroendocrine neoplasm has dispersed single cells as well as loosely cohesive groups of tumor cells.
- Plasma cell neoplasm are dispersed single cells. Perinuclear hof is a characteristic feature (Fig. 12.20).
- Melanoma tumor cells show variation in tumor cells and have binucleation and prominent nucleolus (Fig. 12.21).

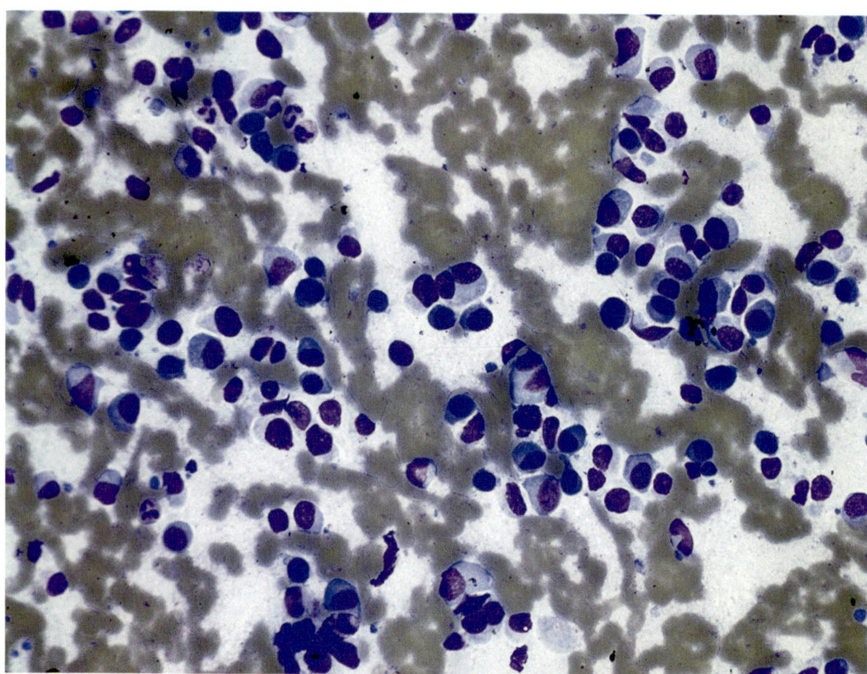

Fig. 12.20 Plasma cell neoplasm. Dispersed single cells with eccentrically located nuclei, perinuclear hof, and occasional binucleation (Diff-Quik stain, ×400)

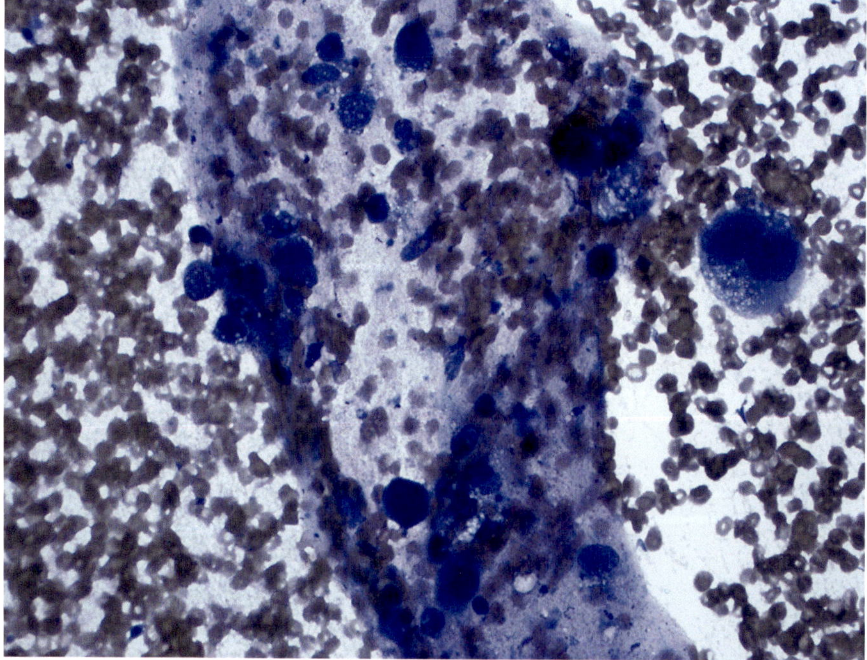

Fig. 12.21 Metastatic melanoma. Dispersed pleomorphic single cells with high nuclear-to-cytoplasmic ratios, conspicuous nucleolus, and rare binucleation (Diff-Quik stain, ×400)

Lesions of Predominantly Lymphoid Cells

When smears show abundant lymphoid cells, the differential diagnosis should include chronic pancreatitis and a lymphoproliferative disorder [76]. Accessory spleen is the rare lesion of lymphoid origin [38, 39].

- The lymphoid cells in chronic pancreatitis are mixed inflammatory cells including lymphocytes, plasma cells, and histiocytes. Reactive ductal cells and acinar cells are most likely present.
- The most common lymphoproliferative disorder involving the pancreas is diffuse large B-cell lymphoma, which shows significant atypia such as variation in size, irregular nuclear contours, and conspicuous nucleolus (Fig. 12.22).
- Accessory spleen or splenule shows large cohesive clusters of lymphoid cells. Interestingly, large aggregates of platelets may aid in the diagnosis (Fig. 12.23).

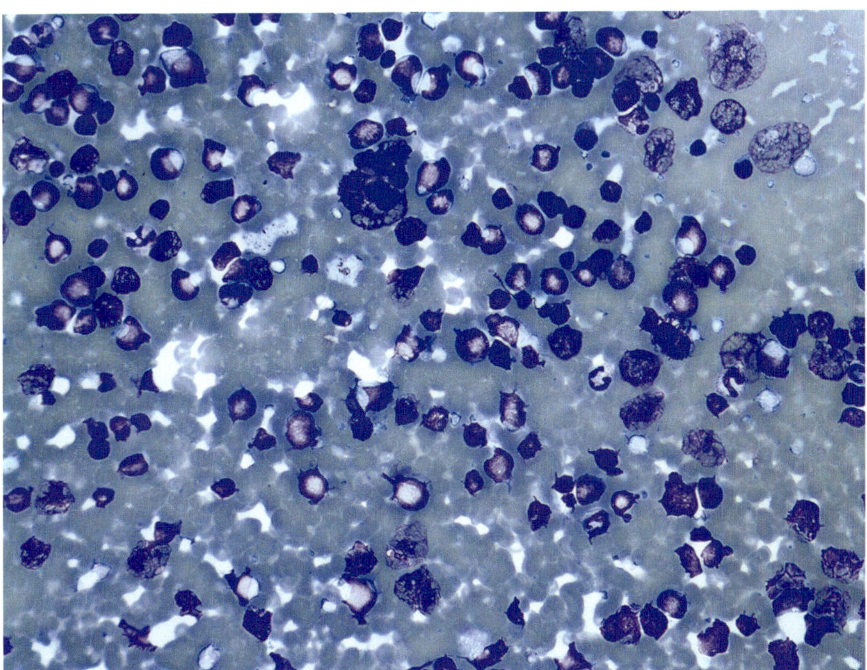

Fig. 12.22 Diffuse large B-cell lymphoma. Dispersed pleomorphic lymphocytes with high nuclear-to-cytoplasmic ratios and irregular nuclear contours (Diff-Quik stain, ×400). Scattered lymphoglandular bodies present

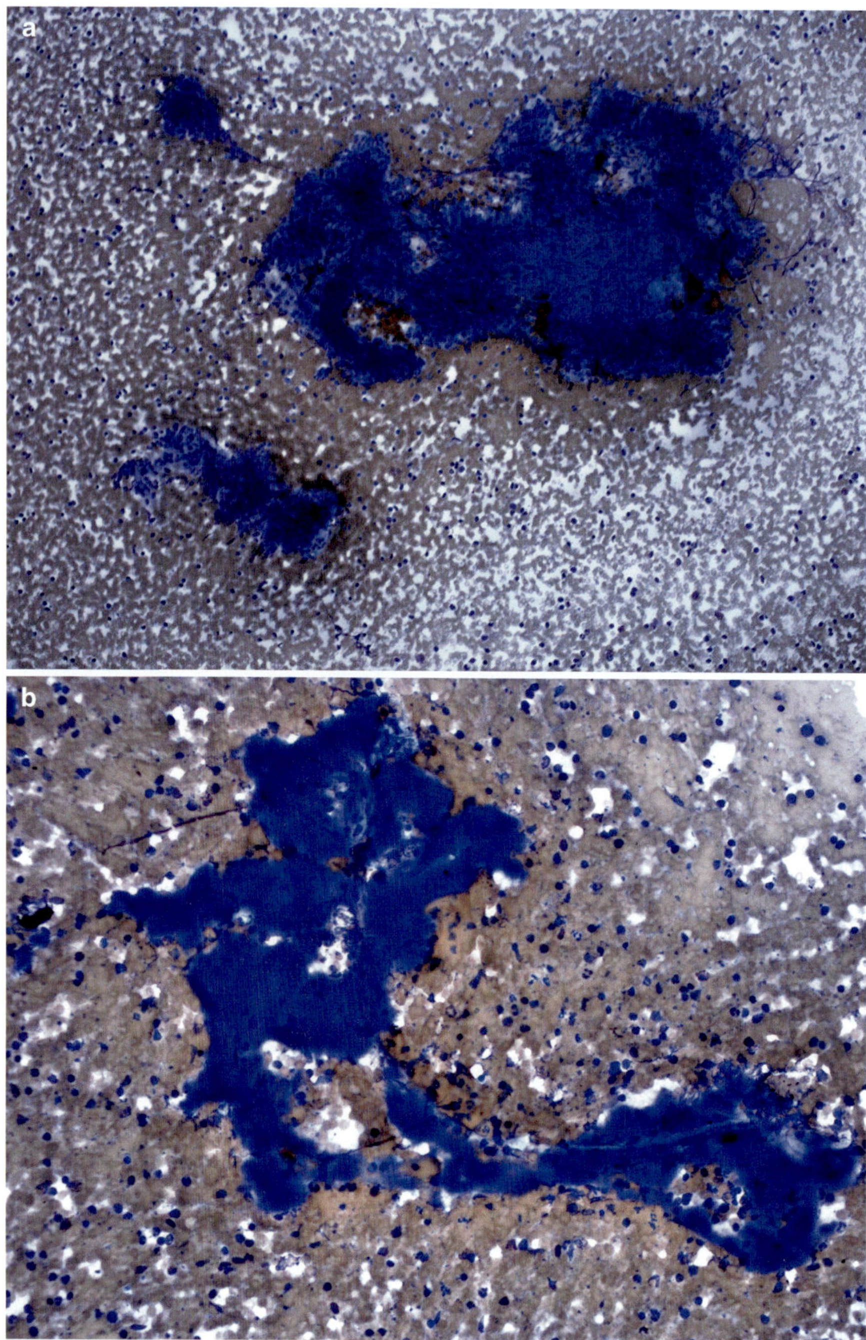

Fig. 12.23 Accessory spleen. Large clusters of lymphoid tissue as well as dispersed single small lymphocytes (**a** Diff-Quik stain, ×100) with large platelet aggregates (**b** Diff-Quik stain, ×200)

References

1. Farrell JJ. Prevalence, diagnosis and management of pancreatic cystic neoplasms: current status and future directions. Gut Liver. 2015;9(5):571–89.
2. Midwinter MJ, Beveridge CJ, Wilsdon JB, Bennett MK, Baudouin CJ, Charnley RM. Correlation between spiral computed tomography, endoscopic ultrasonography and findings at operation in pancreatic and ampullary tumours. Br J Surg. 1999;86(2):189–93.
3. Dumonceau JM, Deprez PH, Jenssen C, Iglesias-Garcia J, Larghi A, Vanbiervliet G, Aithal GP, Arcidiacono PG, Bastos P, Carrara S, Czakó L, Fernández-Esparrach G, Fockens P, Ginès À, Havre RF, Hassan C, Vilmann P, van Hooft JE, Polkowski M. Indications, results, and clinical impact of endoscopic ultrasound (EUS)-guided sampling in gastroenterology: European Society of Gastrointestinal Endoscopy (ESGE) clinical guideline – updated January 2017. Endoscopy. 2017;49(7):695–714.
4. Faigel DO, Ginsberg GG, Bentz JS, Gupta PK, Smith DB, Kochman ML. Endoscopic ultrasound-guided real-time fine-needle aspiration biopsy of the pancreas in cancer patients with pancreatic lesions. J Clin Oncol. 1997;15(4):1439–43.
5. David O, Green L, Reddy V, Kluskens L, Bitterman P, Attal H, Prinz R, Gattuso P. Pancreatic masses: a multi-institutional study of 364 fine-needle aspiration biopsies with histopathologic correlation. Diagn Cytopathol. 1998;19(6):423–7.
6. Shin HJ, Lahoti S, Sneige N. Endoscopic ultrasound-guided fine-needle aspiration in 179 cases: the M. D. Anderson Cancer Center experience. Cancer Cytopathol. 2002;96(3): 174–80.
7. Raut CP, Grau AM, Staerkel GA, Kaw M, Tamm EP, Wolff RA, Vauthey JN, Lee JE, Pisters PWT, Evans DB. Diagnostic accuracy of endoscopic ultrasound-guided fine-needle aspiration in patients with presumed pancreatic cancer. J Gastrointest Surg. 2003;7(1):118–28.
8. Jhala NC, Jhala D, Eltoum I, Vickers SM, Wilcox CM, Chhieng DC, Eloubeidi MA. Endoscopic ultrasound-guided fine-needle aspiration biopsy: a powerful tool to obtain samples from small lesions. Cancer Cytopathol. 2004;102(4):239–46.
9. Bergeron JP, Perry KD, Houser PM, Yang J. Endoscopic ultrasound-guided pancreatic fine-needle aspiration: potential pitfalls in one institution's experience of 1212 procedures. Cancer Cytopathol. 2015;123(2):98–107.
10. O'Toole D, Palazzo L, Arotearena R, et al. Assessment of complications of EUS-guided fine-needle aspiration. Gastointest Endosc. 2001;53:470–4.
11. Tarantino I, Fabbri C, Di Mitri R, Pagano N, Barresi L, Mocciaro F, Maimone A, Curcio G, Repici A, Traina M. Complications of endoscopic ultrasound fine needle aspiration on pancreatic cystic lesions: final results from a large prospective multicenter study. Dig Liver Dis. 2014;46(1):41–4.
12. Klapman JB, Logrono R, Dye CE, Waxman I. Clinical impact of on-site cytopathology interpretation on endoscopic ultrasound-guided fine needle aspiration. Am J Gastroenterol. 2003;98(6):1289–94.
13. Jhala NC, Eltoum IA, Eloubeidi MA, Meara R, Chhieng DC, Crowe DR, Jhala D. Providing on-site diagnosis of malignancy on endoscopic-ultrasound-guided fine-needle aspirates: should it be done? Ann Diagn Pathol. 2007;11(3):176–81.
14. Iglesias-Garcia J, Dominguez-Munoz JE, Abdulkader I, Larino-Noia J, Eugenyeva E, Lozano-Leon A, Forteza-Vila J. Influence of on-site cytopathology evaluation on the diagnostic accuracy of endoscopic ultrasound-guided fine needle aspiration (EUS-FNA) of solid pancreatic masses. Am J Gastroenterol. 2011;106(9):1705–10.
15. Hébert-Magee S, Bae S, Varadarajulu S, Ramesh J, Frost AR, Eloubeidi MA, Eltoum IA. The presence of a cytopathologist increases the diagnostic accuracy of endoscopic ultrasound-guided fine needle aspiration cytology for pancreatic adenocarcinoma: a meta-analysis. Cytopathology. 2013;24(3):159–71.
16. Matynia AP, Schmidt RL, Barraza G, Layfield LJ, Siddiqui AA, Adler DG. Impact of rapid on-site evaluation on the adequacy of endoscopic-ultrasound guided fine-needle aspiration

of solid pancreatic lesions: a systematic review and meta-analysis. J Gastroenterol Hepatol. 2014;29(4):697–705.
17. Collins BT, Murad FM, Wang JF, Bernadt CT. Rapid on-site evaluation for endoscopic ultrasound-guided fine-needle biopsy of the pancreas decreases the incidence of repeat biopsy procedures. Cancer Cytopathol. 2013;121(9):518–24.
18. Pitman MB, Centeno BA, Ali SZ, Genevay M, Stelow E, Mino-Kenudson M, Fernandez-del Castillo C, Max Schmidt C, Brugge W, Layfield L, Papanicolaou Society of Cytopathology. Standardized terminology and nomenclature for pancreatobiliary cytology: the Papanicolaou Society of Cytopathology guidelines. Diagn Cytopathol. 2014;42(4):338–50.
19. Nayer H, Weir EG, Sheth S, Ali SZ. Primary pancreatic lymphomas: a cytopathologic analysis of a rare malignancy. Cancer Cytopathol. 2004;102(5):315–21.
20. Deshpande V, Mino-Kenudson M, Brugge WR, Pitman MB, Fernandez-del Castillo C, Warshaw AL, Lauwers GY. Endoscopic ultrasound guided fine needle aspiration biopsy of autoimmune pancreatitis: diagnostic criteria and pitfalls. Am J Surg Pathol. 2005;29(11): 1464–71.
21. Cai G, Bernstein J, Aslan ian HR, Hui P, Chheing D. Endoscopic ultrasound-guided fine-needle aspiration biopsy of autoimmune pancreatitis: diagnostic clues and pitfalls. J Am Soc Cytopathol. 2015;4(4):211–7.
22. Krishna NB, Mehra M, Reddy AV, Agarwal B. EUS/EUS-FNA for suspected pancreatic cancer: influence of chronic pancreatitis and clinical presentation with or without obstructive jaundice on performance characteristics. Gastrointest Endosc. 2009;70(1):70–9.
23. Siddiqui AA, Kowalski TE, Shahid H, O'Donnell S, Tolin J, Loren DE, Infantolino A, Hong SK, Eloubeidi MA. False-positive EUS-guided FNA cytology for solid pancreatic lesions. Gastrointest Endosc. 2011;74(3):535–40.
24. Hruban RH, Takaori K, Klimstra DS, Adsay NV, Albores-Saavedra J, Biankin AV, Biankin SA, Compton C, Fukushima N, Furukawa T, Goggins M, Kato Y, Klöppel G, Longnecker DS, Lüttges J, Maitra A, Offerhaus GJ, Shimizu M, Yonezawa S. An illustrated consensus on the classification of pancreatic intraepithelial neoplasia and intraductal papillary mucinous neoplasms. Am J Surg Pathol. 2004;28(8):977–87.
25. Aso A, Ihara E, Osoegawa T, Nakamura K, Itaba S, Igarashi H, Ito T, Aishima S, Oda Y, Tanaka M, Takayanagi R. Key endoscopic ultrasound features of pancreatic ductal adenocarcinoma smaller than 20 mm. Scand J Gastroenterol. 2014;49(3):332–8.
26. Khashab MA, Emerson RE, DeWitt JM. Endoscopic ultrasound-guided fine-needle aspiration for the diagnosis of anaplastic pancreatic carcinoma: a single-center experience. Pancreas. 2010;39(1):88–91.
27. Rahemtullah A, Misdraji J, Pitman MB. Adenosquamous carcinoma of the pancreas: cytologic features in 14 cases. Cancer Cytopathol. 2003;99(6):372–8.
28. Sakamoto H, Kitano M, Komaki T, Noda K, Chikugo T, Kudo M. Small cell carcinoma of the pancreas: role of EUS-FNA and subsequent effective chemotherapy using carboplatin and etoposide. J Gastroenterol. 2009;44(5):432–8.
29. Schmidt CM, Matos JM, Bentrem DJ, Talamonti MS, Lillemoe KD, Bilimoria KY. Acinar cell carcinoma of the pancreas in the United States: prognostic factors and comparison to ductal adenocarcinoma. J Gastrointest Surg. 2008;12(12):2078–86.
30. Matos JM, Schmidt CM, Turrini O, Agaram NP, Niedergethmann M, Saeger HD, Merchant N, Johnson CS, Lillemoe KD, Grützmann R. Pancreatic acinar cell carcinoma: a multi-institutional study. J Gastrointest Surg. 2009;13(8):1495–502.
31. Stelow EB, Bardales RH, Shami VM, Woon C, Presley A, Mallery S, Lai R, Stanley MW. Cytology of pancreatic acinar cell carcinoma. Diagn Cytopathol. 2006;34(5):367–72.
32. Sigel CS, Klimstra DS. Cytomorphologic and immunophenotypical features of acinar cell neoplasms of the pancreas. Cancer Cytopathol. 2013;121(8):459–70.
33. Chang F, Vu C, Chandra A, Meenan J, Herbert A. Endoscopic ultrasound-guided fine needle aspiration cytology of pancreatic neuroendocrine tumours: cytomorphological and immunocytochemical evaluation. Cytopathology. 2006;17(1):10–7.

34. Chatzipantelis P, Salla C, Konstantinou P, Karoumpalis I, Sakellariou S, Doumani I. Endoscopic ultrasound-guided fine-needle aspiration cytology of pancreatic neuroendocrine tumors: a study of 48 cases. Cancer Cytopathol. 2008;114(4):255–62.
35. Bernstein J, Ustun B, Alomari A, Bao F, Aslanian HR, Siddiqui U, Chhieng D, Cai G. Performance of endoscopic ultrasound-guided fine needle aspiration in diagnosing pancreatic neuroendocrine tumors. Cytojournal. 2013;10:10.
36. Sigel CS, Krauss Silva VW, Reid MD, Chhieng D, Basturk O, Sigel KM, Daniel TD, Klimstra DS, Tang LH. Assessment of cytologic differentiation in high-grade pancreatic neuroendocrine neoplasms: a multi-institutional study. Cancer Cytopathol. 2018;126(1):44–53.
37. Dodd LG, Evans DB, Symmans F, Katz RL. Fine-needle aspiration of pancreatic extramedullary plasmacytoma: possible confusion with islet cell tumor. Diagn Cytopathol. 1994;10(4):371–5.
38. Tatsas AD, Owens CL, Siddiqui MT, Hruban RH, Ali SZ. Fine-needle aspiration of intrapancreatic accessory spleen: cytomorphologic features and differential diagnosis. Cancer Cytopathol. 2012;120(4):261–8.
39. Schreiner AM, Mansoor A, Faigel DO, Morgan TK. Intrapancreatic accessory spleen: mimic of pancreatic endocrine tumor diagnosed by endoscopic ultrasound-guided fine-needle aspiration biopsy. Diagn Cytopathol. 2008;36(4):262–5.
40. Dinarvand P, Lai J. Solid pseudopapillary neoplasm of the pancreas: a rare entity with unique features. Arch Pathol Lab Med. 2017;141(7):990–5.
41. Law JK, Stoita A, Wever W, Gleeson FC, Dries AM, Blackford A, Kiswani V, Shin EJ, Khashab MA, Canto MI, Singh VK, Lennon AM. Endoscopic ultrasound-guided fine needle aspiration improves the pre-operative diagnostic yield of solid-pseudopapillary neoplasm of the pancreas: an international multicenter case series (with video). Surg Endosc. 2014;28(9): 2592–8.
42. Jahangir S, Loya A, Siddiqui MT, Akhter N, Yusuf MA. Accuracy of diagnosis of solid pseudopapillary tumor of the pancreas on fine needle aspiration: a multi-institution experience of ten cases. Cytojournal. 2015;12:29.
43. Barkin JA, Barkin JS. Pancreatic cysts: controversies, advances, diagnoses, and therapies. Pancreas. 2017;46(6):735–41.
44. European Study Group on Cystic Tumours of the Pancreas. European evidence-based guidelines on pancreatic cystic neoplasms. Gut. 2018;67(5):789–804.
45. Singhi AD, Zeh HJ, Brand RE, Nikiforova MN, Chennat JS, Fasanella KE, Khalid A, Papachristou GI, Slivka A, Hogg M, Lee KK, Tsung A, Zureikat AH, McGrath K. American Gastroenterological Association guidelines are inaccurate in detecting pancreatic cysts with advanced neoplasia: a clinicopathologic study of 225 patients with supporting molecular data. Gastrointest Endosc. 2016;83(6):1107–17.
46. Shen J, Brugge WR, Dimaio CJ, Pitman MB. Molecular analysis of pancreatic cyst fluid: a comparative analysis with current practice of diagnosis. Cancer Cytopathol. 2009;117(3): 217–27.
47. Pitman MB, Lewandrowski K, Shen J, Sahani D, Brugge W, Fernandez-del Castillo C. Pancreatic cysts: preoperative diagnosis and clinical management. Cancer Cytopathol. 2010;118(1):1–13.
48. Reid MD, Choi H, Balci S, Akkas G, Adsay V. Serous cystic neoplasms of the pancreas: clinicopathologic and molecular characteristics. Semin Diagn Pathol. 2014;31(6):475–83.
49. Karoumpalis I, Christodoulou DK. Cystic lesions of the pancreas. Ann Gastroenterol. 2016;29(2):155–61.
50. Ketwaroo GA, Mortele KJ, Sawhney MS. Pancreatic cystic neoplasms: an update. Gastroenterol Clin North Am. 2016 Mar;45(1):67–81.
51. Belsley NA, Pitman MB, Lauwers GY, Brugge WR, Deshpande V. Serous cystadenoma of the pancreas: limitations and pitfalls of endoscopic ultrasound-guided fine-needle aspiration biopsy. Cancer Cytopathol. 2008;114(2):102–10.
52. Collins BT. Serous cystadenoma of the pancreas with endoscopic ultrasound fine needle aspiration biopsy and surgical correlation. Acta Cytol. 2013;57(3):241–51.

53. Lilo MT, VandenBussche CJ, Allison DB, Lennon AM, Younes BK, Hruban RH, Wolfgang CL, Ali SZ. Serous cystadenoma of the pancreas: potentials and pitfalls of a preoperative Cytopathologic diagnosis. Acta Cytol. 2017;61(1):27–33.
54. Crippa S, Salvia R, Warshaw AL, Domínguez I, Bassi C, Falconi M, Thayer SP, Zamboni G, Lauwers GY, Mino-Kenudson M, Capelli P, Pederzoli P, Castillo CF. Mucinous cystic neoplasm of the pancreas is not an aggressive entity: lessons from 163 resected patients. Ann Surg. 2008;247(4):571–9.
55. Stelow EB, Shami VM, Abbott TE, Kahaleh M, Adams RB, Bauer TW, Debol SM, Abraham JM, Mallery S, Policarpio-Nicolas ML. The use of fine needle aspiration cytology for the distinction of pancreatic mucinous neoplasia. Am J Clin Pathol. 2008;129(1):67–74.
56. Sigel CS, Edelweiss M, Tong LC, Magda J, Oen H, Sigel KM, Zakowski MF. Low interobserver agreement in cytology grading of mucinous pancreatic neoplasms. Cancer Cytopathol. 2015;123(1):40–50.
57. Smith AL, Abdul-Karim FW, Goyal A. Cytologic categorization of pancreatic neoplastic mucinous cysts with an assessment of the risk of malignancy: a retrospective study based on the Papanicolaou Society of Cytopathology guidelines. Cancer Cytopathol. 2016;124(4):285–93.
58. Fernández-del Castillo C, Adsay NV. Intraductal papillary mucinous neoplasms of the pancreas. Gastroenterology. 2010;139(3):708–13, 713.e1-2
59. Maire F, Couvelard A, Hammel P, Ponsot P, Palazzo L, Aubert A, Degott C, Dancour A, Felce-Dachez M, O'toole D, Lévy P, Ruszniewski P. Intraductal papillary mucinous tumors of the pancreas: the preoperative value of cytologic and histopathologic diagnosis. Gastrointest Endosc. 2003;58(5):701–6.
60. Emerson RE, Randolph ML, Cramer HM. Endoscopic ultrasound-guided fine-needle aspiration cytology diagnosis of intraductal papillary mucinous neoplasm of the pancreas is highly predictive of pancreatic neoplasia. Diagn Cytopathol. 2006;34(7):457–62.
61. Adsay NV, Merati K, Basturk O, Iacobuzio-Donahue C, Levi E, Cheng JD, Sarkar FH, Hruban RH, Klimstra DS. Pathologically and biologically distinct types of epithelium in intraductal papillary mucinous neoplasms: delineation of an "intestinal" pathway of carcinogenesis in the pancreas. Am J Surg Pathol. 2004;28(7):839–48.
62. Volmar KE, Jones CK, Xie HB. Metastases in the pancreas from nonhematologic neoplasms: report of 20 cases evaluated by fine-needle aspiration. Diagn Cytopathol. 2004;31(4):216–20.
63. DeWitt J, Jowell P, Leblanc J, McHenry L, McGreevy K, Cramer H, Volmar K, Sherman S, Gress F. EUS-guided FNA of pancreatic metastases: a multicenter experience. Gastrointest Endosc. 2005;61(6):689–96.
64. Layfield LJ, Hirschowitz SL, Adler DG. Metastatic disease to the pancreas documented by endoscopic ultrasound guided fine-needle aspiration: a seven-year experience. Diagn Cytopathol. 2012;40(3):228–33.
65. El Hajj II, LeBlanc JK, Sherman S, Al-Haddad MA, Cote GA, McHenry L, DeWitt JM. Endoscopic ultrasound-guided biopsy of pancreatic metastases: a large single-center experience. Pancreas. 2013;42(3):524–30.
66. Waters L, Si Q, Caraway N, Mody D, Staerkel G, Sneige N. Secondary tumors of the pancreas diagnosed by endoscopic ultrasound-guided fine-needle aspiration: a 10-year experience. Diagn Cytopathol. 2014;42(9):738–43.
67. Smith AL, Odronic SI, Springer BS, Reynolds JP. Solid tumor metastases to the pancreas diagnosed by FNA: a single-institution experience and review of the literature. Cancer Cytopathol. 2015;123(6):347–55.
68. Alomari AK, Ustun B, Aslanian HR, Ge X, Chhieng D, Cai G. Endoscopic ultrasound-guided fine-needle aspiration diagnosis of secondary tumors involving the pancreas: an institution's experience. Cytojournal. 2016;13:1.
69. Krishna SG, Bhattacharya A, Ross WA, Ladha H, Porter K, Bhutani MS, Lee JH. Pretest prediction and diagnosis of metastatic lesions to the pancreas by endoscopic ultrasound-guided fine needle aspiration. J Gastroenterol Hepatol. 2015;30(10):1552–60.

70. Varghese L, Ngae MY, Wilson AP, Crowder CD, Gulbahce HE, Pambuccian SE. Diagnosis of metastatic pancreatic mesenchymal tumors by endoscopic ultrasound-guided fine-needle aspiration. Diagn Cytopathol. 2009;37(11):792–802.
71. Samad A, Conway AB, Attam R, Jessurun J, Pambuccian SE. Cytologic features of pancreatic adenocarcinoma with "vacuolated cell pattern." Report of a case diagnosed by endoscopic ultrasound-guided fine-needle aspiration. Diagn Cytopathol. 2014;42(4):302–7.
72. Gilani SM, Tashjian R, Danforth R, Fathallah L. Metastatic renal cell carcinoma to the pancreas: diagnostic significance of fine-needle aspiration cytology. Acta Cytol. 2013;57(4):418–22.
73. Pannala R, Hallberg-Wallace KM, Smith AL, Nassar A, Zhang J, Zarka M, Reynolds JP, Chen L. Endoscopic ultrasound-guided fine needle aspiration cytology of metastatic renal cell carcinoma to the pancreas: a multi-center experience. Cytojournal. 2016;13:24.
74. Safo AO, Li RW, Vickers SM, Schmechel SC, Pambuccian SE. Endoscopic ultrasound-guided fine-needle aspiration diagnosis of clear-cell pancreatic endocrine neoplasm in a patient with von Hippel-Lindau disease: a case report. Diagn Cytopathol. 2009;37(5):365–72.
75. Levy GH, Finkelstein A, Harigopal M, Chhieng D, Cai G. Cytoplasmic vacuolization: an under-recognized cytomorphologic feature in endocrine tumors of the pancreas. Diagn Cytopathol. 2013;41(7):623–8.
76. Sadaf S, Loya A, Akhtar N, Yusuf MA. Role of endoscopic ultrasound-guided-fine needle aspiration biopsy in the diagnosis of lymphoma of the pancreas: a clinicopathological study of nine cases. Cytopathology. 2017;28(6):536–41.

Chapter 13
Gastrointestinal Tract

Rita Abi-Raad and Guoping Cai

Introduction

In gastrointestinal tract, a cytologic sample may be adjunct to a core biopsy, or the sole sample from the lesions [1–7] that may be inaccessible or pose significant risk of complications such as bleeding or perforation from standard biopsy [1], and when other modalities have failed [8]. Rapid on-site evaluation (ROSE) is used to strengthen the cytopathologic analysis. Immediate assessment of cytology specimens by a cytopathologist at the time of the procedure has been shown to reduce the frequency of nondiagnostic specimens regardless of tumor size [9–11] while improving agreement with final interpretation [12].

Material for cytomorphologic examination may be obtained by various means, depending on the location and type of tumors. Endoscopic brushings are particularly useful for strictured lesions as well as broad surface precancerous lesions such as Barrett's esophagus and chronic ulcerative colitis. Esophageal brushings are however mostly performed to exclude Candida infection, gastric brushings are usually performed to distinguish benign from malignant gastric ulcers, and rectal brushings may be performed on a rectal mass to rule out malignancy. Deeper/submucosal and mural lesions may be sampled by fine needle aspiration (FNA) with assistance of endoscopic ultrasound [13]. When a tissue biopsy is taken, imprint cytology is particularly useful as an immediate assessment of adequacy of the biopsy sample and may also be helpful for triaging specimens. Air-dried smears should first be screened at low power to assess background, overall cellularity, cellular preservation, and architectural arrangements. Next, high-power systematic examination should be performed for the presence of cytologic abnormalities.

The cytomorphologic evaluation of gastrointestinal malignancies is highly dependent on the availability of expertise in procuring, processing, and evaluating the cyto-

R. Abi-Raad (✉) · G. Cai
Department of Pathology, Yale University School of Medicine, New Haven, CT, USA
e-mail: rita.abiraad@yale.edu; guoping.cai@yale.edu

G. Cai, A. J. Adeniran (eds.), *Rapid On-site Evaluation (ROSE)*,
https://doi.org/10.1007/978-3-030-21799-0_13

logic specimens. The involved pathologist should be aware of the clinical, laboratory, and imaging data regarding the lesions sampled, and the primary task is to differentiate lesional material from non-lesional native tissue as both may be sampled. It is important to be aware of where and how the lesions are sampled in order to avoid potential pitfalls. Once lesional tissue has been identified, the specimens should be appropriately triaged for ancillary studies, such as culture and flow cytometry, or saved for cell block for potential immunocytochemistry and molecular analysis.

Diagnostic Considerations

Specimen Adequacy Assessment

- There are no well-established criteria for requirement of certain cellularity.
- In general, the specimen is considered adequate when the cells on the smear explain clinical and radiologic findings.
- If the lesion includes a solid component, cyst contents only are considered inadequate sampling; cyst contents only are considered adequate if the lesion of interest is a simple cyst such as duplication cyst.

Approach for Mucosal Lesions

- Mucosal lesions are often sampled by brushing rather than fine needle aspiration biopsy.
- Based on the on-site findings and clinical presentation or impression, the lesion should be classified into a neoplastic and a nonneoplastic process.
- If a neoplasm is suspected, endoscopic tissue biopsy should be recommended due to the difficulty in determining the degree of dysplasia and invasiveness of the lesion on cytological material.
- If a nonneoplastic lesion is favored, such as infection, additional material should be sent for culture or saved for special stains.

Approach for Submucosal Lesions or Lesions Arisen from the Wall of Gastrointestinal Tract

- The lesions may include infiltrating tumors, lymphoproliferative disorders, and spindle cell tumors such as gastrointestinal stromal tumor and leiomyoma, which are best evaluated by fine needle aspiration biopsy.
- It is important to recognize lesional material during on-site evaluation; lymphoid cells from submucosal chronic inflammation or lymph node and spindle cells from gastrointestinal wall may sometimes cause confusion.

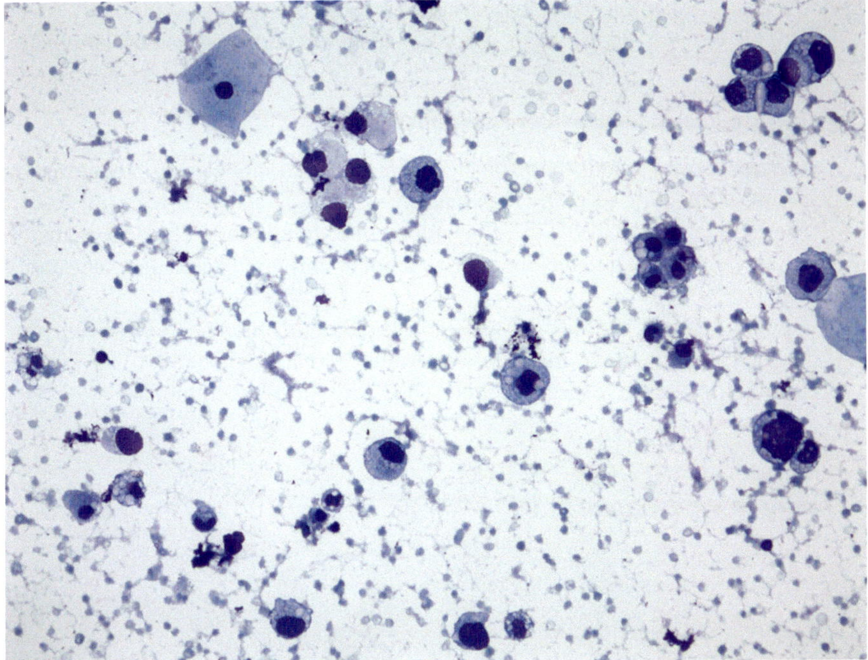

Fig. 13.1 Metastatic urothelial carcinoma to esophagus. Metastatic malignant single cells to the esophagus in a patient with history of urothelial carcinoma (Diff-Quik stain, ×200)

- If abundant lymphocytes are present, additional samples should be obtained and saved in RPMI for flow cytometry study. Excessive samples can also be saved to prepare a cell block for potential immunocytochemical work-up.
- If a spindle cell neoplasm is suspected based on the cellularity or cytomorphology, additional passes should be performed and aspirate material should be saved for a cell block. Diagnosis and classification of spindle cell neoplasm require immunocytochemical characterization.
- An infiltrating tumor may represent a primary neoplasm, metastasis, or directly invading from surrounding organs. In all cases, additional passes should be saved for a cell block for immunocytochemistry to rule out a metastasis (Fig. 13.1).

Esophagus

Normal Elements

1. Intermediate and superficial squamous cells

   - Squamous epithelial cells (superficial and intermediate types) in sheets, clusters, and single cells.

- Parabasal squamous cells may occur as a result of vigorous scraping.
- Round to oval nuclei have a smooth contour and a vesicular chromatin pattern.

2. Columnar glandular cells in distal esophagus

   - Originate from glands in the distal esophagus or from the gastric mucosa as a result of brushing reaching the stomach.
   - Small to large flat sheets of cells with distinct cellular borders, delicate cytoplasm, small round nuclei, finely granular chromatin, and inconspicuous nucleoli.
   - Replacement of the normal squamous epithelium lining the esophagus by metaplastic columnar epithelium (Barrett's esophagus) should always to be taken into account, especially when cells with mucus secretion are present.

Nonneoplastic Lesions [14]

1. Candida: most common esophageal infection

   A. Cytomorphologic features

      - Fungal organisms with yeast forms and pseudohyphae
      - Reactive squamous cells
      - Mixed inflammatory cells

   B. Tips and pitfalls

      - Brushings should be taken from the center of the ulcer and the edges
      - More sensitive than biopsies (oral contamination is not an issue because brush is contained within a sheath)

2. Cytomegalovirus: often seen in immunocompromised individuals

   A. Cytomorphologic features

      - Enlarged cells with intranuclear cytoplasmic inclusions, owl-eye nuclear inclusions
      - Infects epithelial, stromal, and endothelial cells

   B. Tips and pitfalls

      - The large intranuclear inclusions of many viral infections can be mistaken for the macronucleoli of repair or malignancy. Reactive cells can become enlarged and hyperchromatic.
      - The classic intranuclear inclusions are not seen as a reactive phenomenon or malignancy. Additional material for cell block analysis is recommended.

3. Herpes simplex virus

   A. Cytomorphologic features

      - Multinucleation, nuclear molding, chromatin margination (3Ms)
      - Dirty/necrotic background, reactive/reparative squamous cells

   B. Tips and pitfalls

      - The large intranuclear inclusions of many viral infections can be mistaken for the macronucleoli of repair or malignancy.
      - Look for multinucleated cells with nuclear molding.

4. Duplication cyst [15, 16]

   A. Cytomorphologic features

      - Squamous and ciliated cells, hemosiderin-laden macrophages, and detached ciliary tufts
      - Background with proteinaceous material, debris, and crystals

   B. Tips and pitfalls

      - Duplication cysts can sometimes contain solid secretions leading to misclassification of these lesions as soft tissue masses by imaging. The most common differential diagnosis by endoscopic ultrasound is GIST.
      - FNA smears of duplication cysts are paucicellular with only scattered epithelial cells if any.

5. Reparative epithelium

   Mucosal injuries, ulceration, and infections evoke reactive and reparative changes which may be mistaken for dysplasia and carcinoma.

   A. Cytomorphologic features

      - Two-dimensional/flat cohesive sheets with streaming pattern (school of fish), no single cells, uniformly enlarged nuclei, smooth nuclear membranes, fine chromatin, prominent nucleoli, normal mitosis, inflammation.
      - Radiation-/chemotherapy-induced changes produce proportionate cellular and nucleomegaly, multinucleation, cytoplasmic metachromasia, and nuclear and cytoplasmic vacuolation.

   B. Tips and pitfalls

      - Repair, dysplasia, and invasive carcinoma may share some cytomorphologic features including nuclear enlargement and prominent nucleolus.
      - Repair shows cohesive, flat, uniform sheets.
      - Dysplasia shows occasional three-dimensional clusters and/or slightly dyshesive sheets, pleomorphic cells, no/rare single cells, and clean background.

- Invasive carcinoma shows many tight/loose three-dimensional clusters and/or dyshesive sheets with markedly pleomorphic cells with crowding and overlapping, single cells, coarse chromatin, thick irregular nuclear membranes, and background tumor diathesis.

Precursor/Malignant Lesions

1. Barrett's esophagus [17, 18]

   A. Cytomorphologic features

   - Single cells or honeycomb sheet of glandular cells on brush cytology
   - Scattered or admixed goblet cells characterized by single large cytoplasmic vacuole displacing the nucleus

   B. Tips and pitfalls

   - Complimentary to multiple endoscopic biopsies
   - Not specific, can sample glandular cells of cardia with neutral mucin (different from acid mucin)
   - Should be correlated with endoscopic findings

2. Low-grade dysplasia [19, 20]

   A. Cytomorphologic features

   - Cohesive/flat groups, stratification, mucin depletion, mild atypia with slightly enlarged nuclei

   B. Tips and pitfalls

   - Significant intra- and interobserver variation.
   - Low-grade dysplasia is difficult to differentiate from reactive changes and even from high-grade dysplasia.

3. High-grade dysplasia [19–22]

   A. Cytomorphologic features

   - Rare finding in cytologic preparations
   - Clean background, architectural abnormality, crowded groups, rounding of cells, rare isolated cells, higher cellularity, higher N:C ratio, coarse chromatin, mild nuclear membrane irregularity

   B. Tips and pitfalls

   - High-grade dysplasia resembles adenocarcinoma but lacks tumor diathesis, cellular dispersion, and discohesive single cells.
   - It is clinically important to grade dysplasia as the management for high-grade dysplasia differs with either more frequent surveillance intervals or resection.

4. Adenocarcinoma [19–22]

   Often located at mid- and distal third of the esophagus in the setting of Barrett's esophagus

   A. Cytomorphologic features

      - Grungy tumor diathesis, high cellularity, marked architectural abnormality (3D clusters, sheets with overlapping and loss of polarity, loosely cohesive groups and marked dyshesion with abundant single cells).
      - The cytoplasm is variable in amount, delicate, and finely granular and may show vacuolation.
      - The tumor cell nuclei are enlarged with high N:C ratio and pleomorphic, have irregular nuclear membranes and coarse chromatin, and show prominent nucleoli.
      - A background of Barrett's intestinal metaplasia may be present.

   B. Tips and pitfalls

      - Differential diagnosis includes severe repair, high-grade dysplasia in Barrett's epithelium, and poorly differentiated squamous cell carcinoma.

5. Squamous cell carcinoma

   A. Cytomorphologic features (Fig. 13.2)

      - Well-differentiated squamous cell carcinoma: prominent necrosis, variable cell shapes, keratinized cytoplasm, angulated hyperchromatic/pyknotic nuclei

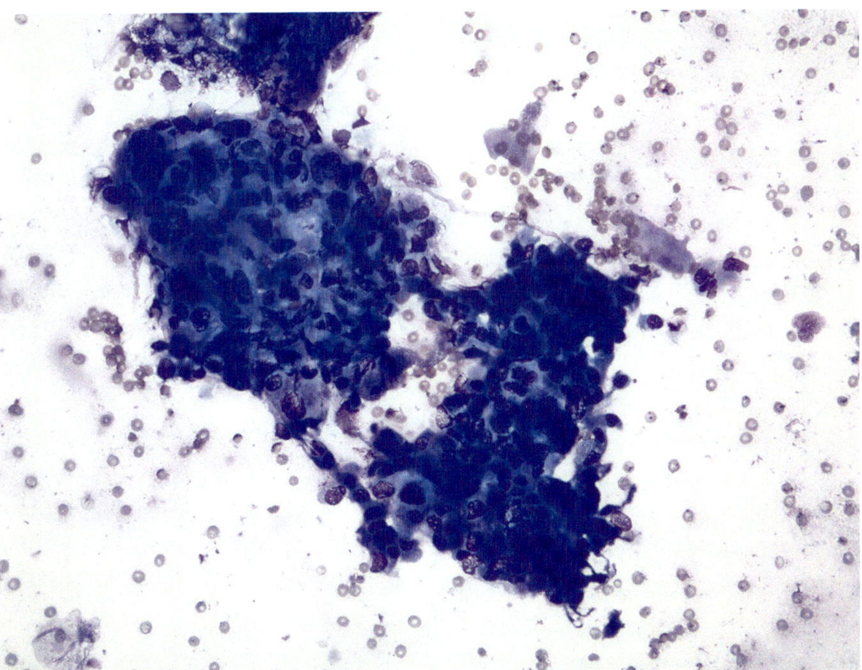

Fig. 13.2 Squamous cell carcinoma of esophagus. Crowded group of malignant cells with overlapping, high N:C ratio (top) adjacent to a fragment of muscularis (bottom) (Diff-Quik stain, ×200)

- Poorly differentiated squamous cell carcinoma: prominent necrosis, isolated tumor cells with increased N:C ratio, dense cytoplasm with sharply defined borders and less keratinization, coarse chromatin with less nuclear angulation, variably prominent nucleoli
- Other squamous cell carcinoma variants: verrucous carcinoma and adenosquamous carcinoma

B. Tips and pitfalls

- Differential diagnosis includes reactive changes, dysplasia (no tumor diathesis), and adenocarcinoma.

Benign Tumors or Tumors with Uncertain Behavior

1. Gastrointestinal stromal tumor (GIST) [23–25]

A. Cytomorphologic features (Fig. 13.3)

- Large tissue fragments of crowded, spindled, or epithelioid cells with wispy cytoplasm, paranuclear vacuoles.

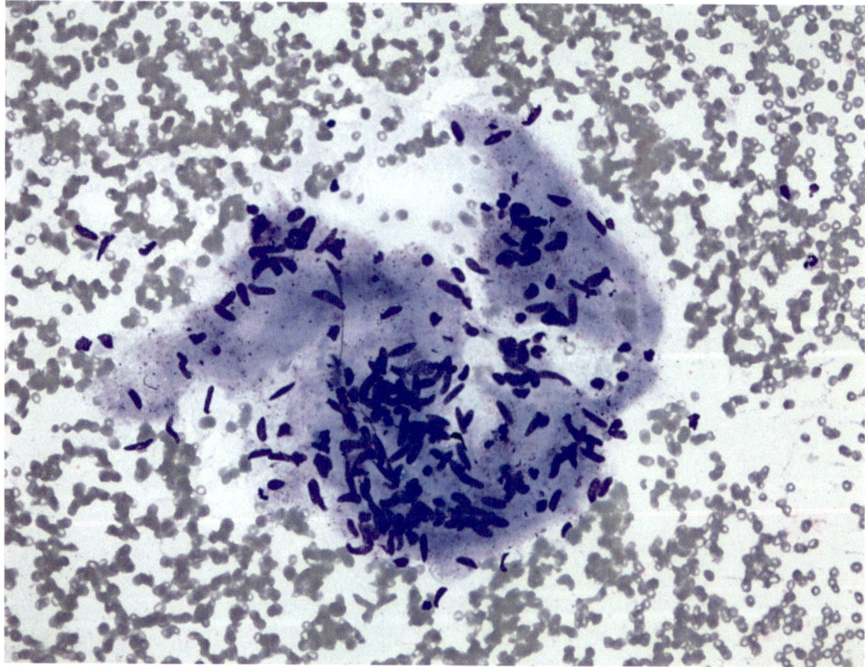

Fig. 13.3 Gastrointestinal stromal tumor of esophagus. Spindle-shaped group of cells with bland chromatin (Diff-Quik stain, ×200)

- Cells may resemble mesenchymal elements of normal esophagus. Rounded epithelioid cells with vacuolated cytoplasm may be present.
- Presence of necrosis or brisk mitosis suggests a diagnosis of malignant GIST.

B. Tips and pitfalls

- Should be sampled by fine needle aspiration; brushing often nondiagnostic.
- Differential diagnosis includes normal fragments of muscularis propria, especially when only rare spindle cell fragments are present. Increased cellularity and nuclear crowding within the fragments favor GIST.

2. Leiomyoma

A. Cytomorphologic features (Fig. 13.4)

- Spindled cells, more common in esophagus and colorectum than in stomach

B. Tips and pitfalls

- Differential diagnosis may include normal smooth muscle cells from gastrointestinal wall. Increased cellularity favors a neoplastic process.
- Metastatic lesions such as spindle cell melanoma should also be in the differential.

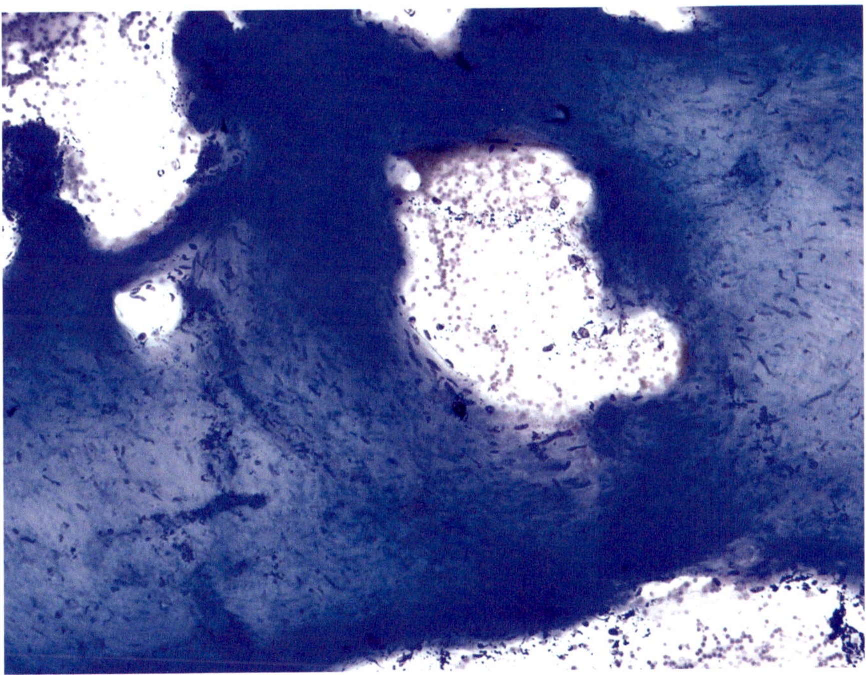

Fig. 13.4 Leiomyoma of the esophagus. Spindle-shaped cells with abundant fibrillar cytoplasm (Diff-Quik stain, ×100)

3. Granular cell tumor [26, 27]
   Rare, incidental, occurs mostly in distal esophagus

   A. Cytomorphologic features

      - Nests of cells with large/round polygonal cells with abundant granular cytoplasm, small pyknotic nuclei, and absence of mitotic figures

   B. Tips and pitfalls

      - The differential diagnosis includes metastatic carcinoma (single cells with high N:C ratio, coarse chromatin) and melanoma (large nuclei with prominent nucleoli and intracytoplasmic melanin pigments).
      - Nucleoli are prominent in melanoma, while granular cell tumor shows only pyknotic nuclei.
      - Malignant cells in carcinoma are usually pleomorphic and more atypical compared to granular cell tumor.

Stomach

Normal Element – Gastric Epithelium (Fig. 13.5)

- Mucus-secreting uniform cuboidal to columnar cells in large cohesive sheets, with a honeycomb arrangement and clean background.

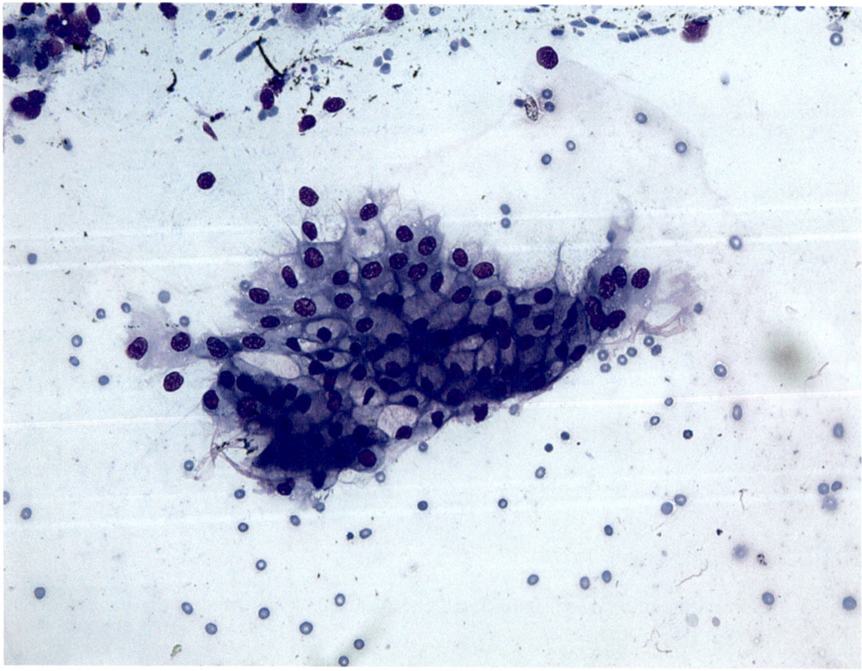

Fig. 13.5 Normal foveolar gastric epithelium (Diff-Quik stain, ×200)

- The nuclei are basally situated and have a fine chromatin pattern.
- Parietal, chief, and neuroendocrine cells are rarely seen in brush specimens.

Nonneoplastic: Infections

1. *Helicobacter pylori* [28, 29]

   Helicobacter pylori infection may be asymptomatic or present with chronic gastritis or ulceration. It is a cofactor in the development of gastric carcinoma and lymphoma.

   A. Cytomorphologic features

   - Short curved or spiral-shaped rods that inhabit the mucus covering the epithelial surface of the gastric mucosa
   - Reactive changes secondary to gastritis and ulceration

   B. Tips and pitfalls

   - Brush cytology: Increased sensitivity compared to biopsy (samples wider area of antral mucosa compared to biopsy)
   - Imprint cytology of gastric biopsy: Increased sensitivity if imprint cytology is combined with biopsy
   - Should be taken from the center of the ulcer and the edges

2. Atypical mycobacteria

   A. Cytomorophologic features

   - Abundant macrophages with abundant vacuolated cytoplasm
   - Reactive epithelial cells

   B. Tips and pitfalls

   - Should be differentiated from granular cell tumor and signet ring cell carcinoma

Precursor/Malignant Lesions

1. Low-grade dysplasia/adenoma

   Often associated with atrophic gastritis

   A. Cytomorphologic features

   - Crowded flat sheets or cohesive 3-dimensional clusters, uniform nucleomegaly, high N:C ratio

   B. Tips and pitfalls

   - Cannot be reliably differentiated from reactive changes and should not be diagnosed definitively

2. High-grade dysplasia [22]

   A. Cytomorphologic features

      - Similar to carcinoma but is less cellular
      - Some irregular cellular arrangement, nuclear atypia, dyshesion
      - No tumor diathesis, no cell dispersion, no marked pleomorphism

   B. Tips and pitfalls

      - High-grade dysplasia resembles adenocarcinoma but lacks tumor diathesis, cellular dispersion, and discohesive single cells.

3. Adenocarcinoma/intestinal type [22]

   A. Cytomorphologic features (Fig. 13.6)

      - Usually associated with intestinal metaplasia of the gastric epithelium and resembles colorectal carcinoma
      - Necrotic background, loosely cohesive three-dimensional clusters with loss of polarity, single malignant cells, cytologic atypia, and pleomorphism

   B. Tips and pitfalls

      - Differential diagnosis includes severe repair and high-grade dysplasia.
      - Single malignant cells are more frequently seen in adenocarcinoma compared to dysplasia.

4. Adenocarcinoma/diffuse signet ring cell type [30]

   Tumor infiltrates lamina propria with less mucosal involvement. Difficult to sample with a brush and higher rate of false negative by surface brushing technique unless ulceration is present

   A. Cytomorphologic features

      - Tumor diathesis
      - Crowded groups, loosely cohesive clusters, and isolated crescent-shaped small cells with vacuolated cytoplasm (large mucin vacuole) and angulated eccentric hyperchromatic nucleus

   B. Tips and pitfalls

      - Signet ring carcinoma can be very difficult to detect on both cytologic and histologic specimens. High degree of suspicion and high-power examination are key.
      - Some signet ring cells may have bland nuclei and be confused with histiocytes. Additional sampling for cell block is recommended to perform immunocytochemistry.

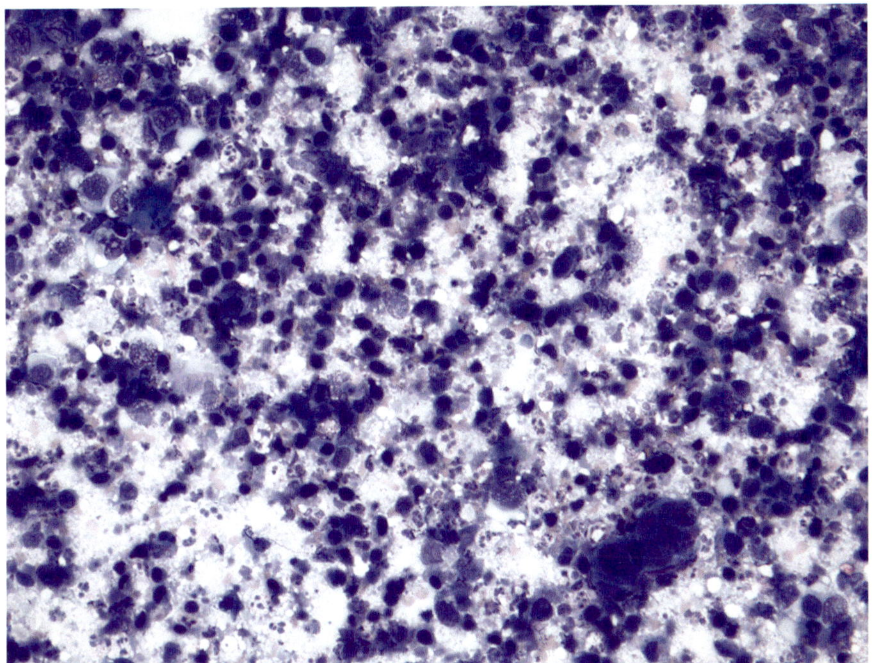

Fig. 13.6 Gastric adenocarcinoma. A group of malignant cells is seen in the lower right with abundant single cells. Note background necrosis (Diff-Quik stain, ×200)

5. Neuroendocrine tumors

   Second most common epithelial tumor of stomach. Presents as polypoid lesion

   A. Cytomorphologic features (Fig. 13.7)

      - Tumor cells are monomorphic, dyshesive, and eccentric, with moderate amount of granular cytoplasm and stippled "salt and pepper" nuclei.
      - Stripped bare nuclei may be present.

   B. Tips and pitfalls

      - Additional material should be requested for cell block preparation and will allow characterization by immunocytochemical stains.

6. Non-Hodgkin lymphoma [31]

   Second most common malignancy of the stomach, accounts for 5% of gastric malignancies. Most common site for extranodal non-Hodgkin lymphomas. Grossly polypoid, fungating, ulcerative, or infiltrative

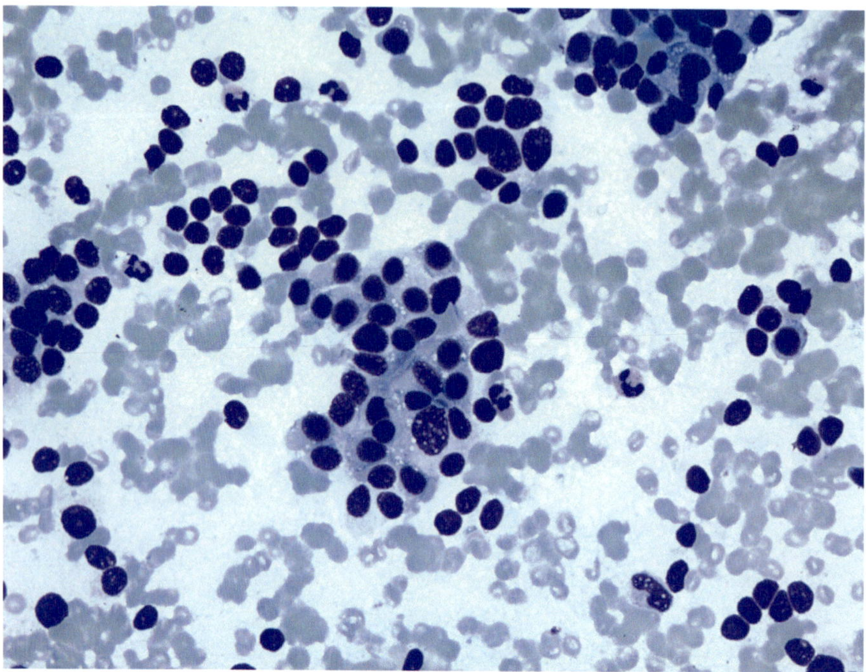

Fig. 13.7 Well-differentiated neuroendocrine tumor of the stomach. Abundant monomorphic stripped nuclei with stippled chromatin (Diff-Quik stain, ×400)

A. Cytomorphologic features

- Single cell population with dispersed monotonous cells and scant cytoplasm and lymphoglandular bodies. The nuclei have a lymphoid chromatin character.
- Classified into low-grade and high-grade lymphomas.
- Low-grade lymphoma includes follicular lymphoma and MALToma showing monomorphic small cells with scant cytoplasm (Fig. 13.8).
- Diffuse large B-cell lymphoma is the most common lymphoma of the stomach showing large pleomorphic lymphoid cells with irregular nuclear contours.

B. Tips and pitfalls

- Low-grade lymphoma should be differentiated from chronic inflammation and neuroendocrine tumor.
- High-grade lymphoma should be differentiated from poorly differentiated carcinoma.
- Additional passes should be performed for cell block preparation, and saved in RPMI for flow cytometry.

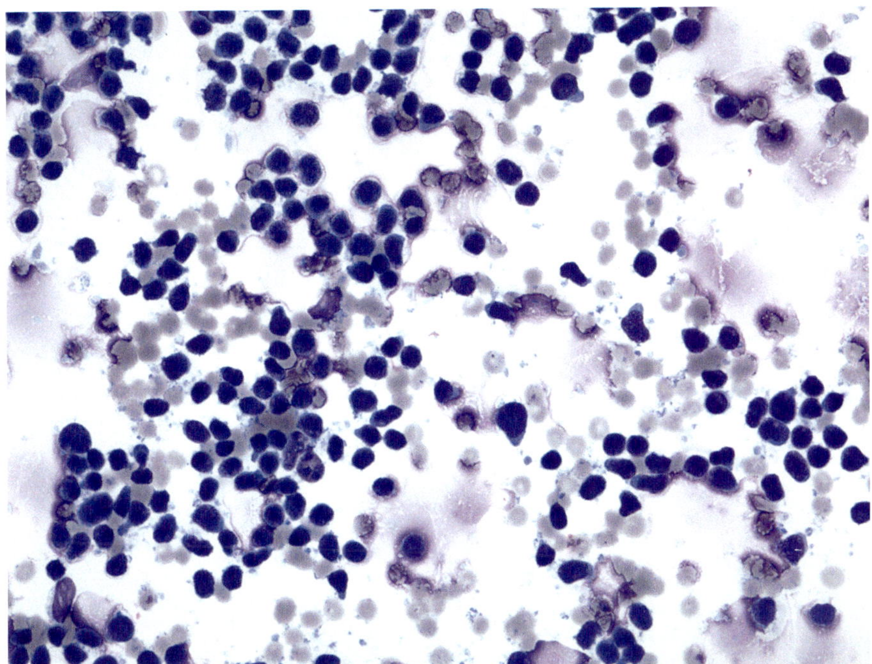

Fig. 13.8 Non-Hodgkin lymphoma of the stomach. Relative uniform single cells with lymphoglandular bodies in the background (Diff-Quik stain, ×200)

Benign Tumors or Tumors with Uncertain Behaviors

- Gastrointestinal stromal tumor and leiomyoma are the two common lesions; see Part 3 for details.

Small Intestine/Duodenum

Normal Elements – Intestinal Epithelium

- Large, flat honeycomb sheets with interspersed mucin-secreting goblet cells, giving a starry sky or "Swiss cheese" appearance.
- Brunner glands may also be present.
- Commonly seen as contaminant in EUS-FNA of the pancreatic head or contaminant in bile or pancreatic duct brushing specimens.

Nonneoplastic Infections

1. Giardia: commonly seen in immunocompetent hosts
   - Gray, pear-shaped, binucleate with four pairs of flagella
   - Reactive epithelial changes
2. Microsporidium: commonly seen in immunocompromised hosts
   - Intracellular eosinophilic rod-shaped/ovoid organisms in apical cytoplasm (1–4 μm)
   - Reactive epithelial changes
3. Cryptosporidia: commonly seen in immunocompromised hosts
   - Round and basophilic on luminal surface of cells (2–5 μm)
   - Reactive epithelial changes

Precursor/Malignant Lesions [32]

1. Low-grade dysplasia/adenoma

   A. Cytomorphologic features

   - Cohesive three-dimensional clusters of crowded columnar cells with increased N:C ratio, absent goblet cells, palisading and molding of elongated nuclei with fine chromatin and absent/small nucleoli.
   - Often associated with an adenocarcinoma.
   - Majority of tumors in the duodenum and periampullary region are well-differentiated adenocarcinomas.

   B. Tips and pitfalls

   - Difficulty in separating these well-differentiated tumors from reactive changes makes the sensitivity of diagnosis relatively low and false negatives frequent.
   - In reactive atypia, cellularity is low with scattered small groups of slightly enlarged, pleomorphic uniform cells with mildly hyperchromatic nuclei, while the presence of papillary fragments with nuclear stratification and peripheral palisading in the absence of cytologic atypia favors adenoma.
   - False-negative diagnoses may also be due to desmoplasia or poor sampling. False-positive diagnoses are rare in experienced hands.
   - The less common moderate to poorly differentiated tumors do not pose major diagnostic problems.

2. High-grade dysplasia [22, 32]

   A. Cytomorphologic features

- Clean background, higher cellularity, crowded groups with nuclear overlapping and loss of polarity, architectural abnormality
- Presence of few isolated cells
- Higher N:C ratio, coarse chromatin, mild nuclear membrane irregularity

B. Tips and pitfalls

- Adenoma with high-grade dysplasia are frequently categorized as malignant.
- High-grade dysplasia resembles adenocarcinoma but lacks tumor diathesis, cellular dispersion, and discohesive single cells.
- The difference between high-grade dysplasia and carcinoma is mostly quantitative.

Adenocarcinoma [22, 32]

A. Cytomorphologic features (Fig. 13.9)

- High cellularity, necrotic background, 3-dimensional cell balls
- Single cells
- Pleomorphism, enlarged nuclei with high N:C ratio, irregular nuclear membrane, and coarse chromatin

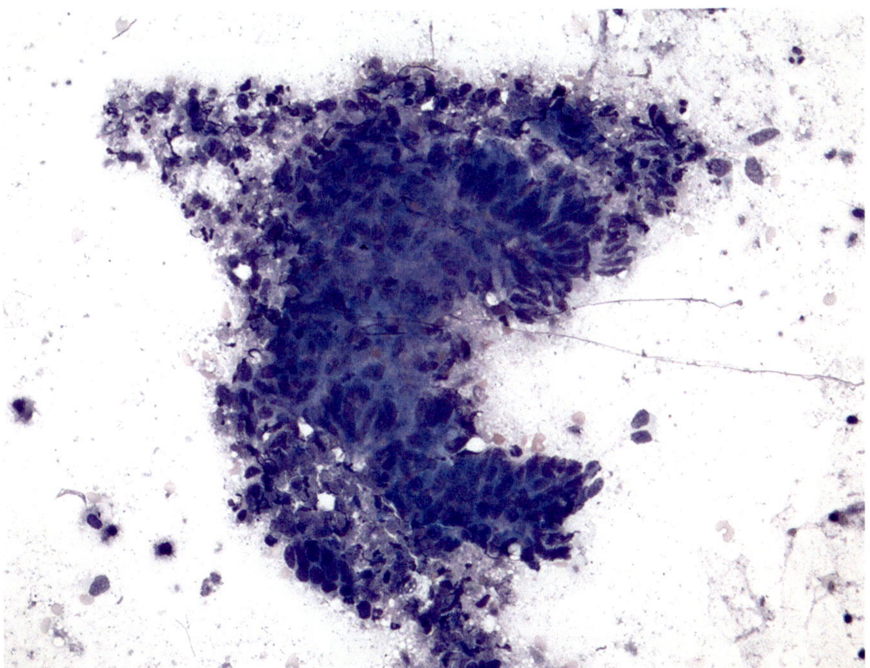

Fig. 13.9 Duodenal adenocarcinoma. Group of stratified disorganized cells with background necrosis (Diff-Quik stain, ×200)

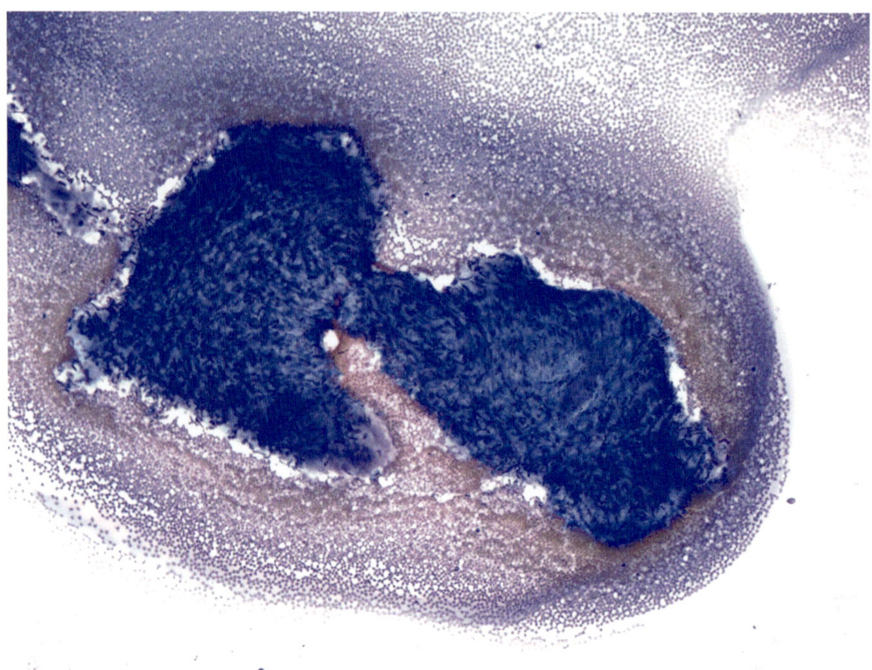

Fig. 13.10 Gastrointestinal stromal tumor of the duodenum. A cohesive group of bland spindle cells (Diff-Quik stain, ×100)

B. Tips and pitfalls

- Brush cytology and FNA cannot always differentiate between high-grade dysplasia and adenocarcinoma (cytologic sampling does not provide any advantage over biopsy diagnosis).

Benign Tumors or Tumors with Uncertain Behaviors

- Gastrointestinal stromal tumor and leiomyoma are the two common lesions; see Part 3 for details (Fig. 13.10).

References

1. Geisinger KR. Endoscopic biopsies and cytologic brushings of the esophagus are diagnostically complementary. Am J Clin Pathol. 1995;103(3):295–9.
2. Batra M, Handa U, Mohan H, Sachdev A. Comparison of cytohistologic techniques in diagnosis of gastroesophageal malignancy. Acta Cytol. 2008;52(1):77–82.

3. Jhala N, Jhala D. Gastrointestinal tract cytology: advancing horizons. Adv Anat Pathol. 2003;10(5):261–77.
4. Cohen J. Successful training in gastrointestinal endoscopy. Boston: Wiley-Blackwell; 2011.
5. Hoda RS, VandenBussche C, Hoda SA. Gastrointestinal tract cytology. In: Diagnostic liquid-based cytology. Berlin, Heidelberg: Springer; 2017.
6. Tummidi S, Kothari K, Sathe P, Agnihotri M, Fernandes G, Naik L, Jain A, Chaturvedi R. Endoscopic ultrasound guided brush/fine-needle aspiration cytology: a 15-month study. Diagn Cytopathol. 2018;46(6):461–72.
7. Chhieng D, Jhala D, Jhala N, Eltoum I, Chen V, Vickers S, Heslin M, Wilcox C, Eloubeidi M. Endoscopic ultrasound-guided fine-needle aspiration biopsy: a study of 103 cases. Cancer. 2002;96(4):232–9.
8. Chen V, Eloubeidi M. Endoscopic ultrasound-guided fine-needle aspiration of intramural and extraintestinal mass lesions: diagnostic accuracy, complication assessment, and impact on management. Endoscopy. 2005;37:984–9.
9. Jhala N, Jhala D, Eltoum I, Vickers S, Wilcox C, Chhieng D, Eloubeidi M. Endoscopic ultrasound-guided fine-needle aspiration biopsy: a powerful tool to obtain samples from small lesions. Cancer. 2004;102:239–46.
10. Klapman JB, Logrono R, Dye CE, Waxman I. Clinical impact of on-site cytopathology interpretation on endoscopic ultrasound-guided fine needle aspiration. Am J Gastroenterol. 2003;98:1289–94.
11. Chang KJ, Katz KD, Durbin TE, et al. Endoscopic ultrasound-guided fine-needle aspiration. Gastrointest Endosc. 1994;40:694–9.
12. Eloubeidi M, Tamhane A, Jhala N, Chhieng D, Jhala D, Crowe R, Eltoum I. Agreement between rapid onsite and final cytologic interpretations of EUS-guided FNA specimens: implications for the endosonographer and patient management. Am J Gastroenetrol. 2006;101:2841–7.
13. Zargar SA, Khuroo MS, Mahajan R, Jan G, Dewani K, Koul V. Endoscopic fine needle aspiration cytology in the diagnosis of gastro-esophageal and colorectal malignancies. Gut. 1991;32:745–8.
14. Cibas ES, Ducatman BS. Cytology: diagnostic principles and clinical correlates. Philadelphia: Saunders/Elsevier; 2014.
15. Napolitano V, Pezzullo A, Zeppa P, Schettino P, D'Armiento M, Palazzo A, Della Pietra C, Napolitano S, Conzo G. Foregut duplication of the stomach diagnosed by endoscopic ultrasound guided fine-needle aspiration cytology: case report and literature review. World J Surg Oncol. 2013;11:33.
16. Eloubeidi M, Cohn M, Cerfolio R, Chhieng D, Jhala N, Jhala D, Eltoum I. Endoscopic ultrasound-guided fine-needle aspiration in the diagnosis of foregut duplication cysts: the value of demonstrating detached ciliary tufts in cyst fluid. Cancer Cytopathol. 2004;102(4): 253–8.
17. Padmavathy F, Siddaraju N, Sistla SC. Role of brush cytology in the diagnosis of Barrett's esophagus: an analysis of eight cases. Diagn Cytopathol. 2010;39(1):60–4.
18. Geisinger KR, Teot LA, Richter JE. A comparative cytopathologic and histologic study of atypia, dysplasia, and adenocarcinoma in Barrett's esophagus. Cancer. 1992;69(1):8–16.
19. Hughes J, Cohen M. Is the cytologic diagnosis of esophageal glandular dysplasia feasible? Diagn Cytopathol. 1998;18(4):312–6.
20. Wang HH, Doria MI, Purohit-Buch S, Schnell T, Sontag S, Chejfec G. Barrett's esophagus. The cytology of dysplasia in comparison to benign and malignant lesions. Acta Cytol. 1992;36(1):60–4.
21. Pan QJ, Roth M, Guo H, Kochman M, Wang G, Henry M, Wei WQ, Giffen C, Lu N, Abnet C, Hao C, Taylor P, Qiao YL, Dawsy S. Cytologic detection of esophageal squamous cell carcinoma and its precursor lesions using balloon samplers and liquid-based cytology in asymptomatic adults in Linxian, China. Acta Cytol. 2008;52(1):14–23.
22. Wang HH, Ducatman BS, Thibault S. Cytologic features of premalignant glandular lesions in the upper gastrointestinal tract. Acta Cytol. 1991;35(2):199–203.

23. Vander Noot M, Eloubeidi M, Chen V, Eltoum I, Jhala D, Jhala N, Syed S, Chhieng D. Diagnosis of gastrointestinal tract lesions by endoscopic ultrasound-guided fine-needle aspiration biopsy. Cancer Cytopathol. 2004;102(3):157–63.
24. Elliott D, Fanning C, Caraway N. The utility of fine-needle aspiration in the diagnosis of gastrointestinal stromal tumors. A cytomorphologic and immunohistochemical analysis with emphasis on malignant tumors. Cancer Cytopathol. 2006;25(108):49–55.
25. Fu K, Eloubeidi M, Jhala N, Jhala D, Chhieng D, Eltoum I. Diagnosis of gastrointestinal stromal tumor by endoscopic ultrasound-guided fine needle aspiration biopsy – a potential pitfall. Ann Diagn Pathol. 2002;6(5):294–301.
26. Wang J, Repertinger-Fisher S, Mittal S, Deng C. A large esophageal granular cell tumor with review of literature. J Cancer Sci Ther. 2011;3(9):213–5.
27. Goldblum JR, Rice TW, Zuccaro G, Richter JE. Granular cell tumor of the esophagus: a clinical and pathologic study of 13 cases. Ann Thorac Surg. 1996;62(3):860–5.
28. Mostaghni A, Afarid M, Eghbaki S, Kumar P. Evaluation of brushing cytology in the diagnosis of Helicobacter pylori gastritis. Acta Cytol. 2008;52(5):597–601.
29. Mendoza ML, Martin-Rabadan P, Carrion I, et al. Helicobacter pylori infection. Rapid diagnosis with brush cytology. Acta Cytol. 1993;37:181–5.
30. Hughes J, Leigh C, Raab S, Hook S, Cohen M, Suhrland M. Cytologic criteria for the brush diagnosis of gastric adenocarcinoma. Cancer Cytopathol. 1998;84(5):289–94.
31. Pugh JL, Jhala NC, Eloubeidi MA, Chhieng DC, Eltoum IA, Crowe DR, Varadarajulu S, Jhala DN. Diagnosis of deep-seated lymphoma and leukemia by endoscopic ultrasound-guided fine-needle aspiration biopsy. Am J Clin Pathol. 2006;125(5):703–9.
32. DeFrain C, Chang C, Srikureja W, Nguyen P, Gu M. Cytologic features and diagnostic pitfalls of primary ampullary tumors by endoscopic ultrasound-guided fine-needle aspiration biopsy. Cancer Cytopathol. 2005;105(5):289–97.

Part VI
Evolving Concepts of Rapid On-Site Evaluation

Chapter 14
Cytological Evaluation During Intraoperative Consultation

Guoping Cai

Intraoperative consultation is a pathology service to provide guidance to surgeons by pathologists through rapid examination of the specimens obtained intraoperatively. A number of questions can be addressed via intraoperative consultation; however, the request for intraoperative consultation should be limited to those that really influence intraoperative patient management. The most common applications include assessment of surgical resection margins and evaluation of sentinel lymph node metastasis. Intraoperative consultation can also be performed to achieve a diagnosis or secure sufficient diagnostic material for a lesion of unknown etiology or undetermined nature in an exploratory surgical procedure [1–3]. The information derived from intraoperative consultation helps surgeons to decide whether additional tissue should be taken to clear surgical margins, whether additional lymph nodes should be removed when metastasis is revealed in a sentinel lymph node, and whether additional surgical procedure should be pursued in an exploratory setting.

Frozen section is the primary means of intraoperative consultation, which is a pathology laboratory procedure to perform rapid microscopic analysis of a specimen. Intraoperative cytological evaluation may provide similar information as frozen section and may sometimes reveal features that are difficult to be recognized through routine frozen section. Therefore, cytological evaluation can be used as an alternative to or used in combination with frozen section to improve the performance of intraoperative consultation. The use of cytological evaluation for surgical margin assessment is controversial [4, 5], but cytological approach has been widely used in intraoperative assessment of the status of sentinel lymph node [6–8] and may help determine the nature of an indeterminate lesion [9–12]. In addition, cytological approach can be performed for intraoperative evaluation of tissue that are not suitable for frozen section such as bony lesions [13–16].

G. Cai (✉)
Department of Pathology, Yale University School of Medicine, New Haven, CT, USA
e-mail: guoping.cai@yale.edu

G. Cai, A. J. Adeniran (eds.), *Rapid On-site Evaluation (ROSE)*,
https://doi.org/10.1007/978-3-030-21799-0_14

As compared to frozen section, cytological approach has a shorter turnaround time and requires less laboratory resources [17]. In addition, cytological approach allows preservation of tissue as much as possible for final histopathological evaluation. Some morphologic features might be better illustrated on cytological preparation [9–11]. However, cytological interpretation may require special competent practice training and experience, and cytological diagnosis could be challenging due to lack of architectural information and inappropriate preparation of cytology specimens.

Cytological Preparations for Intraoperative Evaluation

The most common preparations for intraoperative cytological evaluation include touch imprint and scrape preparation. Touch imprint is most likely used for evaluating status of sentinel lymph node metastasis, while scape preparation is the preferred method for assessment of an indeterminate lesion [6, 7, 9].

Touch Imprint

To prepare a touch imprint, the targeted lesion should be bisected along the longitudinal axis to allow revelation of a maximal cut surface. If the lesion is large, serial sections may be needed to increase the sensitivity of detection and avoid a false-negative diagnosis. When the lesion is sectioned, a glass slide is applied to and kept close contact with the cut surface (Fig. 14.1). The touch process should

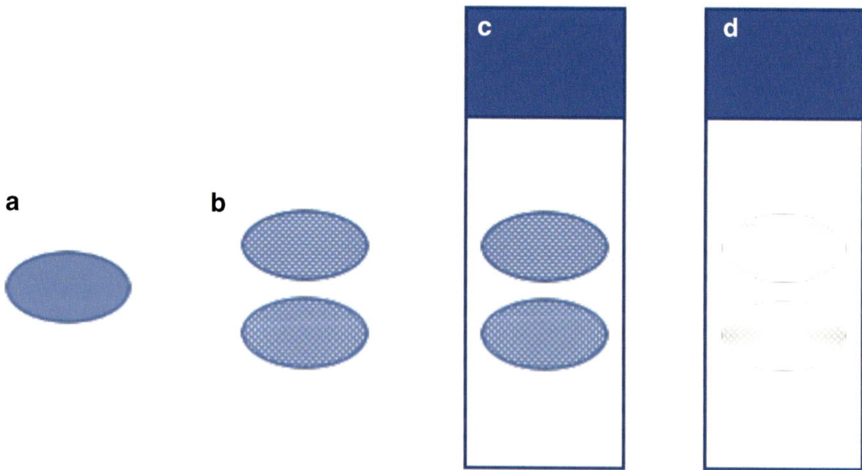

Fig. 14.1 Schematic illustration of touch imprint preparation. (**a**) Dissection, (**b**) bisection, (**c**) touching, (**d**) touch imprint

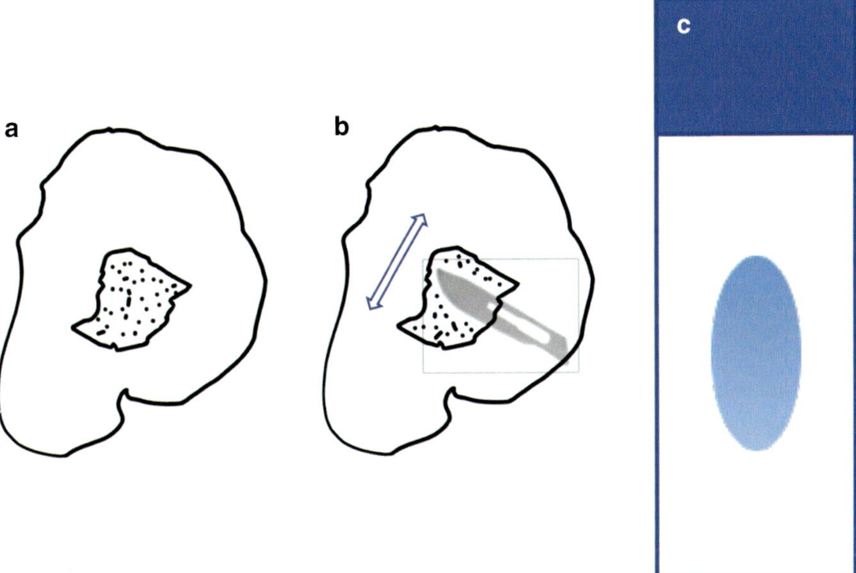

Fig. 14.2 Schematic illustration of scrape slide preparation. (**a**) Sectioning, (**b**) scraping, (**c**) scrape smear

be gentle but the imprint does need to cover the full cut surface. No excessive force should be applied to avoid damage to the tissue.

Scrape Preparation

To make a scape preparation, the targeted lesion should be bisected or sliced. The cut surfaces should be carefully examined and a representative area be chosen. A surgical blade is used to collect cells or/and small tissue fragments by gently moving the blade cutting edge back and forth along the cut surface (Fig. 14.2). The collected material will be transferred onto a glass slide and smeared using another slide. Scraping material from the specimen should avoid areas of necrosis and hemorrhage.

Stains for Cytological Evaluation

Since intraoperative cytological evaluation almost exclusively occurs in frozen section room where rapid hematoxylin-eosin (H&E) stain is routinely performed for frozen section, rapid H&E stain is also no doubt the most common stain used for intraoperative cytological preparations. However, other stains, especially Diff-Quik stain, may be advantageous to the H&E stain in assessment of some lesions such as lymphoid lesions and those matrix-containing lesions.

Rapid Hematoxylin-Eosin Stain

If rapid H&E stain is chosen for cytological evaluation, cytological specimens should be fixed immediately in 95% of ethanol after the preparation. H&E stain is superior for demonstration of nuclear details such as nuclear membrane irregularity, chromatin patterns, and nucleoli. Preparation artifacts, especially drying artifacts, may compromise or hamper accurate interpretation of cytological findings. Care should be taken to avoid drying when preparing a slide. The protocols of rapid hematoxylin-eosin stain may vary slightly at different institutions. The step-by-step protocol at our institution is detailed in Fig. 14.3.

Diff-Quik Stain

Diff-Quik stain is a rapid staining process and requires less than 1 minute to complete (Fig. 14.4). It is widely used for cytological evaluation, especially during rapid on-site evaluation, due to its easiness and quickness of the staining process. For Diff-Quik

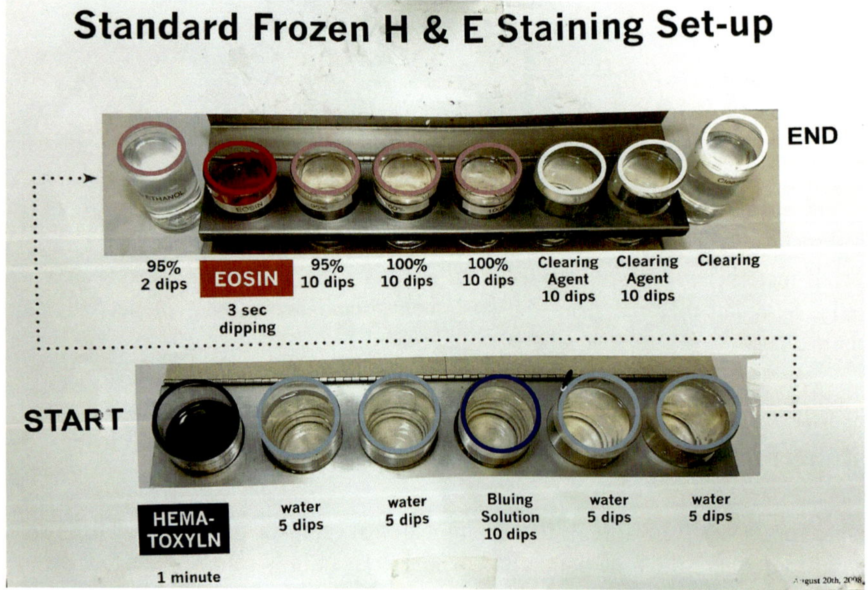

Fig. 14.3 Staining process of rapid hematoxylin-eosin stain

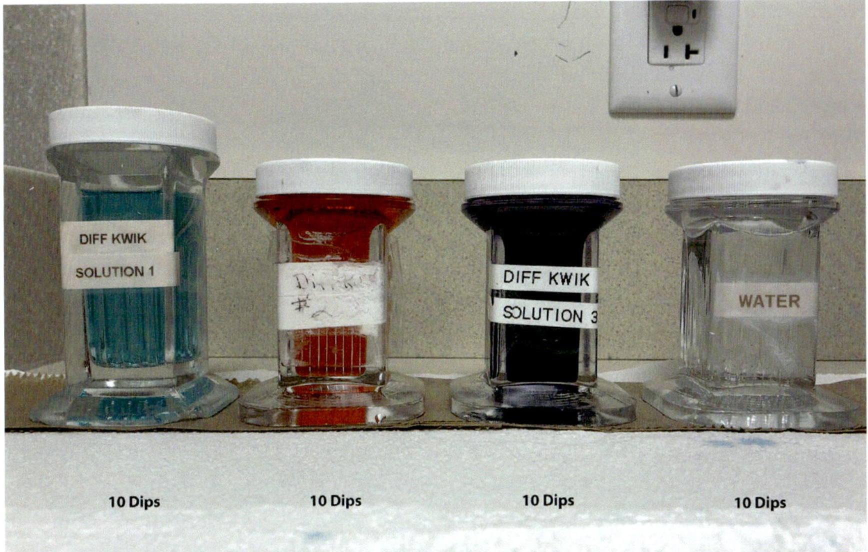

Fig. 14.4 Staining process of Diff-Quik stain

stain, the cytological preparations have to be completely air-dried prior to initiation of staining process. Diff-Quik stain is similar to the Giemsa stain that is widely used in hematology lab and therefore is the preferred stain for evaluation of lymphoproliferative disorders. Compared to H&E stain, Diff-Quik stain is better in illustrating cytoplasmic features such as cytoplasmic vacuoles, granularity, and pigments as well as highlighting background material such as mucin, colloid, and matrix.

Intraoperative Cytological Assessment of Sentinel Lymph Node

The objective for intraoperative assessment of sentinel lymph node is to determine whether the lymph node harbors metastatic tumor, which would necessitate additional lymph node sampling or removal. The sentinel lymph node biopsy is widely used in surgical management of diseases such as breast cancer and melanoma.

Metastatic Breast Carcinoma

Sentinel lymph node biopsy is well established as standard care for axillary lymph node staging in patients with early-staged breast cancers [18]. If the lymph node is found to harbor metastatic disease, axillary lymph node dissection may follow.

Frozen section is often used for intraoperative assessment of sentinel nodal metastatic status in patients with breast cancer. A large number of studies have demonstrated that cytological evaluation is also reliable for intraoperative assessment of sentinel nodal metastasis [8, 19–23]. Touch imprint is the preferred method although some studies have used scrape preparation [23, 24].

Nevertheless, cytological approach is far from being perfect, especially for its false-negative rate with the sensitivity lower than 70% [23, 25]. Also, there are other challenges and issues with cytological approach such as (1) lack of size information for the metastatic focus and higher false-negative rate in micrometastasis [26, 27], (2) the effects of neoadjuvant therapy [28–30], and (3) atypical features of lobular carcinoma [31, 32].

Diagnostic tips and pitfalls (Fig. 14.5):

- The presence of three-dimensional cell clusters on cytological preparations is highly suggestive of metastatic carcinoma since epithelial cells are cohesive and present as cell clusters on cytological preparations. It should be kept in mind that lymphohistiocytic aggregates and granulomas can mimic clusters of epithelial cells. Careful examination of cell morphology helps avoid diagnostic pitfalls.
- The tumor cells of poorly differentiated breast carcinoma can be seen as discohesive or single cells. However, the tumor cells often show significant cytological atypia.
- In most cases of lobular breast carcinoma, the tumor cells are small and uniform. They are present as single cell or loose groups, which may mimic histiocytes on cytological preparations. The tumor cells may display unique cytomorphologic features such as plasmacytoid appearance and intracytoplasmic luminal structures.

Metastatic Melanoma

Although controversies still exist, sentinel lymph node evaluation may be indicated for prognostic assessment of early-staged melanomas based on risk assessment including Breslow thickness, presence of ulceration, high mitotic rate, and/or lymphovascular invasion [33]. Sentinel lymph node status may impact future therapeutic decisions, including recommendations for active nodal ultrasound surveillance or complete lymph node dissection and adjuvant therapy. Complete lymph node dissection following a positive sentinel lymph node has been shown to have a better locoregional disease control [33, 34].

Frozen section of sentinel lymph node has been shown to be able to identify metastatic disease in patients with melanoma, which may benefit surgical decision-making [35–40]. However, relatively low sensitivity and high false-negative rate have become the major argument against the routine use of frozen section for evaluation of sentinel lymph node [40–43]. It has also been noticed that frozen section evaluation may potentially reduce accuracy of pathologic assessment of sentinel

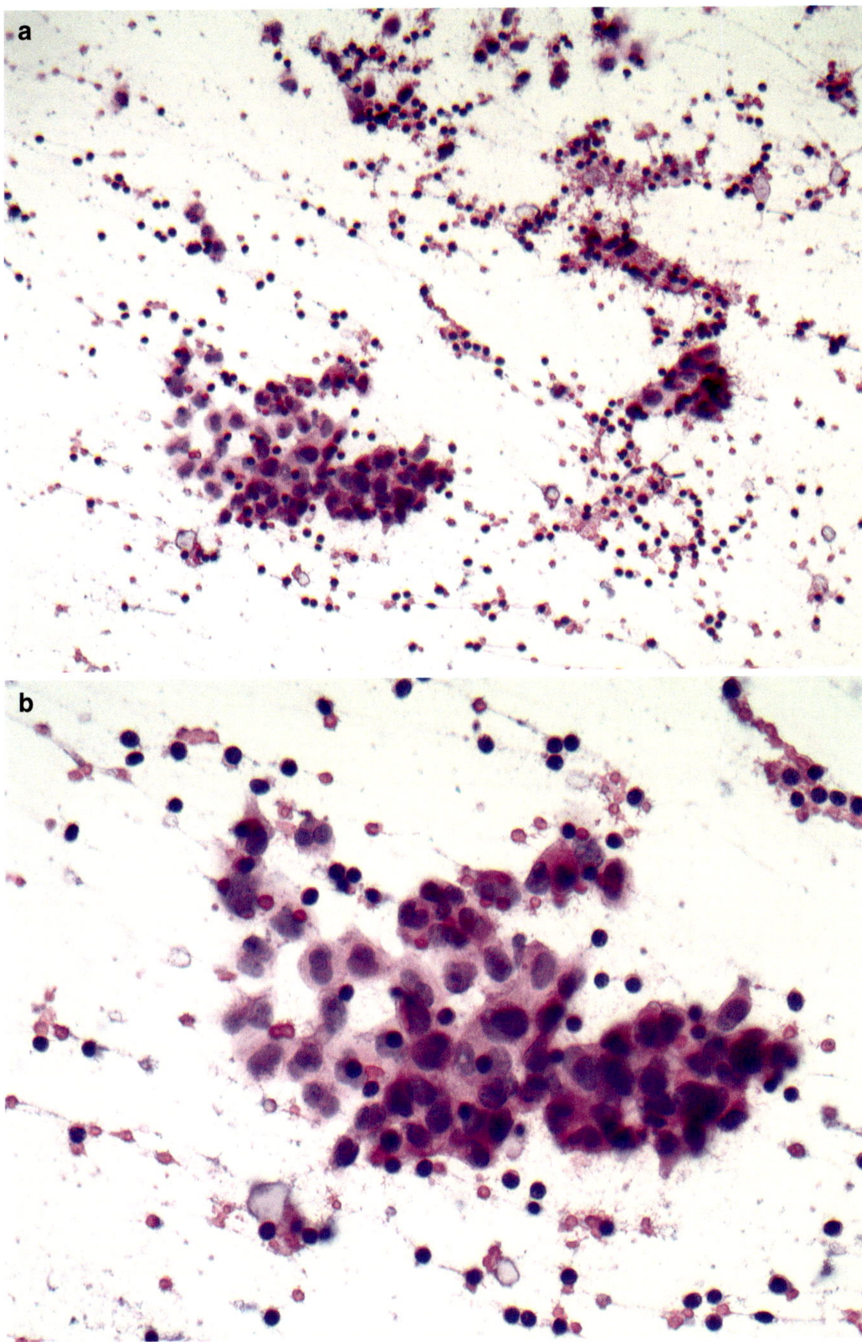

Fig. 14.5 Touch imprint of breast carcinoma metastatic to sentinel lymph node. Clusters of atypical epithelial cells with scattered lymphocytes in the background (**a**. hematoxylin-eosin stain, ×200). The tumor cells show enlarged nuclei with irregular nuclear membranes and conspicuous nucleolus (**b**. hematoxylin-eosin stain, ×400). Some tumor cells are arranged in an acinar pattern (**c**. Diff-Quik stain, ×400)

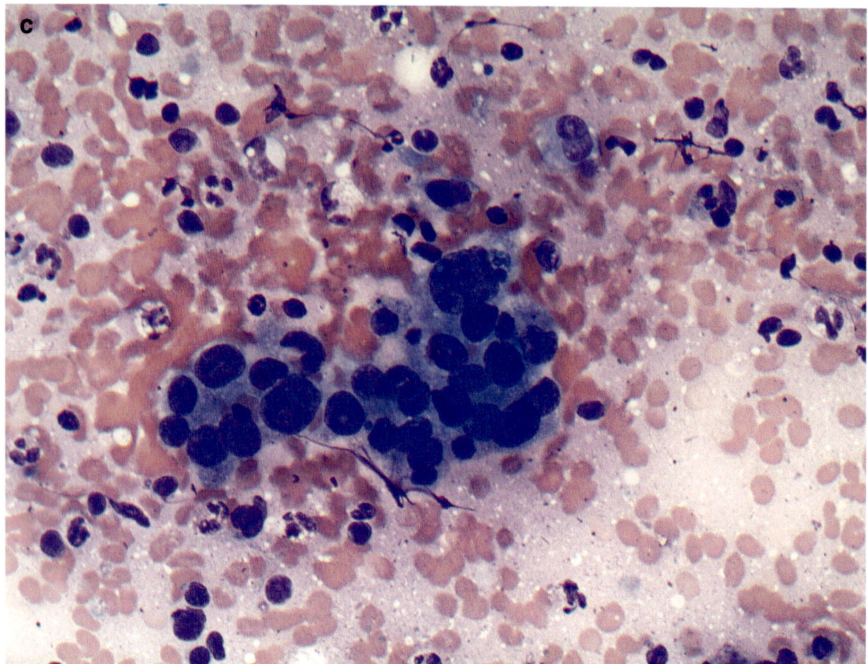

Fig. 14.5 (continued)

lymph nodes [44]. For these reasons, the status of sentinel lymph node assessment may need to be deferred upon routine pathologic evaluation [41].

Intraoperative cytological evaluation, often in the form of touch imprint, has been well documented in the literature [7, 39, 45–48]. Similar to frozen section, cytological approach has high specificity but relatively low sensitivity [45, 48]. Combining cytological approach with frozen section may slightly increase the detection sensitivity; but caution should be taken when rendering a diagnosis in challenging cases to avoid false-positive interpretation [39, 46].

Diagnostic tips and pitfalls:

- Melanoma cells are typically large and have round nuclei with prominent nucleolus, individually intermixed with background lymphocytes. The nuclei are often eccentrically placed, giving a plasmacytoid appearance. Binucleation, multinucleation, and cytoplasmic melanin pigments can be seen in some cases (Fig. 14.6).
- Melanoma cells may lack typical features and present as scattered bland epithelioid cells with inconspicuous nucleoli. In this setting, differential diagnosis may include histiocytes, plump endothelial cells, centroblasts, immunoblasts, and rarely intracapsular nevus cells (Fig. 14.7).
- Spindle cell melanoma is a morphologic variant of melanoma and can sometimes be encountered.

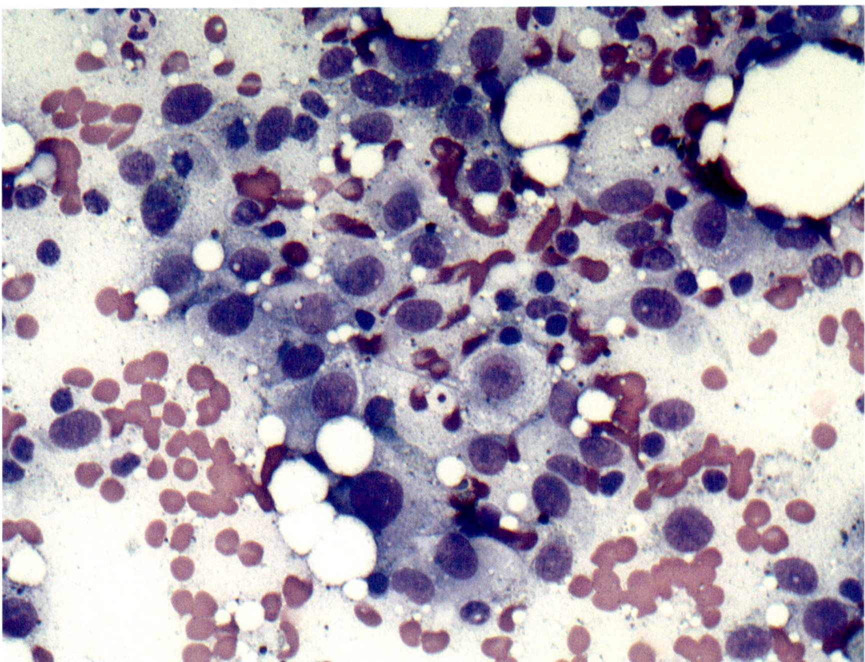

Fig. 14.6 Touch imprint of melanoma metastatic to sentinel lymph node. Dispersed large atypical cells with oval nuclei, prominent nucleolus, and intracytoplasmic melanin pigments are seen with few scattered lymphocytes (Diff-Quik stain, ×400)

Intraoperative Cytological Assessment of Indeterminate Lesions

A definite diagnosis can be reached via frozen section evaluation in most cases. However, diagnosis may be deferred due to the uncertainty about the morphologic features on frozen section. Cytological preparation can sometimes display morphologic features not revealed or subtle on frozen section, and therefore it may help render a diagnosis or at least narrow down differential diagnosis for certain lesions [1, 9–11]. Such lesions are exampled by lymphoproliferative disorders and indeterminate thyroid nodules.

Lymphoproliferative Disorders

When a tumor shows no morphologic features suggestive of cell lineage, its differential diagnosis is usually broad and may include tumors of epithelial, mesenchymal, lymphoid, or melanocytic origin. Diagnosis of such a tumor is quite challenging.

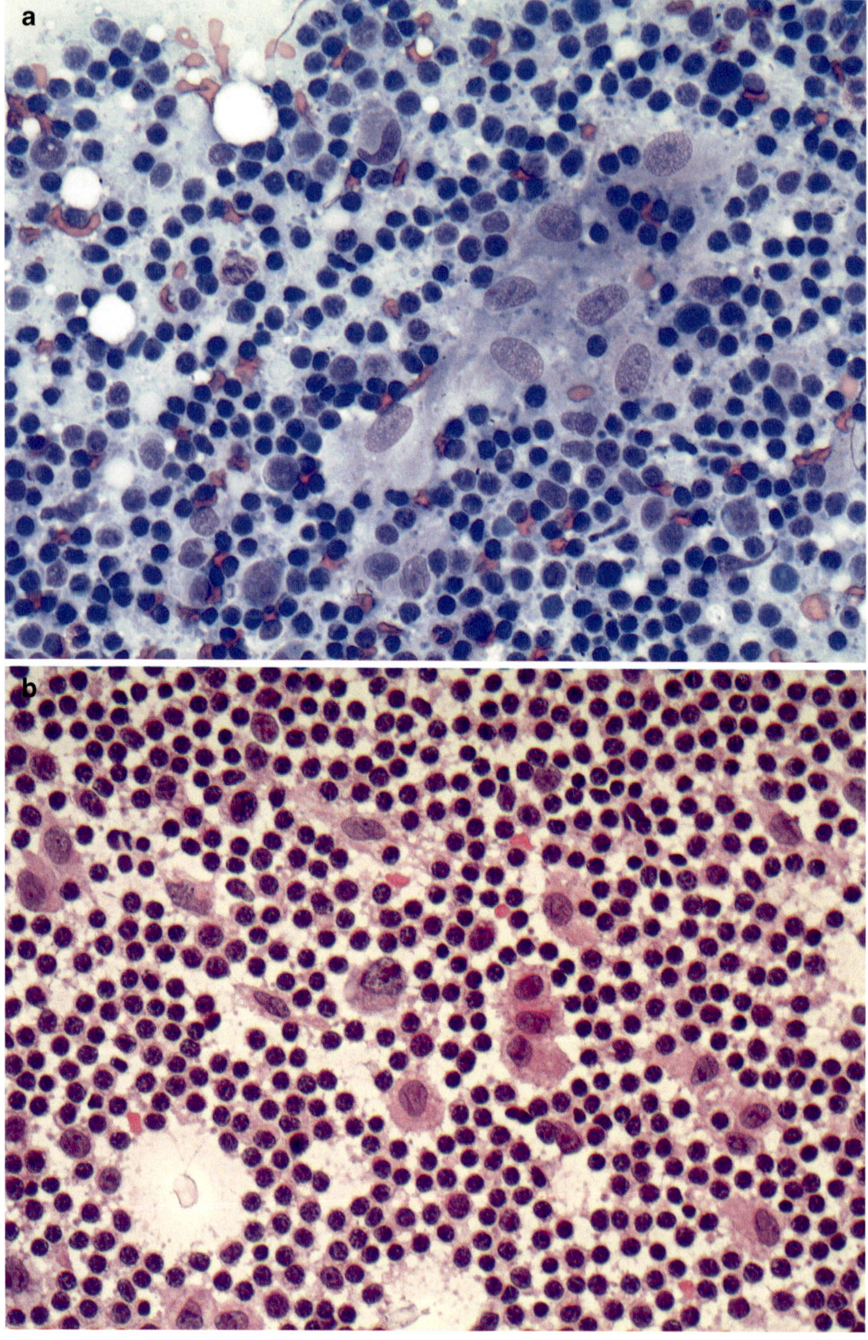

Fig. 14.7 Touch imprint of reactive lymph node. Polymorphous population of lymphocytes with scattered histiocytes that have oval nuclei with small nucleoli (**a**. Diff-Quik stain, ×400). Scattered histiocytes and rare centroblasts are seen with polymorphous lymphocytes (**b**. hematoxylin-eosin stain, ×600)

Not infrequently, frozen section is inconclusive and the case has to be deferred. Separation of lymphoproliferative disorder from other tumors is quite important. A definite diagnosis and classification of lymphoproliferative disorder often rely on the results of flow cytometry analysis performed on fresh tissue. However, the morphologic features of lymphoid tumors could be quite subtle on frozen section and may not be confused with other poorly differentiated neoplasms. Failure to recognize lymphoproliferative disorders on frozen section leads to unable to salvage fresh tissue and thus hamper their diagnostic evaluation. Recognition of lymphoproliferative disorders during intraoperative consultation may also help prevent unnecessary surgery [49–51].

Cytological preparations are superior to frozen section for demonstrating morphologic features of lymphoproliferative disorders, particularly lymphomas [11, 50, 52–55]. Lymphoid lesions can be recognized by the following cytomorphologic features (Fig. 14.8): (1) single dispersed cells, (2) smearing crush artifacts, and (3) lymphoglandular bodies in the background. Lymphoid lesions are diverse and consist of Hodgkin lymphomas and non-Hodgkin lymphomas.

Diagnostic tips and pitfalls (Fig. 14.9):

- Hodgkin lymphomas are characterized by scattered large atypical cells with mixed reactive lymphocytes and should be differentiated with metastatic tumors such as melanoma and poorly differentiated carcinoma.
- Non-Hodgkin lymphomas may show significant cytological atypia which are exampled by diffuse large B-cell lymphoma and anaplastic large cell lymphoma.
- Uniform small lymphocytes may suggest low to intermediate grade lymphomas, which should be differentiated from reactive lymphoid tissue.

Indeterminate Thyroid Nodule

Fine needle aspiration biopsy is a preferred method to evaluate thyroid nodules [56, 57]. However, an indeterminate diagnosis can be seen in some cases, and those patients may be subjected to surgical resection such as lobectomy. If malignancy is confirmed, completion thyroidectomy may be indicated. Intraoperative consultation via frozen section may help reduce the rate of secondary surgery and therefore decrease overall healthcare costs [58–60].

An indeterminate diagnosis of fine needle aspiration includes follicular lesion of undetermined significance, follicular neoplasm, and suspicion for malignancy. The possible entities with such cytological diagnoses include follicular lesions such as adenomatoid thyroid nodule, follicular adenoma, follicular carcinoma, as well as papillary carcinoma [61, 62]. The utility of frozen section in further classifying the follicular lesions is very limited, with a high deferral rate [12, 63–65]. Confirmation of papillary thyroid carcinoma by frozen section is hampered by frozen artifacts, which compromise the nuclear features characteristic of papillary thyroid carcinoma [66, 67].

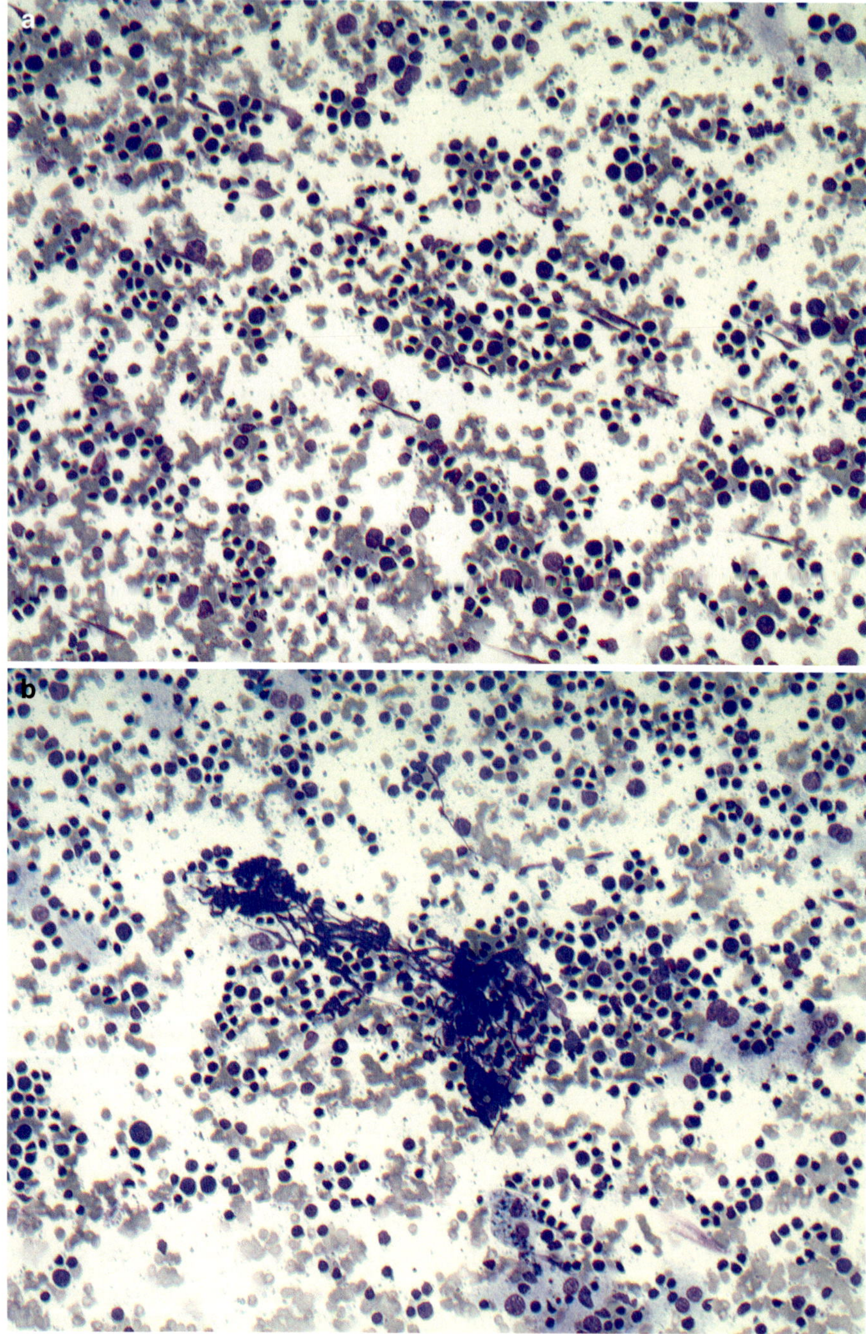

Fig. 14.8 Scrape preparation of reactive lymph node. Cytomorphologic features of lymphoid lesions are characterized by single dispersed cells (**a**. Diff-Quik stain, ×200), smearing crush (nuclear streaming) artifact (**b**. Diff-Quik stain, ×200), and lymphoglandular bodies (variable-sized blue dots) (**c**. Diff-Quik stain, ×400)

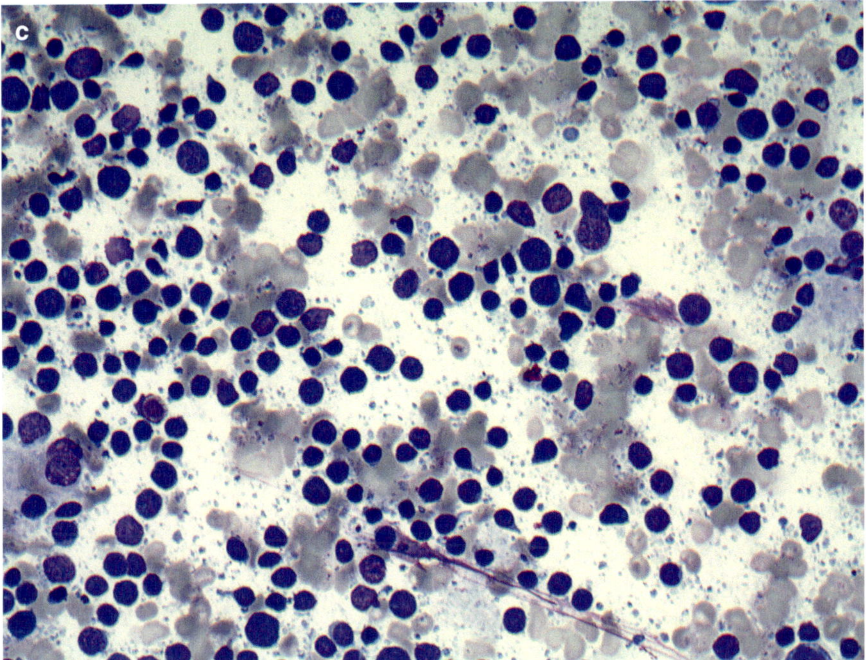

Fig. 14.8 (continued)

Cytological approach, alone or in combination with frozen section, has been used for intraoperative evaluation of thyroid lesions. Similar to frozen section, cytological evaluation has a limited role in the differential diagnosis of follicular lesions since no cytologic features can distinguish adenomatoid nodule or follicular adenoma from follicular carcinoma. The presence of nuclear features shown on cytological preparations does help with the diagnosis, at least in some cases, of papillary thyroid carcinoma [68–71].

Diagnostic tips and pitfalls (Fig. 14.10):

- Papillary architecture and nuclear characteristics including nuclear enlargement, nuclear elongation, nuclear grooves, intranuclear pseudoinclusions, and wash-out/clear chromatin are the cytomorphologic features diagnostic of papillary thyroid carcinoma.
- With the newly introduced entity, known as noninvasive follicular thyroid neoplasm with papillary-like nuclear features, diagnosis of papillary thyroid carcinoma should be rendered with extreme caution in the absence of papillary architecture.

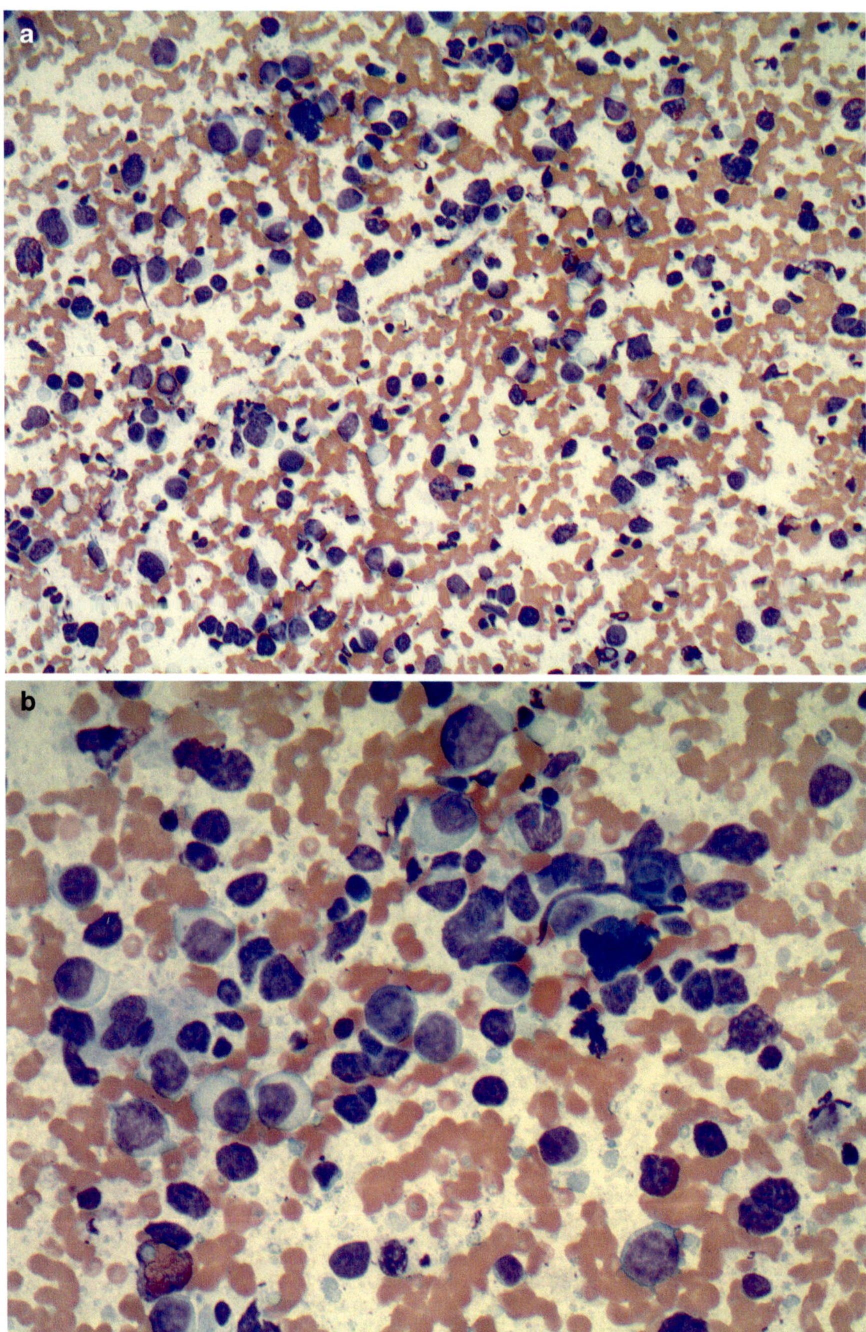

Fig. 14.9 Scrape preparation of diffuse large B-cell lymphoma of the lung. Dispersed large pleomorphic atypical cells intermixed with scattered small lymphocytes (**a**. Diff-Quik stain, ×200). The tumor cells have scant blue cytoplasm and irregular nuclear contours. Lymphoglandular bodies are seen in the background (**b**. Diff-Quik stain, ×400)

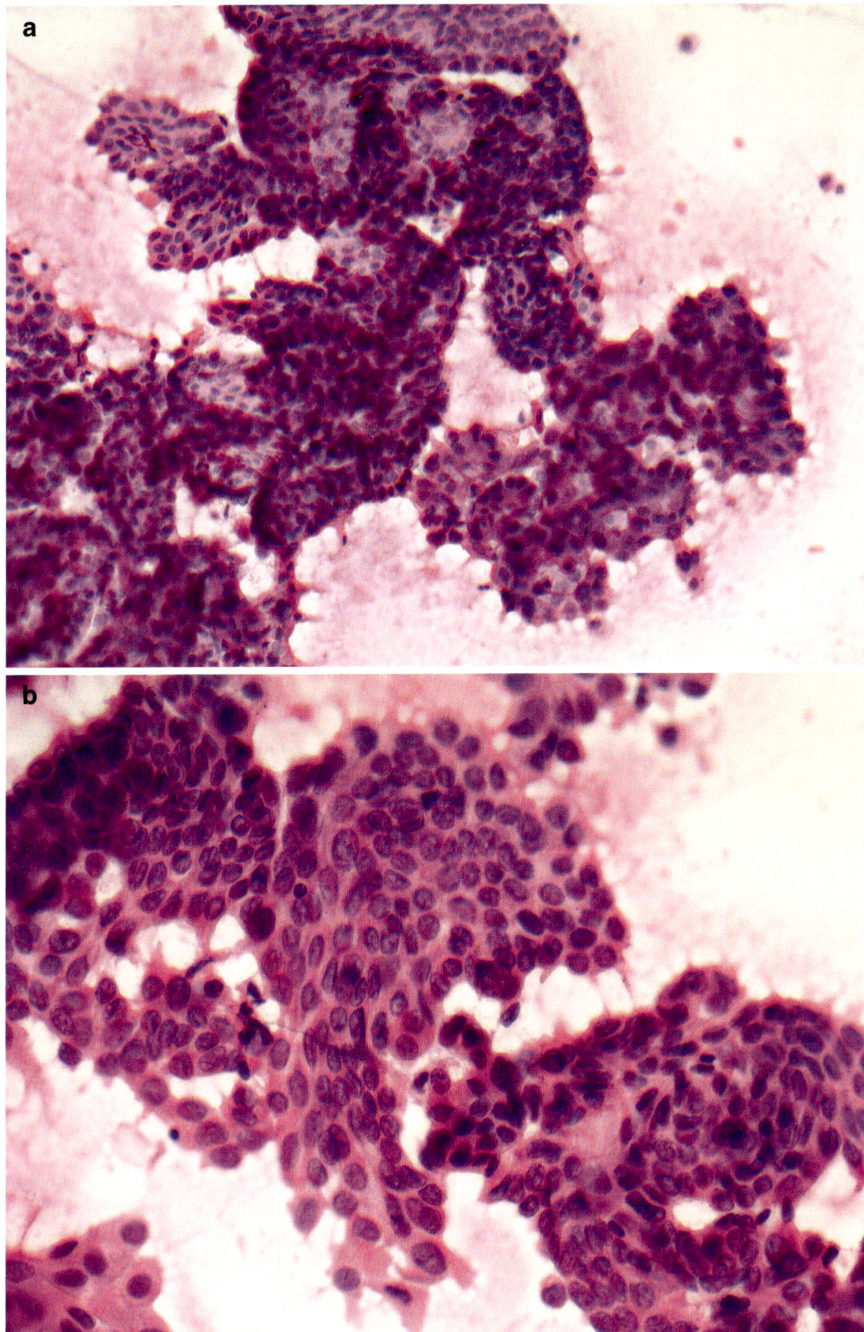

Fig. 14.10 Scrape preparation of papillary thyroid carcinoma. Papillary clusters of atypical follicular cells are seen (**a**. hematoxylin-eosin stain, ×200). The tumor cells have oval enlarged nuclei with pale chromatin and prominent nuclear grooves (**b**. hematoxylin-eosin stain, ×400)

References

1. Acs G, Baloch ZW, LiVolsi VA. Intraoperative consultation: an historical perspective. Semin Diagn Pathol. 2002;19(4):190–1.
2. Gal AA, Cagle PT. The 100-year anniversary of the description of the frozen section procedure. JAMA. 2005;294(24):3135–7.
3. Taxy JB. Frozen section and the surgical pathologist: a point of view. Arch Pathol Lab Med. 2009;133(7):1135–8.
4. St John ER, Al-Khudairi R, Ashrafian H, Athanasiou T, Takats Z, Hadjiminas DJ, Darzi A, Leff DR. Diagnostic accuracy of intraoperative techniques for margin assessment in breast cancer surgery: a meta-analysis. Ann Surg. 2017;265(2):300–10.
5. Esbona K, Li Z, Wilke LG. Intraoperative imprint cytology and frozen section pathology for margin assessment in breast conservation surgery: a systematic review. Ann Surg Oncol. 2012;19(10):3236–45.
6. Gupta PK, Baloch ZW. Intraoperative and on-site cytopathology consultation: utilization, limitations, and value. Semin Diagn Pathol. 2002;19(4):227–36.
7. Soo V, Shen P, Pichardo R, Azzazy H, Stewart JH, Geisinger KR, Levine EA. Intraoperative evaluation of sentinel lymph nodes for metastatic melanoma by imprint cytology. Ann Surg Oncol. 2007;14(5):1612–7.
8. van der Noordaa MEM, Vrancken Peeters MTFD, Rutgers EJT. The intraoperative assessment of sentinel nodes – standards and controversies. Breast. 2017;34(Suppl 1):S64–9.
9. Kolte SS, Satarkar RN. Role of scrape cytology in the intraoperative diagnosis of tumor. J Cytol. 2010;27(3):86–90.
10. Rakha EA, Haider A, Patil S, Fourtan H, Chaudry Z, Soomro IN. Evaluation of touch preparation cytology during frozen-section diagnoses of pulmonary lesions. J Clin Pathol. 2010;63(8):675–7.
11. Kaba S, Tokoro Y, Washiya K, Tokairin T, Ono I, Tsuchida S, Kojima M, Koshikawa T. Cytology of pulmonary marginal zone B-cell lymphoma of MALT type: lessons learned for intra-operative diagnosis. Cytopathology. 2011;22(5):346–9.
12. Roychoudhury S, Souza F, Gimenez C, Glass R, Cocker R, Chau K, Kohn N, Das K. Utility of intraoperative frozen sections for thyroid nodules with prior fine needle aspiration cytology diagnosis. Diagn Cytopathol. 2017;45(9):789–94.
13. Bui MM, Smith P, Agresta SV, Cheong D, Letson GD. Practical issues of intraoperative frozen section diagnosis of bone and soft tissue lesions. Cancer Control. 2008;15(1):7–12.
14. Rahman K, Asif Siddiqui F, Zaheer S, Sherwani MK, Shahid M, Sherwani RK. Intraoperative cytology—role in bone lesions. Diagn Cytopathol. 2010;38(9):639–44.
15. Sezak M, Doganavsargil B, Kececi B, Argin M, Sabah D. Feasibility and clinical utility of intraoperative consultation with frozen section in osseous lesions. Virchows Arch. 2012;461(2):195–204.
16. Tathe SP, Parate SN, Jaiswal KN, Randale AA. Intraoperative crush smear cytology of vertebral chondroblastoma: a diagnostic challenge. Diagn Cytopathol. 2018;46(1):79–82.
17. Adhya AK, Mohanty R. Utility of touch imprint cytology in the preoperative diagnosis of malignancy in low resource setting. Diagn Cytopathol. 2017;45(6):507–12.
18. Lyman GH, Somerfield MR, Bosserman LD, Perkins CL, Weaver DL, Giuliano AE. Sentinel lymph node biopsy for patients with early-stage breast cancer: American Society of Clinical Oncology clinical practice guideline update. J Clin Oncol. 2017;35(5):561–4.
19. Lisa Attebery M, Sieling BA, Ciocca R, Grujic E, Smink R, Frazier TG. Touch prep cytology as a preferred approach for evaluating sentinel lymph nodes in breast cancer. Breast J. 2007;13(1):106–7.
20. Upender S, Mohan H, Handa U, Attri AK. Intraoperative evaluation of sentinel lymph nodes in breast carcinoma by imprint cytology, frozen section and rapid immunohistochemistry. Diagn Cytopathol. 2009;37(12):871–5.

21. Liu LC, Lang JE, Lu Y, Roe D, Hwang SE, Ewing CA, Esserman LJ, Morita E, Treseler P, Leong SP. Intraoperative frozen section analysis of sentinel lymph nodes in breast cancer patients: a meta-analysis and single-institution experience. Cancer. 2011;117(2):250–8.
22. Howard-McNatt M, Geisinger KR, Stewart JH 4th, Shen P, Levine EA. Is intraoperative imprint cytology evaluation still feasible for the evaluation of sentinel lymph nodes for lobular carcinoma of the breast? Ann Surg Oncol. 2012;19(3):929–34.
23. Bruzzone M, Saro F, Bruno S, Celiento T, Mazzarella G, Lanata S, Aquilano MC, Parmigiani G, Pollone M, Gandolfo F, Costigliolo G, Sironi M. Synergy of cytological methods in the pathological staging of breast cancer: axillary fine-needle aspiration and intraoperative scrape cytology of the sentinel lymph node. Diagn Cytopathol. 2018;46(11):919–26.
24. Mannell A, Wium B, Thatcher C. Intraoperative examination of sentinel lymph nodes using scrape cytology. S Afr J Surg. 2014;52(3):75–8.
25. Llatjós M, Castellà E, Fraile M, Rull M, Julián FJ, Fusté F, Rovira C, Fernández-Llamazares J. Intraoperative assessment of sentinel lymph nodes in patients with breast carcinoma: accuracy of rapid imprint cytology compared with definitive histologic workup. Cancer. 2002;96(3):150–6.
26. Dabbs DJ, Fung M, Johnson R. Intraoperative cytologic examination of breast sentinel lymph nodes: test utility and patient impact. Breast J. 2004;10(3):190–4.
27. Cox C, Centeno B, Dickson D, Clark J, Nicosia S, Dupont E, Greenberg H, Stowell N, White L, Patel J, Furman B, Cantor A, Hakam A, Ahmad N, Diaz N, King J. Accuracy of intraoperative imprint cytology for sentinel lymph node evaluation in the treatment of breast carcinoma. Cancer. 2005;105(1):13–20.
28. Jain P, Kumar R, Anand M, Asthana S, Deo SV, Gupta R, Bhutani M, Karak AK, Shukla NK. Touch imprint cytology of axillary lymph nodes after neoadjuvant chemotherapy in patients with breast carcinoma. Cancer. 2003;99(6):346–51.
29. Elliott RM, Shenk RR, Thompson CL, Gilmore HL. Touch preparations for the intraoperative evaluation of sentinel lymph nodes after neoadjuvant therapy have high false-negative rates in patients with breast cancer. Arch Pathol Lab Med. 2014;138(6):814–8.
30. Pétursson HI, Kovács A, Mattsson J, Olofsson Bagge R. Evaluation of intraoperative touch imprint cytology on axillary sentinel lymph nodes in invasive breast carcinomas, a retrospective study of 1227 patients comparing sensitivity in the different tumor subtypes. PLoS One. 2018;13(4):e0195560.
31. Creager AJ, Geisinger KR, Perrier ND, Shen P, Shaw JA, Young PR, Case D, Levine EA. Intraoperative imprint cytologic evaluation of sentinel lymph nodes for lobular carcinoma of the breast. Ann Surg. 2004;239(1):61–6.
32. Caudle AS. Intraoperative pathologic evaluation with targeted axillary dissection: editorial for "intraoperative touch imprint cytology in targeted axillary dissection after neoadjuvant chemotherapy among breast cancer patients with initial axillary metastasis". Ann Surg Oncol. 2018;25(11):3112–4.
33. Swetter SM, Tsao H, Bichakjian CK, Curiel-Lewandrowski C, Elder DE, Gershenwald JE, Guild V, Grant-Kels JM, Halpern AC, Johnson TM, Sober AJ, Thompson JA, Wisco OJ, Wyatt S, Hu S, Lamina T. Guidelines of care for the management of primary cutaneous melanoma. J Am Acad Dermatol. 2019;80(1):208–50.
34. Morton DL, Thompson JF, Cochran AJ, Mozzillo N, Nieweg OE, Roses DF, Hoekstra HJ, Karakousis CP, Puleo CA, Coventry BJ, Kashani-Sabet M, Smithers BM, Paul E, Kraybill WG, McKinnon JG, Wang HJ, Elashoff R, Faries MB, MSLT Group. Final trial report of sentinel-node biopsy versus nodal observation in melanoma. N Engl J Med. 2014;370:599–609.
35. Belli F, Lenisa L, Clemente C, Tragni G, Mascheroni L, Gallino G, Cascinelli N. Sentinel node biopsy and selective dissection for melanoma nodal metastases. Tumori. 1998;84(1):24–8.
36. Gipponi M, Solari N, Lionetto R, Di Somma C, Villa G, Schenone F, Queirolo P, Cafiero F. The prognostic role of the sentinel lymph node in clinically node-negative patients with cutaneous melanoma: experience of the Genoa group. Eur J Surg Oncol. 2005;31(10):1191–7.

37. Morton DL, Thompson JF, Cochran AJ, Mozzillo N, Elashoff R, Essner R, Nieweg OE, Roses DF, Hoekstra HJ, Karakousis CP, Reintgen DS, Coventry BJ, Glass EC, Wang HJ, MSLT Group. Sentinel-node biopsy or nodal observation in melanoma. N Engl J Med. 2006;355(13):1307–17.
38. Alkhatib W, Hertzenberg C, Jewell W, Al-Kasspooles MF, Damjanov I, Cohen MS. Utility of frozen-section analysis of sentinel lymph node biopsy specimens for melanoma in surgical decision making. Am J Surg. 2008;196(6):827–33.
39. Badgwell BD, Pierce C, Broadwater JR, Westbrook K, Korourian S, Davis D, Hiatt K, Lee J, Cheung WL, Klimberg VS. Intraoperative sentinel lymph node analysis in melanoma. J Surg Oncol. 2011;103(1):1–5.
40. Fahy AS, Grotz TE, Keeney GL, Glasgow AE, Habermann EB, Erickson L, Hieken TJ, Jakub JW. Frozen section analysis of SLNs in trunk and extremity melanoma has a high false negative rate but can spare some patients a second operation. J Surg Oncol. 2016;114(7):879–83.
41. Gibbs JF, Huang PP, Zhang PJ, Kraybill WG, Cheney R. Accuracy of pathologic techniques for the diagnosis of metastatic melanoma in sentinel lymph nodes. Ann Surg Oncol. 1999;6(7):699–704.
42. Koopal SA, Tiebosch AT, Albertus Piers D, Plukker JT, Schraffordt Koops H, Hoekstra HJ. Frozen section analysis of sentinel lymph nodes in melanoma patients. Cancer. 2000;89(8):1720–5.
43. Stojadinovic A, Allen PJ, Clary BM, Busam KJ, Coit DG. Value of frozen-section analysis of sentinel lymph nodes for primary cutaneous malignant melanoma. Ann Surg. 2002;235(1):92–8.
44. Scolyer RA, Thompson JF, McCarthy SW, Gershenwald JF, Ross MI, Cochran AJ. Intraoperative frozen-section evaluation can reduce accuracy of pathologic assessment of sentinel nodes in melanoma patients. J Am Coll Surg. 2005;201(5):821–4.
45. Creager AJ, Geisinger KR, Shiver SA, Perrier ND, Shen P, Ann Shaw J, Young PR, Levine EA. Intraoperative evaluation of sentinel lymph nodes for metastatic breast carcinoma by imprint cytology. Mod Pathol. 2002;15(11):1140–7.
46. Hocevar M, Bracko M, Pogacnik A, Vidergar-Kralj B, Besic N, Zgajnar J. Role of imprint cytology in the intraoperative evaluation of sentinel lymph nodes for malignant melanoma. Eur J Cancer. 2003;39(15):2173–8.
47. Nejc D, Pasz-Walczak G, Piekarski J, Pluta P, Sek P, Bilski A, Durczynski A, Berner A, Jastrzebski T, Jeziorski A. 94% accuracy of intraoperative imprint touch cytology of sentinel nodes in skin melanoma patients. Anticancer Res. 2008;28(1B):465–9.
48. Jonjić N, Rajković Molek K, Seili-Bekafigo I, Grbac Ivanković S, Girotto N, Jurišić D, Zamolo G, Pavlović Ružić I, Prpić Massari L. Predictive value of intraoperative sentinel lymph node imprint cytology analysis for metastasis in patients with melanoma. Acta Dermatovenerol Croat. 2017;25(2):99–106.
49. Gupta R, Dastane A, McKenna RJ Jr, Marchevsky AM. What can we learn from the errors in the frozen section diagnosis of pulmonary carcinoid tumors? An evidence-based approach. Hum Pathol. 2009;40(1):1–9.
50. Subik MK, Gordetsky J, Yao JL, di Sant'Agnese PA, Miyamoto H. Frozen section assessment in testicular and paratesticular lesions suspicious for malignancy: its role in preventing unnecessary orchiectomy. Hum Pathol. 2012;43(9):1514–49.
51. Shahraki AD, Mohammadizadeh F, Zafarbakhsh A. Intraoperative diagnosis by frozen section study would prevent unnecessary surgery in ovarian Burkitt's lymphoma. Adv Biomed Res. 2014;3:71.
52. Nishimura R, Tsujimoto M, Kurokawa K, Tsukiyama A, Okuda T, Uraoka T, Gunji Y, Taki I, Yamanishi H, Nakahara M, Nakao K, Aozasa K. Usefulness of intraoperative cytology for the diagnosis of primary pancreatic lymphoma. Acta Cytol. 2001;45(1):104–6.
53. Bandyopadhyay A, Majumdar K, Gangopadhyay M, Khan K, Chakraborty S, Ghosh AK. Primary bilateral small lymphocytic lymphoma of ocular adnexal origin: imprint cytology suggests the intraoperative diagnosis. Saudi J Ophthalmol. 2013;27(1):61–3.

54. Singh C, Krigman HR, Pambuccian SE. Paranuclear and extracellular globules in intraoperative cytology preparations of anaplastic large cell lymphoma. Diagn Cytopathol. 2014;42(8):686–9.
55. Sugita Y, Terasaki M, Nakashima S, Ohshima K, Morioka M, Abe H. Intraoperative rapid diagnosis of primary central nervous system lymphomas: advantages and pitfalls. Neuropathology. 2014;34(5):438–45.
56. Cibas ES, Ali SZ. The 2017 Bethesda system for reporting thyroid cytopathology. Thyroid. 2017;27(11):1341–6.
57. Tang AL, Falciglia M, Yang H, Mark JR, Steward DL. Validation of American Thyroid Association ultrasound risk assessment of thyroid nodules selected for ultrasound fine-needle aspiration. Thyroid. 2017;27(8):1077–82.
58. Berg RW, Yen TW, Evans DB, Hunt B, Quiroz FA, Wilson SD, Wang TS. Analysis of an institutional protocol for thyroid lobectomy: utility of routine intraoperative frozen section and expedited (overnight) pathology. Surgery. 2016;159(2):512–7.
59. Abu-Ghanem S, Cohen O, Raz Yarkoni T, Fliss DM, Yehuda M. Intraoperative frozen section in "suspicious for papillary thyroid carcinoma" after adoption of the Bethesda System. Otolaryngol Head Neck Surg. 2016;155(5):779–86.
60. Bollig CA, Gilley D, Lesko D, Jorgensen JB, Galloway TL, Zitsch RP 3rd, Dooley LM. Economic impact of frozen section for thyroid nodules with "suspicious for malignancy" cytology. Otolaryngol Head Neck Surg. 2018;158(2):257–64.
61. Lumachi F, Borsato S, Tregnaghi A, Marino F, Polistina F, Basso SM, Koussis H, Basso U, Fassina A. FNA cytology and frozen section examination in patients with follicular lesions of the thyroid gland. Anticancer Res. 2009;29(12):5255–7.
62. Zanocco K, Heller M, Elaraj D, Sturgeon C. Cost effectiveness of intraoperative pathology examination during diagnostic hemithyroidectomy for unilateral follicular thyroid neoplasms. J Am Coll Surg. 2013;217(4):702–10.
63. Kennedy JM, Robinson RA. Thyroid frozen sections in patients with preoperative FNAs: review of surgeons' preoperative rationale, intraoperative decisions, and final outcome. Am J Clin Pathol. 2016;145(5):660–5.
64. Trosman SJ, Bhargavan R, Prendes BL, Burkey BB, Scharpf J. The contemporary utility of intraoperative frozen sections in thyroid surgery. Am J Otolaryngol. 2017;38(5):614–7.
65. Bollig CA, Lesko D, Gilley D, Dooley LM. The futility of intraoperative frozen section in the evaluation of follicular thyroid lesions. Laryngoscope. 2018;128(6):1501–5.
66. Furlan JC, Bedard YC, Rosen IB. Role of fine-needle aspiration biopsy and frozen section in the management of papillary thyroid carcinoma subtypes. World J Surg. 2004;28(9):880–5.
67. Baloch ZW, LiVolsi VA. Cytologic and architectural mimics of papillary thyroid carcinoma. Diagnostic challenges in fine-needle aspiration and surgical pathology specimens. Am J Clin Pathol. 2006;125(Suppl):S135–44.
68. Basolo F, Ugolini C, Proietti A, Iacconi P, Berti P, Miccoli P. Role of frozen section associated with intraoperative cytology in comparison to FNA and FS alone in the management of thyroid nodules. Eur J Surg Oncol. 2007;33(6):769–75.
69. Miller MC, Rubin CJ, Cunnane M, Bibbo M, Miller JL, Keane WM, Pribitkin EA. Intraoperative pathologic examination: cost effectiveness and clinical value in patients with cytologic diagnosis of cellular follicular thyroid lesion. Thyroid. 2007;17(6):557–765.
70. Anila KR, Krishna G. Role of imprint cytology in intra operative diagnosis of thyroid lesions. Gulf J Oncolog. 2014;1(16):73–8.
71. Pyo JS, Sohn JH, Kang G. Diagnostic assessment of intraoperative cytology for papillary thyroid carcinoma: using a decision tree analysis. J Endocrinol Investig. 2017;40(3):305–11.

Chapter 15
Economics, Regulations, and Trends in Practice

Angelique W. Levi and Guoping Cai

Rapid on-site evaluation (ROSE) is a service that pathologists perform to assess cellular material and specimen adequacy of fine needle aspiration (FNA) smears and biopsy touch imprints in real-time collaborative patient care, most often at the procedural point of care. ROSE can be used in the setting of pathologist-performed FNA of superficial lesions and ultrasound, endobronchial ultrasound (EBUS), endoscopic ultrasound (EUS), or computed tomography (CT)-guided FNA or biopsy. Depending on the clinical setting including both academic and community-based medical centers and the expectations of the affiliated multispecialty practices, the overall demand for ROSE service and its associated FNA procedure or imaging-guided biopsy type may vary [1–5]. In many clinical settings, EBUS and EUS-guided FNA procedures have increased in recent years and have accounted for the increase in ROSE service requested in our institution and others [3, 5]. ROSE can inform the clinician or pathologist performing the procedure of the need to obtain additional material for diagnostic adequacy and ancillary studies, such as flow cytometry, microbiology cultures, and/or molecular studies.

Many studies have focused on the impact of ROSE on FNA adequacy rates emphasizing how fewer passes are needed to obtain sufficient material from less invasive procedures, and fewer repeat procedures are performed, the advantages being the decrease in risk of complications to the patient and lower overall healthcare costs [6–8]. However, emerging molecular tests in current pathology practice have placed a higher demand on maximizing limited material obtained by FNA or biopsy procedures [1, 5, 9–12]. ROSE is a way to ensure that small samples are handled properly for adequate morphological review, appropriate specimen triage, and accurate diagnosis and ultimately translate into an optimal treatment plan.

A. W. Levi (✉) · G. Cai
Department of Pathology, Yale University School of Medicine, New Haven, CT, USA
e-mail: angelique.levi@yale.edu; guoping.cai@yale.edu

G. Cai, A. J. Adeniran (eds.), *Rapid On-site Evaluation (ROSE)*,
https://doi.org/10.1007/978-3-030-21799-0_15

Cost and Reimbursement

The question of when ROSE is cost-effective is a complicated one and rests on many factors. Because ROSE can reduce the number of needle passes, thereby reducing clinical complications associated with multiple passes and avoid repeat procedures, it has the potential to reduce overall costs [6–8, 13, 14]. However, ROSE increases operational costs to the pathology laboratory because it requires additional personnel and may increase procedure time. Reimbursement for ROSE fails to provide adequate compensation, and in recent years there has been an increase in FNA procedures and time spent providing ROSE further exacerbating the issue of cost-effectiveness [2, 3, 5, 14–17]. In busy practices, the cost of pathologists' time for providing ROSE far exceeds the reimbursement rates because of unreimbursed time spent in the procedure suite waiting for a clinician to provide material, recent CMS changes in allowable billing codes, the steady drop in overall reimbursement rates, as well as a decrease in work Relative Value Units (wRVU). CMS changed billing practice to allow only one unit of CPT code 88172 per specimen site with a separate CPT code 88177 for each additional pass [15–17] (Table 15.1). Compensation for ROSE over the last decade has decreased by about half. Mathematical models have been employed to evaluate which procedures types at specific anatomic sites under a subset of fixed conditions could be cost-effective to use ROSE, but it is very difficult to account for the complete cost of care and potential cost savings to the patient [14]. Given the efficiency and optimal patient care ROSE can provide in the appropriate set of circumstances, ROSE may play an important role in justifying better reimbursement rates at an institutional and national level, as the practice of medicine moves away from volume based to value and patient outcomes based.

Personnel and Regulations

It is a subject of discussion and debate about who is best suited to provide ROSE. Appropriate training and competency to provide assessment is the driving force; however, there are no standards in training or assessment tools. The majority of healthcare professional who have training to provide ROSE include general pathologists, cytopathologists, cytopathology fellows/residents, and cytotechnologists.

Table 15.1 CPT codes for ROSE with fine needle aspiration (FNA) smears and core tissue biopsy touch preparations (TP)

CPT code	Description
88172	On-site cytological examination of FNA smear, first pass
88177	On-site cytological examination of FNA smear, each additional pass
88333	On-site cytological examination of tissue biopsy TP, first area
88334	On-site cytological examination of tissue biopsy TP, each additional area

In academic medical centers, cytopathology fellows and pathology residents in ACGME-approved training programs are an integral part of the FNA team. Under the training and supervision of credentialed, American Board of Pathology-certified pathologists, they may also provide ROSE in a direct and potentially indirect manner. Competency of pathology trainees to provide ROSE in an indirectly supervised manner is at the discretion of the medical directors of each training program, as there are no ACGME procedural requirements [18].

Cytotechnologists train for 1 year in the field of cytopathology. They learn the skills necessary to identify abnormal cells and quickly classify them accurately into an interpretive or diagnostic category. While they may not have extensive experience in FNA for ROSE, it is expected during their clinical rotation training that they will observe FNAs. With hands-on FNA experience and mentorship of supervising pathologists, cytotechnologists become qualified to provide ROSE. After appropriate training, in some institutions, cytotechnologists and pathology trainees may be the only professionals to perform ROSE. Previous studies have evaluated the performances of cytotechnologists versus cytopathologists and found out that cytotechnologists were competent to provide specimen adequacy assessment of FNA biopsy [19, 20]. However, due to inherent constraints and limitations, cytotechnologists may not be able to best fulfill other functions of ROSE service including specimen triage for appropriate ancillary studies and preliminary diagnosis [21, 22].

Controversy may arise when non-pathology medical specialists such as pulmonologists and gastroenterologists perform ROSE, as it may be outside their scope of practice [23–27]. Generally, such training programs do not provide comprehensive pathology training and do not have adequate experience in tissue evaluation or cytomorphology. A strategy could be to train non-pathology clinicians to perform ROSE, but again there are no standards for how they may be trained in ROSE for FNA. Also, the ROSE performed by non-pathology medical specialists is limited to specimen adequacy assessment. Additionally, most non-pathologist physicians cannot bill a professional fee for ROSE, as the Centers for Medicare and Medicaid Services (CMS) classify ROSE as a laboratory test, which falls under the mandates of the Clinical Laboratory Improvement Amendments.

Changing Trends in the Practice

The increased demands of patient care and simultaneous economic stressors force changing trends and ultimately practice patterns. In the era of personalized medicine for targeted therapy, there is more pressure than ever before for pathologists to do more with less. Strategies to cut costs include reorganizing laboratory resources and workflow. Some institutions have decided to only send cytotechnologists and pathology trainees to perform ROSE or let non-pathology physicians to perform their own ROSE, though they cannot bill for ROSE services. In this setting, cytotechnologists or non-pathology physicians can accurately provide ROSE adequacy assessments and save significant pathologist time in order to allow the pathologist to continue to generate revenue in higher reimbursable activities, which seems to be cost-effective in some settings [28].

Other institutions have reported a significant increase in needle core biopsies (NCB) for potential molecular testing and tissue triage, increasing the demand for performing ROSE on touch preparations (TP) [5, 9, 29]. The shift in specimen acquisition requires an investment in time to standardize the procedure and become familiar with the morphological differences in ROSE for core biopsy TP versus FNA smears. Not only is ROSE for TP much less time-consuming than FNA for the pathologist to evaluate, but also the CPT billing code is different (88333 and 88334) (Table 15.1) and reimbursable at a significantly higher rate, approximately double that of FNA.

Another approach to face adversity in challenging times is to embrace innovation and technology in an economically sound way. Telecytology (TC) can be used to provide ROSE services more efficiently, as a single pathologist can accommodate ROSE in multiple locations simultaneously while performing other billable work in between ROSE procedures from a remote office location [30–36]. The emergence of fast and high-resolution digital imaging technologies makes it possible to implement TC for ROSE, and it has been instituted with great success in the transmission of live imaging in a large, high-volume medical center. There are different platforms available for image transmission including static and live video microscopy, as well as whole-slide scanner images as a potential future option [36]. TC FNA ROSE requires an experienced cytotechnologist on-site for slide preparation, staining, and focused morphological review of pertinent regions of interest. In addition to the investment of a cytotechnologist, this type of system requires an upfront investment of infrastructure: an imaging platform, hardware (a dedicated microscope and camera), software, and secure remote access.

References

1. da Cunha Santos G, Ko HM, Saieg MA, Geddie WR. "The petals and thorns" of ROSE (rapid on-site evaluation). Cancer Cytopathol. 2013;121(1):4–8.
2. Tambouret RH, Barkan GA, Kurtycz DFI, Padmanabhan V. FNA cytology: rapid on-site evaluation – how practice varies. CAP Today. May 2014.
3. Collins BT, DuBray-Benstein B, Naik K, Smith MA, Tiscornia-Wasserman PG. American Society of Cytopathology rapid on-site evaluation (ROSE) position statement. ASC Bull. 2015;52(2):I–VIII.
4. Kraft AO. Specimen acquisition: ROSEs, gardeners, and gatekeepers. Cancer Cytopathol. 2017;125(S6):449–54.
5. Gonzalez MF, Akhtar I, Manucha V. Changing trends and practices in cytopathology. Acta Cytol. 2017;61(2):91–5.
6. Nasuti JF, Gupta PK, Baloch ZW. Diagnostic value and cost-effectiveness of on-site evaluation of fine-needle aspiration specimens: review of 5,688 cases. Diagn Cytopathol. 2002;27(1):1–4.
7. Collins BT, Chen AC, Wang JF, Bernadt CT, Sanati S. Improved laboratory resource utilization and patient care with the use of rapid on-site evaluation for endobronchial ultrasound fine-needle aspiration biopsy. Cancer Cytopathol. 2013;121(10):544–51.

8. Schmidt RL, Witt BL, Lopez-Calderon LE, Layfield LJ. The influence of rapid onsite evaluation on the adequacy rate of fine-needle aspiration cytology: a systematic review and meta-analysis. Am J Clin Pathol. 2013;139(3):300–8.
9. Coley SM, Crapanzano JP, Saqi A. FNA, core biopsy, or both for the diagnosis of lung carcinoma: obtaining sufficient tissue for a specific diagnosis and molecular testing. Cancer Cytopathol. 2015;123(5):318–26.
10. Roy-Chowdhuri S, Aisner DL, Allen TC, Beasley MB, Borczuk A, Cagle PT, Capelozzi V, Dacic S, da Cunha Santos G, Hariri LP, Kerr KM, Lantuejoul S, Mino-Kenudson M, Moreira A, Raparia K, Rekhtman N, Sholl L, Thunnissen E, Tsao MS, Vivero M, Yatabe Y. Biomarker testing in lung carcinoma cytology specimens: a perspective from members of the Pulmonary Pathology Society. Arch Pathol Lab Med. 2016;140(11):1267–72.
11. Auger M, Brimo F, Kanber Y, Fiset PO, Camilleri-Broet S. A practical guide for ancillary studies in pulmonary cytologic specimens. Cancer Cytopathol. 2018;126(Suppl 8):599–614.
12. Jain D, Allen TC, Aisner DL, Beasley MB, Cagle PT, Capelozzi VL, Hariri LP, Lantuejoul S, Miller R, Mino-Kenudson M, Monaco SE, Moreira A, Raparia K, Rekhtman N, Roden AC, Roy-Chowdhuri S, da Cunha Santos G, Thunnissen E, Troncone G, Vivero M. Rapid on-site evaluation of endobronchial ultrasound-guided transbronchial needle aspirations for the diagnosis of lung cancer: a perspective from members of the Pulmonary Pathology Society. Arch Pathol Lab Med. 2018;142(2):253–62.
13. da Cunha Santos G. ROSEs (rapid on-site evaluations) to our patients: the impact on laboratory resources and patient care. Cancer Cytopathol. 2013;121(10):537–9.
14. Schmidt RL, Walker BS, Cohen MB. When is rapid on-site evaluation cost-effective for fine-needle aspiration biopsy? PLoS One. 2015;10(8):e0135466.
15. Dhillon I, Pitman MB, Demay RM, Archuletta P, Shidham VB. Compensation crisis related to the onsite adequacy evaluation during FNA procedures-urgent proactive input from cytopathology community is critical to establish appropriate reimbursement for CPT code 88172 (or its new counterpart if introduced in the future). Cytojournal. 2010;7:23.
16. Davey DD, Neal MH. Coding changes in the United States front and center: implications for cytopathology. Cancer Cytopathol. 2011;119(5):310–4.
17. Renshaw AA. 88172 is more than counting cells: ensuring the quality of immediate assessment of fine-needle aspiration material. Am J Clin Pathol. 2012;138(1):27–8.
18. Naritoku WY, Black-Schaffer WS. Cytopathology fellowship milestones. Cancer Cytopathol. 2014;122(12):859–65.
19. Burlingame OO, Kessé KO, Silverman SG, Cibas ES. On-site adequacy evaluations performed by cytotechnologists: correlation with final interpretations of 5241 image-guided fine-needle aspiration biopsies. Cancer Cytopathol. 2012;120(3):177–84.
20. Olson MT, Ali SZ. Cytotechnologist on-site evaluation of pancreas fine needle aspiration adequacy: comparison with cytopathologists and correlation with the final interpretation. Acta Cytol. 2012;56(4):340–6.
21. Mesa H, Rawal A, Gupta P. Diagnosis of lymphoid lesions in limited samples: a guide for the general surgical pathologist, cytopathologist, and cytotechnologist. Am J Clin Pathol. 2018;150(6):471–84.
22. Sung S, Crapanzano JP, DiBardino D, Swinarski D, Bulman WA, Saqi A. Molecular testing on endobronchial ultrasound (EBUS) fine needle aspirates (FNA): impact of triage. Diagn Cytopathol. 2018;46(2):122–30.
23. Savoy AD, Raimondo M, Woodward TA, Noh K, Pungpapong S, Jones AD, Crook J, Wallace MB. Can endosonographers evaluate on-site cytologic adequacy? A comparison with cytotechnologists. Gastrointest Endosc. 2007;65(7):953–7.
24. Harada R, Kato H, Fushimi S, Iwamuro M, Inoue H, Muro S, Sakakihara I, Noma Y, Yamamoto N, Horiguchi S, Tsutsumi K, Okada H, Yamamoto K. An expanded training program for endosonographers improved self-diagnosed accuracy of endoscopic ultrasound-guided fine-needle aspiration cytology of the pancreas. Scand J Gastroenterol. 2014;49(9):1119–23.

25. Bonifazi M, Sediari M, Ferretti M, Poidomani G, Tramacere I, Mei F, Zuccatosta L, Gasparini S. The role of the pulmonologist in rapid on-site cytologic evaluation of transbronchial needle aspiration: a prospective study. Chest. 2014;145(1):60–5.
26. Meena N, Jeffus S, Massoll N, Siegel ER, Korourian S, Chen C, Bartter T. Rapid onsite evaluation: a comparison of cytopathologist and pulmonologist performance. Cancer Cytopathol. 2016;124(4):279–84.
27. Wyse J, Rubino M, Iglesias Garcia J, Sahai AV. Onsite evaluation of endoscopic ultrasound fine needle aspiration: the endosonographer, the cytotechnologist and the cytopathologist. Rev Esp Enferm Dig. 2017;109(4):279–83.
28. Pearson LN, Layfield LJ, Schmidt RL. Cost-effectiveness of rapid on-site evaluation of the adequacy of FNA cytology samples performed by nonpathologists. Cancer Cytopathol. 2018;126(10):839–45.
29. Padmanabhan V, Barkan G, Nayar R. Assessing needle core biopsy adequacy – survey of practice. CAP Today. May 2016.
30. Marotti JD, Johncox V, Ng D, Gonzalez JL, Padmanabhan V. Implementation of telecytology for immediate assessment of endoscopic ultrasound-guided fine-needle aspirations compared to conventional on-site evaluation: analysis of 240 consecutive cases. Acta Cytol. 2012;56(5):548–53.
31. Buxbaum JL, Eloubeidi MA, Lane CJ, Varadarajulu S, Linder A, Crowe AE, Jhala D, Jhala NC, Crowe DR, Eltoum IA. Dynamic telecytology compares favorably to rapid onsite evaluation of endoscopic ultrasound fine needle aspirates. Dig Dis Sci. 2012;57(12):3092–7.
32. Heimann A, Maini G, Hwang S, Shroyer KR, Singh M. Use of telecytology for the immediate assessment of CT guided and endoscopic FNA cytology: diagnostic accuracy, advantages, and pitfalls. Diagn Cytopathol. 2012;40(7):575–81.
33. Bott MJ, James B, Collins BT, Murray BA, Puri V, Kreisel D, Krupnick AS, Patterson GA, Broderick S, Meyers BF, Crabtree TD. A prospective clinical trial of telecytopathology for rapid interpretation of specimens obtained during endobronchial ultrasound-fine needle aspiration. Ann Thorac Surg. 2015;100(1):201–6.
34. Sirintrapun SJ, Rudomina D, Mazzella A, Feratovic R, Alago W, Siegelbaum R, Lin O. Robotic telecytology for remote cytologic evaluation without an on-site cytotechnologist or cytopathologist: a tale of implementation and review of constraints. J Pathol Inform. 2017;8:32.
35. Lin O, Rudomina D, Feratovic R, Sirintrapun SJ. Rapid on-site evaluation using telecytology: a major cancer center experience. Diagn Cytopathol. 2019;47(1):15–9.
36. Lin O. Telecytology for rapid on-site evaluation: current status. J Am Soc Cytopathol. 2018;7(1):1–6.

Chapter 16
Telecytopathology

Adebowale J. Adeniran

Introduction

Minimally invasive procedures such as fine needle aspiration (FNA) and small core tissue biopsy to obtain material for diagnosis are becoming increasingly popular, and with it is rapid on-site evaluation (ROSE). ROSE of FNA specimens by cytopathologists is very important and is increasingly being used to assess sample adequacy, to triage specimens for other ancillary tests, and to establish a preliminary cytologic interpretation [1–4]. Core biopsy can also mandate ROSE for touch imprints to determine cellular content and adequacy [5]. ROSE is also becoming increasingly popular because it improves patient care by reducing the number of repeat procedures and/or more invasive procedures, which ultimately decreases healthcare costs and minimizes potential side effects from the procedures, such as lower rates of infection and hemorrhage [5–8]. Ultimately it expedites care and improves patient satisfaction [9]. A cost and compensation analysis for providing ROSE suggested that, in comparison to the lengthy time spent on providing ROSE, Medicare reimbursement has remained inadequate to support the salary of a staff cytopathologist. As a result, cost-effective alternatives are being increasingly investigated to provide ROSE [10].

In large centers and in this era where institutions acquire multiple small practices and pathologists have to travel to different locations for FNA, the elaborate logistics and difficulty in moving from site to site may prevent a timely immediate assessment and can make on-site evaluation by a pathologist difficult and time-consuming. The advent of telecytopathology has significantly helped with this process, as it enables the electronic transmission of images online for consultation and discussion. Over the years, this method has been in use and is very efficient for intraoperative frozen section consultation [11, 12]. It represents a new option for communication among cytopathologists and between cytopa-

A. J. Adeniran (✉)
Department of Pathology, Yale University School of Medicine, New Haven, CT, USA
e-mail: adebowale.adeniran@yale.edu

G. Cai, A. J. Adeniran (eds.), *Rapid On-site Evaluation (ROSE)*,
https://doi.org/10.1007/978-3-030-21799-0_16

thologists on the one hand and interventional radiologists and clinicians that perform procedures located at different sites on the other hand [1].

Prior to implementation, it is essential that key stakeholders such as cytopathologists, cytotechnologists, hospital administration, interventional radiologists, and clinicians that will be involved with the process and information technology analysts should be engaged so that the need for the technology as well as other issues such as implementation and possible challenges at the initial stages can be discussed [9]. Information technologists need to be involved to optimize data transfer and also ensure the protection of patient-related information, especially if the on-site operator and remote viewer are located in different hospitals, institutions, or outreach settings [2]. It is important to obtain feedback from all individuals involved so as to confirm that there is thorough understanding of the workflow and how this technology will affect all processes and individuals involved [9].

The 2014 American Telemedicine Association guidelines addressed the use of telecytopathology in ROSE, stressing the need for sufficient Internet speed and images resolution as well as the concern regarding security issues when using mobile devices [13]. Overall, the rates of sample adequacy, deferral, and preliminary and final diagnoses for telecytopathology cases have been found to be comparable to the rates obtained by cytopathologists using conventional on-site microscopy. The time required for preliminary telecytodiagnosis is comparable to that for regular on-site microscopy [1, 5, 9]. Misinterpretations in telecytopathology are mainly due to on-site evaluator's insufficient experience as seen in early part of cytopathology training year or in the early part of cytotechnologist's engagement. Hence, cytopathologists may need to spend more time in examining smears when working with a less experienced on-site operator.

Several technology solutions are available for telecytopathology. These include live video streaming, static imaging, robotic microscopy, whole slide imaging, and hybrid devices that offer both robotic live viewing and whole slide imaging. The most important consideration in determining which solution to adopt is whether or not there is a skilled cytotechnologist or cytopathology fellow available to go on-site to handle procured samples, prepare slides, and then show them live to remote cytopathologists in real-time while they screen them on-site using a conventional light microscope [9]. The selection of telecytopathology platform should also be based on the workflow of each individual laboratory and should take into consideration the resources available, both human and technical, as well as image quality, user-friendliness, reliability, and security of the equipment [5, 14].

Process Workflow

Dynamic Telecytopathology

- The telecytopathology system is comprised of a digital camera, monitor, microscope, computer, and Internet connection. Dynamic images of the Diff-Quik smears are captured and processed with a digital camera system and a digital sight series that features a built-in display monitor. This unit can be connected to a personal computer and functions as Web server for image distribution. The microscope uses objectives from X4 to X40 magnification. The images are transmitted via Ethernet and are accessible from any computer with Internet access [1, 5].

- Dynamic telecytopathology allows live images to be transmitted and viewed electronically in real time at a remote site. It represents the most time and cost-effective platform. It allows cytopathologists to review the entire slide [5, 15]. Live image transmissions can be performed with different types of equipment.
- The on-site operators should be professionals with at least minimal experience in cytological procedures such as smearing, staining, and microscopy. They should have the expertise necessary to locate the most representative areas necessary for interpretation [16]. The operator, usually a cytotechnologist or cytopathology fellow, controls the microscope. He or she provides essential clinical information to the cytopathologist and moves the slides on the microscope stage to show the diagnostic fields.
- A cytopathologist interprets the cytologic images on a computer screen in their office in real time while communicating with the operator over the telephone.
- The cytopathologist provides adequacy assessment and preliminary diagnoses to the operator that are then conveyed by the operator to the radiologist performing the procedure and are documented in the requisition form.

Limitations

- Quality of the interpretation depends heavily on the ability of the person who moves the slides and selects the fields of view.
- Potential network issues and quality of image when changing magnifications.
- Required level of security mandated by most institutions makes it difficult to use such applications for clinical purposes [14].

Static Telecytopathology

- Static telecytopathology is a "store and forward" technique whereby only selective representative images of a slide are captured and transmitted via a Web browser either to a designated recipient or to a shared Web site [17]. It is inexpensive and simple as it is easy to send, store, maintain, and retrieve images.
- Images require only a small amount of computer memory; hence they can be readily transmitted and viewed over existing networks. However, it is often a partial representation of the specimen. Also, it appears to be less accurate than dynamic systems in cytology specimens [18]. This is because the cytology specimen is thicker and has an increased depth of focus that would require a similar experience to observing the specimen under a microscope. This can be better achieved with video imaging in contrast to still images. The static systems might not be suited for large-volume settings.

Limitations

- The remote viewer entirely depends on the judgment of the person who captures the images.
- The system does not allow the full review of the slides.
- The speed of scanning of cytologic images is very slow.
- Images may sometimes be insufficient.
- Lack of focus planes and poor quality of images (mostly with thick, crowded groups).
- Images are subject to quality issues with seemingly minor variations in image parameters (e.g., color, contrast) potentially leading to markedly different variations.

Robotic Telecytopathology

- Robotic telecytopathology is considered for adequacy assessments when there is an anticipated low ROSE volume and frequency performed at a satellite station such that the volume and frequency of ROSE cannot justify hiring cytotechnologists on-site [19]. Implementation of a robotic cytology solution requires a multidisciplinary process reevaluation of existing staffing and workflows and the configuration of a dynamic robotic telecytopathology solution [20]. Robotic-controlled slides offer the possibility of real-time simulated microscopy enabling thorough examination of potentially all the material present on the slides [21].
- A robotic digital microscope offers live viewing with a robotic stage that manages up to four slides simultaneously with four interchangeable objectives. The Windows-based user interface application allows the operator to have full control of the slide, including the location of the image, magnification, and focus [20].
- The radiologists perform the smears and stain them. They are trained and tested for their proficiency in preparation of Diff-Quik-stained slides and loading of the slides on the microscope before they can use the robotic microscope for adequacy assessment.
- Cytology staff members are only present on-site for routine visits to audit equipment, stain, and procedure quality and train employees on any new processes.
- Cytotechnologist evaluation of the specimen is performed remotely utilizing robotic microscopy and desktop sharing applications over the institutional intranet. Image viewing and control are remote via the intranet with the use of HD monitors.
- WebEx application enables the interventional radiology team to share the remote viewing session with cytotechnologists. The cytotechnologist is in close communication with the radiologist by phone in order to obtain all relevant information directly from the radiologist as well as communicate the adequacy assessment results [20].
- Remote network testing for readiness is performed daily by cytotechnologists at the main institution.

Limitations

- Remotely controlled robotic microscope has slow image refresh rates and requires a large bandwidth network connection and significant maintenance.
- Reliance on staff without prior cytology training to stain and load slides.
- When there are temporary network issues that lead to inability to access images, this can result in a delay in adequacy assessment.

Whole Slide Imaging

- Whole slide imaging is a digital imaging modality that uses computerized technology to scan and convert glass slides into digital images so that they can be viewed on a computer using viewing software [21–23]. This software allows a user to scan from field to field and increase or decrease the magnification, simulating panning around and zooming in or out with a conventional microscope. The whole slide is available for review by the remote viewer; hence issues of field selection and lack of low-power impression are essentially nonexistent.

Limitations

- Lack of standardization (multiple vendors, software, and lack of interoperability)
- Large file size leading to storage issues
- Limited focusing functions
- Slow speed of scanning of images
- Limited validation studies

Advantages and Disadvantages of Telecytopathology

Advantages

- Elimination of cytopathologist wait time at the site of evaluation and traveling time to various locations to perform ROSE, thereby helping to better manage cytology workflow and also allow the cytopathologist to perform other reimbursable activities concurrently.
- Less overall procedure time for cytopathologists, since on-site personnel can screen slides and show only key passes and regions of interest.
- Allows for multiple on-site operators from different locations. For instance, if an operator is held up at a location and there is a second concomitant procedure at another location that requires immediate assessment, another operator can be dispatched to perform this. Only one cytopathologist can simultaneously perform ROSE at many different locations.
- A cytopathologist may consult a colleague in the same vicinity on a difficult case, during a procedure by inviting them to view the images simultaneously. This helps to reach a consensus, thereby minimizing diagnostic errors.

- This platform also facilitates on-site evaluations at multiple sites by different pathologists, thereby allowing them to use their time more efficiently.
- Considering the low cost of the equipment, telecytopathology is a cost-effective alternative that can be integrated into mainstream diagnostic cytopathology. There is further cost saving as less cytopathologists are needed for ROSE.
- More independence for cytotechnologists, leading to confidence boost for them.
- Ability to remotely offer ROSE and thereby maximize small biopsies by reducing nondiagnostic specimens.

Disadvantages

- Less face-to-face interaction between cytopathologists and physicians who are performing the procedures.
- For streaming of images, skilled cytotechnologists or cytopathology fellows must be competent and confident to talk to clinicians.
- Reliance on others for navigation of slides and display of relevant cytologic material.
- Significant up-front capital investment and ongoing maintenance required [9].
- Initial learning curve, interpretation errors, and technology failures.
- Psychological barriers such as technophobia, fear of making mistakes, loss of control, and frustration [9].

Advent of Low-Cost Telecytopathology

Recently, positive results have been reported from the evaluation of low-cost telecytopathology systems using portable devices and video calls through mobile phones for real-time live transmission of images, and such systems may contribute further to the broad implementation of transmission of dynamic images, especially in remote or low-resource scenarios [24, 25].

Advantages

- The devices are widely available and have built-in, high-resolution cameras that can work as alternatives for expensive, fixed, dedicated microscope cameras.
- Phone can connect to network systems through Wi-Fi and eliminate the need for a hardwired Ethernet connection.
- Portability is a very important benefit of smartphones, thereby bringing technology to remote centers.

Disadvantages

- Need for a stable server connection
- Issues in image focusing
- Requirement of a skilled slide driver [16, 25]

References

1. Alsharif M, Carlo-Demovich J, Massey C, Madory JE, Lewin D, Medina AM, Recavarren R, Houser PM, Yang J. Telecytopathology for immediate evaluation of fine-needle aspiration specimens. Cancer Cytopathol. 2010;118:119–26.
2. Kraft AO. Specimen acquisition: ROSEs, gardeners, and gatekeepers. Cancer Cytopathol. 2017;125:449–54.
3. Schmidt RL, Witt BL, Lopez-Calderon LE, Layfield LJ. The influence of rapid onsite evaluation on the adequacy rate of fine-needle aspiration cytology: a systematic review and meta-analysis. Am J Clin Pathol. 2013;139:300–8.
4. Collins BT, DuBray-Benstein B, Naik K, Smith MA, Tiscornia-Wasserman PG. Commentary: American Society of Cytopathology rapid on-site evaluation (ROSE) position statement. J Am Soc Cytopathol. 2015;4:I–VIII.
5. Lin O, Rudomina D, Feratovic R, Sirintrapun SJ. Rapid on-site evaluation using telecytology: a major cancer center experience. Diagn Cytopathol. 2019;47:15–9.
6. de Koster EJ, Kist JW, Vriens MR, Borel Rinkes IH, Valk GD, de Keizer B. Thyroid ultrasound-guided fine-needle aspiration: the positive influence of on-site adequacy assessment and number of needle passes on diagnostic cytology rate. Acta Cytol. 2016;60:39–45.
7. Ecka RS, Sharma M. Rapid on-site evaluation of EUS-FNA by cytopathologist: an experience of a tertiary hospital. Diagn Cytopathol. 2013;41:1075–80.
8. Ganguly A, Giles TE, Smith PA, White FE, Nixon PP. The benefits of on-site cytology with ultrasound-guided fine needle aspiration in a one-stop neck lump clinic. Ann R Coll Surg Engl. 2010;92:660–4.
9. Monaco SE, Koah AE, Xing J, Ahmed I, Cuda J, Cunningham J, Metahri D, Progar A, Pantanowitz L. Telecytology implementation: deployment of telecytology for rapid on-site evaluations at an Academic Medical Center. Diagn Cytopathol. 2019;47:206–13.
10. Layfield LJ, Bentz JS, Gopez EV. Immediate on-site interpretation of fine-needle aspiration smears: a cost and compensation analysis. Cancer. 2001;93:319–22.
11. Frierson HF Jr, Galgano MT. Frozen-section diagnosis by wireless telepathology and ultra-portable computer: use in pathology resident/faculty consultation. Hum Pathol. 2007;38:1330–4.
12. Baak JP, van Diest PJ, Meijer GA. Experience with a dynamic inexpensive video-conferencing system for frozen section telepathology. Anal Cell Pathol. 2000;21:169–75.
13. Pantanowitz L, Dickinson K, Evans AJ, Hassell LA, Henricks WH, Lennerz JK, Lowe A, Parwani AV, Riben M, Smith CD, Tuthill JM, Weinstein RS, Wilbur DC, Krupinski EA, Bernard J. American Telemedicine Association clinical guidelines for telepathology. J Pathol Inform. 2014;5:39.
14. Sirintrapun SJ, Rudomina D, Mazzella A, Feratovic R, Lin O. Successful secure high-definition streaming telecytology for remote cytologic evaluation. J Pathol Inform. 2017;8:33.
15. Evans AJ, Chetty R, Clarke BA, Croul S, Ghazarian DM, Kiehl TR, Perez Ordonez B, Ilaalagan S, Asa SL. Primary frozen section diagnosis by robotic microscopy and virtual slide telepathology: the University Health Network experience. Hum Pathol. 2009;40:1070–81.

16. Collins BT. Telepathology in cytopathology: challenges and opportunities. Acta Cytol. 2013;57:221–32.
17. Goyal A, Jhala N, Gupta P. TeleCyP (Telecytopathology): real-time fine-needle aspiration interpretation. Acta Cytol. 2012;56(6):669–77.
18. Yamashiro K, Taira K, Matsubayashi S, Azuma M, Okuyama D, Nakajima M, Takeda H, Suzuki H, Kawamura N, Wakao F, Yagi Y. Comparison between a traditional single still image and a multiframe video image along the z-axis of the same microscopic field of interest in cytology: which does contribute to telecytology? Diagn Cytopathol. 2009;37:727–31.
19. Sirintrapun SJ, Rudomina D, Mazzella A, Feratovic R, Alago W, Siegelbaum R, Lin O. Robotic telecytology for remote cytologic evaluation without an on-site cytotechnologist or cytopathologist: an active quality assessment and experience of over 400 cases. J Pathol Inform. 2017;8:35.
20. Sirintrapun SJ, Rudomina D, Mazzella A, Feratovic R, Alago W, Siegelbaum R, Lin O. Robotic telecytology for remote cytologic evaluation without an on-site cytotechnologist or cytopathologist: a tale of implementation and review of constraints. J Pathol Inform. 2017;8:32.
21. Thrall M, Pantanowitz L, Khalbuss W. Telecytology: clinical applications, current challenges, and future benefits. J Pathol Inform. 2011;2:51.
22. Pantanowitz L. Digital images and the future of digital pathology. J Pathol Inform. 2010;1. pii: 15.:15.
23. Gilbertson J, Yagi Y. Histology, imaging and new diagnostic work-flows in pathology. Diagn Pathol. 2008;3(Suppl 1):S14.
24. Costa C, Pastorello RG, Mendonça A, Tamaro C, Morais C, Barbosa B, Ribeiro KB, Caivano A, Saieg MA. Use of a low-cost telecytopathology method for remote assessment of thyroid FNAs. Cancer Cytopathol. 2018;126:767–72.
25. Agarwal S, Zhao L, Zhang R, Hassell L. FaceTime validation study: low-cost streaming video for cytology adequacy assessment. Cancer Cytopathol. 2016;124:213–20.

Index

G. Cai, A. J. Adeniran (eds.), *Rapid On-site Evaluation (ROSE)*,
https://doi.org/10.1007/978-3-030-21799-0

R

GPSR Compliance

The European Union's (EU) General Product Safety Regulation (GPSR) is a set of rules that requires consumer products to be safe and our obligations to ensure this.

If you have any concerns about our products, you can contact us on ProductSafety@springernature.com

In case Publisher is established outside the EU, the EU authorized representative is:

Springer Nature Customer Service Center GmbH
Europaplatz 3
69115 Heidelberg, Germany

Batch number: 10372213

Printed by Printforce, the Netherlands